Epidemiology and the Community Control of Disease in Warm Climate Countries

Epidemiology and the Community Control of Disease in Warm Climate Countries

EDITED BY

Derek Robinson, MD

Senior Lecturer in Epidemiology, Liverpool School
of Tropical Medicine; Associate Clinical Professor
of Community Health, Tufts University, Boston;
Lecturer in Infectious Disease Control, General
Council of British Shipping; External Examiner,
Amsterdam and Antwerp Tropical Institutes; Lecturer
European Course in Tropical Epidemiology

FOREWORD BY

Dr S K Litvinov

Assistant Director-General
World Health Organization, Geneva

SECOND EDITION

CHURCHILL LIVINGSTONE
EDINBURGH LONDON MELBOURNE AND NEW YORK 1985

CHURCHILL LIVINGSTONE
Medical Division of Longman Group Limited

Distributed in the United States of America by Churchill
Livingstone Inc., 1560 Broadway, New York, N.Y.
10036, and by associated companies, branches and
representatives throughout the world.

First edition 1976
Second edition 1985

ISBN 0 443 02655 6

British Library Cataloguing in Publication Data
Epidemiology and the community control in
    warm climate countries. — 2nd ed. —
    (Medicine in the Tropics)
    1. Epidemiology — Developing countries
    2. Public health — Developing countries
    3. Tropical medicines
    I. Robinson, Derek II. Epidemiology
    and community health in warm climates.
    III. Series
    614.4'0913   RA651

Library of Congress Cataloging in Publication Data
Main entry under title:
Epidemiology and the community control of disease
    in warm climate countries.
    Includes index.
    1. Tropical medicine. 2. Epidemiology — Tropics.
    3. Medicine, Preventive — Tropics. 4. Community
    health services — Tropics. I. Robinson, Derek,
    1928–   . [DNLM: 1. Community Health Services.
    2. Developing Countries. 3. Epidemiology. 4. Tropical
    Climate. WA 100 E645]
    RC961.5.E65   1984   614.4'0913   84–9435

Printed in Hong Kong by
Sing Cheong Printing Co Ltd

Foreword

Infectious and parasitic diseases are a major cause of morbidity and mortality in most developing countries. These are, needless to say, closely related to prevailing social and economic conditions, and impede social and economic development. More than 30 per cent of deaths in children in their first five years of life are due to acute diarrhoeas, resulting in as many as three to five million deaths annually. Only about one-third of the people in the world's less developed countries have dependable access to a safe water supply and adequate sanitary facilities. Acute respiratory infections are a cause of high morbidity in the developed world, but in the third world these infections, primarily pneumonias, are another major killer in children, with a worldwide estimate of 2.2 million deaths per year. The common infectious diseases of childhood are still rampant in the developing countries whereas they have been reduced to minor nuisances in the developed countries. Tuberculosis still remains a major public health problem in all developing countries.

Parasitic diseases, in particular, are chronic and debilitating, and are endemic in most poverty-stricken areas. Malaria continues to take its toll, with some 150 million people affected annually, and about one million children dying every year in tropical Africa alone. Probably some 200 million people are infected with one or more of the lymphatic-dwelling filarial parasites, and another 20–40 million suffer from onchocerciasis, and in different ecological zones varying proportions are at risk of blindness. Schistosomiasis is increasingly related to attempts at agricultural and water-resources development schemes.

It was against this background that the social conscience of the WHO Member countries moved them in 1979 within their forum of the World Health Assembly — that is, developing and developed countries alike — to launch a Global Strategy for attaining the goal of 'Health for All by the Year 2000'. Among its main thrusts is the development *by countries* of national health infrastructures, starting with primary health care, for the delivery of country-wide programs that reach the whole population, and include referral level support.

Primary health care is essential health care made universally accessible to individuals and families in the community by means acceptable to them, through their full participation and at a cost that the community and country can afford. It forms an integral part both of the country's health system of which it is the nucleus and of the overall social and economic development of the community.

The launching of the ambitious target 'Health for All by the Year 2000' is tied up with the attempt at breaking the vicious circle of a heavy burden of disease, the meagre resources available, the frustrating struggle to make the slightest dent in morbidity or mortality, and the failure of the health services to participate effectively in helpful social development. It is only by breaking this vicious circle that countries can eventually look forward to promoting health rather than preventing or controlling disease.

Simple effective technologies are available to prevent morbidity and mortality when applied in the community and at home. Effective vaccines are available for the prevention of a number of early childhood killers and maimers — tetanus, diphtheria, pertussis, tuberculosis, measles and poliomyelitis. The introduction of oral rehydration therapy (ORT) has had a dramatic effect on mortality from diarrhoeas. The ease of preparation and administration of rehydrant solutions has taken the treatment of diarrhoea to the household, to enable the mother to attend to her sick child.. There is also a highly promising new drug against malaria, i.e. mefloquine.

Despite the well-known difficulties in research and in delivery systems for new drugs, there are major signs of progress in the chemotherapy of human parasitic infections representing fruitful results of collaboration between the Organization and those specialized sectors of the pharmaceutical industry with parallel interests.

In many diseases and undoubtedly in the case of three main killers in childhood in the developing world — diarrhoea, acute respiratory infections and malaria — case management within primary health care, i.e. within the family, the community (primary health worker's level) and the front-line referral service, is the main intervention providing a relief from suffering and preventing death.

The introduction of highly effective, non-tox'c orally administered drugs has revived interest in the use of population-based chemotherapy for morbidity control in selected parasitic diseases. The employment of new, simple quantitative parasitological examination techniques provides both a quantitative diagnosis and an evaluation mechanism. These technologies can now be delivered at many locations within the primary health care system, for example villages and schools.

Contributions from the health service must come at several levels. The core of the implementation of these technologies is behaviour change and the most crucial group to convince may be health professionals. They need to be interested in the common diseases as public health problems and to put their full weight behind simple interventions. Health workers of all sorts need training and must know how to reach the community to care for the health of all its members. The message to the community must be consistent and continuous.

Cooperation with other sectors outside the health service is essential to provide the flexibility and the resources that widespread promotion of these interventions demands. These might include schools, religious bodies, voluntary agencies, community groups, traditional health systems including midwives and healers, and private enterprises such as pharmacies. The onus is on the health leaders to mobilize community resources, to secure medical support to community action and to maintain a continued epidemiological assessment of the impact of health medical interventions on the disease picture.

Geneva, 1985   S.K.L.

Preface

Compared with both its predecessors and some contemporary tropical texts this volume deals comprehensively with all the important threats to health in warm climate countries. It is arranged in eight sections so that subjects with characteristics in common, especially in transmission and control, are adjacent to each other.

The first section is designed to assist the District Health Officer to investigate the community and wisely to plan the use of the resources available. The next two sections deal with the epidemiologically distinct airborne infections and food and water borne infections. The diseases within each of these groups have a great deal in common in the ways they are spread and controlled. In the fourth section are those opportunistic direct invaders of the body's surfaces which are assisted in their spread by foibles of human behaviour. Next come the vector borne infections, many of them limited to the warm, wet climates their vectors require. In the sixth section are those diseases not intended for Man who has strayed into a cycle of infection intended for other animals. The control of these diseases is bound up with Man's relationships with those animals, especially those kept close. In the next section are grouped the non-infectious illnesses, not a homogeneous group but of huge importance because together they account for more disease and death than all the other sections put together. Finally in this book come those variables in populations which simply cannot be disregarded in any attempt to influence population health.

This is not a textbook of primary universal education or transport technology, applied psychology or marketing, communications technology or individual rights legislation, banking or systems planning, agriculture or ecologically sound primary resources utilization, industrial engineering, ergonomics or urban planning. The reader who wishes to solve the problems of the developing countries will be involved in those activities rather than in health. This is because medicine or sophisticated health care contributes relatively little to social or economic development and is a symptom rather than a cause of affluence. Indeed when applied prematurely to an agriculturally and educationally underdeveloped population both preventive and curative services could have a mischievously unbalancing effect upon population growth. The sensitive humanitarian sees health care in such a society as a short-term means of relieving individuals of the consequences of their poverty and thereby relieving the pain that occasions in the observer. The economist sees health care either as a long term investment designed to avoid the waste of newly trained, potentially productive, young people, or as a means of avoiding that expensive unproductive care of the unnecessarily disease damaged which offends the cost conscious mind. Future enlightened generations may view health care as a responsibility of each informed, equipped and motivated individual. Few in any population are at that self-sufficient stage, and for the primitive present the District Health Officer must be content with the patronizing role of assisting a poor urban or rural population in the process of bettering itself.

The reader who finds this book useful may like to know who deserves the credit. First come the publishers who initially had the good judgement to see that Professor Robert Cruickshank in beginning the progenitor of this text had identified an important gap in the medical literature, then had the courage to accept that for the mid 80s it was necessary to start all over again. It has taken two years, during which my colleagues of the Liverpool School of Tropical Medicine have tolerated an increasing preoccupation. A special debt is owed to students who tolerated a teacher and counsellor apparently always pouring over manuscripts or disobedient typewriters. The only doubts arose from whether it would be possible to get top experts busy in the pride of their careers to write these chapters for future Distirct Health Officers, and this, moreover, to a disciplined format I had thought desirable. In the end they were all persuaded and the reader is left to judge the result. Even so, this book might have ended in the third chapter but for the prompt intervention of my nursing and medical colleagues of the Royal Liverpool Hospital who then tolerated a storm of composition unleashed by the unplanned interval away from teaching. Not least the useful aspects of this volume are owing to the support of friends and family who, though irreverently unimpressed by academia, made life otherwise easier for me during this two years. The reader who finds fault must blame me alone, and should feel obliged to write and tell me how things can be improved next time.

Liverpool, 1985   D.R.

Contributors

M. Abdussalam
Director, International and Scientific Cooperation, Institute of Veterinary Medicine, Robert von Osterag Institute, Berlin, Germany

O. P. Arya
Consultant Venereologist, Royal Liverpool Hospital, Liverpool, UK

Peter C. Bewes
Consultant Surgeon, Birmingham Accident Hospital, Birmingham, UK

Uwe K. Brinkmann
Epidemiological Advisor, GTZ Schistosomiasis Control Projects, Bamako, Mali

Michael L. Chance
Senior Lecturer in Parasitology, Liverpool School of Tropical Medicine, Liverpool, UK

John L. Cox
Senior Lecturer in Psychiatry, Royal Edinburgh Hospital, Edinburgh, UK

Peter Cox OBE
Senior Lecturer, Nuffield Centre for Health Services Studies, Leeds, UK

B. Cvjetanovic
Andrija Stampar School of Public Health, University of Zagreb, Zagreb, Yugoslavia

A. Davis
Director, Parasitic Diseases Program, World Health Organization, Geneva, Switzerland

D. T. Dennis
Filariasis Research Division, Institute Penyelidikan Perubatan, Kuala Lumpur, Malaysia

Nicholas Dodd
United Nations Fund for Population Activities, New York, USA

I. Dömök
Chief, Division of Epidemiology and Microbiology, National Institute of Hygiene, Budapest, Hungary

T. P. Eddy
Retired Senior Lecturer, London School of Hygiene and Tropical Medicine, Hove, UK

Nevzat Eren
Associate Professor, Department of Community Medicine, Hacettepe University School of Medicine, Ankara, Turkey

Paul E. M. Fine
Senior Lecturer. Ross Institute, London School of Hygiene and Tropical Medicine, London, UK

H. M. Gilles
Professor of Tropical Medicine, Liverpool School of Tropical Medicine, Liverpool, UK

David R. W. Haddock
Senior Lecturer in Tropical Medicine, Liverpool School of Tropical Medicine, Liverpool, UK

Sixten R. S. Haraldson
Retired Director, Nordic School of Public Health, Traslovslage, Sweden

D. A. Henderson
Dean, Johns Hopkins School of Hygiene and Public Health, Baltimore, Maryland, USA

Margaret D. Janes
Senior Research Assistant, Alder Hey Childrens Hospital, Liverpool, UK

T. Kereselidze
Medical Officer, Bacterial and Venereal Infections, World Health Organization, Geneva, Switzerland

L. Leowski
Medical Officer, Tuberculosis and Respiratory Infections, World Health Organization, Geneva, Switzerland

W. H. R. Lumsden
Professor Emeritus in Medical Protozoology, London School of Hygiene and Tropical Medicine, London, UK

W. W. Macdonald
Dean, Liverpool School of Tropical Medicine, Liverpool, UK

James A. McFadzean
Director of Research, May & Baker Limited, Dagenham, Essex, UK

Sir Ian A. McGregor CBE
Professorial Fellow, Liverpool School of Tropical Medicine, Liverpool, UK

I. F. Maitchouk
Ophthalmologist, Program for the Prevention of Blindness, World Health Organization, Geneva, Switzerland

J. W. Mak
Head, Filariasis Research Division, Institute Penyelidikan Perubatan, Kuala Lumpur, Malaysia

P. D. Marsden
Professor of Medicine, University of Brasilia, Brazil

David C. Morley
Professor of Tropical Child Health, Institute of Child Health, London, UK

C. S. Muir
Descriptive Epidemiology Program, Division of Epidemiology and Biostatistics, International Agency for Research on Cancer, Lyon, France

D. M. Parkin
Descriptive Epidemiology Program, Division of Epidemiology and Biostatistics, International Agency for Research on Cancer, Lyon, France

Wai-On Phoon
Professor of Social Medicine and Public Health, National University of Singpore, Singapore

J. Ponnighaus
LEPRA Evaluation Project, Chilumba, Karonga District, Malawi

Irene M. L. Pugh
Research Directorate, May & Baker Limited, Dagenham, Essex, UK

Derek Robinson
Senior Lecturer in Epidemiology, Liverpool School of Tropical Medicine, Liverpool, UK

David A Robinson
Medical Officer, Expanded Program on Immunization, World Health Organization, Geneva, Switzerland

Jon E. Rohde
Haiti representative, Management Sciences for Health, Port-au-Prince, Haiti

J. Rotta
Director, WHO Streptococci Reference Centre, Institute of Hygiene and Epidemiology, Praha, Czechoslovakia

H. B. L. Russell
Retired Senior Lecturer, Edinburgh University, Edinburgh, UK

G. R. Serjeant
Director, Medical Research Council Laboratories, University of the West Indies, Mona, Kingston, Jamaica

A. G. Shaper
Professor of Clinical Epidemiology, Royal Free Hospital, London, UK

David H. Smith
Senior Lecturer in Tropical Medicine, Liverpool School of Tropical Medicine, Liverpool, UK

T. Strasser
Medical Officer, Cardiovascular Diseases, World Health Organization, Geneva, Switzerland

Marigold J. Thorburn
Director, Caribbean Institute on Mental Retardation, Kingston, Jamaica

B. Thylefors
Program Manager, Prevention of Blindness, World Health Organization, Geneva, Switzerland

G. B. Wyatt
Senior Lecturer in Tropical Medicine, Liverpool School of Tropical Medicine, Liverpool, UK

A. J. Zuckerman
Professor of Microbiology, University of London, London, UK

Contents

1
D. Robinson

Epidemiology defined

INTRODUCTION

The art of epidemiology can be applied for several distinct purposes. Though all the practitioners are epidemiologists the tasks they are set to do differ one from the other. Though the custody of the principles and the analysis of population data can be left to the original academics, more and more there are needs to intervene in or to influence events. More and more these active intervenors are becoming distinct practitioners. In this chapter the purpose and the language of each of these groups is summarized. After that what most of this book is about is the practical application of epidemiology in the investigation, prevention and control of sickness in the population of warm climate countries.

THE ART OF EPIDEMIOLOGY

The occupation of the working epidemiologist parallels that of the general medical practitioner. Fortunate is the woman or man whose time can be organised to practice both. The wise practising physician uses established methods appropriate to the complaints of the patient. He or she is obliged to base many judgements on sometimes conflicting experiences and puzzling data and advises on the remedy apparently best matching the circumstances. He or she maintains surveillance of the patient to note quickly changes in the complaint, condition or data and is ever ready to modify the original decision. The practising physician is not a scientist, though he or she uses scientifically based and, hopefully, proven methods, does not use patients as experimental objects and only at his or her peril employs eccentric remedies. The physician is practising a subtle art. The few medical scientists privileged to probe the frontiers of current knowledge do not change the art but only add to the tools at its disposal. The science of epidemiology is a relatively small thing. Some new methods of forming, processing, storing or interpreting data are tried out, new models are devised to forecast events or to plan future programs, new mathematical formulas are suggested to explain events, new ideas are produced in the attempts to explain human fallibility. In an era of expanding communications developments can be expected. But mostly epidemiology, like its parent medicine, is an art, the practise of long established principles, the application of proven scientific methods.

This is not a textbook of epidemiologic methods or principles. Instead it returns to basics, the prevention of unnecessary illness, disability and death. As it is concerned with that vast majority of the human population not yet protected by northern affluent life styles and technology it will dwell longest upon the communicable diseases. It will also remind the reader that human corruption, folly and self indulgence affect health in the emerging societies just as they do in those more fortunate. So too do the vast problems of genetic and functional disruption for which medical science has as yet produced little benefit.

One definition of art (*Oxford English Dictionary*, 1971) is of human weakness opposed to nature. Medicine, including epidemiologic prevention, is opposed to those causes of sickness and decay which may be said to be 'natural'. The early churches were not entirely unjustified in concluding that all sickness was a punishment for sin — which we would now call folly. The religious philosophy failed because it could not distinguish between those illnesses in which man has a part by reason of neglect or ignorance and those which visit individuals by accident of place, time, family, occupation or, to add a modern rubric, immune deficiency.

Unfortunately medicine and epidemiology, by the success of their 'unnatural' battles against natural disease and decay, and aided by the agricultural engineering and social sciences, have tampered with the controls normally limiting population expansion. These 'natural' controls were, for populations, famine, plagues and conflict and, for individuals, errors of decision, an inability to compete, poisoned food and water and aging. The consequent expansion in human numbers has been at the expense of other higher life forms. It seems destined to consume the resources upon which the ecology was painstakingly balanced by Creation. It is irrational to accept, on the one hand, that 'unnatural' medicine is a good thing but, on the other hand, to do nothing to restrain the population growth which results. Having had a part in creating this paradox epidemiology must also share in seeking the solution — or share in the eventual apocalypse.

Just as epidemiology must share man's medical guilt for unbalancing nature, so also epidemiologists, the practitioners of the art, are responsible for the observer's or student's confusion about the nature of the art itself. Increasingly divided by their use of their own special language or jargon epidemiologists of the different kinds are coming to know less and less about each other.

Methodologic epidemiology

This is epidemiology as understood in the schools and universities. It is also the basis of most textbooks of epidemiology. The academically inclined epidemiologist studies the health characteristics of populations and their constituent sub groups, and notes the changes, often subtle, which occur in the health and well being of those populations. Gradual changes, for example a progressive decline in the proportion of newborn babies who die shortly after birth, will be called a *trend*. As most methodologic epidemiology is practised in the high technology 'northern' societies its interests, latterly, have been in the degenerative changes which plague aging populations. In particular, the methodologists have been concerned with the causes of premature aging, for example coronary disease in males under 40 or cervical cancer in females. The methodologic epidemiologist relies very much on the inflow of information and upon its accuracy. This *data* provides a basis to decide what is *normal*. It is any change in this normal pattern of sickness in a population which these epidemiologists hope to spot quickly and if possible to explain. The objective, if practicable, is to suggest ways of encouraging the change if it is favourable or of limiting the damage if it is unfavourable. An example of a very small, but important, change in population health detected by comparing data on deaths year by year was the, at first, unexplained rise in frequency of mesothelioma, a fatal cancer of the liver. The epidemiologists finally traced the cause to occupational exposure to certain types of asbestos.

The methodologic epidemiologists have traditionally been the guardians of epidemiologic method and language. It is the methodological approach to disease investigation and control and the methodological steps to deal with community health emergencies which are most useful to the individual responsible for disease control at District or Regional level in a developing country.

To the academic epidemiologists goes the privilege of looking inwards on the art of epidemiology itself, defining the ways in which raw data may be stitched into lessons useful to their clinical and managerial colleagues. Academics are separated from the clinical world, its distracting demands and prejudices, in order to form hypotheses or credible explanations for health or disease differences in different individuals or groups. They then plan the step by step analysis of old or new data which will test that hypothesis and will demonstrate whether it was right or wrong.

The work of methodologic epidemiologists over generations of observing and testing populations has produced what is often called *descriptive epidemiology* of which more later. Sufficient now to state that descriptive epidemiology has drawn attention to the many influences, they tend to be called *variables*, within a population. These variables determine collectively the *risk* that individuals in particular situations will or will not fall victim to sickness, and at what degree of severity. The presence of a toxin, stress or infectious agent is not the sole variable determining that exposed individuals will actually become sick or even die. The influences which modify the susceptibility of individuals to disease can be favourable or unfavourable. They are discussed later in chapter two.

Though this book is not devoted to epidemiologic method, its readers will benefit if they possess at least a passing familiarity with the basic tools which are used to study the distribution of disease and its change in populations. Man is born, suffers and dies. Hopefully in between the beginning and the ending of this life there is some reward, pleasure and contentment. Rightly or wrongly high technology man has assumed that total freedom from sickness or disability is essential to this contentment. Epidemiology is in part devoted to obtaining this freedom. Vitality, health and contentment though are very hard to measure. Instead epidemiology usually replies on measuring the degree to which they are absent. That is ill health and death and patient complaints which are easily defined. Ill health is called *morbidity* and death is known as *mortality*. Complaints are 'symptoms'. To these important informational tools the epidemiologist adds birth which is also easily quantifiable.

Because there is no such thing as an exactly 'normal' or ideal population the epidemiologist, in measuring the degree of departure of a particular population from what is the desirable pattern of health, is obliged to devise a *standard* population which becomes the basis for the comparisons. Simply to report that 131 babies died of diarrhoea in population A while 35 babies died of diarrhoea in population B suggests nothing about the relative risks to which the babies in either community are exposed. To compare the two populations requires that the period of time over which the deaths took place is known as well as the numbers in each population at risk — that is the babies alive at the beginning of the observation period. In order to compare population with population or to compare the experiences of the same population at different periods of its history we refer to the *incidence* of disease, that is the number of illnesses beginning in a particular time period, most commonly a year. We express that as a *rate*, that is the frequency of the event in a standard unit of population at risk. It is useful to know the incidence of disease in a population year by year as a program to control that particular disease is put into operation. If the program is effective the frequency with which new cases occur will decline. In the case of long lasting diseases, like leprosy or filariasis, the *prevalence* of the disease, that is the proportion of people in the population who suffer it at any one time, will never change all that rapidly. This is so even if a successful control program effectively reduces the number of new cases added, in a particular year, to the large bank of old ones and which die off only a few at a time. Though the prevalence tells little or nothing about the success of a control program it does indicate the load of patients requiring treatment.

Similarly in studying birth and death it may be interesting and even useful to know what the quantity is in any community — the total of new babies, the total of deaths — but what really matters is the rate or frequency of these events in, say, each average 1000 of the population. These frequencies are respectively the *birth rate* and the *death rate*. They will be described as *crude* because they take no account of differences in the populations, such as a lot of young or a lot of old people, which would respectively result in a lot of births or a lot of deaths. In order to make comparisons of health data between different populations which probably differ in their age, educational and occupational groups and which differences might affect collective survival, the epidemiologist *standardises* the data. Unfortunately such standardization can only be performed if there is reasonably accurate information about the numbers of individuals in the different age, educational and occupational groups which make up the population. As such data is rarely obtainable in developing countries the 'crude' figures of birth, sickness or death are all that may be available and great caution is needed in interpreting them. By contrast specialised data processing and information gathering centres are being set up or proposed for many developing countries. An example is the Cancer Registries whose academic nature contrasts, at times oddly, with the dearth of reliable information about presently treatable or preventable disease in the community.

Research epidemiology

Methodologic epidemiology sometimes appears at pains to distance itself from clinical research. Traditionally the one conducts its research on populations the other on specific groups of individuals already set apart, usually by reason of illness, from their fellows. In practice such distinctions are artificial. For research epidemiology is nothing more than the application of investigative techniques. The chief differences lie in the population studied. Research populations are carefully defined and their health is changed by the intervention of the researcher. The objective is not to know about the population in detail but about the effect of this intervention.

The data may be collected in *retrospective* or in *prospective* studies. Retrospective data is that sought about the subject after the event being studied has already occurred, for example death. It relies either upon existing accounts or records which were not formed with the particular research in mind. Or it relies upon the memory of persons concerned in the event. Prospective data begins with the event which identified the subject to be studied, such as the onset of illness, and then follows each individual as the effects of a new treatment are noted: it may follow the progress of those individuals until death finally occurs or complete recovery is confirmed. Prospective studies are usually very time consuming and require great patience and often much expense. In general though they provide a far greater degree of protection against error than can be afforded in retrospective studies. In, for example the original studies of the factors causing the epidemic of lung cancer it was suggested that one cause might be cigarette smoking and this was reinforced by a large scale retrospective survey of cancer patients (Doll and Hill 1950). It was not, however, until a large number of British physicians of already known smoking habits were followed prospectively for some years that excessive death rates were confirmed in those who smoked most heavily (Doll and Hill 1956). That is there was a *causal relationship* between cigarette smoking and cancer of the lung, though the exact carcinogen has yet to be identified. Similar confirmatory prospective studies cannot always be performed because of ethical reasons. For example the apparent association of mental damage with high environmental lead levels in preschool children has to rest on retrospective data. It would be unreasonable to leave a group of such children in a probably damaging high lead level environment in order to test the hypothesis.

Sometimes in epidemiologic research it is convenient to study particular *cohorts* that is groups of individuals sharing a common historical event or experience. If their health differs from that of other groups of individuals identical except for a particular event or experience it suggests that the event or experience was responsible for the health difference — good or bad. Inevitably there are catches in making comparisons of cohorts. For example it might be possible to compare the subsequent health of two cohorts both drawn from villagers born in the same year in Indo-China. One cohort would be those still living there while the other would be of those who became refugees. The refugees finally settled in an affluent society may or may not be subsequently found to live longer than their reflatives who stayed at home. Some of any difference there might be could be related to the different conditions under which they subsequently lived and the different health services they might enjoy. The groups are, however, *self selected*. One chose to leave their villages whatever the risk, one chose to stay behind whatever the consequences. Making even such a choice divides people into different personality types, behavourial characteristics, survival instincts or ambitions which may themselves be large determinants of *longevity*.

Except when there is a sensational promise of cure relatively little attention is paid to that segment of research epidemiology concerned with the trials of drugs, vaccines or other treatment such as surgery. Unfortunately some clinicians and surgeons undertake such *trials* without appropriate planning or care so that a majority of those which are published in the medical journals, and presumably the best ones are chosen from among those submitted, are invalidated by omissions, errors or contradictions. (Ambroz et al 1978). Research epidemiology is usually expensive and sometimes, as in the Framingham, USA studies of causation and heart disease, takes a very long time to reach any conclusion.

Outcome studies of even quite commonly prescribed treatment schedules have often never been made or pursued with any seriousness. Clinical medicine has a great deal of catching up to do before physicians or surgeons can be scientifically sure that one treatment really is superior to another. At risk are such procedures as intensive neonatal care for low weight newborns for which there is much enthusiasm but little evidence of cost benefit (Steiner et al 1980). Many past studies carefully designed to avoid all possible confusing influences on the results may now be invalidated. This is a result of the growing appreciation of the inherent differences in survival between those individuals who are conscientious and cooperative and those who comply with treatment or advice poorly. This difference has nothing to do with the actual treatment or advice which was given. (The Coronary Drug Project Research Group 1980).

Some research into populations is relatively simple. Many characteristics of man may be described as 'normal'. That means no more than that in a relatively large group of reasonably healthy people those whose anatomical or physiological measurements come close to the high central point on a *normal curve*, that is the arithmetic *mean* or *average* of the whole group will be the healthiest. The further away from the mean and the less desirable the implication for the individual. Such a departure from the group ideal is seen in the excess mortality in individuals at the extremes of body mass as calculated by the formula in which the weight is divided by the height squared (Garrow 1979). This is also the basis for some calculations of risk and for such standard measurements as the *centile charts* used to check childrens' growth and development. Departures from the 'normal' can also be expressed in terms of the *standard deviation* which mathematically describes the extent to which individual measurements differ from the group mean. The smaller the deviation, the narrower the curve, the more important the mean.

Care should always be exercised in interpreting normal curves and means taken from group measurements in part because being normal is not the same as being 'ideal', in part because we are not privy to what ideal standards the Creator was working and in part because in the developing countries conditions may be so different to those enjoyed by the original test population that to apply the same standards may be nonsensical. As an example the typical high carbohydrate diet and acceptable intestinal parasite load of a tropical population is unlikely to yield the same mean levels of haemoglobin as would be found in the population of a cold climate country with high proportions of animal protein in the diet. Frequent pregnancy and endemic malaria may further reduce haemoglobin levels but the giving of iron by mouth to bring the population up to the cold country standards may not be of unequivocal benefit. For such a population the epidemiologist will have to use a more appropriate standard or construct one. There will be more on the setting up of such a field survey study in chapter twelve.

Biostatistical epidemiology

The analysis and interpretation of data is as much a practise of mathematical as of epidemiologic arts. The relatively simple arithmetic used in analysing the results of population surveys or the ratios and proportions used by the methodologic epidemiologist now give way to more sophisticated techniques in planning prospective trials and in interpreting the *significance* of research findings. Any one of the biostatistical texts such as that by Bradford Hill

(1977) will guide the reader through this subject. Any hopeful researcher should first be familiar with the meaning of significance in its statistical sense and with the ways in which it may be tested. Such tests will show whether the findings of the researcher show real differences between different groups or whether, on the contrary, the differences could have occurred by chance.

Certainly it is the mathematical planning errors which spoil the greater number of individual research or study programs. Such errors can only be avoided by involving the biostatistician from the outset and again when the data are being processed and interpreted. The use of portable computers has brought *information storage and retrieval* and complex processing through preset programs into the hands of researchers with relatively little statistical knowledge. As a consequence sophisticated techniques are being applied to data regardless of whether they are appropriate. As an example the *chi*^{2} test will be used because that is the only one the researcher can process on the computer though it may be quite the wrong test for the particular situation. The consequence of the spread of statistical technology without statistical expertise has added a new danger in medical research. Readers of published reports can too easily reach false assumptions on the basis of data which appears respectably analysed but whose findings are actually invalid. Inevitably in this age of communications the relatively cheap technology will spread quickly throughout the developing world. The information such analyses produce can be no better than the reliability of the source of raw data allows. To this must now be added the possible uncertainties of the persons who will operate and service the equipment.

Anxieties will be raised on information storage and especially on who will have access to *confidential* health information in years to come. As the realisation dawns on aspiring national leaders that the indescretions of their youth are tidily docketed in computer information banks they will act with more haste than does a generation whose past is mercifully indistinct. The protection of confidentiality, including protection of the individual from either governmental or society's tyranny will be one of the major concerns in the last part of the twentieth century.

Administrative epidemiology

Governments, especially the agencies of government responsible for education, social security, employment, pensions, transport, agriculture and health care services have a burning need to know where populations are, how many *dependants* or workers there are now and will be in future years and what services the population or its sub groups will need. Parallel actuarial calculations are used by insurance and assurance companies, by banks in considering investment and by industrial producers in planning to produce and market goods saleable and attractive to a particular population. There is no point in building new schools and training new teachers in a population with a declining birthrate. Conversely a population with a large proportion of young adults will be highly mobile and an easy market for luxury consumables. A hospital manager will want to know just what resources will be needed to meet seasonably predictable demands. As an example, the admission rates for respiratory infections and for sickle cell crises may be expected to be high in the cold season while the diarrhoeal infections will increase with the heat.

The administrator-epidemiologist planner relies, like his colleagues, on the customary data of birth, sickness and death with additional data about population movements in or out. The *demographer* specialises in such population information. The administrator-epidemiologist, though invariably working in governmental or industrial planning agencies will, from time to time, need to contact field personnel to obtain information. At the time of a national or regional *census* of the population the entire emphasis will be upon field data gathering. At other times governments and international agencies produce forecasts or comparative *life expectancy* tables. They can only have any validity if they are based on a population in which the proportion of people dying in each age group, known as the *age specific mortality rate* is known with reasonable accuracy. From the data at each age is constructed a population *Life Table*. This is no more than a systematic vehicle for calculating how many days, months or years are left to the average member within each age group. As the calculations are based on the latest available death rates they do not forecast what the average length of life will actually be but only what it would be if everything remained exactly the same as on the day the measurements were made. The calculations are also misleading in developing countries as high death rates in infancy exaggerate the risks which those who survive infancy face in such countries.

Cohort Life Tables, by contrast, are constructed prospectively as the lives of those in the cohort proceed and finally terminate. They are difficult, expensive and time consuming to construct but they show in real terms the average length of life which can be expected under particular circumstances. They are particularly useful in comparing the long term outcome of different treatments.

Economic epidemiology

As the medical industry has come, at least in the developed world, to be one of the major employers and consumers of national resources, epidemiologic study methods have been applied to the alternative, and possibly cheaper, forms of medical service which may be available. Costs of these services are being compared with outputs or benefits. Where there are several different ways of achieving the same objective the most *cost effective* is likely to be chosen. The method will be required to produce a reasonable outcome at an acceptable cost. It will not necessarily be either the best in outcome or the cheapest in cost. As an example the outpatient treatment of active pulmonary tuberculosis was found to be more cost effective than that provided by the previously sacrosanct sanatoria. Home dialysis is a better use of resources than dialysis in hospital units for the care of chronic renal failure. Renal transplantation, however, is more cost effective than either though it is limited by the number of available donor kidneys. In consequence of these sometimes unpopular analyses of *cost benefit* the coalition of epidemiologists and program planners present the decision makers with the task of choosing between methods of care which will each have their proponents often with a personal interest in the outcome. In the Eastern block Socialist countries such program planning methods are used in drawing up five year or other period plans for using resources (WHO 1980).

Management By Objective (MBO), that is the establishment of exactly what a service or industry is intended to achieve before considering what, if any, service or industry to provide or fund, has come as an unpleasant shock when applied to health care. Health professionals are unused to be questioned on the purposes or worthwhileness of health care. District Health Officers may be unwilling to accept that their possession of professional credentials does not automatically best equip them to manage resources or manpower.

The Program Planning and Business Systems (PPBS) approach has proved especially useful in analysing the various components of a health care system including the alternative ways and costs to achieve the same objective. More often it is a specific program, such as tuberculosis control, which will be analysed in this fashion. Where ongoing evaluation rather than alternate cost analyses is required the Program Evaluation and Review Technique (PERT) is particularly useful. It is the adapted business method probably most frequently used by the international health agencies in deciding how best to allocate funds and to measure the results.

An obvious example of the clash of the resource planner with the popular sensationalism of the day is in the matter of cardiac transplants. Some far more expensive, because far more widespread, new techniques get less publicity but are equally agonized over by those responsible for scrutinizing the value, say of a pre school immunization program against the value of bypass surgery for coronary artery disease (European Coronary Surgery Study Group 1980). In developing countries those responsible for governmental resource allocations have an even more urgent need to examine cost benefit for everything they propose to fund. It is not necessary to repeat every exercise for every country.

Interest in recent years in developing countries has focused on the competing claims of high cost hospital versus low cost, primary health care in the community. The international agencies too have been analysing program costs and possible outcome. As an example the World Bank studied the alternate programs proposed for control of onchocerciasis in the Volta Rivers area of Africa (WHO 1972). The Rockefeller Foundation has also funded a series of analyses of different forms of primary health care in developing countries (Walsh and Warren 1979).

The part played by the epidemiologist in such analyses, more especially in the political skirmishing which sometimes follows, can be an uncomfortable one. To make objective analyses of costs and outcome and to measure health given or life lost are difficult enough. The analyst is also expected to be obliged to explain and to defend, under considerable political pressure, the methods of data collection and analysis and the conclusions reached. The process is, nevertheless, an important one in the age of competing services, and sometimes underemployed professionals, and with technical developments seeking applications.

Practical epidemiology

Here epidemiologic theory and discipline are applied to ongoing *endemic* disease in a community and to any sudden increase in the numbers of those affected which may be termed an *epidemic*. The rules are the same as in the other forms of the epidemiological arts. It is the practitioners themselves who tend to differ. There is a large overlap between all the branches of epidemiology and an epidemiologist may in a single career practice them all. Perhaps though more often than his colleagues the practical epidemiologist will have worked his way into the art from an original interest in clinical or laboratory medicine. She or he often maintains a primarily clinical or research base and sees in epidemiology the opportunity to go further than simply diagnosing and treating individual sickness. A researcher may come to epidemiology to gain expertise in planning and analysing his programs. A medical practitioner whose work and interest are absorbed by a particular disease will seek in epidemiology the means to limit the misery caused by that disease which the treatment of individual patients may not have provided.

It requires some adaptation for the clinician, often working intuitively with individual patients to learn and to practice the systematic methodological approach of academic epidemiology. Merely to become familiar with the sources of infection, the modes of transmission and the distribution of a particular disease does not convert the clinician into an epidemiologist. It is gratifying when epidemiologic information is so valued, but epidemiology is not just information but a discipline. Its value for the clinician lies in its systematic approach to investigation and control of disease and in the relative balance which it demands between treatment of the individual and dealing with the population at risk as a whole.

Ironically at the beginning of her or his career the District Health Officer in a developing country will also be obliged to assume the double role of clinician and epidemiologist. Perhaps too without the conviction that what happens in the community deserves a deliberate slice of time and effort. The daily queue of sick persons can quickly become a prison wall. Individuals may be cured and freed only to return to the same hazards which made them sick and probably will again. The tasks of the practising epidemiologist are to find out:

Who has apparently been affected by disease

What is the nature of the sickness or the manner of death

Where did the events occur or begin

When did the unusual sickness or death begin to be noticed

Why did the events occur as they did, why were those particular victims involved and what common factors united them.

All practical investigations begin by seeking Cause, though not necessarily the exact agent or coincidence of events which led to the particular Effect — the apparent sickness or death. Always the ultimate objective is to remove the cause, to interrupt transmission or to stop further damage by removing those at risk from danger.

In attempting to deal with endemic disease the District Health Officer/Epidemiologist may first have to decide exactly what the principal health problems of a particular population are. Then he or she must decide which problems, given existing resources, can be tackled to give the maximum benefit to the local community.

Always the practising epidemiologist keeps in mind the underlying purpose of a particular disease specific program. Is it to *eradicate* the disease or *control* it? Eradication implies that all active cases plus all new sources of infection have been eliminated. Alternatively in the case of the non infectious disease it implies that all the adverse circumstances which could produce the disease have been permanently removed. These are ambitious objectives. They are practicable only for those infections in which man is the sole reservoir of new infection and for which there exists a means of thoroughly protecting the entire population immunologically with a cheap, stable and reliable vaccine. In theory eradication can also come through simultaneous treatment of an entire population but this is practicable only for small, isolated population groups and is unlikely to be permanent.

Most disease programs have to be content to attempt to control the local problems. That is to reduce the number of those individuals affected to an acceptable number. Inevitably new cases will occur from time to time especially in those individuals who expose themselves to unnecessary risks. Measures to limit the size of outbreaks have to be maintained as long as the hazard persists.

Chapter three will discuss the systematic approach to the investigation and control of disease. The later chapters devoted to particular disease will describe in more detail the individual steps which can be taken to deal specifically with those problems. Chapters six and seven will deal with the ways in which decisions on priorities can be made at district or regional level.

TERMINOLOGY

Age specific mortality rate. See 'rate'. A crude death rate differing from the general population death or mortality rate in that it limits the calculation to the persons dying within a particular age range which is also the population at risk.

Arithmetic Mean. The sum of the units of measurement of all the individuals in a particular population divided by the number of persons in that population.

Average. Widely used to imply the same as the 'arithmetic mean' but in biostatistical language the 'average' includes both the 'mode' and the 'mean'.

Birth rate. See 'rate'. A crude proportion obtained by dividing the total number of live births in a population by the total number of persons in that population. Conventionally the resulting fraction is then multiplied by 1000 so that the rate is expressed per 1000 in the population.

Causal relationship. The degree of association between particular circumstances or events and their eventual apparent consequences. When the influence is a bad one it can be arithmetically calculated as the degree of 'risk'.

Causation. Assignment of the blame for a particular effect noted, especially in health in individuals, back to the true cause or causes. Some epidemiologists refer to the 'web of causation'. That is the unwitting progress of the victim through a series of events or circumstances which when all added together lead almost inevitably to the victim's sickness or death.

Census. A counting of the numbers of individuals in a particular population. Usually additional detail is also collected, such as age and sex. When especially detailed information is needed, such as on housing, occupation and income, a sample census will be more practicable.

Centile or percentile. Usually taken from a chart upon which lines will join the point at which specific proportions of the population have arrived at specific stages of development. On a growth for age chart, for example, the 10th percentile line is the point which 10 per cent of that population has not yet passed, be it height or weight. At the other end of the scale above the 90th centile line are the 10 per cent heaviest or tallest children at the different ages. In practice it is not the relative position on such a chart which matters but whether an individual child progresses with age without falling below its own particular centile level.

Chi^2. A test of the likelihood that two quite different factors or 'variables' could in fact be inter related or whether any apparent relationship, for example between normal individual skin colour and the risks of acquiring leprosy, could really have occurred by chance. It just happens that skin decolouration, a useful sign of leprosy, is more easy to detect in those individuals with a normally heavily pigmented skin.

Cohort. A group of individuals sharing a common feature — usually born at the same time. Other beginning shared events can also be used such as all the persons injured in a particular year. Recently the term has also been used to create groups with a shared experience of hazard, such as exposure to asbestos at work, but not necessarily within the same span of time.

Cohort life table. A specialized form of Life Table. Measures survivorship not in a total population but in a specific sub group or cohort. Used in this context the cohort is most commonly a group of persons with the same sickness. A comparison of mean survival in sub sections of such a cohort treated in different ways is the basis of trials and of therapy outcome studies.

Confidential. To be kept secret except to the individual being investigated or treated and to the person responsible for the investigation or treatment.

Control. Keep the numbers of persons with a disease or the dangers from a known hazard within reasonable limits with the resources available. A control program often aims progressively to reduce the number of persons who become sick or are at risk. In a seperate sense also used to describe the 'normal' population with which an experimental group or with which patients under treatment will be compared.

Cost Benefit. A pricing system for each item of desired outcome. Cost benefit analysis looks at different viable alternatives in program planning and calculates the cost of each. The total program cost to achieve, for example the vaccination of a population is divided by the total number of persons who will benefit by the procedure, in this case the number of persons who would likely have become sick without the vaccination. The examination of the different possible strategies may show that there are cheaper or more acceptable ways of achieving the same objective. In the example given it might be cheaper, especially if infection causes little early fatality, to introduce an early case-finding system and then to treat those infected. If the objective were to eradicate rather than to control the disease the more expensive vaccination program might be of greater cost benefit because it removes the pool of new infection by stopping further transmission.

Cost benefit analysis is designed to enable the planner to choose the strategy which achieves the maximum benefit using available resources.

Cost effective. A standard of efficiency. Usually the cheapest way to achieve a particular objective. Whereas 'cost benefit' calculates the good effect of spending a particular unit of resources, cost effectiveness studies measure how well the resources are being used to achieve a desired goal.

Crude. Uncorrected. When applied to data implies that though a rate can be calculated no account has been taken of peculiarities of that population which may produce a misleading figure.

Data. Aggregations of recorded measurements of individuals or events reported to a central collecting agency. Calculations from these data describe in arithmetic terms the population from which they were derived. The results of such calculations can be misleading if used to compare different populations unless the results are corrected to take into account differences in the make up and circumstances of those populations.

Death rate. See 'rate'. Unless 'standardized' a crude figure relating the total number of deaths in a population to the number of persons in that population. The population size is best counted at the mid point of the period, usually a year. By multiplying the fraction by 1000 expresses what proportion of the population died in a particular year.

Demographer. Usually a biostatistician specializing in the analysis of size and make up of populations and the influences which change them.

Dependant. In demographic terms usually a person either incapable of or distracted from earning his or her own living. For simplification whole age groups are classified as being likely or unlikely to be dependant. This provides in crude terms an indication of what proportion of a population could be working and what proportion is unlikely to be making much contribution to population wealth.

Descriptive Epidemiology. The analysis of who is well and who is sick in a population. Usually broken down into such characteristics as age, sex, occupation and education as a way of showing who is most at risk and if possible why.

Endemic. The level of a particular disease to which a particular population is accustomed.

Epidemic. Any substantial increase in the number of cases of a disease above the level to be normally expected in that population.

Eradicate. Eliminate, usually a disease or health hazard. Hopefully permanent as in the case of smallpox or on a local basis destroying the breeding site of a disease vector.

Hypothesis. An untested idea, theory or tentative explanation of why events occur as they do.

Incidence. The frequency with which a particular event occurs or a particular finding is made in a population during a specific time span — usually a calendar year. As it would mean nothing to state it as so many events occuring without also taking into account the number of individuals at risk the incidence is usually expressed as a proportion per standard unit of population, most often per 100 000. The mortality rate is one of several special kinds of incidence. Incidence most frequently is used to express sickness frequency and then will be limited to sickness occuring for the first time.

Information storage and retrieval. Can mean any system of recording data systematically and so cataloguing it that details of individual events can quickly be found and repeated. Generally used to mean data on a computer.

Life expectancy. The remaining years of life to be enjoyed by the average person within a group of the same age. Most commonly taken to mean life years on average at birth. Unfortunately in the latter context it can be very misleading as many life years are lost if there is an excess of infant deaths.

A better indicator of the relative hazards to adults in any population would be the Life Expectancy at, say, 18 years.

Life table. Also known as the 'Demographic Life Table'. The arithmetic model for calculating the proportion of persons in each age group in a population who will survive for the one year, five years or whatever the age range of the group is. From this is calculated the number of life years which will be accumulated by the group. By adding the different age group accumulations together it is simple arithmetic to calculate the life expectancy for each age group. It has, however, limited usefulness as a forecasting tool as it does not describe what actually will happen but what could happen if all indices, the age specific death rates at all ages, remained stable, an unlikely event.

Longevity. The mean length of life to be expected in a particular group, usually, of adults. Also commonly used as indicating a favourable trend toward longer life in a population.

Morbidity. Sickness levels in a population. Usually expressed as a proportion or rate, that is so much sickness per 1000 or per 100 000 of the population.

Mortality. Death. Can be expressed as to cause and by different, specific groups of the population. Usually expressed as a proportion or rate, the Death Rate.

Normal curve. A diagramatic expression of the frequency of a particular event or finding in a particular population. To be 'normal' this frequency falls off symmetrically on either side of a small, almost plateau, plunges steeply and then gradually flattens out at the extreme readings either side of the arithmetic mean. The mean or average reading will be at the exact centre of the curve. In the case of the normal curve this is also the 'median' and will be recorded from the largest sub group of subjects, that is also the 'mode'. These mid point averages must not be confused with the ideal for the individuals measured. For example a dental survey will reveal a range of decayed or absent teeth from all to none with a normal curve of pathology inbetween. The ideal though is at one extreme end of the curve, all teeth sound and present.

Normality. A standard for a population by which its individual members or other populations can be judged. In general it assumes that what happens to the greatest number is what should happen though this is not necessarily the same as what is desirable. In some contexts it is taken to be the opposite of 'risk'.

Outcome studies. Usually extensive, prospective trials of one form of treatment against another. Only tell the whole story if they continue far beyond the treatment and recovery period and into the subsequent remaining life of the patient. The objective is to calculate what the real contribution the treatment gave to extending and improving the life of the average patient in the treated group as compared to the standard untested or alternatively treated group.

Prevalence. Expresses how common or scarce a particular event or finding is in a population at a particular 'point' in time. So that two populations can be compared it is calculated as a proportion or rate, most commonly per 100 000 population. Also most commonly used to describe the quantity of disease, old or new, in a population at any particular time.

Prospective. Beginning with a particular event, such as being born or falling sick, follows the consequences as time unfolds. The beginning is usually during the time of the study with events taking perhaps years to reach a termination and in this is the most accurate and controllable form of study or trial. Can, however, begin with events long past and rely on reconstructing events as they were subsequently recorded.

Rate. An arithmetic way of describing the frequency at which events occurred in a population during a particular time, or alternatively the proportion of that population affected by some single event. Most useful when the total number of events occuring in the population during the time span chosen, usually a year, is divided by the number of persons 'at risk'. Often the latter cannot be calculated so that the rate will be based on the total population. As such divisions always lead to awkward fractions it is conventional to multiply the answer by 1000 or 100 000 so giving a rate of events per so many population. Occasionally where the event is a common one it is convenient to use 100 as the multiplier and the resulting rate is then also a percentage, that is a rate per 100 population.

Retrospective. Usually an analysis of the circumstances which preceded whatever event is being studied. Best constructed from reports or routine records available on the persons being studied. May be obliged to rely on the memory of the subject or of persons close or involved in the earlier care. In these respects far more subject to error than 'prospective' studies but much quicker and cheaper to perform than the latter.

Self selection. In the past commonly meant 'volunteers'. Subtle biases may exist in choosing a survey or standard population so that particular kinds of person may be encouraged or discouraged to agree to participate in a study or the entrance criteria may unwittingly exclude important sub groups.

Significance. The degree of certainty that a statistical finding, for example differences in mean measurements between two groups represent real differences and not chance variations which would not be repeated if a sufficiently large number of readings were taken. In general it is the range of observations and the number of persons being tested which influence the calculation of significance, the smaller the former and the larger the latter and the more likely is any difference between two populations likely to be a real one. The wider English language usage as alternatives to 'important' or 'meaningful' are avoided by epidemiologists and biostatisticians.

Standard deviation. In terms of the units used for measurement expresses the limits on either side of the mean and within which the population would be regarded as 'normal'. Mathematically describes the degree of scatter from the mean or the relative width of the 'normal curve'. The more subjects there are, the smaller the range over which the findings vary and the more precise is the definition of normality. The observer has a choice of how far to go in deciding that in a trial of two different treatments there really was a significant' difference in the effect on two groups. Conventionally taking 2 Standard Deviations as the minimal improvement to be regarded as significant the new treatment group's mean, say, survival, would have to be shifted outside the range of survival times of 95 per cent of the untreated standard group. Frequently the reason why trials cannot be proved statistically significant is not because a new treatment is not effective but because the numbers of subjects in the trial are too small. To be calculated the variation from the mean of each subject must be known as well as the number in the group.

Standard population. A substitute for the ideal, normal or exactly representative population which hardly exist in practice. May be a real population or an imaginary one. The total population, if accurately recorded, would also be synonymous with the normal.

Standardization. The processing of crude data so that differences in two populations being compared, such as unequal proportions of different age groups, are mathematically neutralized. Difficult to do in most developing countries where the absence of a reliable data base about the total population greatly reduces the worthwhileness of the exercise.

Trend. A consistent change, as shown by serial observations from what has been the previous normal or mean for a population. Can be good or bad.

Trials. Tests usually involving two or more population groups each given a different treatment or exposed to different conditions. At some point in time the investigator will assess how far the groups differ presumably as a result of the different conditions created for them.

Variables. Measurable influences which may be inbuilt by the investigator, such as drug dose and the measurable consequences such as the proportion of patients who survive. The former are 'independent' the latter are 'dependent' variables.

REFERENCES

Ambroza A, Chalmers T C, Smith H, Schroeder B, Freiman J A, Shareck E P 1978 Deficiencies of randomised control trials. Clinical Research 26: 280A
Bradford Hill Sir A 1977 Short textbook of medical statistics. Lippincott London
Doll R, Bradford Hill A 1950 Smoking and carcinoma of the lung. British Medical Journal 2: 739–748
Doll R, Bradford Hill A Lung cancer and other causes of death in relation to smoking. British Medical Journal 1956 2: 1071–1081
European Coronary Surgery Study Group 1980 2nd interim report: Prospective randomised study of coronary artery bypass surgery in stable angina pectoris. Lancet 2: 491–495
Oxford English Dictionary 1971 The Compact Edition. Clarendon Press Oxford
Steiner E S, Sanders E M, Phillips E C K, Maddock C R 1980 Very low birth weight children at school age: comparison of neonatal management methods. British Medical Journal 281: 1237–1240

The Coronary Drug Project Research Group 1980 Influence of adherence to treatment and response of cholesterol on mortality in the coronary drug project. New England Journal of Medicine 303: 1038–1041

Walsh J A, Warren K S 1979 Selective primary health care. An interim strategy for disease control in developing countries. New England Journal of Medicine 301: 967–974

WHO/FAO/IBRD/UNDP 1972 Onchocerciasis control in Volta river basin area. WHO Geneva.

WHO 1980 The Gabrovo health services model in the people's republic of Bulgaria. Regional Office for Europe. Copenhagen. pages 30–35

The threats to health

Microorganisms and parasites which can first infect man and then cause sickness and death are present virtually everywhere that human life itself can be supported. The higher animals, including Man, carry about with them, especially in the gastrointestinal tract, a host of organisms many harmless but many also *pathogenic* and a few, though not necessarily the same ones which are highly *virulent*. In nature and at all levels of development the primary objective is that of genetic survival and, as a corollary, survival of the species. For the microorganisms and other parasites this necessitates a constant, if automatic, search for new victims. Time is very short except for the relatively few pathogenic microorganisms which can survive outside host tissues for very long.

This suggests that Man, like other higher animals, is constantly under siege, constantly peppered by attackers. The next chapter will describe the different ways in which these attacks can be effected. This chapter will look at the factors which predispose to actual sickness. Why do some individuals succumb to sickness when others, in apparently identical circumstances, remain well?

SICKNESS PREDISPOSING FACTORS

The spread of sickness in an epidemic form, rolling over a whole population, or selecting the obviously weak or feeble, is easy to understand. All defences are overcome though the severity of the disease will still vary from individual to individual. Endemic disease occurring here and there in an otherwise unaffected young adult population or seeking out particular individuals in otherwise unaffected families is harder to understand.

Measures to protect populations from endemic disease may be relatively expensive for the benefit expected precisely because it is rarely clear who exactly is at risk and which individuals are likely to be the next victims. As our knowledge of immunology increases we shall more certainly be able to identify who is at risk — the likelihood that the particular individual meeting the particular microorganism will fall victim.

It has long been apparent that immunity, whether through circulating antibodies or through previously alerted T lymphocytes, is increased each time the body overcomes the same antigen types of invading organisms. The opposite is true for the non infectious causes of sickness. Exposure to and damage from the toxins and microtoxins of nature and the environmental hazards of high technology produce additive damage and increased susceptibility to further damage. Already the highly developed 'northern' countries have moved away from many infectious dangers only to find that much less clearly defined and much more insidious hazards of diet, environment and life style accelerate physical and emotional decay faster. in some individuals than in others.

The factors which modify or collectively upset the balance between Man's resistance and the power of the attacker can be classified into four principal groups.

1. Host — Parasite relationships

(a) The parasite.

Of the apparently endless lists and distinct species of microorganism only a relatively few have the ability to infect higher animals. Even for a high proportion of the infecting types the ability to produce actual sickness, that is their pathogenicity, is quite limited. In all the family of the Streptococci only the Group A beta hemolytic variant is truly important to man. Disease producing microorganisms may be highly virulent, dangerous to those of a particular species of animal whom they successfully parasitise, like cholera in Man, and be virtually harmless to other species of animal. Some invaders, like the Lassa virus, initially virulent in human victims then either fail to be transmitted or to be pathogenic to later potential human hosts.

The ability of an organism to parasitise new victims in a population will obviously be modified by any circumstance which affects its usual transmission pathway. Fortunately few microorganisms are as enterprising as the anthrax bacillus which can not only invade through the air and into the lungs, through infected food into the gastrointestinal tract and through infected inanimate objects into the lightly damaged skin but can also form spores capable of remaining inert through years of waiting for a new warm blooded victim. Moreover the anthrax bacillus attacks warm blooded animals indiscriminately. Most viruses and bacteria are quite limited in their invasive ability while others, especially the tropical parasitic infections, depend upon a complex cycle of alternate hosts and vectors and are limited to particular stages of development in different hosts.

The speed with which an infection can produce sickness, that is the incubation time is epidemiologically important only in keeping track of a spreading disease. Of more importance is the epidemiologic *generation time*, that is the interval between the initial infection of the new victim and the production of transferable organisms ready for the next victim. An outbreak is most difficult to control when individuals, infected but not yet sick, are mobile and transmitting the infection to others. This is particularly the case in the airborne infections of childhood.

Clear waves of secondary and tertiary infection can best be identified in a disease like typhoid in which infectivity comes relatively late in the sickness. In theory at least such long generation time diseases should be easy to control but in practice many of those infected and eventually transmitting in their turn to others never experience the clinical illness which could alert the health authorities to remove them from contact with potential new victims. Similarly in amoebic dysentery though trophozoites can be found early in the stool of the new victim it is not until the recovery stage that the disease transmitting cysts appear in the stool.

The peculiar degree to which the relationship between host and parasite can develop is shown in the tolerance of the human body for certain microorganisms, especially those of the gastrointestinal tract. On recovery from an infection of the bloodstream, with or without the development of serious sickness, the host allows the parasite to persist. So the host becomes a *carrier* apparently healthy but able to transmit the infection to new victims. Long term silent carriers are the principal sources of infections like typhoid. Healthy, apparently unaffected, but short time carriers, are important in infections like poliomyelitis in which many individuals are quickly infected but in which few become sick.

Finally in all the relevant parasite factors that of dose may be paramount. A native of Paris will rarely encounter a leprosy bacillus and the chances of a single encounter producing disease are probably quite small. A single bacillus is no more likely to be successful in Dar-es-Salaam but the number of such encounters may be enormous. So the chances of acquiring the infection are much greater. Similarly family or other close contacts of infectious individuals are at danger because of the frequency with which they are bombarded with microorganisms. What part is played by the number of microorganisms in each contact is less certain. In the gastrointestinal infections at least it seems clear that the chance of sickness is related to the size of the dose.

(b) The host.

The potentially invasive organism, the damaging toxin or the destructive agent of the non infectious diseases, must usually first overcome the *natural* or primary barriers which protect the higher animals from the majority of pathogens. These natural barriers will be described in the next chapter. Those thrown up by the potential victims include the skin, the mucous barrier of the nasopharynx, the ciliated epithelium of the respiratory tract, the small limiting aperture of the terminal bronchioles, the acid in the stomach and the normal flora and ph values of the gastrointestinal tract. Certain especially vulnerable points, like the conjuctiva, mouth and anus are protected by tears, saliva and oily secretions which dilute as well as wash away potential invaders. Once the natural barriers are breached the body must fall back upon its macrophages and the memory accelerated reactions of the T and B lymphocytes and other cellular and serological defences as yet incompletely understood. From an epidemiologic viewpoint immunity may be classed as of three types. They are as follows:

(*i*) *Innate or species specific.* Each warm blooded animal is susceptible only to a limited number of microorganism types. Resistance to the rest is absolute under ordinary conditions. Either nothing at all occurs or, as in the case of human *Toxacara canis* infection, the development is limited though some ill effects, in this case granuloma formation in vital areas, may ensue.

(*ii*) *Disease specific.* This provides a normally susceptible animal with a degree of resistance which can vary from slight to virtually complete. Disease specific resistance depends either upon the presence of antibodies in the serum or upon the cell mediated immunity conferred by alerted T lymphocytes. In some infections, like *S. typhi* both mechanisms probably play a part in host resistance. As the process is influenced primarily by the antigens at the surface of invaders it follows that effective resistance to one organism type will provide some protection from other organisms which have a similar surface antigen. This would be the basis, for example, for some resistance to leprosy being conferred by BCG vaccination. It also follows that any organism which has the ability to mutate or periodically to vary its surface antigens is best suited to evade the body's immune mechanism. This is the problem experienced, for example in the development of resistance to trypanosomiasis, especially the African variety.

Disease specific immunity is often subdivided in two ways, first into Active or Passive. In 'active immunity' the host body has done the work as a result of previous infection which it has successfully overcome. It has produced anti-bodies or now has alerted T cells. In 'passive immunity' the body has made no effort. It has either acquired antibodies from its mother across the placenta or in the mother's milk or the antibodies are given, injected, as part of a disease prevention campaign.

Some epidemiologists also prefer further to break down the classification into whether the immunity was acquired by 'natural' or by 'artificial' means. The important distinction though is whether the immunity is active or passive. For immune globulins however acquired, if from another source than the host's own body, are fairly quickly broken down by the host so that the immunity they confer lasts at most for a few months. By contrast the active immunisation produced by live vaccines, even though the process is an 'artificial' one can work just as well as a real attack by pathogens in stimulating long lasting immunity.

(*iii*) *Herd.* There is nothing mysterious about the high resistance which certain groups of people have to particular diseases. It is a consequence of long continued exposure to a particular infection in any stable, relatively isolated community. A substantial proportion of the members of such a group will be resistant or tolerant to disease which might seriously affect or kill outsiders introduced into the same environment.

Herd immunity results from three mechanisms and in two of them the essential element is the ability of certain individuals to survive sickness. The third mechanism is unpredictable — the chance distribution throughout the community of a non pathogenic but infecting organism which will produce cross immunity to pathogenic strains. It is, for example, alleged that in the past children were naturally vaccinated against pulmonary tuberculosis forms through drinking M. bovis infected milk. Wild strains of enterovirus have protected against subsequent epidemics of poliomyelitis. Generally though herd immunity is a survival phenomenon. It may occur through survival of individuals from endemic infections like the diarrhoeas or survival of epidemics like measles. In both cases there will be a high cost in the numbers who do not survive. A community perpetually faced with the need to produce survivors is obliged to produce a large excess of babies in order to counteract the losses.

Herd immunity acquired after an epidemic is more notable by its absence than its presence. The sweeping of an epidemic through an unimmune population soon draws attention. When such an epidemic selects only the young who were not alive in previous epidemics it confirms the long lasting nature of naturally acquired active immunity. It was such an episode which was noted by Panum in the Faroe Islands in 1846. This confirmed both the infectious nature of measles and the immunity to it conferred by previous infection.

It is not necessary for every person in a community to become sick or to acquire immunity for disease transmission to cease. Immunisation levels, though, have to be high totally to prevent new cases from occurring (See Henderson Chapter 19). Community vaccination and immunisation programs are aimed at achieving the results of natural infection but without its casualties. Nature can sometimes aid Man in accentuating the gain from a compaign. A live vaccine given by mouth, like poliomyelitis, will spread throughout the community by the usual faecal-oral routes.

Unfortunately many infectious agents have so many antigenic variations that immune survivors from one population will fall victim to the same morphologically identical but antigenically variant infection of another population. Examples are seen in the high rates of Streptococcal and Meningococcal infections experienced when new army recruits from different areas of a country are first mixed together.

Finally there is the kind of herd immunity which comes from generations of reproduction from within a population and which is obviously much more likely to occur among individuals with high innate resistance and high survival chance than among those immunologically less fortunate. The innate immunity is genetically transferred and gradually enhanced. Such herd immunity is more notable when it is absent as in the apparently tuberculosis prone original inhabitants of the Americas and the Pacific

Islands. It is also seen in the Sickle Cell trait particularly common in individuals of West African origin and apparently confers increased likelihood of surviving malaria. Unfortunately only the heterozygotes benefit and the herd immunity to malaria is maintained at the expense of the early death of the homozygotes. Genetically derived herd immunity continues automatically in subsequent generations of a population while the acquired forms last only as long as the survivors of infection remain dominant in the population. Once new non immune individuals are added by birth or immigration the herd immunity begins to wane and with each passing year the likelihood of a new outbreak increases.

2. Individual host factors

Surveys into what is often termed 'descriptive epidemiology' are frequently designed to quantify the relationship, if any, between disease and early death and those factors which affect the individual because she or he is who they are. This section is devoted to those relationships. Reliable information about the total precedents of sickness is limited by the expense and necessarily prolonged nature of the studies needed (Dawber et al 1963).

Though fascinating to study there is an inevitable negativism about the personal factors which put certain individuals at higher risk of disease or decay, especially if the course of the disease is unalterable. What is the profit for example in identifying individuals with creases in their ear lobes, alleged to indicate increased risk of coronary disease, if there is nothing which can yet be done to reduce the risk? Obviously very young or very old people are more susceptible than others to normally minor infections. Only women are affected by cancer of the cervix. Yet the documented progressive rise of cancer of the lung in women provides useful evidence of an adverse and reversible change in female life style. The analyses of age and social class specific mortality figures for cancer of the cervix suggest that here too there may at least be a component of life style with increased risk for the girls who early engage in sexual activity and who come from homes with poor standards of hygiene (Dunn and Martin 1967). A program to discourage young mothers from smoking on whatever pretext may reduce cancer of the lung but campaigns to voluntarily curb adolescent precociousness are much less likely to be productive.

If, as previously suggested, there is a genetic link to disease specific resistance it follows that the reverse will also be true. In effect some children will actually acquire a susceptibility from their parents in their chromosomes. This was shown to be the case in tuberculosis (Kellman and Reisner 1943). Such information is useful if only to indicate those individuals deserving priority in disease prevention and surveillance.

A different mechanism of inheriting susceptibility is of particular practical importance for many developing countries. It is demonstrated by the relationship of cancer of the liver in adults and the acquisition of hepatitis B virus from the mother occurring many years before (See Zuckerman chapter 26).

Stress, and its many variations including both trauma and fatigue, also victimizes individuals and apparently increases their susceptibility for a time to some infectious diseases as well as causing premature degeneration. Presumably stress either imposes some kind of unbearable load upon the immune system or activates inhibiter mechanisms. Physical effects such as gastrointestinal ulceration associated with emotional stress are as yet unexplained. A remarkable study begun prospectively in the United States forty years ago has shown that mental health, measurable in adolescence, is one of the principal determinants of physical health in later life (Vaillant 1979). The devastating effects of the 1919 *influenza pandemic* were explained as a consequence of chronic fatigue because that outbreak did not affect the normally susceptible, the very young or elderly, but the young working adults in a war devastated world. Stress-linked high infection rates can be seen today in some refugee groups though it appears that a population under conditions of disruption fairly soon learns to cope with the stress. Civil disruption can become so institutionalised in a population that the herd acquires an indifference to it which might appall an outsider. Indifference to stress, including the constantly repeated infections inherent in some life-styles and the abuse of drugs, may however exhaust the immune system producing the acquired immune deficiency syndrome (AIDS) ie Kaposi's sarcoma, lymphadenopathy and opportunistic infections in the sexually promiscuous (US.DHW ii 1981) later found in other individuals (US.DHW iii 1982).

Finally there is that group of potentially high risk factors related to deprivation or peculiarities of group behaviour. Measles and the diarrhoeas are the consequence of such problems in many warm climate countries because they impose themselves upon nutritionally weakened populations. The adversity may sometimes be self imposed by the community. Whole populations may be held back in development by bizarre dietary beliefs, taboos and destructive customs. Affluent societies too aberrate from healthy standards by consumption of the wrong foods, alcohol and drugs, by indolence and in the real or simulated pursuit of exciting pleasures (US.DHW i 1979). Each has its price in terms of ill health or the danger of infection or violence. Sadly these high technology pleasure-pursuing dangers have already been introduced into the developing countries also.

3. External discrimination

The previous section was concerned with those adversities or risks in which the individual has an element of choice. By contrast the external dangers or pressures upon the individual are largely imposed by the chance circumstances of the group into which the individual was born or has come to live. Such hazardous circumstances will exert their adverse effects unequally on the members of that group. Populations living in a year-round warm moist climate will inevitably be at greater risk from vector borne infections. The health benefits of a warm climate are also often negated by poverty and the risks, expecially from faecal-oral infections, which almost invariably accompany it. By contrast the colder the climate, the more likely is Man to crowd together and the greater the chance of airborne infections. The individual may run the additional hazards of being obliged regularly to travel to work in crowded discomfort. Or she or he may be obliged to work under hazardous conditions or exposed to gradually accumulative poisons or gradual destruction of the body.

Most societies exercise some form of social or class distinction or reward some individuals with special privileges. In an egalitarian society the distinctions may be as inapparent as the preference to be in the company of individuals with like jobs or educational background. The inevitable consequence is the increased likelihood of self destructive behaviour, such as excess drinking, in the self selected groups with least sensitivity to their own needs. In many developing countries the distinctions may be long institutionalised, as in the Hindu caste system of India, thus removing many elements of self choice though not necessarily eliminating equally destructive patterns of behaviour. In all either overt or concealed class systems the most poor become the worst educated, are forced into the meanest jobs and life styles and have the least knowledge to protect themselves from health dangers. In the United Kingdom, despite two generations of a health service which provides equal access and equal levels of service to all, the class differences in the likelihood of survival at birth and at later ages persist.

It can even be argued that the maintenance of the liberal class structure while permitting, as in Western Europe, an upward mobility for talented individuals actually deepens class differences in health. The previously ameliorating mixture of capable 'have-nots' when propelled into more privileged classes leave behind neighbours who are increasingly likely to constitute a large section of genetically perpetuated 'cannots'. The creation by the high technology society of a permanent technocracy at the top and of a permanent aggressive proletariat at the bottom is something many epidemiologists observe with anxiety. Any health care system itself is damaged as the more knowledgeable and more privileged seek private alternatives. This leads inevitably to deteriorating standards in the care provided for those less able to discriminate between what is and what is not an acceptable standard of service.

The effects of class are not simply economic or educational. Attitudes are fixed, practices are condoned which may be good or bad for the individual. The hazard, for example, of being a regular soldier originates not so much in the danger of being killed by an enemy as in the self destructive behaviour of alcohol and tobacco indulgence and violence which come from boredom. So much information is now becoming available about how individuals could, if they wished, improve their chances of health and survival that it has even been suggested by Stokes (1983) that health insurance charges should be related to risk.

Family risks are largely a compendium of what have already been described as potential hazards to each individual. They range from the immunity the individual inherits, the nutrition and intellectual stimulation of the infant and child, the standards of self discipline acquired, the dose of met infections endured — the dose being related to the number of individuals inhabiting a particular volume of space — the food and water storage and supply of the household and the attention and support, or antagonism and aggression, within the family unit. Even in the creation of the new family by marriage or life-sharing the individual enters into a relationship which will either be supportive of good health practices or, especially if disliked or stressful, is likely to lead to ill health. Though the arranged partnerships of Hindu India may appear remarkably trouble free the facts are that Indian women after marriage suffer far more hysterical and emotional illness than do women of other countries (Dube 1970). The health problems which tend to dog students in developing countries removed from the security of their family will be referred to in later chapters. In the developed societies similar ill health trends have been noted in individuals removed from a normal pattern of life sharing (Berkman and Syme 1979). Males rather than females seem to require a caring stable family environment for survival (House et al 1982). Care must always be exercised in interpreting such data. Comparisons made between cohorts of individuals based upon one facet of their lives, such as success or failure in marriage, take no account of differences in personality, education or original family background which inevitably push the individual to behave or react to circumstances in one way or another.

Even religious practices have profound effects upon the health of some individuals. These vary from the stress induced by moral rigidity or intolerance to the physical mutilation of female circumcision which is still widely practised in many African societies. Religious taboos against, for example, the eating of pork or shellfish might have a very sensible origin in a prehistory observation that such foods could be hazardous. Unfortunately the perpetuation of such taboos long after the hazard has been controlled may deprive growing children in those societies of good and relatively cheap sources of much needed protein. Marriage strictly limited to adherents of the same religion leads to concentration of defective genes in particular populations, for example of Tay-Sachs disease in Ashkenazy Jews.

4. Community shared hazards

With these the individual is like a helpless cork tossed on the sea of chances, victim of where she or he is. They are perhaps the hardest to change because community attitudes often conspire against the reformer. Generations of slow acceptance of new ideas and norms may be required to effect change, for example, birth spacing, or change may only come when a reasonable level of economic development and increased literacy creates the impetus for change within the society itself.

Individuals must suffer when born into a society with too many young dependents and too few opportunities. High levels of endemic illness or parasitism permit Man to remain fertile but sap the work capacity thus condemning the society to poverty continued. The rules or expectations of that society may force the individual into a hopelessly inappropriate role with inborn talents entirely wasted. The stress and deprivation tend to be all the greater when the individual is part of a minority group or has no local group affiliation.

Rigid societies dissipate individual abilities. Half the talent of intellect bound by chance into female bodies may be utterly discounted. It has been alleged that it is modern technology including preventive and curative medicine, which has created many of the ills in developing societies, when undeveloped they were in demographic balance with nature but now attitudes, aspirations and population numbers seem out of control.

In the high technology society too the community shared hazards seem to leave the individual dangerously adrift. From the threat of nuclear warfare to the frustration of the individual unable to attain the beckoning standards of happiness seen on the video screen the community has come to be a threat rather than a protector. The extension of controls over individuals and over their choices through centralised information systems looms every nearer with the society now the efficient if well-meaning tyrant. The profound simplicity of slogans which call for health (?care) for all fail to take into account that health is not something which can be bought or passively provided for each individual. Health is an extraordinarily complex amalgam of good fortunes, matching expectations. Medical care can never assure, rarely completely restore health in its widest sense once spoiled. This is in part because the factors which lead to sickness and to decay are far more complex than the mere meeting of microorganism or toxin and victim.

TERMINOLOGY

Carrier. In epidemiology an apparently healthy individual who not only has a reservoir of live organisms in his or her body but also possesses the accidental capacity to transmit them and infect new victims. The carrier may or may not have suffered the disease previously. In practice, through food handling it is the food spread infections in which the carrier state plays so important a part in the repeated cycles of diarrhoeal disease within family and community groups.

Generation time. Epidemiologically the interval between initial infection of a new victim and the beginning of the capability of this victim to further transmit the infection to new victims. Bacteriologically the mean interval of time for a particular type of microorganism to reproduce itself by division.

Incubation time. The period between the initial infection of a victim and the onset of recognisable sickness. In old parlance the Incubation Period was sometimes taken to be the same as the Quarantine Period. That is the entire period from the exposure to possible infection until the end of the possibility of further transmission taking place, taken originally to mean the end of the convalescent period.

Natural barriers. The mechanisms which nature has devised, such as the mucous membranes of the respiratory tract, or which happen to be part of the environment, such as the ultraviolet component of sunlight, which prevent most microoganisms and parasites from reaching the interior tissues of the body or which kill them before they can even reach a new victim. Further described in chapter three.

Pandemic. An epidemic spreading across all continents, worldwide. The virulence of the organism type sometimes wanes during repeated passage. The air-spread diseases are the most likely ones to be successfully transmitted throughout the world because of their short generation time, because of the difficulty in controlling them unless an effective, stable vaccine is available, because of the speed of Man's international travels and because some of the organisms, like the influenza virus, are particularly adept at changing their surface antigen and thus evade the normal braking mechanisms of an immunologically resistant population.

Pathogenic. Ability to cause actual disease in those a microorganism infects.

Virulence. Ability of a microorganism to cause serious or fatal illness in those in whom it causes disease.

REFERENCES

Berkman L F, Syme S L 1979 Social networks, host resistance and mortality: a nine-year follow-up study of Alameda County residents. American Journal of Epidemiology 109: 186–204
Dawber T R, Kennel W B, Lyell L P 1963 An approach to longitudinal studies in a community: the Framingham study. Annals of the New York Academy of Science 107: 539–556
Dube K C 1970 A study of prevalence and biosocial variables in mental illness in a rural and urban community in Uttar Pradesh — India. Acta Psyciatrica Scandinavica 46: 327–359
Dunn J E, Martin P L 1967 Morphogenesis of cervical cancer. Findings from San Diego County cytology register. Cancer 20: 1899–1906
House J S, Robbins C, Metzner H L 1982 The association of social relationships and activities with mortality: prospective evidence from the Tecumseh Community Health Study. American Journal of Epidemiology. 116: 123–140
Kellman F J, Reisner D 1943 Twin studies on the significance of genetic factors in tuberculosis. American Review of Tuberculosis 47: 549
Panum P L 1846 Observations made during the epidemic of measles on the Faroe Islands in the year 1846. Reproduced 1940 in Panum on Measles. American Public Health Association. New York

Stokes J 1983 Why not rate health and life insurance premiums by risk? New England
Journal of Medicine 308: 393–395

US.DHW i 1979 Healthy People: the Surgeon General's report on health promotion and
disease prevention. Washington DC. Government Printing Office (DHW publication
number (PHS) 79–55071)

US.DHW ii 1981 Kaposi's sarcoma and *Pneumocystitis* pneumonia among homosexual men
— New York City and California. Morbidity and Mortality Weekly Report. 30: 305–308

US.DHW iii 1982 Update on Kaposi's sarcoma and opportunistic infections in previously
healthy persons — United States. Morbidity and Mortality Weekly Report. 31: 294 and
300–301

Vaillant G E 1979 Natural history of male psychologic health. Effects of mental health on
physical health. New England Journal of Medicine 301: 1249–1254

Disease transmission and control

The first objective of the practical epidemiologist, it is agreed, is to limit disease spread. Total permanent eradication is rarely practicable. Control measures to be successful must be appropriate for the disease being transmitted. Once transmission is interrupted the task remaining is to concentrate on treatment of those already infected. Planning to interrupt the transmission of the infectious diseases is made simpler by the limited numbers of ways in which these disease are spread. Control is also simplified by the clues which most disease gives in its effects on its victims. Long before a specific diagnosis has been confirmed the correct transmission controls can be in place. Most infections fall clearly into one of four transmission types.

1. AIRBORNE INFECTIONS.

Generally these are caused by the viruses and bacteria able to infect from wet droplet aerosols produced by the coughing or sneezing patient. The droplets may also remain infectious as they dry to become droplet nuclei small enough to remain floating in the air until breathed in by a new victim. In order to launch themselves the diseases must cause a throat irritation or cough, a nasal irritation or sneeze. The mechanism is simple and the already infected victim actively connives in the spread of the microorganisms. The most likely target is the respiratory system of whoever is susceptible. It is also advantageous to the airspread invaders if each new generation is ready to travel before the first victim becomes sick and so removed from active circulation and contact with fellow men and women. For this reason the epidemiologic generation time of the airborne infections tends to be short.

The natural barriers against airspread infections are formidable. Few organisms can withstand drying — dessication — for long. Most are quickly killed by the ultra violet component of sunlight especially strong in most warm climate countries. Once fallen to the ground as fine dust most organisms also quickly lose their pathogenicity or die. Even if they remain floating in the air alive for a time they are so diluted by the atmosphere that their survival depends upon their ability to infect at very low dosage.

The conjunctiva is a vulnerable target especially for an aerosol of viruses but the barrier of tears with its potent IgA is able to deal with most microorganisms. IgA is the immune globulin found in body secretions, especially in the respiratory and gastrointestinal tract, which is usually able to deal with such organisms as the influenza virus or the cholera bacillus.

In the respiratory passages the invader must elude the sticky secretions and trapping hairs of the nasopharynx and trachea and the ciliated epithelium of the lower air passages. Finally invaders may be stopped by the small aperture of the terminal bronchioles which effectively prevent most particles over ten *microns* in diameter from reaching the vulnerable balloon-like alveoli where blood gases are exchanged. In effect this rules out colonisation of the alveoli except by those microorganisms which even when grouped together make only small particles — the viruses if they can stay in there despite the constant air currents — and the single cell invaders — the mycobacteria and deep mycoses. Infections like psittacosis, anthrax, plague and brucellosis can also successfully invade by this mechanism. The fungal or mycotic infections pose a special menace to man in the ability of their spores to remain viable for long periods either in dust or suspended in the air and additionally, especially in the case of coccidioidomycosis (Flynn et al 1979), to be transmitted over long distances by winds. The mycoses are not epidemiologically important in that man is usually the *end-point* host but the pulmonary forms can be especially dangerous for individuals exposed to bird or bat droppings. The mycoses are widely spread throughout the tropics and are of special danger to travellers through dry areas and conversely to workmen clearing forests (Lacuz 1980).

The control of the more common airborne infections is at once simple and difficult. In practice the diseases are unlikely to be transmitted by food, drink, inanimate objects, or even by direct contact with the victim — the oro-pharynx excepted. But also in practice it is almost impossible to change human behaviour to the extent of safely disposing of nasal secretions and of coughing, spitting or sneezing safely away from others. Any indoor habits of potential victims are helpful to infection, sunlight is excluded, air interchange is limited and victims are close to those already harbouring the microorganisms. Modern technology with the creation of airconditioning systems has even assisted in the dispersal of these diseases. Not surprising then that the crowded institutions, meeting places, buses, army and refugee camps are particularly vulnerable points for airborne disease transmission. Given equal resources, the inhabitants of warm climate countries with less need to stay indoors should be at less risk from this group of infections than inhabitants of less hospitable climates. It does indeed seem evident that the decline in the incidence of airborne diseases like tuberculosis or rheumatic heart disease owe more to economic advancement with consequent improvements in housing and nutrition than to any deliberate disease control programs.

Attempts to interrupt disease transmission by preventing individuals from gathering into groups during *epidemics*, by flooding buildings with fresh air and by making the infected wear surgical masks have been of limited success. For very special purposes air can be cleansed but at very great cost (Meers 1983). It is obviously sensible in designing a new hospital which will provide care for some patients with airborne infections to ensure that their used air is not then ducted to other patients. The use of ultra violet light, special measures for dust suppression and the physical segregation of patients from each other and from staff seen not worth the cost.

In practice the control of some airborne infections has been fortuitously assisted by the development of reliable immunising agents and by the sensitivity of the bacilli to relatively inexpensive antibiotic therapy. For the many common cold viruses and the various mutations of the influenza virus, control is much less practicable though the chances of being infected are obviously reduced by maintaining a safe distance between susceptibles and those showing symptoms.

2. FOOD AND WATER BORNE INFECTIONS.

There is no important epidemiologic distinction between those diseases most commonly spread through foods and those through water or water based drinks. Most depend upon the faecal, less commonly vomit or urinary, contamination of whatever other potential victims consume by mouth. In most cases the transmission is simple, man to man, though a few of this group of infections are primarily of animal origin and a few are passed to man when he eats another animal, its milk or its eggs.

The size of the infecting particle is no longer critical so that pathogenic organisms from tiny enteroviruses to the large eggs of parasites are equally well borne into the human gut. As the vehicle is food or water it follows that the diseases must include a mechanism by which the food or water of others can be contaminated liberally by excretions from the gastro-intestinal tract. Explosive diarrhoea or vomiting efficiently scatter the contained pathogens over the food or into the drainage leading to the water supply of the next victim. It follows that the food and water spread diseases will usually cause diarrhoea or at least some gastrointestinal irritation. Fortunately the urine, which would be an excellent vehicle for onward transmission, has only been adopted by a small proportion of these infections. Notable outbreaks of typhoid have been attributed to this method of spread. A secondary mechanism is a more direct faecal-oral spread without contamination of food. Such infections spread primarily within families like hepatitis A rather than in epidemic forms and diarrhoea does not need to occur. Reference has already been made to the particular importance of symptomless carriers in this whole group of infections.

The natural barriers against these organisms are, in environmental terms, less formidable than those ranged against the airborne pathogens. Certainly water, rather less food, tends to dilute the dose. But humans tend to live closely together and to share food and water more intimately than they share air. The multiple uses to which water is put, drinking, washing, irrigation and recreation also add to the hazards. Once inside the human body the natural barriers include the acidity of the stomach and the digestive juices. The relatively effective barrier of the lining of the intestinal tract with its potent IgA may also be why the minimum infecting dose of the food and water spread pathogens is surprisingly high. (See Rohde chapter 20 and Robinson chapter 22.)

The control of the food and water borne infections is, at least in theory, relatively easy. While freeing air of pathogens on any scale is impracticable, the means of sterilisation or pasteurisation of fluids and foods are relatively simple. The fact that the human hand also commonly acts as the vehicle between the anus of the first and the food of the second victim should also facilitate interruption of transmission. The hand is relatively easily cleaned of pathogens, at least in the numbers required to cause sickness. Cross infections to man of animal type salmonellae will obviously be related to the consumption of high risk foods such as duck eggs for *typhimurium*. Controls are more expensive when they involve foods which are not usually cooked such as milk and its products.

In practice the food and water transmitted infections, especially in malnourished groups, are the principal causes of both sickness and premature death in the world. Both immunising agents and currently available antimicrobials are relatively ineffective in preventing outbreaks and even in treating those infected. It follows that the only reliable way to interrupt transmission of the man to man infections is to change human behaviour and to keep the victims alive until their own immune mechanism can deal with the invader. In the first case it is necessary to improve standards of hygiene and food storage, in the second it is necessary to restore fluid balances which are especially unfavourable to the very young. Unfortunately to improve hygiene, especially in food preparation, requires more than health education. It seems to require not so much a perfectly safe supply of water but one which is so available in each home that it will be used for washing (Cairncross and Feachem 1978).

3. DIRECT CONTACT INFECTIONS.

This is the smallest group of infections but contains some frightening diseases. The group has only one characteristic in common. In some way each succeeds in penetrating the outer envelope of the body. The group includes the relatively mild coccal diseases of the skin most commonly associated with warm moist climates and poor nutrition. Of the several invaders of the conjunctiva trachoma is the most important. Some rely on an ability to invade mucous membranes rather than the intact skin and this is the particular transmission pattern of the venereal infections. Others including hepatitis B and Kuru viruses spread through direct tissue transfer, respectively active secretions such as tears and mothers milk and human brain eaten raw.

Only a few members of this group have the power to penetrate the undamaged skin but they include the cercariae of schistosomiasis, the larvae of ancylostomiasis and the free living forms of the leptospires. As a sub group they are particularly insidious because they leave behind no obvious skin damage.

Other members of the group depend for their penetration into the living tissues under the epidermis upon some interruption in that cover. This characteristic of infections like anthrax, tetanus and fungi can be provided by even minor trauma in a non furred animal such as man. Or it can come through the bite of an infected animal, the mechanism for rabies. There will always be a history of trauma but this may be forgotten during the long incubation periods of several of these diseases.

The group as a whole is epidemiologically daunting because the natural barriers prove ineffective. There is a climatic barrier for those parasites which like schistosomiasis depend upon a warm moist environment but this is not easily manipulated. Anthrax and tetanus depend for their peculiar power not on any actual facility to penetrate the skin but on their propensity to lie around for years as inert spores on the chance that some accident will get them in. They are also highly resistant to normal decontamination procedures and appear to be able to produce disease with very small doses.

The control of this group of infections depends primarily upon limiting Man's intimate contact with the hostile environment, protecting the skin, especially the feet, eliminating zoonotic sources of infection and taking good care of wounds. Eradication of the sexually transmitted disease is technically possible and tetanus and hepatitis B could be eliminated by universal, maintained vaccination.

The epidemiologist is faced, in attempting to control these infections, by two almost impossible tasks. The first is that of eradicating the sources of infection in nature, the second is that of radically changing preferred patterns of human behaviour. Cannibalism at least has virtually ceased so presumably ending the chances of Kuru tranmission.

4. VECTOR SPREAD INFECTIONS.

Most of the tropical fevers will be found in this group. Their particular association with warm and especially with wet climates, stems from the temperature sensitive nature of most of the vectors as well as the part played by water in the life cycles of both vectors and parasites. Not all the vectors are warm climate dependent. Even malaria and arbovirus transmitting mosquitoes can survive in highly seasonal climates with transmission limited to a few months each year. The flea borne plague and louse born rickettsiae seem actually favoured by climates that encourage Man to huddle in unwashed groups. Both have a potential for explosive outbreaks especially under conditions of social disruption. Tularemia is virtually limited to cold climates.

For most of the epidemiologically important vector spread diseases the problem as seen by the District Health Officer will be one of the ebb and flow of *endemic* or *holoendemic* disease. The susceptibles will be the youngest members of the population. For those infections of zoonotic origin the problem will occur as spills-over from the zoonotic reservoir. In several of the group including leishmaniasis, plague and other arboviruses, any monitoring of environmental hazard levels is best performed at the animal source. As this level rises spill-over into the human population can be anticipated.

Control of many of the vector borne infections should, theoretically, be relatively easy. The vectors of the common rickettsiae are easily eliminated or avoided. Man can be isolated from the sylavatic sources of fleas, phlebotomus, reduviid bugs and glossina. The dose of simulium bites can be reduced through changes in agricultural practices while Aedes breeding can be controlled where it occurs close to Man. Malaria should also be controllable. Man is the sole important reservoir of infection. But the heroic WHO eradication campaigns aimed at the vector proved largely temporary in benefit and at unacceptably high ecological cost.

While much can be done in changing Man's environment, especially his housing, though an expensive investment for poor countries, control of the principal vectors seems unlikely to be the answer for disease like malaria. For the temporary visitor into a malarious area chemoprophylaxis is at least a part solution. It can be used also for some rickettsiae, plague and African (gambiense) trypanosomiasis, but resolution of the problems for the indigent, repeatedly exposed population seems more likely than anything to come through immunologic techniques.

DISCUSSION

At District level the Health Officer/Epidemiologist will find, hopefully, that the ways in which the infectious diseases present are not, in practice, as complex as the variety of morphologic details might suggest. In any area there is generally a fairly steady incidence of the same type of disease. Even in the case of unexpected outbreaks there will often be obvious clues in the common symptoms which will indicate what epidemiologic precautions should be taken to prevent further spread. It is the sheer quantity of endemic sickness, especially the diarrhoeal type diseases, which can be discouraging especially to a physician or nurse practitioner frequently preoccupied by surgical and obstetric emergencies.

The hard pressed District Health Officer would do well to remember that the control of most of the infectious diseases can only be effective and permanent if there is coincident economic and educational advancement in the community. It is a tragic irony that much can already be done using available technology. But the shortfall in resources or unreliability of supplies, the reluctance to change lifestyles, completely confound the inappropriate skills taught in medical and nursing schools. They require instead infinite patience and political aptitude. There is even an ethical argument against allowing disease control programs to develop if dependent upon the vigour and determination of one person. Will the program continue when that individual is gone from the area? To deal effectively with disease outbreaks in epidemic quantity the requirement is speedy response and the rapid mobilisation of available resources without being wasteful. There is a generic pattern of actions which can be applied to most disease outbreaks, modified by local circumstances. Proceed step by step as follows:

1. Make sure that the report is true. As far as possible verify that the reported symptoms, or any tentative diagnosis made by field personnel, fit the facts. Much effort and unnecessary alarm have been wasted on false reports or on the panic of an inexperienced individual.

2. Having confirmed that the disease, possibly tentatively identified, exists make sure that the number of cases really is far in excess of normal. Once this is confirmed the need for epidemiologic skills is established. It is only at this point that the Health Officer should consider going personally to the area or sending other valued professionals.

3. The epidemiological investigation begins by seeking the common factors which link the cases. It documents the numbers of individuals affected, where they live or work and establishes a schedule or time pattern of when each individual began to be sick. As well as the 'Who-When-Where' it may be profitable briefly to consider the age distribution of cases, sex, culture, recent ceremonial or population movements and any recent environmental events.

4. Identify the type of outbreak. By now it should be clear whether there is a 'point-source' or whether infection is being propagated in a series of cycles with outbursts of new cases. Cyclical effects are soon lost after the first part of an epidemic. Be prepared to consider multiple sources of infection. The time scheduling of the original cases is important because once widespread the origin of any infection becomes completely obscured.

5. Now define the population which is not yet sick but which is at risk. These individuals require protection but they will also carry the infection if they travel to other areas. If this is a man-to-man type infection it is likely that this presently well but at-risk population also contains the original reservoirs or carriers. If the disease is of probable animal origin, a zoonosis, the veterinary or agricultural experts should now be involved in control attempts.

6. By now the epidemiologist should be in a position to suggest a likely cause for the epidemic. Its type, air borne, food or water borne, contact or vector borne should be apparent. So also its nature, probably infectious if fever is a common symptom, probably toxic if there are few cases with fever. Anticipate that patients sick from quite unrelated infections will mix into

and confuse the case load. And of course it is not unknown for two unrelated epidemics to coincide in the same population.

7. The search for additional unreported cases will now be important if the infection is life-threatening but treatable or if each untreated case must be dealt with before the spread can be contained. Total case control is particularly important in some airborne infections, like the meningococcus and in the flea and louse borne infections, plague and typhus. By contrast the food or water borne infections will usually already have been widely dispersed in a community before any control measures can be imposed. In such circumstances it may be better to attempt to contain it to the population originally at risk and allow it to burn out, removing the original source of infection, and concentrating on rehydration if diarrhoea is the main symptom.

8. Interrupt the infection cycle if this has not already been done. This is the stage of active intervention and its nature will be dictated by the type of infection, its likely source and the population at risk. First the probable reservoir of infection will have been removed or isolated be it human or animal or the source of a toxin will have been sealed off. Second if the new cases are also highly infectious they will be treated or isolated. Third the mechanism of further transmission will be interrupted by whatever control is possible on suspect food, water, vectors or population behaviour. Fourth the susceptibility of those yet unaffected will be reduced by immunising procedures or by chemoprophylaxis. Fifth the infection will be limited to where it began. The assistance of authority will be useful in preventing individuals from highly infectious communities travelling to others not yet affected. Mixing of cases and unaffected persons within communities is more difficult to control.

9. Maintain observation or surveillance for the expected late cases. Only in a point source epidemic related to a particular water supply or to a particular batch of contaminated food can an epidemic be expected to terminate abruptly.

10. Assess what was done, its apparent effectiveness and consider the likelihood that given similar circumstances a similar later epidemic is likely. Will some permanent preventive measures be necessary or was this a chance occurrence?

11. Institute whatever permanent environmental or immunologic corrections are necessary and as fast as possible. Eliminate a probable *microclimate* danger source. Once a community senses that the danger is past it becomes very difficult to overcome the normal inertia to change anything.

12. Keep in contact with the community, train local individuals to act as observers and early reporters of future health changes.

Four simplifications, or over-simple assumptions, have been made in the suggestions so far. These are that infectious illness in populations can be classified by type, that the type indicates the transmission pattern, that the application of the measures indicated to interrupt transmission can be expected to stop the spread if not eradicate the disease and that government, employers, landowners and even community leaders will act in the best interests of the community.

In practice some diseases, especially those with long incubation periods like typhoid, trypanosomiasis or viral hepatitis creep upon a community by stealth. Or the transmission pattern may simply not be certain, for example the perpetuation of a simple zoonosis like some forms of leishmaniasis without any apparent animal reservoir. The third and most serious oversimplification comes through viewing human populations, especially in developing countries, as passive 'herds' willing to respond as advised or as ordered. No individual, however well educated, likes to make an effort for which there is no apparent purpose especially if the effort also costs money and has to be kept up over a long period of time. The diarrhoeal diseases for example will be controlled only when people wish to be clean and to dispose of their faeces safely because that is seen as socially desirable and when such habits as hand washing before preparing food are deeply ingrained from infancy. It is similarly difficult to persuade village ladies to use a new well rather than to go down to the Glossina infested river bank for their water and gossip.

Finally the frequent failures of the establishment to respond to the health needs of communities when these involve investing scarce capital, or forcing unpopular changes in local habits, can be understood. Sadly aid from outside intended to effect such changes is sometimes diverted or frittered away.

The Health Officer must also be careful to ensure that the correction of one evil does not increase another, for example the proliferation of filariasis vectors in open sewerage drains. Where any real permanent improvement in the health of the community can only come through correction of poverty and ignorance the will of the people to change must be aroused. This requires the skills of the propogandist and the mass media. After that they will need not the skills of the physician but those of the politician, economist, agricultural and industrial developer and the environmental engineer. Only then will the major infectious diseases be controlled.

TERMINOLOGY

1. *End-point host.* In human terms an individual infected with a disease which is unable to complete its life cycle in Man but may cause damage in the meantime. Also used to indicate an individual infected with a disease whose onward transmission requires a vector which is unlikely to feed on Man.

2. *Holoendemic.* Used most frequently in the description of the prevalence of malaria where it implies that at least 75 per cent of younger children have enlarged, palpable spleens. In such communities with virtually

universal repeated malaria infections the surviving adults will have high resistance to the disease and relatively few will have a palpable spleen.

3. *Microclimate.* A local reversal of ecology which allows an unexpected vector to prosper and presents an unexpected pattern of parasitism in the human population. The microclimate may be man made, for example discarded cans which retaining the occasional rain in a dry climate make it possible for Yellow Fever carrying Aedes mosquitoes to breed. Or the microclimate may be nature made, for example the termite hills of East Africa which harbour the moisture-seeking, leishmaniasis-carrying Phlebotomus.

4. *Micron.* The single unit of this linear measurement is one thousandth part of a millimetre. Usually expressed as a 'μ'.

5. *Point source epidemic.* A brief exposure of a group of susceptibles to the same infection or toxin source at the same time. The effect will be a sudden peak of cases and no more. A 'common source' epidemic is similar except that the single origin of sickness may continue to affect others in the same area for some time.

6. *Pasteurisation.* Heat treatment, most frequently of fluid to be taken by mouth, sufficient to kill all important pathogens but not to cause a taste change. (See Abdussalam Chapter 39)

7. *Propagated epidemic.* Spreading from case to case with increasing numbers until the susceptibles have mostly been affected when numbers of new cases will then decline.

8. *Sterilisation.* Heat, chemical or radiation treatment designed to kill all living organisms. Essential in medical procedures as well as in food canning and bottling. As it causes an undesirable taste change in many foods and liquids, especially milk, pasteurisation is often preferred.

REFERENCES

Cairncross S, Feachem R 1978 Small water supplies. Ross Institute Information and Advisory Service. London.
Flynn N M et al 1979 An unusual outbreak of coccidioidomycosis. New England Journal of Medicine 301: 358–361.
Lacuz C, Da Silva 1980 Deep mycoses in tropical countries. From Health policies in developing countries. p 109–111. Royal Society of Tropical Medicine. London.
Meers P D 1983 Ventilation in operating rooms. British Medical Journal 286: 244–245.

Immunization

INTRODUCTION

The spread of some diseases, such as yaws, brucellosis and rabies, can most effectively be suppressed by a strategy which prevents transmission from the source host. Some infections, such as cholera, typhoid and urban yellow fever can be controlled by attacking the causal organism during its passage through the environment from one host to another. The third major approach is to induce immunity in the potential recipient, thus protecting him from infection and, at the same time, hindering the spread of the agent through the community.

The fact that immunity often follows attacks of disease was recognised many centuries ago, and led to the practice of variolation, the deliberate induction of smallpox in healthy individuals by innoculating them with infective material from mild cases. The risks of this procedure, although great, were considered to be less than that incurred from naturally occurring smallpox.

When Jenner observed that milkmaids stayed pretty because their exposure to cowpox protected them from smallpox, he introduced the idea of immunising agents whose dangers were greatly less than those of the diseases against which they offered protection. What he did was to recognise in vaccinia a virus whose ability to produce disease in man was low but whose antigenic structure was sufficiently similar to that of the smallpox virus to induce an immunity against both infections.

Jenner employed a naturally occurring virus, but the principle of immunisation that he introduced continues through all vaccines to the present day — that of administering a substance which is capable of inducing a protective immunity against a specific infection or disease, without itself producing that disease.

During the last 80 years this principle has been applied in vaccines which contain deliberately modified live organisms (e.g. Measles, BCG), unmodified but killed organisms (e.g. pertussis, typhoid), treated toxins produced by virulent organisms (e.g. tetanus, diphtheria) and, more recently, specific antigens obtained by splitting virulent organisms (e.g. meningococcal vaccine).

Immunisation is generally a simple, straightforward procedure, and programmes of immunisation offer countries the opportunity to effect radical improvements in the health of their populations more rapidly, safely and cheaply than using any other single approach. They have become the foundation upon which the development of wider health care services has been possible in many developing countries.

BACKGROUND TO IMMUNIZATION — ACTIVE AND PASSIVE IMMUNITY

Active immunity

Active immunity is the response by the immune system to the presence of a specific antigen. The serological response in previously unexposed individuals is usually in two phases. The immediate response is the production of macroglobulin (IgM), which is often measurable as complement fixing antibody and which may last for a few weeks only. Under cover of this defence there starts the production of specific gamma globulin (IgG), which is often detectable as neutralizing antibody. If the site of entry involves mucous membrances, as in the gut or the pharynx, there may also be a local response shown by the appearance of secretory IgA.

The production of IgG follows the learning by the immune mechanisms of the appropriate pattern of the specific antibody to be manufactured to neutralise the antigen. Once this pattern has been learned it is usually remembered for many years, if not for life. The significance of this is that the response to challenge by natural infection or vaccine at any time after this immunological memory has been established will be the production of large quantities of specific IgG in time to neutralise the infecting agent before it can invade. This is the secondary (booster) response.

Active immunity can follow exposure to either naturally occurring or artificial (vaccine) antigens.

Passive immunity

Antibody produced by active response to an antigen will provide protection against challenge by the same antigen. If this antibody is transferred to another individual it will provide similar protection until it is used up or catabolised.

The transfer of ready-made antibody can occur naturally or artificially. Specific protective IgG formed against a variety of infectious agents crosses the placenta from mother to foetus during the last trimester of pregnancy. This antibody acts to protect the infant against the appropriate antigens. The level of antibody so given wanes with a half life of about thirty days. The duration of protection depends on the original antibody titre and the level necessary for protection, varying from three to five months for poliomyelitis up to nearly a year for measles.

The role of this passive antibody is to give the infant a chance to survive the difficult first few months without being overwhelmed by the more common infections. At the same time, however, the antibody will act against vaccine antigens, and vaccines will tend to be less effective if given at a time when the infant still has circulating maternal antibody.

Not all infections induce transferable antibody. Pertussis is not only common but severe in the first three months of life, because no protective antibody comes from the mother, even if she is herself immune.

Preparations of specific antibodies — antisera — are still used for the management of tetanus and in the post exposure prophylaxis of rabies, but except in these infections, this approach is now less commonly used than formerly.

VACCINES

The purpose of vaccines is to induce an active, artificial immunity without

Table 4.1 Summary of characteristics of live and non-live vaccines

	Live	Non-live
Efficacy	Full range of immune response, as to natural infection.	More limited range of immune response
Number of primary doses	One dose usually enough	Multiple doses usually needed
Duration of immunity	Longlasting or lifelong	Usually needs reinforcement
Safety	Risk of reversion to virulence. Biological risks of infection	No risk of causing specific disease. High antigen mass may cause hypersensitivity/immune complex problems
Storage	Most are heat labile	Less heat labile. Long shelf life

Table 4.2 Table of classification of important vaccines

	Viral	Bacterial
Live	Measles Poliomyelitis (Sabin) Yellow Fever Rubella Mumps Smallpox	B.C.G. (tuberculosis)
Killed	Rabies Poliomyelitis (Salk) Influenza	Pertussis Typhoid Cholera
Toxoids	—	Diphtheria Tetanus
"Split antigens"		Meningococcus Pneumococcus

the risks attending the natural infection. The choice lies between vaccines with live or non-live components (see tables 1 and 2)

Live vaccines

If an infective agent is appropriately treated, its virulence can be reduced while its antigenic potential remains intact or only slighty lowered. This process of attenuation can be achieved by repeated culture of the agent in conditions which tend to select out less virulent strains.

A strain so produced will colonise, multiply and induce an immunological response in the host in much the same way as its more virulent cousins. If it is introduced into the host by the natural route it will induce an immunity that is qualitatively similar to that following a natural infection.

It must be remembered, however, that infection, be it with natural or attenuated strains, is a biological interaction between two or more types of organisms, and the outcome is never totally predictable. Two of the possibilities to be considered are that an atypical host may react in an abnormal, and possibly deleterious fashion, or that the attenuated organism may revert in the host to a virulent form which may be dangerous to the recipient or his contacts.

A further important aspect of live vaccines is that they must remain alive in order to be effective. This entails special care in both transport and use.

Non-live vaccines

a. Killed vaccines

If a virulent organism is killed, its ability to infect, and thus cause its specific disease, is eliminated. At the same time, if the organism is killed gently it may be possible to retain its antigenic structure, and thus produce an effective vaccine.

Although this principle has worked for many infections, such as pertussis and typhoid, it does not always work as well as it might, for the lack of ability to infect may imply a lowered antigenic potential. Whereas a live vaccine organism may work its way into the body, stimulating the immune defenses at various points and multiplying to many times its original number, a preparation of killed organisms can only go where it is put and cannot multiply. The efficacy of killed vaccines is often qualitatively and quantitatively less than that of their live counterparts.

The intensity of the primary immune response is proportional to the size of the antigenic mass. A live vaccine, introduced in suitable dosage, will multiply up to the appropriate mass, and therefore produce a durable response from a single dose. Because the killed antigen cannot do this, it is necessary to inject large masses of antigen and to repeat the dose in order to ensure an adequate response.

b. Toxoids

Some infectious diseases, such as tetanus and diphtheria, are caused not through invasion by the agent but by the action of the toxin that it produces. If the bacteria causing these diseases are cultured in a suitable medium, it is possible to extract the toxin and to render it harmless but still antigenic. Toxoids are among the safest vaccines. Because their inherent antigenicity is low they are usually adsorbed onto metallic adjuvants.

c. Purified antigen preparations

The antigens which are responsible for stimulating the production of protective antibody make up a small proportion of the total mass of the bacterium or virus. The remainder may at best be dead weight as far as a vaccine is concerned and at worst, by producing hypersensitivity reactions, be actively harmful. The identification and extraction or synthesis of specific antigens can lead to the production of precisely effective vaccines. Vaccines which contain purified polypeptides and polysaccharides are now becoming available. Meningococcal vaccine is an example. Vaccines of this type promise much for the near future.

VACCINES IN COMMON USE IN DEVELOPING COUNTRIES

Vaccines are available against many human infections of public health importance, but only a few are very widely used. The diseases against which most developing countries aim to protect their children with the use of vaccines are:

Diphtheria	Measles
Pertussis	Poliomyelitis
Tetanus	Tuberculosis

Some characteristics of these vaccines are given in table 3 for ease of reference. Important aspects other than these will be described individually.

1. Diphtheria

Diphtheria is probably not a major problem in most developing countries, although it is undoubtedly underdiagnosed and under-reported. Surveys show a high prevalence of naturally acquired immunity, which probably arises from opportunistic skin infections rather than faucial diphtheria.

The toxoid, which is given by intramuscular injection, gives solid immunity after two doses, but most programmes include a reinforcing dose at school entry. It is almost always given as a component of the Diphtheria-Pertussis-Tetanus "triple antigen" vaccine. The side effects of this combination usually amount to no more than mild fever and soreness at the injection site. The very occasional serious effects that do occur are attribut-to the pertussis component (see over)

Table 4.3 Characteristics of some commonly used vaccines

Vaccine	Type	Route	Minimum Starting Age	Doses	Duration of Immunity	Storage Life 2–8°C	37°C	Price* US$
Diphtheria	Toxoid	Intramuscular	2–3 months	2 +	5 years +	2–6 yrs**	2–6 mths	.04 (DPT)
Tetanus	Toxoid	Intramuscular	2–3 months	2 +	5 years +	2–6 yrs**	2–6 mths	.04 (DPT)
Pertussis	Killed	Intramuscular	2–3 months	3 +	5 years +	18–24 mths**	4 weeks +	.04 (DPT)
Measles	Live	Intramuscular	9–12 months	1	Life	1 yr +	2–28 days	.10
BCG	Live	Intradermal	Birth	1	15 years	1 yr +	2 weeks +	.02
Polio (Sabin)	Live	Oral	3 months	3 +	Life	3 mths–1 yr	1–2 days	.02
Polio (Salk)	Killed	Intramuscular	3 months	3 +	Life	2 yrs +	4 weeks	1.0
Yellow Fever	Live	Intramuscular	9 months	1	Life	1 yr	1–2 days	0.10

* The prices quoted are minimum prices obtainable by very large bulk purchase in 1981 (except Killed Polio vaccine — 1982 price estimated for 'low antigen' vaccine)
** Diphtheria–Pertussis–Tetanus combined vaccine must be kept *above* –5°C, at which temperature it freezes and denatures.

2. Tetanus

Tetanus is a major contributor to neonatal mortality, accounting for 40 per cent or more of all deaths in this age group in some developing countries. The most important cause is contamination of the newly cut umbilical cord. The practices which lead to this are not easily changed, but the infant can be protected by stimulating maternal antibody production to ensure that protective quantities of IgG are transferred to the foetus. Two doses of vaccine separated by six weeks during pregnancy are recommended for this purpose.

Tetanus is also a problem in older children and adults. Immunity does not develop in response to natural exposure to *Clostridium tetani* or its toxin, even after an attack of tetanus, and the only way to ensure protection is therefore with the use of toxoid. At least two doses in infancy followed by a reinforcing dose on school entry will induce long term protection, but the opportunity should be taken to offer further doses after injuries.

Tetanus toxoid is given by intramuscular injection. It is safe, cheap and effective, with only the same minor side effects as are seen with diphtheria toxoid, plus a very occasional urticarial reaction and an even rarer 'serum sickness' type of response.

3. Pertussis

Whooping cough is common in all developing countries and ranks as the most important specific infection of childhood in some. In epidemic waves the case fatality rate may exceed one per cent.

The vaccine contains whole, killed *Bordetella pertussis* organisms. Like diphtheria and tetanus toxoids it is given by intramuscular injection, usually in the form of triple antigen. Its efficacy is estimated to be between 60 and 80 per cent, but when it fails to protect vaccinees completely, it appears to reduce the severity of the disease. This vaccine has been at the centre of controversy recently because of its rare association with screaming attacks, convulsions and permanent neurological damage. In developing countries particularly, these small but real risks must be set against the serious nature of the natural disease.

The disease is most severe in children below the age of six months, which allows little time for the required minimum of three doses of vaccine. The protection of slightly older children, however, may delay infection in their younger siblings to a less hazardous age, by reducing transmission of the organism within the family.

A more effective and safer pertussis vaccine is high on the list of requirements for immunisation programmes everywhere.

4. Measles

Because of poor nutrition, measles poses a large threat to the health and life of many children in developing countries, where the case fatality rate may be 5 per cent or more. Measles holds a dominant place in the vicious circle of infection, diarrhoea and malnutrition, so that the effective use of vaccine will reduce morbidity and mortality not just from measles but also from other associated causes.

For maximum effect in developing countries, measles vaccine needs to be given between the ages of nine months, when passive immunity is waning, and about eighteen months, the modal age for infection. On operational grounds, many countries' programmes tend to go for an earlier rather than a later dose, offering the vaccine at nine to twelve months. The overall protective efficacy is about 85 per cent.

Measles vaccine is given by the intramuscular route. It is a safe vaccine, but mild febrile reactions are not uncommon. Encephalitis is the only serious side effect, occurring in association with about one in a million doses. Modern measles vaccines are more thermostable than their predecessors (see table 2), but they will not withstand exposure to sunlight.

As is the case with all live vaccines, a pre-existing infection or poor state of nutrition in a child who is to receive measles vaccine does increase the worry of an atypical reaction. However, because a child in this condition is likely to be made even worse if he should contract measles, there is a good argument for not withholding the vaccine.

5. Poliomyelitis

Evidence from surveys carried out in the past few years has shown that the incidence of polio in developing countries may reach 40 per 100 000 total population, representing a prevalence of lameness in schoolchildren of one per cent. The majority of clinical poliovirus infections occur in the first two years of life. Maternal antibody offers some protection against infection for the first three to four months, and reduces the efficacy of vaccine given in that period.

Oral poliomyelitis vaccine (Sabin type)

OPV contains live, attenuated strains of poliovirus. It is usually given as a preparation containing a balanced mixture of all three serotypes. Because of interference between the types it is necessary to give at least three doses to be reasonably sure of achieving seroconversion to all three serotypes. The first dose may be given at three months, and three doses should be given before the end of the first year. If possible, a minimum interval of six weeks should be left between doses, to allow for the cessation of excretion of virus following the previous dose.

For a number of reasons, including enterovirus competition, persistent maternal antibody and intercurrent infective diarrhoea, OPV induces seroconversion less reliably in hot countries with poor sanitation than it does in developed countries. Attempts to overcome this problem have included repeated mass campaigns and pulsing strategies which depend on the proven principle that when a high proportion of children in a community are fed OPV at the same time, the 'take' rates are markedly improved. This probably occurs because of cross infection with the vaccine virus and because the competing enterovirusus are overwhelmed. The same principle underlies the value of OPV in the control of epidemics of poliomyelitis.

The storage and transport of OPV demands efficient refrigeration, which is the main drawback of the vaccine. The success of a programme in administering OPV is a measure of the effectiveness of its cold chain.

OPV is a very safe vaccine. The only side effect is the occurrence of paralytic disease in vaccinees or their contacts. This occurs about once for every million children fully immunised, and is usually associated with vaccine serotypes 2 or 3.

Inactivated (injectable) poliomyelitis vaccine (Salk type)

The first poliomyelitis vaccines used were prepared from killed virulent polioviruses. The newest vaccines, licensed in 1982, are not radically different from those early vaccines, but contain a greater mass of antigen. IPV is a highly effective and extremely safe vaccine which was responsible for most of the decline of poliomyelitis in developed countries. Although it has not yet been widely used in developing countries, the results of field trials and the fact that it is much more heat stable than OPV, promise that IPV will be a very useful addition to the vaccine armoury, particularly as it offers the chance of achieving lasting immunity with only two doses. The outstanding problem is the price, which is considerably higher than that of OPV.

6. Tuberculosis (BCG)

Tuberculosis is endemic in every country. Surveys in some developing countries have revealed active pulmonary tuberculosis in two per cent of the population. It is a disease of underdevelopment, responding rapidly to improvements in nutrition, housing and environment. The use of BCG is a useful adjunct to this, but used as the only control measure it is unlikely to bring the disease under control.

The vaccine contains live attenuated bovine mycobacteria. It acts by inducing a local cell-mediated response which is analagous to the primary complex and which is detectable by the tuberculin reaction. It can be used effectively at any age from birth.

Field studies have shown protection rates from BCG against pulmonary tuberculosis which vary from 80 per cent waning over 15 years in Europe, to no protection at all in south India. Protection against disseminated infection in infancy, and particularly meningitis, appears to be more clear cut.

BCG is given by intradermal injection. When it 'takes', a small nodule appears at the site of the injection within a few days. This usually breaks down to an ulcer which heals over the next 4 to 6 weeks, leaving a permanent scar. This is normal and cannot be looked upon as a side effect, but occasionally, and particularly if the vaccine is administered in too large a dose or too deep, large ulcers may result. Regional lymphadenopathy may develop and, very rarely, disseminated infection may occur. The management of these atypical reactions may call for antituberculous therapy.

In those developed countries where BCG is used in adolescents rather than infants, the vaccine is offered only to those found to be tuberculin negative. This is not applicable where BCG is used in an infant schedule, and most developing countries find the two stage operation involved in tuberculin testing too costly to be workable, even when the vaccine is being used in older children.

BCG is freeze dried and has a good storage life at refrigerator temperature, but it cannot tolerate sunlight.

VACCINES WHICH ARE LESS USED IN ROUTINE PROGRAMMES

a. Yellow fever

In countries in the yellow fever belt, vaccine may be included in the infant schedule. A single intramuscular dose of the highly effective live vaccine will give long term, probably lifelong protection. It is not recommended for children below six months of age because of an increase in the very small risk of encephalitis.

b. Typhoid

Typhoid vaccine contains whole, killed organisms. It confers approximately 75 per cent protection after two intramuscular or intradermal doses, but the protection does not last more than a year or two and this vaccine is therefore most appropriately used as a personal protection for travellers and others at special risk, and as a second line measure in epidemic control. A new, live oral vaccine is showing great promise under test.

c. Cholera

Cholera vaccine contains whole killed organisms, is administered intramuscularly and induces reasonable levels of circulating antibody for periods of up to nine months. This antibody is largely inappropriate because cholera is caused not by invasion by the vibrio but through the local action of exotoxin on the bowel. The vaccine offers about 60 per cent protection after two doses, but is of no value in controlling epidemics or international spread as it does not affect the incidence of asymptomatic excretion.

CONTRAINDICATIONS

Contraindications are formulated either for the protection of the vaccinee or to ensure the full efficacy of the vaccine. In most developing countries the risk from the target diseases far outweighs any risk from the vaccines, and a health worker who turns a mother and her child away from an immunisation session on the grounds of a minor illness, when they may have spent all morning getting there, risks never seeing them again.

A guideline which may be appropriate in much of the developing world is that any child in the target age group who attends, for any reason, a health facility other than a hospital should be considered eligible for immunisation unless the clinical condition necessitates referral to hospital. In such cases a decision on immunisation can be taken by the hospital medical officer. Hospital authorities may want to offer vaccine to newly admitted children in order to prevent the spread of infectious diseases within the hospital.

SIMULTANEOUS ADMINISTRATION OF VACCINES

Concern is sometimes expressed over the simultaneous administration of different vaccines. Two reasons might be proposed for avoiding this; first that the risk of side effects might be increased, and second that the vaccines might lose effectiveness. Neither is valid. Mixing of vaccines in the same container or syringe, except where they are specifically formulated like this (e.g. DPT), may introduce problems of reactions between additives, but there need be no hesitation in giving a range of vaccines in different sites at the same encounter with the child.

BENEFIT AND RISK

All vaccines constitute some hazard to the recipient. The size of the risk in terms of severity and frequency of associated morbidity must be balanced against the probability of the individual (whether or not he is immunised) contracting the natural infection, and the likely outcome if he does. When the target disease is serious and common, a vaccine with appreciable dangers may be deemed acceptable, as was the case when smallpox was endemic. When the naturally occurring disease becomes rare, the dangers of the vaccine grow in significance, and very small risks, such as that from oral polio vaccine, may become unacceptable.

Even when 'immunisable' diseases are still a major problem, these ethical considerations must not be neglected by programme planners. The parents of a child have the right to know of any side effects to which their offspring is to be exposed, and the smooth running of a local programme can be seriously hampered if this is not considered.

IMMUNIZATION PROGRAMMES

The choice of infant immunisation as a public health intervention must imply a national commitment of resources for an indefinite period, for the practical aim of any immunisation programme in a developing country must be long term control, not eradication, of the target diseases. This commitment to the success of the programme is the decisive factor. With it, a way will be found round all difficulties, without it the enterprise is doomed to stagnation and failure.

This chapter is not long enough for a detailed discussion of programme development and implementation, but the headlines can be considered.

1. Determining the size of the problem

The commonest childhood infections amenable to vaccines are the six discussed above; pertussis, diphtheria, tetanus, measles, poliomyelitis and tuberculosis. An estimate of the incidence and social importance of these diseases and an indication of the age at which they commonly occur may be obtained by anecdote, by special surveys or by estimates based on the experience of other countries. Reliable field survey techniques exist for poliomyelitis, neonatal tetanus and measles, and should be used. There is little place for serological surveys.

2. Priorities

Child care is high on the list of health priorities for most developing countries, and immunisation is usually seen as a relatively cheap and effective intervention. The social and political importance of the diseases susceptible to immunisation are the main determinants of of the priority accorded to them, but the practicalities of their control must be considered. Thus, despite its recognition as an important cause of long term morbidity, poliomyelitis is sometimes given low priority because of the extra delivery problems inherent in the thermolability of OPV.

3. Programme management structure

Immunisation is the most effective, visible and accountable facet of primary maternal and child health care. Organised as such it can be used as a spur to primary health care development, and at the same time can itself benefit from a milieu in which mothers and children are accustomed to receiving care and support. An immunisation programme needs strong management through a structure which gives a clear definition of roles and responsibilities throughout, from the programme manager to the vaccinator in the field. This structure must be designed at the planning stage, and training and retraining of personnel must be a major component of the plan.

4. Vaccine storage and transport — the cold chain

The effective life of all vaccines is dependent upon their being stored within specified temperature limits (see table 3). This requires the development of a chain of refrigerated stores and transport containers stretching from the vaccine manufacturer to the child. This has been made possible by the development of refrigeration and transport equipment which is reliable in tropical developing country conditions. Cheap and effective temperature monitors have also been produced which give a warning if vaccines have been exposed to unsuitable temperatures, and at the same time provide a marker of the efficiency of different parts of the chain.

Despite all this, the chain depends on every link being maintained adequately and under supervision, and on the precise control of ordering, stocktaking and deliveries. The logistic details must be worked out in detail before a major programme is embarked upon, and the need to provide relevant and continuing training to personnel in the techniques of the cold chain are paramount.

5. Programme targets and objectives

In order that a programme may have a yardstick against which it may measure its progress and costs, realistic and quantified goals must be set:

Targets should be in terms of the coverage of the target population with a specified number of doses of each vaccine

Objectives should be of stated reductions in incidence of the target diseases.

Both targets and objectives should be set within a realistic time structure.

6. Immunization schedules

Within the immunological requirements of each vaccine, the age at which doses are given, the number of doses and the intervals between them are to some extent determined by operational constraints such as communications, accessibility of mothers and children at different ages, and the capabilities of the cold chain. The guideline that must prevail is that the schedule should achieve protection with each vaccine before the age at which the child is at major risk from the disease. In practical terms in developing countries this means full dosage of all vaccines before the end of the first year of life — three spaced doses each of DPT and polio vaccines and one dose each of BCG and measles, if all six antigens are to be used.

7. Strategies

The design of mechanisms by which an effective schedule is implemented can follow no fixed rules, but any strategy must take into account:

— The demands of the epidemiology of the target diseases e.g. age of attack, seasonality, epidemic periodicity
— The demands of the vaccine e.g. storage and transport requirements
— The demands of the recipients of the programme e.g. distance to travel, work patterns, harvest times
— The capacity of the logistics and delivery system e.g. resources, personnel, transport, cold chain

A most important feature is that the strategy must be suitable for a long term, if not permanent programme. Flash-in-the-pan programmes do more harm than good.

Programmes may be based on fixed centres, may be fully mobile, or may have features taken from both approaches, with a fixed centre serving outlying areas through outreach clinics. All can be effective in the right conditions, but delivery through fixed units does offer unique advantages of stability and mutual support from the other facets of primary health care, as well as more economical use of staff. Most countries are attempting to channel their primary health care through static centres wherever feasible.

8. Surveillance

As an indicator of progress towards objectives, surveillance of the target diseases is essential. Various approaches to this can be suggested, the local circumstances dictating the method(s) chosen.
— Notification by health units. Data collected this way are notoriously unreliable, but may be of value in indicating trends.
— Sentinel health units. Full reporting may be limited to a few reliable and appropriately placed health units.
— Specialised health units. Cases of particular diseases may gather in specialised units, which are then in a position to gauge their incidence over a large area. This has worked well for poliomyelitis reporting by physiotherapy/rehabilitation units,
— Incidence/prevalence surveys. Periodic surveys of sample populations may provide useful information for special purposes and can provide correction factors for other methods of data collection.

9. Community participation and health education

The selection of priorities and target diseases must take place in the light of the wishes as well as the needs of the potential recipients of the programme. The design of schedules and strategies must take account of the preferences and practicalities of everyday life of parents and children. If these things are not considered, the programme risks having low attendance and poor results. The delivery of successful immunisation services to a community and the maintenance of community interest are not only a matter of posters and loudspeakers but also of consideration and attention shown in the clinic and an attitude of caring reflected in the advice and support coming from it.

10. Evaluation

It is essential that the activities and progress of the programme be evaluated continuously and at intervals. With all functions fully described, it is possible for each level of the programme to be assessed in relation to the achievement of its defined objectives and targets. The value of evaluation as a means of providing information for management cannot be overstated.

11. Vaccine testing

In a perfect programme all vaccine would be administered in mint condition. However, for those occasions when breakdown in the cold chain is suspected, when there is epidemiological evidence of ineffective vaccine being used, or for the occasional checking of vaccine that is close to its expiry date, vaccine testing facilities should be available, either in the country or through international cooperation. The results must be made available as rapidly as possible if they are to have any practical value.

THE WHO EXPANDED PROGRAMME ON IMMUNIZATION (E.P.I.)

In 1974, the World Health Assembly, recognising the value of immunisation programmes in reducing morbidity and mortality in childhood, committed WHO to a programme to develop immunisation services. EPI has set itself the target of making immunisation against the six target diseases discussed in this chapter available to all children in the world by the year 1990.

The chief areas of activity of the programme are management advice, training at all levels, the development of cold chain equipment and techniques, assistance with programme evaluation and, in collaboration with other agencies such as UNICEF, the provision of vaccines which conform to the WHO requirements.

A central tenet of E.P.I. is that immunisation programmes are a national responsibility, and that although they can be supported by external financial assistance (particularly for those capital items requiring 'hard' currency, such as vaccines), at least two thirds of the cost must be met from national budgets for an indefinite period.

The WHO Expanded Programme on Immunization is an example of the sort of international collaborative effort that can only really effectively be mediated through international organisations. Its progress and successes to date suggest that its medium and long term impact on child health throughout the world will be very large indeed.

The District Health Officer

To most people brought up in traditional Western medicine, public health, community medicine and epidemiology are compulsory chores to be signed off as quickly as possible so that the 'real medicine' of surgeon, physician and gynaecologist can be studied. Indeed anyone who does not adopt this practice will undoubtedly fail his examination. This is a pity because everyone who has served in a developing country where health services are run on a few pounds per capita per year will know that much of the knowledge that he painfully acquired is irrelevant and most of the problems have their roots in the very parts of the course that were glossed over or neglected. The District Health or Medical Officer in such an area has a unique opportunity for solving clinical problems, benefitting a community and contributing to the general epidemiological knowledge of the country.

BACKGROUND INFORMATION

Before any meaningful medical policy can be formulated the physician must get as much information as possible about
   a) The area and physical environment
   b) The people and their customs.

The area and environment

1. It is essential to obtain an accurate *large scale map* of the district. Mark in every health facility, hospital, health centre and even visiting point of the mobile unit. Round each one draw a 5 or 10 mile circle — to show the present stage of health coverage and indicate the areas for development.

Mark in important roads, tracks, air-strips, schools and administration centres, and water sources. Note that certain rivers may isolate a large area if they flood, and that construction of an air-strip might ensure access in an emergency.

The altitude may vary by 500 or 750 m in different parts of the district — which in turn affects the vector population and disease pattern. In some

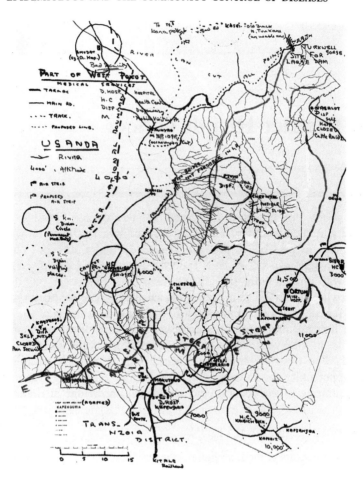

Fig 5.1 An example of a large scale map

districts with steep escarpments, the variation is so acute that it is possible to identify the patient's village by his condition. (Cox 1973)

2. As rainfall and temperature are rarely recorded in different parts of a district, check with the local department of agriculture, who often keep detailed records, and if they are not available, invest in a few wedge rain gauges and maximum/minimum thermometers. A member of staff in each sub-centre can then be taught to use them. This information is important in assessing the vector population and in any future cooperation with agriculturalists in the challenge of malnutrition.

The people and their customs

The customs and beliefs of the people are even more important to an under-standing of health problems — and usually much harder to uncover. It is essential to find out what the local people believe about disease and particularly what *they* regard as problems, if we are to get co-operation in what *we* think are the priorities.

To this end, find out all local names for diseases — and if possible the usual treatment. Occasionally this may be helpful — but often it is not, working on the principle that the disease is something to be expelled by purgation or emesis or driven out by sacrifice.

Find out what people eat and how often and how the diet varies in different seasons. Pay particular attention to the customs regarding food taboos in pregnancy and weaning customs, because these often lie at the back of the prevalence of Kwashiorkor and other problems of malnutrition.

The attitude to curses and evil spirits may often provide an explanation for the undiagnosed condition or mental abnormality.

Just as the disease pattern may vary within a district — so customs and way of life may vary between Urban, Farming and Nomadic communities and any preventive measure will have to be presented in a completely different way in each situation.

For instance, it is of little use advocating latrine construction for Nomads; washing for people with a three miles' walk to a water hole or regular checkups for people 30 or 40 miles from a dispensary. Nor is it much use advocating a high protein diet in pregnancy when eggs are taboo, unless careful thought is given as to the exact food that is not only available but also acceptable.

The classic investigations into Kuru and its connection with cannibalism (Matthews, Glass and Lindenbaum 1968; Hornabrook and Moir 1970) and Pigbel with pig-feasting (Murrell, Roth, Egerton, Samuels and Walker 1966) — both in the Highlands of New Guinea show the importance of custom to the epidemiologist. Another example is that of the Pokot tribe of Kenya whose women believe the possession of a tape worm will enhance the chances of pregnancy — thus giving a false prevalence to males in the dispensary returns (Cox, 1972) as women do not seek treatment.

ESTABLISHING BASELINES

No progress can be measured in any health situation unless there are records with which to compare the current situation. (L. Blanc and M. Blanc 1981).

1. Collate and codify all existing records, reducing attendances and certain disease incidences to graphical form.

2. Observe upward or downward trends or changes from the norm — particularly looking for slow changes or cyclical changes in incidence, which may enable one to predict epidemics, as in the case of Poliomyelitis in Kenya. (Fendall, 1960; Metselaar and Nottay, 1974).

3. In assessing seasonal change, add the same monthly figures for several years together and plot on a graph.

4. Use your local knowledge to 'translate' these trends for the Ministry.

For instance, a sudden rise in attendance at a dispensary may merely indicate the removal of an unpopular staff; the rise of Sexually Transmitted Disease, the opening of a new 'bar'; or the sudden advent of Brucellosis, the start of the use of the Rose-Bengal test in the laboratory, rather than the start of an epidemic.

One of the most useful tools for establishing baselines is the 'Mini Survey'. This technique consists of getting all staff with primary patient contact to elicit one fact, measure one parameter or note one characteristic during the normal day's work. It costs nothing and the cumulative information is invaluable — even if it is in no way a proper random sample.

1. Use a specially designed tally sheet for each investigation (Fig. 5.2)
2. Use the issue of the sheet as an opportunity to educate the staff, inform them of previous results and generally enthuse them over the task of gathering information.
3. Make instructions simple and unambiguous and the question to be asked or measurement to be made, capable of being carried out in a few seconds.

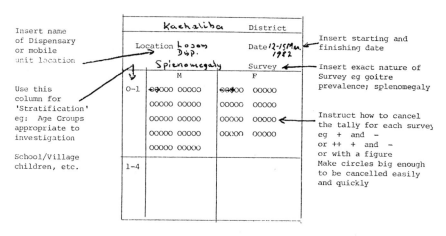

Fig. 5.2 Example of Tally Sheet

4. Apart from the specific instruction give general rules for all investigations. For example:

Once started — see *every* consecutive case. Record all cases, negative or positive. Continue until about 50 consecutive cases have been seen, etc.

The design of the tally card is very important:-

Use circles arranged in groups of 5 which can be crossed through or filled in with a + or – . Make sure they are sufficiently widely spaced to allow easy and rapid marking and unambiguous counting.

Divide the sheet vertically for Male and Female; and horizontally for stratification into age groups, occupation or other characteristic as necessary.

In an investigation into infant mortality use a simple squared sheet, which can take 2 numbers separated by an oblique stroke — thus 2/5 signifying two children have died out of a total of five deliveries.

The Mini Surveys can be used simultaneously over the whole district during one week. It is a flexible tool and ideally suited to mobile work. An example of its use would be to estimate prevalence of splenomegaly, goitre, eye disease, varicose veins, etc. Or to establish the infant mortality rate, stillbirth rate or abortion rate — although this line of questioning takes longer and might be confined to the clinics — only asking the normal outpatient workers to question a much smaller number of patients. (See Fig 5.3).

With modern filter-paper techniques samples of blood can be collected in a similar way and sent to larger laboratories where anti-body levels can be estimated, the details of the individual being recorded in pencil on the filter paper itself. Any new ELISA test can also be carried out by this technique (Volles and de Savigny 1981).

RETURNS AND REGISTERS

The record clerk is a key man and should be personally supervised by the D.H.O. Try to cut out useless or reduplicated information. Registers are basically summaries from which broad general statistics are drawn: patient's notes are personal documents that link diagnosis and treatment to an individual.

Thus registers should be drawn up to show:

1. Age/Sex distribution
2. Approximate locality
3. Tribal and ethnic category
4. Preliminary diagnosis
5. Rising or falling attendance
6. Rising or falling incidence of specific conditions

It is not necessary to record names or exact addresses and much can be done by a tally-sheet kept by the outpatient officer himself.

The diagnosis in a register is rarely more than a first impression and is hardly ever changed as a result of tests — so the headings given can be

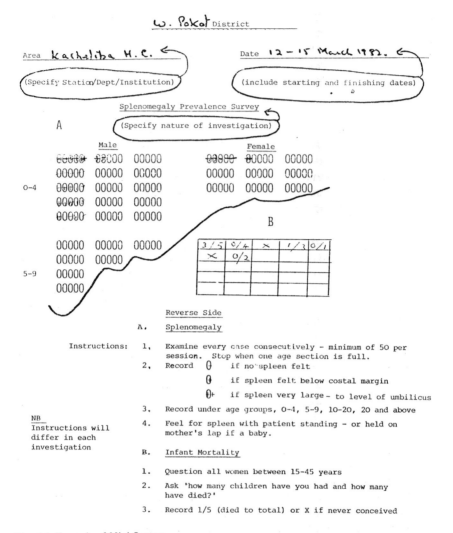

W. Pokot District

Area Kachaliba H.C.

(Specify Station/Dept/Institution)

Date 12 – 15 March 1982.

(include starting and finishing dates)

Splenomegaly Prevalence Survey

A   (Specify nature of investigation)

Male			Female		
00000	00000	00000	00000	00000	00000
00000	00000	00000	00000	00000	00000
00000	00000	00000	00000	00000	00000
00000	00000	00000			
00000	00000	00000			

0-4

B

| 00000 | 00000 | 00000 |
| 00000 | 00000 |
| 00000 |
| 00000 |

5-9

3/5	0/4	✗	1/3	0/1
✗	0/2			

Reverse Side

A.   Splenomegaly

Instructions: 1.   Examine every case consecutively – minimum of 50 per
              session. Stop when one age section is full.
          2.   Record   0   if no spleen felt
                        0   if spleen felt below costal margin
                        0+ if spleen very large – to level of umbilicus
          3.   Record under age groups, 0-4, 5-9, 10-20, 20 and above

NB
Instructions will   4.   Feel for spleen with patient standing – or held on
differ in each   mother's lap if a baby.
investigation
          B.   Infant Mortality

          1.   Question all women between 15-45 years
          2.   Ask 'how many children have you had and how many
              have died?'
          3.   Record 1/5 (died to total) or X if never conceived

Fig. 5.3 Example of Mini Survey

limited to broad disease classification or even a record of symptoms, which
the D.H.O. can interpret from his detailed local knowledge, or by the
simple expedient of getting all cases of 'General Malaise', for instance,
referred to him for a few days, so that he can run laboratory tests and
examine them properly.

Inpatient and laboratory records are the receptacles of accurate diagnosis
and are used to fill in the detail of the general pattern of the disease.

Special registers for Tuberculosis, Leprosy, Cancers and any notable disease
can usefully be kept — usually by the Medical Officer. The main point here

is that all staff must be aware of their existence and refer all cases to be recorded. These registers — or files — are detailed and are used to identify individuals for treatment, follow-up or future research, and are particularly useful in observing patients' progress in chronic conditions or where treatment regimes are varied, and the patient's own notes habitually lost.

SIMPLE INVESTIGATIONS

The planned investigation follows from the perusal of the records and results of the mini-surveys outlined above. Problems should be listed, given a priority and arrangements made to investigate as opportunity allows.

1. The D.H.O. can mount a properly executed survey using his own personnel and perhaps a central laboratory if the local laboratory is too small.

2. A team can be brought in by interesting the national teaching hospital or an international health organization. If possible, this team should be persuaded to use local workers and staff and join in with the day to day work of the hospital, as this will establish their credibility with the local people and also educate the local workers.

Valuable information can be obtained from immigrants in these surveys as their entry into the district can be accurately known and a good idea of incubation times and pattern of transmission obtained — either in imported disease or incidence of local disease in the new population, as in the incidence of Buruli Ulcer in Rwandans in Uganda (Morrow, 1975).

As an example, the writer found that after one year's work in the Pokot area of the Kenya-Ugandan border the problems were:

1. A virtually 100% prevalence of eye-disease — due to trachoma.

2. A high prevalence of gross splenomegaly — thought to be due to Malaria, Kala Azar and/or Brucellosis.

3. A painful hip syndrome.

4. Procidentia in low-para females in the 20–30 age group.

In the circumstances of a semi-nomadic pastoral people and a small mission hospital the following decisions were taken:

(a). To treat the eye conditions as they occurred — prevention being very difficult in view of the habits of keeping cattle near the houses, shortage of water for washing and putting oil on the skin thus attracting flies.

(b). To carry out a series of tests, using a Rapid Agglutination method to diagnose Brucellosis — and later to test these results against the tube agglutination. This yielded the information that about 30 per cent of the spleens and 40 per cent of the hips had a titre greater than 1:240 (Cox, 1966 and 1968).

(c). To carry out a postal survey of the procidentia in the same way as Burkitt worked on the lyphoma (Cook & Burkitt 1970) which eventually showed the condition to be uncommon in E. Africa and very rare in the age groups that we were seeing — the aetiology probably being the result of determined fundal pressure by the local midwives! (Cox and Webster, 1975).

Other investigations carried out in the district by outside teams included a WHO Malaria Survey; the Makerere investigation into the Tropical Splenomegaly Syndrome; various stool surveys on school children; and a long investigation into the sandfly population financed by U.S. aid. (Wykoff, Barnley &Winn, 1969)

The general principles of surveys are well described in the text books, but the following points may be of use:

1. Define the area to be studied.

2. Make sure that every individual or properly random sample is studied.

3. Stratify the population to include educated and uneducated; nomadic, farming and urban; indigenous and non-indigenous; and all age groups.

It is a good discipline to prepare every investigation for publication and it is a regrettable fact that very few Ministries of Health either encourage investigation or give a forum where these important papers can be discussed.

EPIDEMICS AND CONTROL

Most major control schemes such as mollusciciding and treating the local rivers with insecticide or spraying houses are policy decisions handed down from Ministry level — although the D.H.O. should be involved in both the planning and the execution. Epidemics, however, often rest entirely with the D.H.O. in the vital few days between diagnosis of the first cases and mobilization of the national machinery.

1. The outcome of the epidemic depends almost entirely on the speed with which the index cases are dealt with, for if it is a longer time than the incubation period a second generation of cases will appear. (Cox 1970). Thus every member of the health team must be alert to diagnose and be fully aware of exactly what he or she has to do or to whom to report.

2. Have standing orders ready for the eventuality and a committee of local officials and community leaders designated for an emergency. When the alarm is given — treat as top priority and go personally to check the diagnosis and also the fact that it is of epidemic proportion. Take specimens from cases or bodies, if deceased.

Alert the Ministry, request air transport, if appropriate, for the specimens, and keep the authorities informed of your whereabouts.

Arrange quarantine for cases, give instructions to schools and call the local committee to close roads, limit population movement, etc., if this is deemed necessary.

Request vaccines for immunisation and drugs for treatment and prophylaxis. Start vaccinating staff and workers and immediate contacts. Then vaccinate from the centre and aim to form a cordon sanitaire. In certain diseases like cholera and meningitis, give prophylactic treatment to everybody living within a 100 metre radius or every person in an institution if applicable.

Trace movements of cases for the period equivalent to the incubation of the disease (Cox, 1970). Pinpoint and remove the cause if possible — for instance, an infected cow giving Brucellosis; treating or closing a well or shutting up a restaurant.

Lastly make sure that the records of the epidemic are written up from a local standpoint, as well as from the official or scientific point of view. Obviously much of this exercise depends on organisation and logistics and particularly the alertness of the staff — and this can only be obtained by the teaching and example of the D.H.O.

REFERENCES

Blanc L and Blanc M 1981 The Role of utilisation studies in the planning of Primary Health Care, World Health Forum 2 (3): 347–349
Cook P and Burkitt D 1970 An epidemiological study of seven malignant tumours in East Africa, Med Res Council
Cox P S V 1966 Brucellosis — A survey in South Karamoja, E Afr Med J 43.2: 43–50
Cox P S V 1968 A Comparison of the Rapid Slide and Standard Tube Agglutination Tests for Brucellosis, Trans Roy Soc Trop Med & Hyg 62.4: 517–521
Cox P S V 1972 The Disease Pattern of the Karapokot, M D Thesis, London University
Cox P S V 1972 Cholera in Northern Kenya, E Afr Med J 49.6: 440–447
Cox P S V 1973 Geographical Variation of Disease in a Single District, E Afr Med J 50.12: 713
Cox P S V and Webster D 1975 Genital Prolapse among the Pokot, E Afr Med J 52.12: 694–699
Fendall N R E 1960 Poliomyelitis in Kenya, E Afr Med J 37.2: 89–103
Hornabrook R W and Moir D J 1970 Kuru: Epidemiological Trends, Lancet ii 1175
Matthews J D Glass R and Lindenbaum S 1968 Lancet ii: 449
Metsalaar D and Nottay B K 1974 Poliomyelitis, Health and Disease in Kenya, Ed Vogel Muller Odingo Onyango and de Geus, p 255–260 E Afr Lit Bureau
Morrow R H 1975 Buruli Ulcer, Uganda Atlas of Disease Distribution, Hall & Langlands, E Afr Publishing House
Murrell T G C Roth L Egerton J Samuels J and Walker P H 1966 Pigbel — Enteritis necroticans, a study in diagnosis and management, Lancet i: 217
Volles A and de Savigny D, 1981 Diagnostic serology of tropical parasitic diseases. Journal of Immunological Methods 46(1) 1–29
Wykoff D E Barnley G T and Winn M 1969, E Afr J Med 46.4: 1

Disease distribution and program priorities

Whether at district, regional, national or international level what the epidemiologist seeks is information — and reliable information at that. The greater the area and population covered, the more remote is the epidemiologist's contact with the citizens and primary health workers in that population and the greater is the likelihood of missing significant events whose progress might have been changed if they had been noted in the early stages. Given time, interest and some minimal resources it is at district level that the most exciting opportunities exist for gathering information about ill health experiences and for intervening to meet the population's needs.

The information required is concerned principally with the volume of sickness broken down, as far as possible, by type and by the proportion of those who die. In fact death is of all events in the existence of an individual the one most likely to be reported and to be described with some accuracy. Sickness from which recovery takes place is much less likely to be reported, especially when it is the kind of sickness to which the local population is accustomed.

International comparisons of morbidity, the frequency of certain sicknesses in different populations, are often more truly comparisons of the effectiveness of the particular disease reporting system. National data can be no more reliable than the crude information by which it is fed in from the health regions and districts. The less well informed the original informant and the more likely is she or he to misunderstand what information is actually required.

One of the traps to making valid international comparisons lies in the unwillingness of some governments to publish information which would encourage an enemy to think it temporarily weak because of sickness, which would raise awkward questions from its internal political opponents or which would frighten off potential investors or tourists. In the past information has often been suppressed concerning plague, typhus, yellow fever, smallpox and endemic or epidemic famine. Today governments might be more likely to suppress information relating to salmonella type outbreaks, hepatitis, zoonotic events such as anthrax and violence.

As sickness is important primarily because it threatens or shortens life it follows that a simple way to compare the ill health in different populations would be to observe at what average age the members of those populations died. Such comparisons have the disadvantage that they take no account of non-fatal chronic diseases, such as onchocerciasis, which may make life miserable but do not necessarily prematurely terminate it.

Comparisons of the crude death rates in different countries are invalidated by the different age distributions in the populations. A population of young persons, however ill served, will tend to survive. A population with many very young children or elderly persons will be highly sensitive to sickness. A death rate specific to a particular age group would be somewhat less vulnerable to false assumptions. The one most frequently chosen for comparisons is the *infant mortality rate*. Even this though is potentially misleading as it gives no impression of what occurs in other age groups of the population. Useless to be satisfied with a low infant mortality rate if the same infants later die of malnutrition, gastrointestinal infections or measles in the post weaning period. In so far as reliable information exists to support its calculation, the *life expectancy* at birth taking into account the specific mortality of each age group would better indicate the chances of survival of the newborn. Figure 6.1A shows the results of such calculations. The darker the shading, the more likely is a newborn infant to survive into old age.

On figure 6.1B will also be observed the two parallel lines on either side of the equator — 23° 27' North and 23° 27' South. These are the tropical latitudes between which the sun wanders and returns each year. Outside these lines the maximum strength of sunlight declines. The further outside the tropical latitudes and the colder is winter. Climate, and its relative hospitableness to human development, is also influenced through high air currents which, generally rotating from west to east across the world, bring clouded, humid climates to western coasts and leave eastern coasts dry, cold in winter and hot in summer. Seasonal hot summers even well outside the tropics are favourable to the spread of tropical-like infections through the agency of vectors able to adapt to the seasonal swings.

The area subject to tropical-like infections is also wider than the tropics because the principal insect vectors, the main agents of this extra disease load, can withstand all but freezing temperatures. The area free of severe winter frost is shown by the dotted lines between which lie the 'warm climate countries'. This is not to say that populations outside the frost free regions will be entirely free of the vector borne diseases. Flea and louse borne infections have already been noted to prosper in the coldest of climates. Some malaria and arbovirus carrying mosquitoes can survive inside the frost zones and leishmaniasis is very adaptable. Many populations, like those of north Africa, Pakistan, north India, Bangladesh, south Argentina, Chile and Australia live well outside the tropics but nevertheless are at high risk, even if on a seasonal basis, of vector transmitted disease.

If, as figure 6.1A suggests, the populations who live in the warm climate countries tend to have shorter lives than those in the temperate and cold

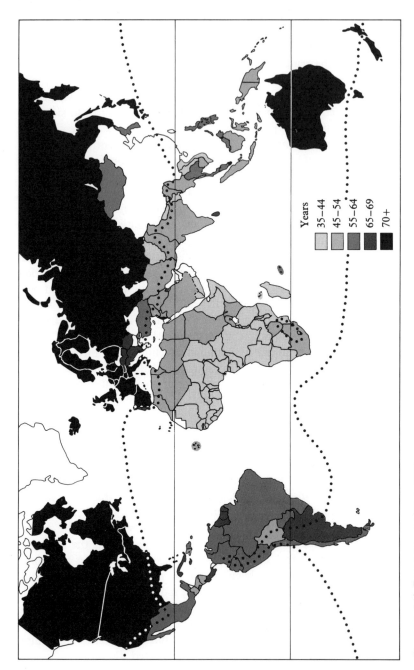

Fig. 6.1A Life Expectancy at birth in 1975
Source: United Nations Population Division

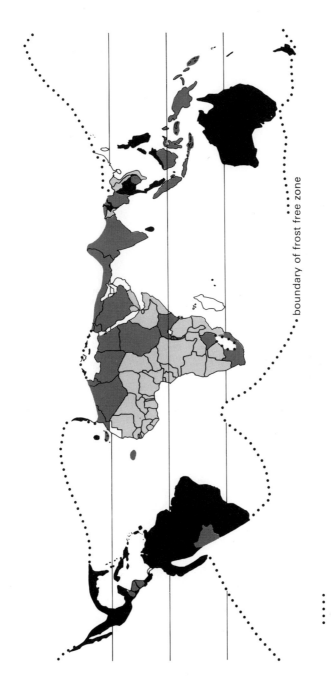

Fig. 6.1B The warm climate countries

boundary of frost free zone

Table 6.1 Birth and death data for twelve warm climate countries

	Fiji 80	Singapore 81	Australia 80	Thailand 80	Cuba 81	Kuwait 79	Mauritius 80	Sri Lanka 80	Ecuador 78	Egypt 81	Guatenala 80	Mali 76
Birth Rate per 1000	29.4	17.0	15.4	23.2	13.9	37.9	26.1	27.6	29.1	37.6	41.8	43.2
Death Rate per 1000	6.4	5.3	7.4	5.3	5.9	4.0	8.1	6.1	7.2	10.1	9.8	18.1
Natural Increase %	23.0	11.3	8.1	17.9	8.0	33.9	18.0	21.5	21.9	27.5	32.0	25.1
Infant Mortality Rate/1000	9.9	10.8	10.7	13.3	18.5	31.1	32.2	37.1	64.4	73.5	85.9	120.9
DEATH RATES/100, 000												
All infections + parasites	37.4	21.5	3.5	48.3	15.4	115.7	45.6	19.4	186.0	31.6	397.8	—
Diarrheal disease	17.8	2.3	0.6	11.7	5.5	65.2	31.3	49.7	106.2	7.5	190.7	—
Respiratory tuberculosis	4.7	12.3	0.4	14.6	2.8	15.2	2.6	10.5	14.7	5.4	14.1	—
Tetanus	0.2	0.2	—	1.9	0.2	2.6	1.8	—	9.9	6.7	2.6	—
Measles	0	0.1	0.1	0.2	0.5	3.2	—	0.5	25.6	2.6	105.6	—
Cancer	32.8	103.5	153.5	21.0	106.3	72.9	46.8	29.5	37.9	19.9	27.8	—
Mental + epilepsy	1.8	1.0	7.0	0.5	1.6	1.4	5.7	—	9.4	2.1	9.8	—
All cardiovascular	157.2	170.6	385.3	43.2	237.7	225.9	250.0	71.5	92.1	205.7	48.4	—
Pneumonia	28.4	40.4	13.9	10.1	41.4	—	28.3	—	49.5	45.1	96.3	—
Pregnancy + childbirth	3.0	0.7	0.3	4.0	1.9	2.8	5.4	4.5	11.8	6.7	12.5	—
All accidents	35.1	45.3	44.4	36.0	57.0	148.1	53.0	35.3	66.2	49.1	264.7	—
Malaria	—	0	—	8.2	—	—	—	3.6	—	—	—	—
Other arthropods	—	—	—	—	—	—	—	—	—	—	—	—
Diabetes	30.2	14.3	10.3	2.7	11.1	12.4	29.8	9.2	5.4	6.2	4.7	—
All nutritional	4.9	1.6	0.4	3.5	1.2	1.0	6.5	14.2	17.1	2.0	40.8	—

calculated by the author from data in World Health Statistics Annuals for 1981 and for 1982. National statistics and causes of death. 1981 and 1982 editions. WHO. Geneva.

climates where do the problem lie? In Table 6.1 are the *disease specific death rates* for a number of the common causes. In the technologically developed countries, with their relatively ageing populations, the principal causes of death are, as would be expected, cardiovascular disease and cancer. There is, however, little point in making comparisons between the young populations of warm climates and the elderly populations of cold climates. Consequently Table 6.1 is concerned only with 12 representative populations in the warm climate zone. As reasonably good data reporting is an obvious prerequisite for being included in the reports from which such tables can be constructed it could be that the 12 countries chosen, being relatively well organised, are not truly representative of those in warm climates.

The first three horizontal columns, the *birth rate*, the *death rate* and the rate of *natural increase* confirm that these are all growing populations. The figures of the fourth column, the infant mortality rate have been used to place the 12 countries in order from most to least favoured. It is evident that there is a rough direct relationship between birth rate and infant mortality.

It also appears from the disease specific columns of Table 6.1 that the higher is the infant mortality and the more frequent are the deaths at all ages reported as due to 'all infections and parasites' and most specifically to the diarrhoeal diseases, tetanus, measles and pneumonia. The eccentric data for tuberculosis suggests that many deaths from this disease are not correctly ascribed to it. In any case as tuberculosis, in its pulmonary forms, will mainly cause death in adults it can be expected to appear as relatively less important in populations, such as those of Egypt and Mauritius which consist largely of children and young people.

Death from accidents is seen to be appallingly frequent in most of these warm climate countries. As in Lagos, Nigeria (Ayeni 1980) road accidents have become the principal cause of death in young adults in those countries in process of economic development. By contrast, at least as far as the official notifications are concerned, death from the tropical diseases occurs less frequently than might be expected. Deaths ascribed to nutritional causes are also not especially frequent. This is not surprising as the malnourished life is usually ended by an infectious episode.

In Table 6.2 are the results of extracting data from the notifications to WHO of the occurrence frequency of the principal diseases in twelve small or medium sized countries in the warm climate zone. In this case the countries are arranged by the incidence of tuberculosis. Such calculations, based upon reports of new incidents of sickness are suspect even when taken from the technologically developed nations. Typically, and at best, they only reflect the true frequency of such major infections as tuberculosis, leprosy and syphilis in which the major components of care are provided by the government as part of a regulatory program. Sickness incidence data tend also to be eccentric from year to year. Exaggerations of frequency occur when an infection is at epidemic levels and there is often an exaggeration

Table 6.2 Infectious disease notifications for twelve warm climate countries*

	Fiji 78	Australia 78	Cuba 79	Thailand 79	Ecuador 79	Sri Lanka 78	Singapore 79	Guinea Bissau 79	Sudan 78	Saudi Arabia 78	Swaziland 78	Guatenala 79	Mean
Dysentery-Enteritis	0.18	0.10	1.42	4.94	—	8.44	0.49	48.7	192.98	13.42	4.05	3.14	53.55
Malaria	—	0.02	0.03	1.68	1.05	5.16	0.09	291.01	153.12	13.81	1.49	10.43	43.44
All Venereal infections	—	1.10	1.42	—	0.68	0.47	5.59	15.09	6.20	0.48	0.18	0.51	3.17
Influenza	0.003	—	—	0.72	1.92	3.79	—	7.41	1.88	—	0.19	9.18	3.14
All Helminths	0.002	0.02	0	3.07	—	3.07	—	—	6.36	—	0.04	—	1.90
Schistosomiasis	—	—	0.0001	—	—	—	—	1.51	5.66	4.70	0.20	—	1.84
Measles	0.003	0.10	0.77	0.29	0.54	0.43	—	6.78	0.95	2.36	1.67	0.51	1.66
All tuberculosis	0.05	—	0.12	0.30	0.40	0.45	1.23	1.39	1.60	1.11	2.72	4.49	1.26
Whooping cough	0.003	—	0.02	0.11	0.25	0.05	—	2.49	6.21	0.01	0.03	0.22	1.15
Dengue-encephalitis	0.002	0.003	7.78	0.30	0.002	0.10	0.07	—	—	0.32	0.10	0.01	0.83
Infectious hepatitis	0.01	0.19	2.26	0.28	—	0.72	0.11	0.92	2.37	—	0.11	0.25	0.68
Filariasis	0.005	—	0.001	—	0.41	0.26	—	2.12	—	—	0.004	—	0.48
Cholera-Salmonella	0.005	0.15	0.02	0.24	—	0.67	0.09	0.01	0.32	0.08	0.15	0.19	0.19
Leprosy	—	0.004	0.04	0.01	—	0.05	0.03	0.70	0.30	0.01	0.17	—	0.14
Tetanus	0.002	0.001	—	0.04	—	0.14	—	0.52	0.11	0.01	0.05	—	0.12
Diphtheria	—	<.001	0.001	0.04	0.003	0.02	0	0.01	0.10	0.02	—	0.001	0.03
All poliomyelitis	—	<.001	<.001	0.02	0.001	0.01	<.001	0.02	0.03	0.03	0.01	0.01	0.01
All rickettsiae	—	<.001	—	0.001	0.008	—	—	—	—	—	0.002	0.002	0.002
Leishmaniasis	—	—	0	—	0	—	—	—	0.16	—	—	—	?
All trypanosomiasis	—	—	0	—	—	—	—	0.01	—	—	—	—	?

calculated by the author from data in World Health Statistics Annual 1980–1981. Infectious Diseases Cases. 1981, WHO. Geneva.
* rates per 1,000 population

of the decline in numbers of new cases as interest is lost. With these limitations such figures do provide the only basis for making international comparisons, short of mounting expensive sample surveillance or case finding surveys in two or more countries simultaneously. In Table 6.2 the data is cited in disease frequency per 100,000 population.

Disease related data can be used in four different ways. First to note the progress of frontier crossing epidemics or pandemics, second to note possible *cyclic variations* in disease, third to make comparisons between populations, fourth to note what particular diseases are of special importance in the individual countries.

The progress of disease across continents is obviously useful to the countries in the path of an epidemic as they can prepare for it and because travellers can be warned to take precautions when planning to go into high risk areas. Recently the progress of both dengue and yellow fever was monitored across South America and the Caribbean. Also in the Americas the progress of sometimes devastating outbreaks of arbovirus encephalitis provided useful advance warning for the mounting of such campaigns as horse vaccination. More traditionally the progress of cholera from South-east Asia along its usual route to Africa alerted governments to that danger. The customary reactions, the tightening of quarantine regulations and insistence on cholera vaccination certificates in arriving travellers, were probably less effective than might have been the long term improvements in hygiene which would have minimised the danger.

Cyclical patterns of disease have been more of academic interest than of practical usefulness. They originate in the exhaustion of the proportion of susceptible individuals in a population so that the number of new cases declines. In following years new susceptibles enter the population by birth or immigration. Though sporadic cases will occur the pool of susceptibles is at first too small to permit wide transmission. As the pool of uninfected susceptibles gradually builds up transmission becomes more likely and eventually a fresh widespread epidemic occurs. This is the pattern seen best in those infections with relatively simple antigenic characteristics and in which a single attack confers long lasting immunity, such as poliomyelitis. By contrast in diseases like malaria, with only imperfect immunity conferred by each new infection, rheumatic heart disease with several antigenically distinct Streptococci contributing, and in influenza with its ever changing antigenic structure, the cyclical patterns will be much less obvious. In recent years attempts to predict the likelihood of an increase in influenza cases and to deal with the susceptible population with vaccines matching the prevalent antigenic strain have not been especially successful.

Cyclical variations occur also in non infectious diseases. There is, for example, an increased likelihood of sickle cell crises occurring in individuals with Sickle Cell disease and who live in countries in which there may be occasional exaggeration of the normal relatively cool season, such as in the Caribbean. Cyclical variations may also occur in infectious diseases as reflections of unrelated adversities. For example a poor harvest, with increased malnutrition may lead to a rise in the death rate from measles.

The drawing of comparisons between different countries based on the diseases each has notified to WHO is not an especially useful exercise except in so far as it confirms a common pattern of sickness in countries with similar population, geographic and climatic conditions. The effectiveness of the respective reporting systems are too subject to variation. Individually they do, however, highlight the principal sickness problems as they are perceived by the inhabitants of those countries. The mean figures for the twelve different countries given in the final vertical column of Table 6.2 confirm the diarrhoeal diseases as the principal problems even though the likelihood of underreporting of such 'normal' type sickness episodes is very high. This tendency to underreport is confirmed by comparing the figure of 19 298 diarrhoeal events per 100 000 population in the Sudan with the 10 per 100 000 in Australia. The latter is a most unlikely figure however favourable the environment. The high figures reported generally for sickness incidence in the Sudan suggest not so much that this is an especially unhealthy country but that its reporting services are more active than in others with similar problems.

After the diarrhoeal infections comes malaria as a cause of sickness in the twelve warm climate countries of Table 6.2. Overall there was a mean of 4344 episodes per 100 000 inhabitants in a year but the cases were concentrated in Guinea Bissau and the Sudan. This suggests that malaria is not perceived as so great a problem as the diarrhoeas in some tropical countries regardless of its actual frequency. No other typically tropical disease appears prominently in the mean incidence listing of Table 6.2. This may in part reflect the low grade, if chronic nature, of diseases like schistosomiasis and filariasis, though it will be noted that the Sudan reports a high frequency of the former.

Looking at the problems as they are individually apparent to the twelve countries reported in Table 6.2 diarrhoea is not always the principal reported sickness. Malaria was ahead in both Saudi Arabia and in Guinea Bissau. In Swaziland tuberculosis was second only to the diarrhoeas. Ecuador had a problem with influenza while in Cuba in 1979 the challenge came from the arboviruses. Guatemala had a high incidence of malaria and higher than average frequencies of influenza and tuberculosis. In Singapore the perceived problem was not the diarrhoeal infections but venereal diseases and tuberculosis. Thailand with remarkably low notifications in all the infections adhered in pattern to the conventional, diarrhoeas first, malaria second. So did Sri Lanka though here there were added problems from the cholera-salmonella infections. infectious hepatitis, the venereal diseases and influenza. The Pacific countries, Fiji and Australia, had some gastrointestinal problems though for Australia the major concern was the venereal infections.

The non tropical diseases which occur most frequently appear to be the venereal infections, influenza, measles, tuberculosis, whooping cough and infectious hepatitis. Such disease distribution trends have been used to argue that the load of sickness in the developing countries is not so much a function of climate as of poverty, ignorance and low standards of hygiene. Some care must though be exercised in reaching such conclusions. The nature of the governmental regulatory processes plus the local interpretation of what is normal or acceptable may considerably distort what is actually reported. The importance of the venereal infections is confirmed by their frequency among university students (Jain and Abengows 1978).

Undeniably though when the morbidity data of Table 6.2 is combined with the mortality data of Table 6.1 the importance of the traditional tropical diseases as population health hazards is somewhat undermined. Sadly though, the survivors of the diseases of poverty face death by violence while cancer and the degenerative diseases gain ground even as quite moderate economic development proceeds.

One inference to be drawn is that there is no such entity as a typical 'developing' or 'warm climate' country. The vector borne or parasitic diseases are present in different proportions as additions to the major burden of diseases which is common to all economically underdeveloped, educationally neglected populations regardless of climate. Additional burdens have been added to those populations in recent years as 'unnatural' medical care has fostered a growing imbalance in populations leading to land and resource pressures which accelerate poverty and deprivation. The beginnings of economic development have additionally threatened previously stable rural populations and have fostered the formation of unstable urban communities with all their attendant high risks to life and wellbeing.

As development proceeds the health pattern of a country changes gradually toward that of the technologically developed society. There remains, nevertheless, a great deal to be done in controlling the diseases of poverty. This action has scarcely begun in many warm climate countries.

REFERENCE

Ayeni O. Causes of mortality in an African city 1980 African Journal of Medical Science 9: 139–149
Jain P S, Abengows C U 1978 Disease pattern among university students in Savanna region of Nigeria. Public Health 92: 131–135.

TERMINOLOGY

Birth Rate. Expressed as the formula:

$$\text{Birth rate} = \frac{\text{Number of live and stillbirths} \times 1000}{\text{Total mid year population}}$$

Cyclic variations. A fairly regular sometimes predictable increase and then decrease in frequency of a particular, usually infectious, disease. The cycle may be an annual one, for example high frequency of upper respiratory infections in cold climate winters. Or the cycles may be prolonged over several years, for example the dozen or so years oc cholera, though in such cases the exact length of the cycle, from minimal frequency back to minimal frequency again is not always the same.

Death Rate. Expressed as:

$$\text{Death rate} = \frac{\text{Number of deaths in the community in the year} \times 1000}{\text{Total mid year population}}$$

Disease Specific Death Rate. In all respects except one the same as the Death Rate. The exception is that the deaths which count are limited to those ascribed to a particular cause. This is not the same thing as the *Case Fatality Rate* in which the denominator is not the total population but only those at risk of dying from a particular disease, that is those who fell sick with it. Expressed usually as a percentage or rate per 100, that is:

$$\text{Case Fatality Rate} = \frac{\text{Number of deaths from the disease} \times 100}{\text{Number of cases of the disease}}$$

Infant Mortality Rate. A variation on the Age Specific Death Rate. The denominator population is as usual the population at risk, in this case the number of infants born in the year under investigation. The formula will then be:

$$\text{Infant Mortality Rate} = \frac{\text{Number of deaths in infants under one year} \times 1000}{\text{Total number of live born infants in that year}}$$

Rate of Natural Increase. The difference between the Birth Rate per 100 and the Death Rate per 100 thus being expressed as a percentage.

Use of epidemiologic information in developing countries

Need is the only relevant consideration in planning new health care or treatment services or in evaluating old ones. The need may be felt or perceived by the community itself. Or the need may be hypothesised on the basis of current information about the disease patterns and environmental hazards in a particular community. Services should never be based on the 'need' of health professionals to exercise personal skills or to satisfy personal interests, however idealistic may be the motives. Nor should they be planned on the blind assumption that what is good for country X must also be good for country Y.

Need defined on the basis of actual conditions, on the numbers at risk of disabling or killing diseases, is probably the most frequent justification used in pleas for funds for new services. The sources of information in the community which would be helpful in defining the problems requiring solution are the subjects of chapters 9 and 10. It is, however, important to emphasise that information limited to what diseases are suffered by a population is not sufficient in planning a community health service program. This is especially true if the poplation has not previously been provided for. As well as epidemiologic data the District or Regional Health Officer will need to know the geography and climate of the area, the size, stability and distribution of the population, its age and sex ratios, the travel and communication resources, occupations and industries, the extent of spendable income, sources of food and the accessibility of existing indigenous native or western type health resources inside or outside the area. The traditional beliefs and customs of the population, particularly in regard to childbirth and child rearing, should also be ascertained together with local behavioural patterns with regard to drug and alcohol abuse, crime, violence and traffic accidents. For all levels of planning or decision making information, reliable information, is the essential basis. This is true whether arranging for the visits of a mobile immunisation team or deciding what drugs to stock in a primary health care centre. Ideally no new district health program should be planned until all this information about the community is available.

The need as the population perceives it is almost equal in importance to that which can be justified on the basis of facts. Sometimes it is overriding regardless of scientific wisdom. Ascertaining what the population seeks or desires in the form of medical care is more difficult than the rough measurements of the problems which can be made by the trained observer. What the population seeks may also be limited by what it concludes it can expect of the new health team including their probity, trustworthiness and respectability. Unfortunate as it may be the success of a health team brought into a community from outside may depend more upon its acceptability by local standards of appearance and behaviour than upon its scientific skills.

Personnel trained in tropical diseases must also be prepared to discover that what their new clients seek is care for the same mundane things as will be found in the slums of Rio de Janeiro or the villages of eastern Turkey. The common complaints which will bring inidviduals into care will be skin infections and injuries, especially of the feet, sore throat, cough, earache and toothache. Dying old people, for which confirmation is sought rather than cure, occasional obstructed labour and some very sick, often dehydrated infants will provide the medical 'stimulation'.

Participation of the community in the planning of their health care services is complicated by the deep division between what the health professional regards either personally or as a result of training as being intolerable and what the community accepts as tolerable or inevitable, for example, the haematuria experienced by adolescent males in schistosomiasis endemic areas. In the event most health care programs begin as patronising services with the providers deciding what to offer.

In affluent societies health education can create a demand for such services as screening for cervical cancer or eye glaucoma. The demand is based on a deliberately stimulated anxiety about what might occur if hidden abnormalities are not corrected. Such programs inevitably suffer in impact by the difficulty they have in reaching the highest risk members of the population, those least concerned to preserve their health or to change damaging behavioural patterns. In developing societies public antipathy can also be the end product of previous health exercises in the area. These may have sought information without bringing subsequent treatment or may have failed to provide continuity of care or to satisfy public standards and expectations. The organisation of population screening programs solely for the purpose of establishing a data base and without following with treatment wherever necessary has been a sad misuse of epidemiology in some developing countries.

Much epidemiologic information is used in deciding how scarce resources can best be used or in measuring how well existing spending achieves its objectives. Population health is also epidemiologically monitored in order to detect early changes in the patterns of sickness. Any such sickness early warning system is incomplete without details of the potential sources of new infection whether this be in human carriers, the local animal or insect population or from environmental toxins.

Long term forecasts or predictions of what is likely to occur in the future must obviously take into account likely population growth. They will also take into account the rising proportion of susceptibles in any community whose immunity has not been properly maintained either by the total lapsing of a program or by desultory coverage of high risk groups. Trouble can certainly be expected if a known typhoid carrier goes into the business of manufacturing flavoured ices for children. Legal authorities do not like to impose sanctions on the basis of what might happen. The health officer more often than not is left waiting unhappily for developments which he can reasonably expect but which he cannot control.

Prediction in epidemiology is a valuable adjunct to long range planning but is requires accurate information to begin with. It is, for example, possible to calculate the number of persons who will be infected and later severly damaged by trypanosomiasis as a group of individuals, such as slash and burn agrarian peasants, move into virgin land in South America or Africa. Arbovirus infections can equally well be anticipated along with leishmaniasis and perhaps even plague as city suburbs edge into warm damp forest areas. The driving of new roads through jungle, the stringing of power and telephone lines, the bulldozing of new sites for industrial and housing developments all require the predictive skills of the epidemiologist. All too often, even on massive public works programs, possible health hazards are not anticipated and the employment of expatriate teams unfamiliar with local conditions merely exacerbates the risks. Contractors and authorities at best satisfy themselves that medical care is available to deal with the inevitable accidents, drunkenness and veneral infections. At its worst this lack of planning can lead to the abandonment of projects or of new housing as panicked workmen or newly imported population get back to where they came from as fast as possible.

The art of prediction, using epidemiologic models which allow each possible contributing factor to be taken into account cannot be dealt with here in depth. It can prove eminently practicable under the right circumstances. As an example, an African government desiring to increase its hard currency income might propose to open up its beaches to foreign tourists. It would first be wise to make advance calculations on the health consequences of such action. One consequence is that many tourists might become sick or even die with malaria. Even safe chemoprophylactic programs, once advised but rarely adhered to, tend to discourage tourists and foreign investment.

The problem could equally well be one of typhus on a Pacific island, plague in South East Asia or typhoid in India. The factors which must be taken into account, assuming that the disease is an inevitable part of the local ecosystem, are all those which increase the likelihood of transmission to a susceptible individual. Each individual hazard can be quantified. Then all the hazards joined into a mathematical formula, produce the predictive likelihood, the degree of chance, that a susceptible individual when exposed to the local conditions will become sick.

The planners can now decide whether the risk is a reasonably small one which can be ignored, whether it is large enough to warrant a warning, whether the project can only be continued with expensive safeguards including environmental modifications or whether it should be abandoned altogether. If the problem were one of malaria, probably the commonest in new tourist areas, the epidemiologist would require the following data in constructing a prediction of risk:

1. The ration between the numbers of the populations of mosquitoes and humans.

2. The proportion of the local female mosquitoes which actually select to bite Man rather than other animals.

3. The proportion of mosquitoes which survive each day after they themselves have been infected by taking blood from a malaria case.

4. The chance that the newly infectious mosquitoes will survive that additional day necessary for them to transmit the parasites to a new human victim.

5. The proportion of the bites of an infected mosquito which actually succeed in inoculating the parasites into the potential victim.

6. The speed of recovery of the next victim, that is the number of days he or she will retain parasites in the circulating blood available to be picked up by an uninfected mosquito.

Such predictive epidemiologic models are a relatively recent innovation. Computerisation will help in making the collective calculations but the results can never be better than the epidemiologic and other data on which they are based. Predictions are also more certain if there is relative stability in the environment, in human behaviour and in the levels of disease reservoir and insect vectors. Other variables can be taken into account in making predictive calculations. For example a sickness risk can be calculated for the different seasonal conditions to be expected in a particular area. Cyclical susceptibility of the human population could be predicted on the basis of immunity level screening. These variable 'scenarios' are already used by epidemiologists employed in program planning to allow them to indicate what is likely to happen under a whole range of different circumstances. As the actual circumstances are monitored the epidemiologist can give advance warning of likely changes in or threats to population health.

In practice the decisions about what services deserve priority in the allocation of resources from the district to the international level are most frequently based on the volume of disease and the quantity of death in populations. It is assumed that this information will indicate the proportion of individuals in a population needing help and such calculations are most persuasive in obtaining funds.

The volume of sickness in the world is not known with any accuracy. In so far as it is possible to construct the likely figures from the reports of sickness and death, but with corrections based on periodic sample surveys, the calculated information has three principal uses.

First in any population it is salutary to face the main treatable or preventable hazard to health. Second, as resources are very limited it is wise to spend them on those health threats which pose the greatest risk internationally. Third, the success of any international control program should be demonstrable in falls in the incidence of new cases and deaths.

Table 7.1 was constructed for the first purpose. It lists the diseases in order of importance as causes of death. Clearly the diarrhoeal infections dominate all other hazards to life. In chapter three it was suggested that these typically 'food and water' transmission infections could be relatively easily controlled through community and family hygiene. The technology is already available. By contrast corrective measures to deal with the toll of respiratory infections are both complex and prohibitively expensive.

Malnutrition appears as the third most frequent cause of death. It also plays a part in the deaths actually ascribed to childhood infections like measles. Malnutrition too is relatively easily corrected, at least on an individual basis. In practice in dealing with malnutrition in whole populations a peculiar amalgam of politics, economics and corruption can largely negate efforts from outside to relieve the situation. Indeed immediate passive solutions, the giving of food to the hungry or improperly fed, may be less valuable than reaching long term solutions. These include correction of imbalance in population growth, poor and wasteful food distribution systems and inefficient agricultural practices. Some communities cheat themselves by selling nutritious foods for cash which will then be used for luxury goods. It cannot be assumed that, given a choice, the needs of children will be considered first.

The most important 'tropical' disease in the world is malaria. Schistosomiasis, tuberculosis and the childhood infections, the latter eminently preventable, follow in the number of deaths which they cause. In determining how resources should be spent and what diseases should be dealt with at highest priority high death rates are not the only factors to consider. Some infections, like onchocerciasis and poliomyelitis cause, immediately or directly, relatively little death. Their case fatality rates are low. They cause instead severe disability and one which for individual, family and community can occasion more suffering and waste than death itself. It is possible to measure both death and disability and to compare the different diseases to find which is the most damaging.

The costs of death or the measurement of life lost can be made by sharing the risk among the whole population or among those who become sick. The calculation is similar in either case. Shared per head of population it dramatically demonstrates the cost to every individual in a community. It probably is more realistic to relate death costs to those who actually become sick. This also highlights the differences between individuals who are protected and those who remain susceptible.

For this second type of calculation all that are needed are the case fatality rate of the particular infection in that particular population and the mean

Table 7.1 Endemic Disease in the Developing Countries
The following are based either on figures given in the following disease specific chapters or on official WHO notifications as modified by research extrapolations and are probably underestimates. Data given are for actual disease — not the numbers infected which in most cases is a much higher number.
The infections are arranged in their importance as bringers of death.

Epidemiologic Control Category	Infection	Clinical Disease Incidence	Deaths per year	Disability Potential	Life Shortening per survivor
B	Diarrhoeas	3–5 000 000 000	5–10 000 000	1	3–5
E (+C)	Respiratory infections	?	2 200 000	2	5–7
C	Malnutrition	?	2 000 000	3	?
B	Malaria	150 000 000	1 200 000	2	3–5
A	Measles	80 000 000	900 000	2	10–14
A	Neonatal tetanus	1 000 000	900 000	0	7–10
B	Schistosomiasis	20 000 000	0.5m–1 000 000	2	600–10
A	Whooping cough	20 000 000	250–450 000	1	21–48
C	Tuberculosis	7 000 000	400 000	2	200–40
D	Chages'	1 200 000	60 000	2	600
A	Diphtheria	700–900 000	50–60 000	1	7–10
D	Hookworm	1 500 000	50–60 000	0	100
D	River blindness (oncho)	200–500 000	20–50 000	3	3000
D	Meningitis	150 000	30 000	4	7–10
D	Amoebiasis	1 500 000	30 000	1	7–10
C	Typhoid	500 000	25 000	0	14–28
D	Ascariasis	1 000 000	20 000	0	7–10
A	Poliomyelitis	2 000 000	10–20 000	4	3000
C	Anthrax	100 000	10 000	1	?
D	Leishmaniasis	400 000	5 000	2	100–200
D	Afr trypanosomiasis	10 000	5 000	3	150
C	Leprosy	10 500 000	low	3	500–3000
D	Trichuriasis	100 000	low	0	7–10
D	Filariasis	2–3 000 000	low	2	1000
D	Dengue	1–2 000 000	100	0	5–7
B	Trachoma	25 000 000	very low	3	?
D	Giardiasis	500 000	very low	0	5–7

Control Categories — amenability   Disability Potential untreated survivo

A Effective and feasible Disability unlikely	0
B Effective but expensive Slight restriction possible	1
C Complex — eradication unlikely Moderate disability	2
D Difficult Considerable disability	3
E None practicable Completely disabling	4

Source: Robinson D. Lecture notes in epidemiology and communicable disease control. 2nd edition. 1981. Liverpool School of Tropical Medicine. Liverpool
*based on Rockefeller Foundation estimates

age of those who die from it. It might, for example, be found that a particular infection killed one in ten of those infected and that the mean age of death was five years. If, in that particular population, a five years old child might otherwise expect on average to live for another 47 years that is the quantity of life which has been lost. It must be shared between the ten sick persons who produced one death so that each sickness, on average, shortened life by 4.7 years. Though this is not a true life situation it allows the disease to be put into perspective and the damage it causes to be costed. For those infections which are highly life shortening such as tetanus the aim must be to treat thoroughly if therapy is available or to raise immunity levels in those who are susceptible.

By contrast some diseases, like the diarrhoeal infections and malaria, have relatively low case fatality rates. It is the frequency with which the infection is repeated which undermines health in many warm climate countries. For such diseases the priority will go to reducing the load of infections rather than in attempting to deal with each individual episode. Indeed, too vigorous attempts to eradicate such infections locally without improving the immulogic efficiency of the susceptibles might prove to be of disservice in the long run. The creation of enclaves of unexposed groups with no useful level of naturally acquired immunity is a very hazardous procedure.

One further way to measure the relative destructive importance of diseases is that of the disability which they cause. A monetary value can be placed on a life as it relates to income producing potential of each individual — modified by skill and age. No simple reporting systems exist to provide such data. While for the individual death is the ultimate disaster for the family and community it is the loss of working capacity and independence in those disabled and the cost of providing to rather than receiving services from them.

In the most technologically developed countries with sickness. care demand constantly filling each newly available, usually expensive, module of care resources the benefit of saving this life as opposed to that one has to be calculated if the maximum benefit is to be derived from finite resources. Such calculations are highly emotive. In the developing countries there is an echo of this controversy in the arguments and competing claims for one kind of care as opposed to another. Usually the argument concerns the cost benefit of high technology hospital versus low technology primary care. There are additional facets to this argument, the central hospital is needed for personnel training but it only serves the population around it, primary community services are cheap and bring a lot of care to many people but they are only effective if there is a referral superstructure for the severely sick.

Such cost benefit comparisons have been made (Walsh 1979) also by calculating the cost of each child life saved by different forms of medical intervention. They show, for example, the excellent economy of episodic primary care, including immunisation, versus the gloomy expensiveness of

Table 7.2 Model Costs

Primary Health Care
  Population 100 000
Health Care provides:
  Basic care for children under 5 (17 000)
  Tetanus toxoid, iron and folic acid for all pregnant women (4000)
  Contraceptive advice and supplies for 30% of fertile women (5100)
  Drugs and supplies for diarrhea
                          acute respiratory infection
                          malaria
                          intestinal parasites

costs (1977) in US dollars	Total	Per capita
Personnel	105 000	1.05
Commodities including vaccines	35 000	.35
Capital costs annuitized (0.33 recurrent)	50 000	.50
Totals	190 000	1.90
Additional possible costs		
Basic food supplementation at 30% malnourished	71 000	.71
Rural water supply (at US$26 per capita)	500 000	5.00
Totals	761 000	7.60

  * Source Gopaldas T et al. Project Poshak. Vol 1. New Delhi. CARE INDIA, 1975
   All other material from World Health Organization. Community water supply and sanitation: strategies for development. (Background document for UN Water Conference). London: Pergamon Press, 1977.

providing a community water supply or correcting malnutrition. Earlier and by a different route calculations (Gopaldas et al 1975) in India similarly presented planners with the alternatives of cheap but limited primary health care services versus the relative high expenses of providing a safe community water supply. Extrapolations of these and WHO material (1977) form the basis for Table 7.2

While the worldwide monetary costs of disabling sickness are relevant to priority decisions the quantity of misery endured can only be guessed at by estimates such as those in Table 7.3. The WHO calculation (1976) suggests that almost 10 per cent of the world's population is disabled. By that is meant that the ability of these individuals to earn a living or to look after themselves is in some way impaired — often totally. The actual extent to which independence is lost will vary not only with the kind of impairment to function but also with the society in which the disabled person lives. Full physical 'normality' is not necessary for many jobs in the industrial societies. By contrast the agrarian peasant family in a developing country may soon be reduced to starvation if the father loses full strength and mobility.

In terms of quantity the data in Table 7.3 suggest that the principal costs put onto individuals, their families and the community are imposed by the congenital problems, the non communicable diseases such as cancer and degenerative conditions and by malnutrition. Together they account for 58.5 per cent of the world's disabled. Following close behind violence accounts for 15.1 per cent of the disabilities while the communicable diseases account for a relatively small 10.8 per cent. Shifting the figures around the

Table 7.3 World Disability Estimates
Based on 4,000 million population

Medical Cause	Number disabled (millions)	Proportion of all disabled
Congenital disturbances		
Mental retardation (all causes)	40	7.7
Somatic hereditary defect	40	7.7
Non-genetic disorders	20	3.9
Communicable diseases		
Poliomyelitis	1.5	0.3
Trachoma	10	1.9
Leprosy	3.5	0.7
Onchocerciasis	1	0.2
Others	40	7.7
Noncommunicable somatic disease	100	19.3
Functional psychiatric distrubances	40	7.7
Chronic alcoholism and drug abuse	40	7.7
Trauma/Injury		
Traffic accidents	30	5.8
Occupational accidents	15	2.9
Home accidents	30	5.8
Other	3	0.6
Malnutrition	100	19.3
Other	2	0.4
Totals	516	100
Correction for possible double accounting	−129	
Net total world disabled	387 000 000	

Source — Reports on specific technical matters, Disability prevention and rehabilitation, 1976, 29th World Health Assembly WHO, Geneva. Table 1, page 17.

analyst is faced with the startling conclusion that the largest contribution to world disability is the consequence of brain injury or deficit at birth, to later psychiatric disturbances and to the self inflicted damage of alcohol and drug abuse. This group accounts collectively for 23.1 per cent of the disabled human population and many of them are young.

When taken together with the data describing the quantity and distribution of episodic sickness and death these figures provide a severe dilemma for health resource planners. In a relative sense it is humbling for health care professionals, including practical epidemiologists, to realise that the contribution which conventional medical care can make can have only a marginal effect on human health and misery. Further humbling half or more of the health care need, especially in the warm climate developing countries, is for mentally rather than for somatically related disease. What favours the allocation of resources to the conventional medical services, even though they deal with a small minority of the health problems, is that the somatic illnesses, the communicable ones in particular, are often preventable or treatable. Appropriate medical care could also reduce the volume of brain damage caused both by poor obstetric care and by diseases in children such as malaria and meningitis.

Health planners also pin hopes on the contribution wise birth spacing could have on the problems of malnutrition and economic development in many developing countries. Somewhat less certain is the part yet to be played by health education and behavioural repatterning in preventing or delaying the onset of the non communicable somatic diseases and in preventing trauma. Unfortunately we have not yet discovered how to persuade individuals that the preservation of health is not only a desirable thing in itself but is also worth effort and the sacrifice of some immediate pleasures.

Choice in what health care services to concentrate upon would be a luxury for the average District Health Centre in a developing country. An endless succession of the sick already exists. When new funds are being sought or new services planned there is, for a time, an opportunity to consider how best to obtain the maximum effect at the lowest cost. The international agencies have the unenviable task of deciding on the global scale exactly what diseases deserve priority. The final decision on where funds are used from such sources as the World Bank may, in the end, depend more on political than epidemiologic considerations. Periodically the World Health Organization publishes a list of the communicable diseases which should have priority in funding from international sources. They are not intended to suggest that other diseases should not be controlled or their victims not treated.

The criteria for placing an infectious disease in the highest priority grouping for the funding of control programs are simple. They are that the disease should be highly prevalent, should cause many deaths and should be relatively easily controlled. In Table 7.1 both Control category A and some B diseases would be part of the group including the following:

(a) the diarrhoeal infections — more because of the effectiveness of rehydration techniques than because of the likelihood of rapidly improving hygiene standards.

(b) the childhood infections in which there is an effective vaccine and including measles, diphtheria, whooping cough, poliomyelitis, tetanus and soon hepatitis B.

(c) malaria because it is both preventable and treatable.

At community level it does not require a highly sophisticated primary health service to deal with the above common infections. Certain over simplified assumptions might have to be made, for example, that all high fever is due to malaria in areas where the disease is prevalent.

The next group of diseases in priority for funding would include those which are highly prevalent and dangerous as in the first group, but for which control is more difficult. Roughly they coincide with Control category C. The difficulty may be related to a huge expense in treatment or environmental engineering, to the long period of time required to effect a change in transmission patterns or to the underlying requirement than success can only be achieved with a considerable change in human behavioural patterns. The group would probably include schistosomiasis, tuberculosis, viral hepatitis and the salmonella infections including typhoid. The airborne infections might in part be committed to this group not because control is easy but because chemoprophylaxis and chemotherapy are available for some of them. Leprosy might be included on the grounds that treatment is practicable though effective control is apparently not. Hookworm might be added to this list but only if a control program were also to correct any nutritional imbalances. The wide nature of the presenting signs dictate that this second group would also require far more sophisticated primary diagnostic and referral services than the first group.

In the third and relatively low priority group the international agencies, in planning fund allocations, would likely place those infections which hazard relatively few individuals or for which there is either no effective control/treatment or in which such programs would either be disproportionately expensive or require vast capital investment on population relocation or rehousing. Such diseases include both African and American trypanosomiasis and it has been argued that leprosy belongs here. The group would also probably include leishmaniasis (except man to man forms), filariasis, dengue, amoebiasis and ascariasis. Most of these low priority diseases, it has been suggested, will be controlled as economic standards and education are advanced so that funds might be better invested in economic development than on attempting to ameliorate the effects of the symptoms of poverty which these diseases to some extent are.

The lessons learned from the malaria eradication program of the last generation have considerably cooled enthusiasm for speculative widespread control programs. Now when these are planned they tend to be limited to particular high risk populations especially those isolated in some natural way from continuing sources of reinfection.

REFERENCES

Gopaldas T et al 1975. Project Poshak. Vol 1. Care India. New Delhi.
Walsh J A, Warren K S 1979. Selective primary health care. An interim strategy for disease control in developing countries. New England Journal of Medicine. 301 967–974
WHO 1979. Reports on specific technical matters. Disability prevention and rehabilitation. Document WHA29/24. Geneva

International health agencies

INTRODUCTION

International agencies are those established under the Charter of the United Nations. The principal international health agency is the World Health Organization (WHO). Others having an interest in aspects of health are the United Nations Childrens Fund, (UNICEF), the Food and Agricultural Organization (FAO) and the International Labour Organization (ILO). In addition there are other agencies such as the Relief and Works Agency for Palestine Refugees in the Middle East (UNWRA), the Drugs and Narcotics Bureau and the High Commission for Refugees (UNHCR) whose work frequently touches on health problems.

HISTORICAL BACKROUND

Conseil Supérieure de Santé de Constantinople

Internationally controlled epidemiological reporting of diseases has a respectable tradition, dating from the establishment about the end of the third decade of the 19th century of the Conseil Supérieure de Santé de Constantinople to provide a quarantine service for ships entering and leaving ports in the Ottoman Empire. The Conseil functioned remarkably successfully considering the almost total absence of any fundamental knowledge of the diseases — mainly cholera and plague — which it was set up to control. About the same time attempts were made to set up quarantine agencies in Egypt, Iran and Morocco. Only the Egyptian agency made any headway, and it progressed to become the Egyptian Board of Health based in Alexandria.

The establishment of the Conseil Supérieure was followed up by the convening of a series of eleven International Sanitary Conferences. These were initially called into being by European powers, conscious of the success of the Conseil Supérieure and apprehensive at the ever-increasing inroads made by cholera. The Conferences aimed at establishing minimal essential maritime quarantine arrangements which could be accepted by the convening powers. The first such conference was held in Paris in 1851, the eleventh also in Paris in 1903.

Until the end of the 19th century little technical progress had been made by the conferences because of the lack of scientific knowledge about diseases and their transmission. The turn of the century witnessed the first major technical breakthrough in disease control with the discovery of the mode of transmission of yellow fever. This was followed in 1902 by the setting up of an International Sanitary Bureau for the Americas dedicated to the eradication of yellow fever from the two continents. In 1903, the 11th International Sanitary Conference succeeded in welding the four sanitary conventions resulting from the previous ten Conferences into one instrument dealing with cholera and plague but surprisingly, not with yellow fever. It also recommended the establishment of a new international organization, wider in scope and extent than the Conseil Supérieure, and in 1907 this recommendation was implemented by the establishment in Paris of the 'Office International d'Hygiène Publique'.

Office International d'Hygiène Publique (OIHP)

Although this organization was primarily one of European countries, it was joined by the United States of America. It commenced an organized study of a wide range of subjects related to communicable diseases and their transmission and disseminated the reports to member governments. These early studies laid the foundation for much of the international work which was to follow under successive organizations.

The outbreak of war in 1914 amongst its member states halted the work of the OIHP, but it resumed its functioning after the Armistice although its activities were largely taken over by the League of Nations Health Organization (LONHO) until its work was brought again to an abrupt halt by the outbreak of war in 1939 followed by the military occupation of Paris. As an international organization, OIHP never resumed its functioning after the termination of hostilities.

League of Nations Health Organization (LONHO)

The establishment of the League of Nations at the end of the First World War was followed by the formation of a League of Nations Health Organization. Although the nearest possible to a really international health organization, its membership was still not global, some States continuing to be members of OIHP only. Both organizations therefore continued to function until 1939. LONHO, being based in neutral Switzerland, was able to function throughout the Second World War despite its staff being reduced at one time to two officials, and it succeeded in bringing out a weekly epidemiological report and distributing it throughout the whole period.

United Nations Relief and Rehabilitation Agency (UNRRA)

The ending of the Second World War saw the establishment of the United Nations and the setting up under its aegis of UNRRA, a temporary organization responsible for fighting epidemics, administering the international sanitary conventions and providing urgent assistance to governments in health matters. In this way UNRRA provided continuity between pre- and post-war international health work, but it was never intended to continue as a permanent organisation. It continued to function however until superseded by the World Health Organization.

The World Health Organization (WHO)

In 1949, 'Health' was by unanimous consent inserted in the United Nations Charter as one of the subjects within its purview. In 1946 the New York International Health Conference agreed to set up a single Agency for Health, designated it 'The World Health Organization' and agreed a constitution for it under which it absorbed the surviving functions of OIHP, LONHO and UNRRA. Today, WHO is the principal international organization for health and functions as a decentralized body having its headquarters in Geneva and regional offices in Alexandria, Brazzaville, Copenhagen, Manila, New Delhi and Washington. In Washington it operates alongside the Pan-American Sanitary Bureau (PASB). This was formerly known as the International Sanitary Bureau for the Americas but its name was changed in 1923, in keeping with health developments in the region. The agreement to establish the WHO Regional Office for the Americas in close association with the Pan-American Sanitary Bureau was concluded in June 1949 and it endowed the Pan-American Sanitary Bureau with additional functions to enable it to operate as the WHO Regional Office. Today the two organizations exist side by side and carry out a unified programme of work covering all States and Territories in the content of which there is no fundamental difference between the PASB and the WHO elements.

The work of WHO in respect of epidemiology and disease control

WHO inherited from the past a traditional responsibility for the control and prevention of disease and the promotion of health. Until recently this has been largely concerned with communicable diseases but now embraces non-communicable disease problems as well. The Organization encourages international co-operation in solving problems, promotes research into the causes of diseases and their transmission and into ways of reducing incidence where, as in the case of most non-communicable diseases infection does not at first sight appear to play a part. WHO aims at present in the case of non-communicable diseases to provide, in the words of the Director-General, a 'neutral platform to validate information and ensure its international exchange, to promote newer directions for research such as the elucidation of environmental factors in cancer or studies on the prevention of cardio-vascular disease on a community scale.'

In the field of epidemiology, techniques to supplement the classical methods of investigation have been devised for both communicable and non-communicable diseases. In the case of the latter, a whole new battery of techniques has been developed to facilitate the study of conditions in which the probable causes seem to be multifactorial rather than primarily related to infection. These diseases have a global interest. Information suggests that rural communities which are overtaken by urbanization and industrializ-ation tend to react by assuming a pattern of morbidity and mortality akin to that exhibited by the older industrialized nations. Industrialization is in most developing countries the avowed aim of economic policy. WHO assists interested countries in studying the problems in their own social and cultural context. For example , the disease problems of the European region are different from those of the South-east Asian or Western Pacific regions.

International quarantine

In the early years of OIHP the rapid dissemination of plague was a matter of great concern particularly to maritime nations and studies were made on the control of this disease and of a number of communicable diseases amongst which yellow fever and cholera were considered to be serious risks to trading nations. The international sanitary convention of 1912 defined plague, cholera and yellow fever as major epidemic diseases capable of attacking without warning large groups of people and it set up an infor-mation system requiring those nations who ratified the convention to notify all cases as they occurred to OIHP which then telegraphed the details to all countries whose geographical or maritime relations placed their peoples at risk.

After the war of 1914–1918, epidemics of communicable disease occurred on a vast scale. During 1919, Poland suffered over a million cases of louse-borne typhus while in Russia over a million and a half cases were reported, and this disease continued to give rise to epidemics during succeeding years. Epidemics of smallpox also occurred after the war ended and so it was that the international sanitary convention of 1926 added louse-born typhus and smallpox to the list of major epidemic diseases. Relapsing fever was added to this list after the second world war.

By this time the system of operating international quarantine through a series of conventions requiring ratification had become rather an unwieldy method of dealing with disease control problems that required a flexible approach and on occasions instant action, so in 1951 the conventions were replaced by the International Sanitary Regulations which consolidated, amended and up-dated the contents of the conventions which they replaced and put the quarantineable diseases in the perspective of air travel as well as travel by land and sea routes. Smallpox eradication appears to be a fact at the time of writing and louse-borne typhus and relapsing fever are no longer internationally notifiable although still subject to surveillance. Apart from smallpox, all the diseases which have at one time or another been listed as quarantineable remain a threat to non-immune members of communities under certain catastrophic conditions such as war, natural disasters and famine. In addition to reporting on the quarantineable diseases WHO today organises the surveillance of a wider group of communicable diseases of contemporary importance, reporting on these regularly in the appropriate publications.

Disease surveillance

WHO has a disease surveillance unit in the Division of Communicable Diseases. Surveillance requires that there be a systematic collection of all information on the occurrence of a disease including morbidity and mortality data, information from bacteriological and virological laboratories, on the prevalence of insect vectors, on the use of vaccines and in the case of zoonotic diseases, movements of animals acting as hosts. The WHO unit is particularly concerned with the surveillance of diseases common to a number of neighbouring states. Surveillance takes different forms; for example, the type of surveillance needed when a disease is thought to have been eradicated differs from that which is monitoring the behaviour of current diseases.

Expert committees and scientific groups

In order to keep itself up-to-date with every aspect of health throughout the world WHO established an Expert Advisory Panel consisting of specialists in all the important fields of activity. Members are called to Geneva head-quarters to sit on expert committees and scientific groups. These were called into being to advise on progress in a large number of fields. In the case of epidemiology and disease control they may be single-disease bodies, for example Malaria or Rabies, or may relate to a particular group of conditions, or a particular group of micro-organisms or macro-organisms. Meetings may consider new developments in epidemiological or laboratory techniques and some committees are concerned with the basic and postgraduate training of all health workers in which teaching in epidemiology and in disease control is considered. The reports of the committees and groups provide a most useful indication of the situation in a given field at a point in time and are of the greatest value to health workers. Although WHO does not bind itself by their recommendations, they nevertheless form the basis on which much WHO policy is built and indeed the work of Expert Committees and Scientific Groups is perhaps one of WHO's most valuable contributions to Health.

WHO collaborating centres

Several hundred national institutes, laboratories and university departments have been formed by WHO into a network of centres which receive micro-organisms and macro-organisms from laboratories all over the world for study and classification. They were formerly known as 'reference laboratories'. Over the years, the experience gained and the data collected by them have made them centres for epidemic and endemic intelligence. The best known of these centres are probably the international influenza centres. These keep continual track of the influenza virus, note any changes taking place in its antigenic structure and assess the risk of future epidemics. The information which they provide enables governments to ensure that effective vaccines are available in the next influenza 'season'. Lists of the Collaborating Centres can be obtained from WHO Headquarters or from any of the regional offices.

Dissemination of information by WHO

Dissemination of information on health matters is one of the most important functions of WHO. Reference has already been made to the reports of expert committees and scientific groups which are published as technical reports in the *Technical Reports series*, each having a serial number. The *Monograph* and *Public Health Papers* also contain expert reports on various subjects. More recently, a series of *off-set publications* have been issued. The *Bulletin of the World Health Organization* contains original papers written by individuals or groups of individuals on the more technical aspects of health work. The *WHO Chronicle* provides more general information for health workers on the work of WHO, and the *World Health Statistics Annual* gives invaluable information of a statistical nature on morbidity and mortality in reporting countries. The *Weekly Epidemiological Record* details the incidence of the internationally notifiable diseases and also summarizes morbidity and mortality trends in a wider range of important diseases. Certain regional offices of WHO produce regional publications on a wide range of subjects important to member states of the region.

While WHO publications are produced mainly in English and French, other working languages of the Organization are also used when appropriate. These are Arabic, Chinese, Russian and Spanish. The European office for example publishes in English, French, German and Russian while the American office publishes mainly in English and Spanish.

WHO programme

Source of Funds WHO's work is funded by a regular budget made up of assessed contributions by member states. In addition it receives considerable funds from the United Nations itself through its Development Programme

(UNDP), the Environmental Programme (UNEP), the Fund for Drug Abuse Control (UNFDAC), the Fund for Population Activities (UNFPA) and also the World Bank and the World Food Programme. Generally speaking, WHO's resources are, as the Director-General recently put it, 'a mere drop in the ocean' compared with world needs, hence the need to husband them carefully and to ensure that member states have the necessary trained personnel and all the necessary information to enable them to undertake important health work within the limits of their own resources wherever possible.

Annual Programme and budget The annual programme and budget provide an insight into the priorities allocated to the work of the Agency. In the 1980/81 proposals 3.57 per cent of the total budget was allocated to the control and prevention of non-communicable diseases while 27.85 per cent — by far the biggest of all individual allocations — was set aside for communicable diseases. This reflects the continuing importance of transmissable disease to most member states. Examination of the itemised budget showed that out of the 3.57 per cent allocated to non-communicable diseases, 2.02 was for cancer and 0.47 for cardiovascular diseases. Of the 27.85 per cent allocated to communicable diseases, 10.37 went to a special programme of research and training in tropical diseases and 8.03 to malaria and other parasitic diseases.

Organisation of WHO To deal efficiently with the problems set out in its work programme requires an organizational structure designed to facilitate the work of the technical and administrative services in as economical a manner as possible. In its Geneva headquarters WHO has a number of divisions made up of units concerned with various action programmes in the field of Health; in the case of disease control there are expert technical units dealing with specific diseases, groups of diseases, epidemiology, surveillance and research. For example, the division of communicable diseases is made up of units dealing with the epidemiological surveillance of communicable diseases, smallpox eradication, tuberculosis and respiratory diseases, bacterial and venereal infections, the diarrhoeal diseases control programme, virus diseases, leprosy, veterinary public health, the prevention of blindness and the special programme on safety measures in microbiology.

The overwhelming importance of malaria has necessitated the splitting of the former division of malaria and other parasitic diseases into two separate programmes. The malaria action programme is made up of units concerned with epidemiological methodology and evaluation, programming and training, and research and technical intelligence. The parasitic diseases programme has units for schistosomiasis and other helminthic infections, trypanosomiasis and leishmaniasis, and filarial infections.

The division of non-communicable disease control and prevention is made up of units concerned with cancer, cardiovascular diseases, oral health, human genetics, immunology and occupational health. Being a decentralised organization, much of WHO's work is carried on through its regional offices working through committees of member states of the regions and maintaining close contact with government departments and individuals on a day-to-day basis. Country programmes make up a very large part of the field work of WHO and are supervised from the regional offices which also undertake their planning.

Regional offices have a director in administrative charge and a staff of experienced specialist regional advisers covering various fields of work supplemented in the more highly specialised fields by visits from headquarters staff or by consultants specially recruited for the purpose. Important epidemiological and scientific studies are carried out at regional level. If requested, WHO will often provide expert international staff for an assisted project to work alongside and train the national staff. A high proportion of projects are assisted in this way but WHO field staff are not always essential provided that the national staff are well trained and the projects can be properly supervised from the regional offices.

Other Agencies Concerned With Health

The United Nations Childrens' Fund (UNICEF)

UNICEF is an agency concerned with health, education and nutrition which means that it works closely with FAO, WHO, and UNESCO (the United Nations Educational, Scientific and Cultural Organization). By virtue of its mandate, UNICEF's particular concern is for the welfare of children, mothers and the family. Through this concern it has been possible for WHO and UNICEF to tackle jointly in many countries the problems of communicable disease control.

WHO stands in an advisory capacity to UNICEF on health matters and the two agencies have a Joint Committee on Health Policy (JCHP) which discusses UNICEF assistance to health projects and defines the criteria governing it. The general pattern is that WHO supplies technical expertise and UNICEF material assistance in the form of equipment and supplies. UNICEF may supply material assistance with WHO technical approval to country programmes which are not being assisted by WHO except that such programmes may be technically appraised from time to time by appropriate regional office staff.

UNICEF's material assistance in a joint project represents an additional source of funds for WHO. Although they do not appear in the WHO budget many important projects would be unable to start without them.

The Food and Agricultural Organization (FAO)

WHO is concerned with the diseases and disorders which arise from faulty or mal-nutrition. FAO is concerned with the general state of nutrition of populations. It attempts to ensure that everybody receives, within their own cultural and social environment, a balanced diet; and in the case of special groups such as pregnant women and nursing mothers that they receive a supply of nutrients sufficient to cope with their special needs. The work of the two agencies in the field of nutrition could be described as inter-locking; they work closely together and collaborate through joint Expert Committees on such subjects as Food Additives, Energy and Protein Requirements, Microbiological aspects of Food Hygiene, Pesticide residues in Food and the Codex Alimentarius.

The International Labour Office (ILO)

The International Labour Office (ILO) was established in 1919 under Part XIII of the Treaty of Versailles and was included in other peace treaties in 1919 and 1920. The preamble to its constitution mentions among other essential tasks 'the protection of the worker against sickness, disease and injury arising out of his employment'.

While a good deal of work in support of this obligation was carried out between the two wars, it was not until 1950, following a number of meetings and discussions that the Governing Body of ILO set up a committee to examine the work programme of the organisation in the sphere of industrial health and safety and to define the particular aspects of the health of workers in dangerous or unhealthy occupations at which inter-national regulations ought to be directed In 1953 the Governing body approved a systematic programme of work for ILO in the field of industrial health and safety, and the International Labour Conference adopted a recommendation containing a comprehensive series of measures to protect the health of workers in their place of employment. As regards Safety, the problems were originally defined as long ago as 1925 and certain conventions were adopted in this field, particularly in 1929 the Convention for the Protection of Dockers and in 1937 the Convention for the Protection of Workers in the Building Industry. Over the years, model codes of safety regulations for different industrial groups have been developed which are now issued in the form of handbooks under the general title of 'ILO Codes of Practice'.

ILO is a Standard-producing body, and arising from its work it draws up (I) Conventions or (2) Recommendations on particular matters. *Conventions* are measures requiring ratification by governments which are then committed to taking action on the matters contained therein in the form set out in the convention. *Recommendations* are passed to member governments and are intended to be drawn to the attention of national parliaments or whatever is the ruling body for guidance in formulating national legislation on the subject matter.

Today, ILO is the principal United Nations Agency concerned with prob-lems of occupational health and the safety and welfare of workers in industry. Apart from conventions covering general conditions of employment a large number of conventions have been adopted over the years concerned with such matters as industrial health, the employment of children, young persons and women, social security (including medical care and sickness benefit) maternity benefit, invalidity benefit, health and welfare of seafarers, indigenous and tribal populations and general social policy.

The impact of ILO activities is widespread throughout the industrialised as well as the developing countries of the world. ILO's work has influenced the legislation on Health and Safety at Work of many countries including the United Kingdom's Committee on Safety and Health at Work which was appointed in May 1970 under the chairmanship of Lord Robens and on the recommendations of which the Health and Safety at Work Act (1974) was based.

CONCLUSION

The continuing work of the international agencies concerned with health is essential to the modern community of nations. They disseminate essential information, provide a global forum for considering disease problems, review current research and deliberate on suitable courses of action in a global manner which could not be undertaken in any other way. In health matters, WHO is an essential organization without which the health and wellbeing of the world community would be much less advanced than it is. For example, it is hardly possible to believe that global smallpox eradication could have been conceived and carried through without the existence of WHO to formulate and guide the programme to its successful conclusion. Voltaire once wrote 'Si dieu n' existait pas, il faudrait l'inventer' ('If God did not exist, it would be necessary to invent him'). Perhaps we, on a less lofty and more mundane level may be permitted the thought that if WHO did not exist it would now be necessary to invent it.

REFERENCES

Russell H B L 1974 The World Health Organisation. In: Passmore R and Robson J S (Ed) Companion to Medical Studies, Blackwell Scientific Publications Edinburgh vol 3 part 2 ch 77

Voltaire François Marie Arouet 1694–1778 Épîtres, xcvi. A l'auteur du livre des Trois Imposteurs

World Health Organisation 1978 Summary by category and object of Expenditure Official Records of the World Health Organisation No 250 WHO Geneva

World Health Organisation 1978 Introductory chapter by the Director-General Official Records of the World Health Organisation No 250 WHO Geneva

Sources of information

Unless by chance an earlier exercise has gathered together all the available information about a particular population it will have to be sought out from wherever it is held. In the United States the recent dismantling of programs under earlier congressional legislation to gather such data about each population planning unit suggests that no great value was ever attached to this information by the populations and health professionals it was intended to guide. The cost of constantly updating each data base, essential for its usefulness, proved very expensive.

In most warm climate countries there is likely to be no such data base for the guidance of the newly appointed Health Officer. That does not prove that information has not been gathered either systematically or episodically from the population. Nor fortunately, are conventional health data gathering and recording systems the only sources of guidance.

This chapter will take a journey from the centre to the very edge of a typical warm climate country in the process of economic development. It will observe what information might be gathered along the way. The journey will wind through the countryside and will tap at both conventional and unconventional sources of data and information. Hard data, that which is objectively collected, verified and satistically processed will be scarce. But of information there will be plenty and it will not necessarily be less valuable or reliable because it comes from untrained observers.

An expatriate health officer or employee of an international agency arriving at the airport of a developing country will, if wise, already have tapped the sources of comparative data provided by WHO and other agencies. Most major libraries in any country carry encyclopaedias describing the geography, climate, economy and peoples of the different countries. Excellent and periodically updated reports about individual countries and their populations and governments are produced also by the US Department of State. More popular reviews are also published, though less systematically by geographical, banking and educational publishers. Particular care should be exercised in reading literature from developing countries designed for potential tourists.

WHO publications are also available in most medical school libraries. The principal ones useful for a Health Officer are mentioned by Russell in chapter eight and are listed in the references at the end of this chapter. Many technologically advanced countries also publish regular epidemiological summaries and will note anything of particular interest which has been documented by another country. Unfortunately the 'Morbidity and Mortality Weekly Reports' from the United States are no longer provided free though the equivalent British publication, Communicable Disease Report, still are.

WHO also publishes public health papers in its 'World Health Forum' and single problem reports in 'WHO Features'. In addition 'World Health' is produced for non-medical readers in a popular format. WHO also produces annually its 'Demographic Year Book' summarising whatever information is available about different populations. Few of the WHO publications are free.

Other international organisations which provide regular reports about conditions in developing countries include the International Labor Organization, the International Planned Parenthood Federation and the Commission of the European Communities in its monthly 'Courier'.

Annual reports or year books are published by both developed and developing countries and are often available in overseas libraries. These reports, though tending to be somewhat delayed in publication, summarise the respective government's reports on the economy, trade, education and population trends.

Finally there are also commercial publications such as 'World Almanac' which together in one fat volume publish in abstract form the principal data about populations, trade and government and also briefly describe each of the countries in the world down to the most minute. It goes without saying that the wise traveller will arm him or herself with all the information which can be obtained before departure, about the political constitution of the destination country, about the forces of influence within it and with the names of whatever individuals may be contacted for assistance or advice.

a. CENTRAL GOVERNMENT

Here will be found, hopefully more up to date than that already published, the conventional data collected by most governments of countries, states, provinces or regions. The government's main interest, apart from avoiding unrest among its subjects, is to know how many people there are and where, what is their potential as producers, taxpayers and soldiers and what demands are they likely to make for education and employment. It will have gathered whatever data it can about vital events such as birth or death and may be able to provide them broken down by small population or tribal groupings. The population may have been counted in a National Census. This may be performed regularly or may have been attempted once after independence is gained and not since.

To achieve an accurate census count of the number of individuals in a population, let along their age, sex, occupation, housing, education, ethnic or family relationships is vastly expensive. Local political and tribal interests tend to exaggerate the numbers, while family reticence and fears of taxation and conscription tend to minimise them. Official apathy tends to result in the omission from a census of migratory peoples and those living in isolated areas. In developing populations at least, the actual current numbers will usually be considerably greater than those reported in the most recent census. Sample censuses, if practicable, are cheaper, faster and can be more accurate.

The following less conventional but still relevant information should also be requested. It falls roughly into four categories.

1. Taxation

The taxation departments should have information about the occupation distributions within an area, the likely spendable incomes of wage earners, size of families and the relative affluence or poverty of different areas of the country. The information will probably be limited to wage earners principally government, professional and industrial workers.

2. Social spending

The extent of this information will depend upon the sophistication of the governmental services at local level. At least the central departments should have the breakdown of budget allocations made to health regions and districts plus any special program-centred or special assistance grants. It should also be able to indicate the quantity of spendable social security or pension money going into an area, and the proportion and distribution of families judged as at or below poverty levels. Data from an unemployment payment or job creation scheme will indicate the extent of joblessness.

3. Land

Governments are usually eager to record the ownership of land because of its tax potential and may have conducted surveys and valuations in the Districts. The existence of farming co-ops and communes may also be carefully recorded. He who owns the land locally also frequently exercises the most influence on the way local government functions so that details on major property owners should also be requested.

4. Capital Investment

Central government will certainly be involved in the provision of local schools and roads and should know the amounts spent, the building completed, proposed or under way. It will be involved in industrial development, land settlement or reclamation and in rehousing or creation of new communities in underdeveloped territory.

b. THE CITY

It may be in the national capital, or with autonomous states or provinces in the regional capital, that all information is to be found about supply and distribution systems and about how money is actually used and for what. The commercial banking system will have information on the proportion of wealth being diverted into individual consumption or corporate spending. By contrast the city will also be the focus of the development of shanty towns and disestablished, disaffected populations. Three types of information should be sought.

1. Communications

How far are radio and television distributed and do telephones, newspapers and scheduled public transport reach the distant health districts? What kind and method of official propoganda or health education is produced centrally directed at peripheral areas and what evidence is there on general literacy levels and the consumption of reading matter?

2. Money

Where is the private wealth held, what influence on capital spending is exerted by private banks and insurance companies, foreign-based banks and international corporations. It is from the city that food stocks and distribution will be controlled and it is here that any large scale local corruption will likely most freely be discussed.

3. Population

The city may indeed be the final destination of the new health appointee. Even if it is not the city population is well worth investigating. Evidence of immigration of trained or educated individuals from the peripheral districts suggests that local resources are being starved of service for whatever reason. Conversely the concentration of poor from the rural areas in the shanty towns suggests that tribal or occupational stresses will be found on arrival in the distant area — or that economic conditions are so harsh that the inhabitants are fleeing away from them. It is also in the city that evidence of violence in the population will be most evident and it might be possible to relate this to particular immigrant groups.

c. THE UNIVERSITY

Here is the intellectual elite of the country and the information it has is from two sources.

1. The students themselves

They will not be representative of the general population. A favoured minority, information on their respective origins within the country will show the relative strengths of local educational services. As by and large it is the children of the local elite who go to the University any report of poor nutrition or health in students coming from a particular area is a very ominous sign. Even if there is no routine physical entrance examination there should be records of health breakdowns or the relative prevalence of problems like pulmonary tuberculosis, frequency of mental ill health, drug or alcohol abuse, the frequency of academic failure, violence or suicide in a particular tribal or geographical group and the experiences of unwanted pregnancy or other reasons for abandoning education. It is relevant to enquire about where graduates go after University, their employment experiences, what proportion return to tribal lands or rural towns and finally what is the international standing of the qualifications obtained by these leaders of the future.

2. Research records

Much valuable information about peripheral areas of a country is often locked away or simply forgotten in the files of the central university. It may be here, for example, that a central bacteriology or parasite reference laboratory is placed. It will have the records, or they can be constructed from the reports filed away, of laboratory specimens sent in from the different parts of the country. They may indicate, for example, where cases of trypanosomiasis, arbovirus infections, or drug resistant organisms are most likely to be found. The medical school is almost certain to have conducted, even if only in pilot form, some local disease investigations. Research may be currently under way into precisely the problems of the inhabitants of the district about which information is being sought. Equally valuable information can be obtained from the university veterinary or agricultural departments about animal or plant diseases in different areas of the country, about toxins, poisonous snakes and insects, potential disease vectors and on positive local assets such as unused fertile land or untapped mineral resources. Finally it may be at the university medical school that international health agencies have placed their own special health teams which may already have visited distant areas. It may be here too that special registries, for example of cancer, will have been sited. Such registries may not be particularly valuable sources of information about local disease patterns but they will at least show how interested local health personnel are in providing data.

d. THE HOSPITAL

Data derived by analysing the inpatient and outpatient loadings of major hospitals and from the causes of illness and death, including post mortem examinations, in hospital patients is of great value but is often misused. It will indicate the kinds of cases being dealt with but more relevantly indicates the ability of the hospital to provide the service for which it was originally intended. Hospital data in its limited applicability to the community provides some measure of the value put upon the hospital by the local populations.

What cannot be done with hospital data in developing countries is to assume that what are reflected are the needs of that community. Hospitals, especially their outpatient services, tend to serve in depth only the immediately surrounding population. The interests and partiality of the hospital staff and the nature of its equipment will largely influence what kind of patients are seen. Hospital mortality lists will simply reflect the kind of cases allowed to terminate there. Morbidity listings of outpatients count numbers and types of visits, say nothing about the actual individuals served or the final outcome of treatment. Because of its role as a referral centre the hospital will inevitably record higher than real frequencies of complications in such normal processes as childbirth or infant rearing.

Despite all these reservations there are four kinds of information, indicative of community health patterns and needs, for which the hospital may be the only source.

1. Laboratory referrals

Central or regional reference laboratories may be set up in the principal teaching hospitals instead of at the University. As specimens are clearly labelled and recorded by origin they permit, for example, a fine picture of country wide resistance to drug therapy to be drawn up.

2. Medical supplies

The principal hospital may also be the main supplier of specialist items such as blood, vaccines, antitoxins and drugs kept in reserve for specially authorised cases. Even simpler supplies like rehydration kits may be made up using hospital components. To where, in what quantity and for what purpose such supplies are made is potentially valuable information. Moreover if there is a blood collection program involving rural populations it can be made to provide continued surveillance data for such diseases as syphilis, hepatitis B and American trypanosomiasis.

3. Emergencies

It is occurrences and conditions in the city itself which are reflected in the individuals brought into care after a disaster, like a fire, an episode like the overturning of a crowded bus or violence such as shooting between political or tribal rival gangs. Analysis of such emergency admissions may be the first noticed indication of a hazard in the community. For example a sudden rise in the frequency of severe child casualties may be the first indicator of the opening of a new road through a village or of a new refreshment stop for truck drivers.

4. Staff

The central hospital staff is likely to be the largest medical elite group in the country. If the hospital is overloaded with physicians, nurses and technicians there is some hope that similar professionals may be working out in smaller towns, perhaps even in rural areas. A staff-short hospital offers poor hope for the rest of the country. The competence of staff reflects competence levels outside unless physicians are obliged to choose between hospital and private practice. The physician to nurse ratio is also a sensitive indicator of balance in health care staff throughout the country. If the proportion of nurses is low there is very likely to be a crippling shortage of trained nurses in the country as a whole. Finally, though the information is of more political than epidemiologic value, the rural health officer will want to know how much the hospital costs and what proportion of the country's health budget is consumed by its high technology care as opposed to rural primary health care.

e. INDUSTRY AND ELECTRIC POWER

Of the world's 65 urban industrial manufacturing conglomerations 40 are in the developing countries. The picture of the typical developing country as being predominantly rural is a false one. Countries such as India are among the leading industrialised societies though the benefits produced by that industry are diluted by the unproductivity of the huge rural section of the economy. Even developing countries which are not intensively industrialised have some factories. All countries produce electric power, print newspapers and run transport with all the attendant support engineering such activities require. These industrial units are valuable and usually untapped sources of information on the health of the populations from which they draw their employees. Three classes of information can be drawn from them.

1. Employee data

In most warm climate countries industrial workers are a relative elite, often literate and rarely a representative sample of local tribal or religious group-ings. Their health experience, if it can be tapped, will indicate the health standards of the somewhat more fortunate. Sickness absences may be recorded. In more mature industries the mean length of working life may be a good indicator of population health. Remember though that the life experiences of 'survivors' do not mirror those of the population in general. The preference of many new industries to recruit and train only young persons can confuse the picture but the reasons for and frequency of rejec-tion of the unfit can be highly instructive.

2. Environmental data

While management will emphasise its economic contribution to the community the Health Officer must still find out what is being produced and with what hazardous materials, what the possible hazards are in the end products and wastes of that industry, how safe is disposal and storage and what drain on local resources results from this industry.

3. Social data

The effects of the development of industry in previously agrarian popu-lations can be devastating. Stress is produced by recruitment policies which employ the children and not their fathers, women rather than men, which undermine the previously labour intensive traditional industries and which produce an influx of new often alien workers into the community. The discarding of older or sick workers now accustomed to a cash income becomes a community problem reflected inevitably in high rates of alcoholism and family abuse. The Health Officer in a rapidly changing rural area may not be able to stop the spreading roots of social disaffection and revolution but to be aware of the hazards is to anticipate the consequences.

f. SPECIAL POPULATION GROUPS

In most populations there are sub groups, usually young males, selected or self selected primarily because of physical eliteness.

1. Sports and athletic teams

Those drawn from the less privileged local population are the most valuable study. A population which can produce young fit looking adults eager to expend energy in sports is almost certainly healthier than a population whose young people are physically apathetic. What matters is not which young people do or do not participate in unessential physical activity for the pleasure of it but how well they can compete with similar groups from other areas. As they are eager to be fit it is especially valuable to learn how frequently, on average, these young participants will be prevented by sickness from participating in their games and how many drop out through sickness and death. In some South American communities it is the frequency with which apparently fit young men die on the soccer field which suggests the prevalence of trypanosomiasis in the community. The frequency of indifference to injuries to the feet of amateur sportsmen in south east Asia may be an indicator to the Health Officer that the prevalence of leprosy had best be investigated.

2. Police

Here the selection again is by self. Characteristically, the hopeful recruit to the police is an establishment oriented literate young male eager for upward social movement, but not eager to leave his tribal area. The records of the screening procedures which young applicants for police training must get through are one of the most careful and useful sources of health information if they can be analysed. The reasons for rejection can be valuable. It is, however, the way in which new recruits stand up to training demands and their subsequent health and sickness records which are the best indicators of parallel health and sickness trends in their families and fellow citizens. The carefully maintained records of many police forces should not be despised.

While extracting data from police records the Health Officer will not neglect the relevant information about the health and well being of the community itself. The police maintain the records, detailed by person, type, place and time of violence, acute family disharmony, drug and alcohol abuse and the number of citizens requiring to be carried by police vehicles as cases of medical emergency.

3. Army

These are potentially some of the best records of all especially if there is a mandatory recruitment policy for all young males (young females are rarely obliged to join the Armed Services). Here is an opportunity to see a cross section of the male population at what should be the fittest time of life. The delicacy of the screening program will obviously differ from country to country and not too much importance should be attached to differences between countries in the proportions of their young men found fit to serve in the Armed Services. In highly technologically developed countries rejection rates, characteristically in the fifty per cent range, have mirrored the insistance of service chiefs that all their subordinates should be able to read, run fast and remain emotionally stable under stress. Armies are not equally scrupulous in their standards but they will all have some screening process and the reasons for rejection, and the proportion found unfit in different health areas, are grist to the epidemiological mill.

g. CAPTIVE GROUPS

Every country imprisons offenders and they are seldom elitist in origin. They are also attractive to investigators because they are relatively easy to study. They have little or no say in the matter. In the past they have been used as investigatory groups for sometimes unethical medical experiments and are eagerly cooperative to gain special rewards and privileges. Such experiments should have ceased. Prisoners as a group no more represent the population from which they have been extracted than the elitist police officers who apprehended them. Most long term stay prisoners at least go through some rough screening process on first admission to prison. The purpose is to determine their work capacity, the likelihood that they will be a menace to staff and other prisoners and as a means of ensuring that venereal infections, tuberculosis or insect infestations are not introduced into the closed community. Where some rough psychological screening is performed this may also produce information about the level of literacy or mental retardation, epilepsy or emotional disturbance. Prisoners are of course at high risk of being disabled or having faulty judgement — perhaps why they were apprehended. Prison populations tend to be highly damaged ones with the added chronic effects of unwise behaviour, self neglect and abuse of alcohol and drugs. As carriers of sickness they exaggerate but reflect the health problems of the community from which they come. When a prison population appears relatively intelligent and physically fit the suspision must be aroused that incarceration is taking place for other than customary anti-social behaviour.

Parallel circumstances will be noted in refugee groups especially when these are restricted to certain fenced in camps. The reasons why families or individuals become long term refugees are rarely as simple as fund raising agencies and politicians would have their supporters believe. The element of opportunism on the one hand or of passive indifference to circumstances on the other tends to distinguish refugees from the general population from which they originated. Even when a total population becomes disrupted, as after a natural disaster, health problems in the survivors can be surprisingly few. The health officer will want to be satisfied that refugees coming into an area or being resettled do not carry diseases which could affect the general populaton but such infectious hazards are rare. The long term hazards from such population movements are more social and economic than health related.

h. ACCIDENTS

These have a special value as sources of epidemiological data because they tend to be better recorded than other localised disasters or personal emergencies. The analysis of time and contributory cause will be an indicator of education and attitudes, especially of young people, towards machinery, the safety of others and the uses of alcohol.

Similar trends can be recognised in the misuse of sporting firearms and defence equipment. The careless use of tools and machinery, and the poor maintenance of safety features in high technology equipment are all too common in some developing countries. In the case of road vehicles screening programs have been introduced in some countries to test, for example, that an applicant for a driving licence has adequate vision. Such mandatory screening programs produce excellent information. For the drivers of buses or trucks the Health Officer may wish to know even more. The careful marriage of regulation and data collection will eventually permit the Health Officer not only to insist upon a widespread system of screening applicants for such posts as emergency vehicle operators but also provide mandatory training for persons likely to be involved in dealing with emergencies.

i. LOCAL GOVERNMENT POPULATION CENTRES

Six sources of information can be indentified in most rural district centres of population.

1. Governmental

It is probably from this level that central government collects its own data related to births, deaths, divorce, taxation, and trade. The data to be found at the local centre may be raw but is recent. It may also be at this level that local health regulations are promulgated and variably enforced. The information on housing standards and on water safety and waste disposal programs will be here as will also any government paid staff to operate them. The government's postal employees will know about communications and transport in the district and where the population actually exists in the outlying rural areas.

2. Local leaders

Identification of who these are is an urgent task of the newly appointed Health Officer. Timing is important as to neglect them even for a short time is to reduce the potential for later help and information. Local leaders and policy makers, tribal, religious, political or land-owning, by virtue of protecting their own position and property, will be highly subjective in describing the needs and attitudes of the community. Their potential influence over local officials, the introductions they can effect and the cooperation they can encourage in rural areas makes them worth cultivating.

3. Local professionals

Local lawyers and physicians in private practice are a rich potential source of information, if they can be presuaded to part with it. More certainly informative will be the local veterinary or agricultural experts, the meat inspectors, butchers and collectors of produce from distant farms. Here are reservoirs of information about the health of domestic and wild animals in the district, about the health and well being of the rural peoples they contact and about the quantities and wholesomeness of food coming into the town from the rural areas.

4. Primary health care centre

Here the usefulness of available information depends upon the degree to which staff have investigated local health needs rather than simply counting demand. It should be possible to extract something useful from the records of local morbidity and mortality but whether that will reflect the experience of the entire population or just that adjacent to the health centre depends upon the energy of its staff and upon the resources available for extending service to rural populations. Immunisation coverage in more peripheral communities should be reasonably evident from work output records. The centre may also have data on mean family size and birth spacing at least in the urban areas. Staff will be aware of the types of disaster which call for obstetric, surgical or epidemic control intervention by workers in the rural areas and will be able to describe how secondary referral is obtained to the regional or capital city hospital.

5. Schools

Here is probably the only source of information about the health and well being of school age children. It will be most valuable if there is a mandatory and enforced requirement that all children receive primary school education. Otherwise it will tend to exclude both poor and rural children. The analysis of school attendance, allied to the observations of the school teacher, is a rich source of information about morbidity causes and frequency. Even the most simple of school health services should be able to identify the existence of malnutrition or other bars to growth and development. The school-teachers should know the degree of literacy in the community, the proportions of motherless or fatherless families, the nature and quantity of family life disruption and the extent of child abuse or unreasonable labour. The best of all information is that about children who fail to attend school.

6. Churches and mosques

Neither religious leaders nor the devout can be taken as representative of any population. They can, however, provide reliable information on the numbers of hurried rituals held over dying babies or mothers, the frequency of out-of-wedlock pregnancy, the break up of families and the numbers and ages of those who are buried in the local graveyard. The churches may be more aware than are the local professional health workers of persons crippled by disease or needing constant care. Religious leaders may also be heightened in their sensitivity to, and therefore more aware of, customs and traditions inimical to health and hidden within rural and poorly educated sections of the population.

j. LONG TERM CARE INSTITUTIONS

These still exist in most countries as wharehouses for the human unwanted. Their very existence and the attitude of the outside population towards the inmates tells much about the understanding, caring attitudes and fears of the outside population about crippling leprosy, drug resistant tuberculosis, psychiatric disturbance, severe retardation and disabling old age. They reflect the patterns of medical failure in the different areas from which they draw patients and it is important to identify where and of what nature such failures are. The experiences of the managers of the institutions are also a valuable guide to the Health Officer on the reliability of governmental funding and supplies and especially of essential drugs. Their records may also supply evidence of foci of health damage in a rural area of which staff on the spot may be unaware.

k. THE RURAL VILLAGE

There is a profound distinction between the relative sophistication of the district town with its governmental services and an educated segment of the population and the relative isolation of the village. The isolation may not so much be from outside contact as from new ideas and from changing ways of life. Objective data may be unobtainable not just because the services which might engender it are non existent or feeble but because the village structure is protective of its families and individuals. Once a primary school is established or a bus service becomes available the manners and desires of the outside world creep in but the four sources of influence and information summarised below will remain little changed.

1. Headman

Without the competition of governmental officials and the educated bourgeoisie of the small towns the village headman or equivalent will serve not only as the principal source of information, if he chooses, but also as the catalyst or brake on the other potential informants. As would be expected the information will be highly subjective and biased by personal or family interests. The principal villager will know about the number of families, their land, possessions and resources and the problem individuals, as they judge them, in the population. They will have opinions about government services or the lack of them, they will comment on changes as they see them in family patterns and lines of authority, they will attempt not to discuss local rituals and unorthodox beliefs, will deplore the increasing indiscipline of young people and the changing ways of life and at the same time will press for better road and bus service, subsidies for crops, fertilizer and insecticides and more veterinary care for their animals. They might even ask for a clinic to be established but with only a vague idea as to its usefulness. The Headman if amenable will open doors into individual families, will allow access to local graveyards and other protected places and will attempt to get the members of his family exclusively either appointed to any new health positions or selected for training courses.

2. Local midwife

If not the Headman's wife she is at least likely to be closely related by family ties. She will be similarly subjective in reporting or commenting on circumstances to make them as favourable as possible to herself. She may have already have had some minimal government sponsored training in basic hygiene and in the recognition of the signs of abnormality in pregnancy and delivery. She has information about the number of pregnancies in the village, the frequency of stillbirth, infant and maternal death and of congenital defects. She might eventually be willing to discuss abortion practices, birth spacing, child rearing and circumcision customs and any new problems such as the introduction of venereal infections into the village. She will know all the family interrelationships and may know a good deal about the health of most members of the community and the remedies and resources the sick or anxious customarily fall back upon.

3. Local or traditional healer

The range of healer types throughout the developing countries complicates any systematic approach to the health information they may possess. In the same village there may be herbalists, bleeders, mystics, magicians, or individuals who have inherited a special limited skill, like curing warts or female sterility and do nothing else. The potential for gaining useful information about the health of the community is likely to be greatest when there is a single all-purpose herbalist type village healer. If confidence can be obtained, and this is difficult at best, the Health Officer may find lodged in the healer's memory the data about principal sickness or behavioural disturbance in the villagers, the principal remedies used and for what, the frequency and range of new disease imported into the village and the details and consequences of secret rituals performed at the principal events of life especially coming-of-age. In general though not too much hope should be built up about this potential source of information. The lack of any education, the eccentric nature of their services and their suspicions of the health professional who is ultimately a competitor militates against a successful tapping of the information they may possess and of whose significance they may be quite unaware.

4. Family heads

If these can be gathered together and persuaded to express an opinion they may present a more objective viewpoint on health care needs and services than their official spokesman, the Headman. They are certainly the source of information about individual family supplies of drinking water, defaecation habits, nightsoil disposal, food storage and the details of crops and animal husbandry. Their attitudes to women and women's role, to family authority, education of their children and how to spend any available cash will be illuminating. More important is the access they provide in many communities to their wives. For it is here that the pertinent health information lies, where the life or death decisions are made and where the levels of family nutrition are determined.

l. THE MARKET

Any place where individuals gather to relax, mix with different age groups and with other communities, exchange goods and information is a rich mine for the observant. Crowds attending sports, political or religious events are too self selected to be representative, too preoccupied by the event itself to reveal their interests and anxieties. By contrast marked places throughout the world have a common purpose of exchange, the process itself is generally enjoyable and relaxed and in most countries both sexes and all ages are involved. The very crowding also allows the observer to be unobserved. Three classes of information can be gleaned.

1. The people

(and their animals). Note their vigour, age range, nutrition, cleanliness, skin scars, disabilities and attitudes toward each other. Observe behavioural patterns, ease of communications, good humour, drunkenness, ability to count (numeracy) and read notices or advertisements.

2. What is being bought and sold

Observe the ability to purchase or barter with cash or goods. In agrarian communities especially a surprising range of goods can be consumed even though cash income per head is very low. Note what the relative costs of different items are — for example, the price of a litre of petroleum fuel, or a goat, of a kilo of sweet potatoes, of a sheaf of dried tobacco leaf, of soap and drugs. Farming products may also be bought in quantity by traders.

If so note what prices are being paid. As well as noting the range of goods available assess their quality, the safety of foods, drugs, tools and electrical products. Attempt to gauge priorities in spending, such preferences as for packets of infant food, adult trash foods and sweets, alcohol, tobacco and luxury items.

3. What is being discussed

This has an important bearing on the health and well being of the community. Unfortunately even when local languages are understood local dialects may render gossip and brief interchanges unintelligible to the outsider. Intermediaries may be necessary. Or simple displays can be used to attract the curious who can then be engaged in banter or conversation. Most peoples are eager to talk about property anxieties — taxes, land disputes and about the deficiencies of the governmental services. It takes somewhat more intimacy to learn about local deaths, births, and sickness, recent violence or drunken episodes and the complexities of marriage and birth.

m. AGRICULTURE AND LOCAL FAUNA

Only by high cost fencing and stock rearing methods inapplicable to most developing countries can man's domestic and farming animals be kept isolated from the zoonoses and epizootics occuring in the animals of the savannah, bush or jungle. The farm animals are indeed a valuable indicator, when disease breaks out in the sylvatic animal population, of danger to man himself. The Health Officer must always be attentive to and encourage information from farmers and any local veterinary personnel. To keep the information flowing can involve difficult choices. The Health Officer has to appear sympathetic to the farmers' problems but must not interfere unnecessarily otherwise the information will cease. Disaster occurs if potentially hazardous diseases, such as an outbreak of anthrax in a local goat herd or the death of some local horses from an arbovirus encephalitis, are concealed. Some specific points of health information related to agriculture and to the sylvatic animal population are as follows.

1. Agriculture

First find out what is being produced on the farms and using what potentially hazardous machinery, chemicals, fertilizers or storage systems. The hygienic standards of foods to be sold to the public will obviously be of concern as will the quality of that food, the health of meat and milk animals and the results of routine meat inspections of the carcasses. What is the source and safety of water used and what happens to animal wastes and slurries and discarded supplies. The episodes of sickness in both the farmer's family and his stock are of equal relevance. The latter may only be evident in an unexpectedly rapid turnover in the stock, including the mysterious disappearance of animals — especially of anthrax and trypanosomiasis prone herbivores. Note too if the farmer grows saleable cash crops, such as tobacoo, in preference to the food essential for his family. The general productivity and efficiency of a farming unit is difficult for the outsider to measure but the neatness of fields and their crops, the timeliness of planting, irrigation and harvesting. the nutritional level of farm animals and their general vigour and cleanliness, including that of their quarters when confined, tell a great deal about an agricultural community and about the health of those who labour in it.

2. Sylvatic animals

Where diseases transmitted to man come primarily from wild animal sources, for example leishmaniasis, plague, typhus, trypanosomiasis and yellow fever, the importance of monitoring health in the wild animal population is obvious. This can be at a simple level, such as observing the frequency with which carcasses or recent skeletons of dead rodents are to be found. Or it can be part of a planned surveillance program in which, for example, predators of the cat family would be regularly trapped and bled for antibody levels. Both such types of surveillance would be appropriate in a community anticipating an upsurge from time to time in plague. The disappearance or death of domestic cats can be significant in such a community. The health of human predators should also be monitored. Hunters or their wives who skin the carcasses may be the first to be affected by zoonotic disease. A change in the types of local fauna or an unexpected decline in the numbers of wild animals should also be taken as cause for further investigation. The crossing and mixing points where wild and domestic animals meet are sensitive areas for diseases such as rabies, tuberculosis and the spirochetal infections en route for man himself. The fouling of agricultural water supplies by wild animals cannot be prevented but knowing where it occurs will enable the Health Officer to deal more rapidly with sickness from such diseases as leptospirosis.

n. THE FRONTIER

This journey ends as it began, attempting to tap official data, information routinely collected by governmental agencies which, if properly interpreted, can be most valuable to the District or Regional Health Officer. Information about the movements of people and goods across the unguarded borders of a health region or district is rarely available. The single exception is school attenders registering for the first time in the local school system. Whether or not a mandatory health screening program for such new arrivals is worthwhile will depend upon local circumstances. It might be considered when such movements take place from a high parasitaemia to a low parasitaemia population.

Official mapped and guarded frontiers are the collecting points for much potentially valuable data and in the following eight categories.

1. Imported disease

Many countries insist on some form of health assessment or screening for prospective immigrants, for refugees and for temporary workers requesting permission to stay. Often the objective of such assessments is to keep out non productive immigrants. They will tend to exclude disabled rather than infectious individuals. Sometimes a procedure such as a chest X-ray examination is part of the immigration control program. The Health Officer should attempt to obtain information about all individuals admitted to the area as foreign immigrants and would certainly want to follow up all persons who might be infected. The parallel to this is the importation of disease by returning travellers or tourists. The Health Officer is obliged to rely on the punctiliousness of immigration personnel and upon the vigilance of airline staff, railway inspectors, bus drivers and frontier guards. An alert local primary health care staff will notify the onset of illness in a recently returned traveller.

2. Health personnel

Though of more interest to the epidemiologist-planner than to the local Health Officer the movements in or out of health personnel have obvious relevance to the future of health care services in any district. The outward trade of health personnel from a particular area of a country has similar implications for local programs. The direction of these inbalances is one of the most difficult problems facing many countries and is not as simple as providing more money.

3. Health supplies

It is on the frontier that information is collected about the drugs and equipment coming into the country. The Health Officer may not be able to divert it away from its ultimate destination in the capital city but knowing that the supplies exist is a strong bargaining counter for a share of them. Imported proprietary medicines will also be listed so that the extent of self, and perhaps unwise, medication can be estimated. The appropriateness of imported supplies might be considered as well as the condition and their being still 'fresh'.

4. Consumable trade

Here will be the data on food importations and on quantities of alcohol and tobacco. The internal taxation system will have information about consumption of internally produced alcohol and tobacco.

5. People

Not only the deficit or inbalance of population produced by immigration and emigration but the kinds of people gained or lost and their likely effect on health care services can be ascertained. The addition of ethnic minorities provides additional possible indirect health hazards and future stresses as will special importations of individuals such as following overseas adoption of refugee children. Refugees can of course travel in either direction though the Health Officer will primarily be concerned with those entering. The reasons for local citizens to escape outward over the frontier, fear of epidemics, authoritarian government, neglect of basic population needs, violence in the community are also of great concern to the Health Officer though usually outside her or his power to correct.

6. International assistance programs

Aid coming into the country may be tapped for local benefit for supplies or staff or the organisers may be persuaded that an ongoing service program should be set up in the area. Conversely the Health Officer may wish to oppose proposed data finding programs for which no ultimate service element is planned.

7. Illegal importations

Official figures will be limited to seizures of smuggled goods such as illegal drugs. The value of such figures is to indicate any demand which in turn implies a hazard to the population. The existence of a 'black market' in illegal goods in an area not only provides distribution of potential health damagers but also drains family resources.

8. Duties and trade

Health Districts cannot be run in isolation from the economic realities of the country. The balance between exports and imports will be perhaps the principal determinant of whether a health program can be expanded or be abandoned or whether necessary supplies can be obtained. It is wise to examine these financial statements before planning future health services. It is also wise to ascertain the duties imposed on any items which must be imported and the likely delay in importation formalities at the frontier.

Similar care should be exercised when it is proposed to import personnel — what will be the likely problems and what procedures must be gone through patiently in order to obtain what is needed? While such information may seem a long way from epidemiology, if not gathered and acted upon wisely there may be no local epidemiology or disease control program.

REFERENCES

Bulletin of the World Health Organization (2 monthly). WHO Geneva
Communicable Disease Report (weekly) Public Health Laboratory Service, Communicable Disease Surveillance Centre, London, NW9 5EQ
The Courier-Africa-Caribbean-Pacific-European Community (monthly) Commission of the European Communities. Brussels
Demographic Year Book (annual) WHO Geneva
Morbidity and Mortality Weekly Reports (weekly) Center for Disease Control, Atlanta, Georgia 30333
United States Department of State. Bureau of Public Affairs
   Background Notes. US Government Printing Office. Washington DC 20402
World Almanac (annual) Newpaper Enterprises Association Inc. New York
World Health (monthly) WHO Geneva
World Health Forum. An International Journal of Health Development (quarterly) WHO Geneva
WHO Chronicle (2 monthly) WHO Geneva
WHO Features (2 monthly) WHO Geneva
WHO Technical Report Series (periodic) WHO Geneva
WHO Monograph Series (Periodic) WHO Geneva
WHO Weekly Epidemiological Record. (weekly) WHO Geneva

Measurements of population health

Need in any general population, as expressed in a demand for health and related services, appears to be a pot with no bottom. Service, and supporting resources, however grandly poured in, never satisfies demand: indeed they grow together. Faced with the necessity of using scant resources wisely the District Health Officer must decide which of the needs of the community should receive priority. One way to do this is to compare the specific 'health related indicators' of different but generally comparable communities. This will highlight both the particular weaknesses and the relative good fortune of different communities of the same type and the susceptible groups of individuals within those communities.

The difficulty lies in obtaining data which is both comparable, one population with another, and which does indeed indicate where corrective service could be effective. Health care planners are not alone in laboring over the task of finding appropriate data. 'Systems analysis' is the methodological approach, designed originally for management in industry, which displays the ways in which manpower, machines and buildings function as productive or unproductive units. Its analogy in clinical practice are the several investigative modes used by the physician to reach a diagnostic conclusion in a puzzling case. Both population needs and the effectiveness of exisiting services can similarly be analysed.

Reference has already been made to the part the epidemiologist should play in making these management and resource allocation decisions. Like the planning agencies in national health care systems considerable attention has been paid to the applications of systems analysis by the international health agencies (WHO 1976).

At a much smaller population level too similar, though perhaps less detailed analyses can measure, for example, the accessibility of existing hospital services to a distant rural population, or can assess the expected benefit of a proposed vaccination program. Such analyses, performed for a specific purpose, will of course not reveal the full picture of strengths and needs of a population. A collection of final reports of such small scale analyses was published fairly recently by WHO (1979).

In practice when comparisons are made between populations it is the different mortality rates which are most commonly compared. Hopefully these will, at the very least, have been standardized as described in chapter one. Especially sensitive indicators of community need are the *maternal mortality rate* and the *perinatal mortality rate*. A particular advantage attached to the use of data about deaths associated with childbearing is that all societies recognise this as an undesirable event or outcome and it is unlikely to be quickly forgotton or ignored. For the Health Officer it should not be too difficult to estimate the number of pregnant women in the population and to gather information about those who fail to survive it. Made at regular intervals such calculations will both monitor the population 'health' and will detect the favourable influence of improved obstetric care.

Though at best a crude indicator the length of life which a newborn baby can, on average, expect to live is a measure of how favourable conditions, including health care, are to long term survival in a particular population. Figure 6.1 in Chapter six showed such an international comparison. This particular indicator, though very commonly quoted, can be somewhat misleading. Early infancy is particularly sensitive to environmental, nutritional and infectious hazards so that life wastage can be high even in those communities for which conditions are reasonably favourable for survival and development in later periods of life. A better indicator of survival potential in the general population would be life expectancy calculated from the end of early chilhood. Such calculations generally suggest that the longer an individual survives into young adulthood and the more likely is the eventual span of life to be of reasonable length whatever the nature of the society and its health services (Swaroop 1960).

Not all health related indicators are based upon information about disease and death. Certain factors, like the absence of an adequate, convenient water supply in each home appear inevitably associated with high frequencies of diarrhoeal disease in a community. Poor infant survival rates can be expected in populations in which the mothers cannot read, especially if they no longer live within traditional tribal or extended family protection. Health is likely to suffer if malnutrition is common. Such factors, descriptive of a population, do not prove that a health problem exists but do clearly indicate a health hazard. An overloaded farm cart may reach its journey's end safely but it is much more likely than is a properly loaded one to be overturned along the way.

Some of the more frequently used health related indicators, including descriptive ones, are given in Table 10.1 and are derived from World Bank analyses which excluded both China and India. Countries have been gathered into three groups according to their *Gross National Product* per capita. Under the respective columns it will be seen that in all their health related indicators the poorest countries suffer the most disadvantage. The poorest populations produce the greatest proportion of new births, the greatest proportion of infant wastage and have the lowest levels of literacy in the parents. The poorest have the worst nutrition and the least access to safe water. Perhaps the most remarkable contrast between the different national groupings is in the survival of children from one to four years of age. Very few die in the industrialized countries.

Table 10.1 Health Related Indicators

Indicator	Year	Low income countries*	Middle income countries	Industrialized countries
Gross national product per capita (US dollars)	1979	240	1420	9440
Crude birth rate (births per 1000 population)	1979	42	34	15
Crude death rate (deaths per 1000 population)	1979	16	10	10
Life expectancy at birth in years	1979	51	61	74
Infant mortality rate (deaths per 1000 liveborn	1978	49–237	12–157	13
Child mortality rate (deaths per 1000 1–4 years of age)	1979	18	10	1
Access to safe water % of population	1975	25	58	100
Daily per capita calories μ % of requirement	1977	96	109	131
Adult literacy rate %	1976	43	72	99

* excludes India and China
μ based on estimates of UN FAO
Sources: World Development Report 1981. Washington DC. World Bank, August 1981

Differences between the groups in levels of nutrition may be unexpectedly small. The principal problem in most poorer countries lies not in a gross deficiency of food but in the equitable distribution of what is available to the whole population, and evenly over the year. Even without much total increase in the quantity of food available the improvements in storage and distribution which occur in middle income countries, remove at least widespread malnutrition and the fragile dependence upon unpredictable harvests.

The ranges of such an indicator as infant mortality reinforce the point already made in Chapter six that preconceived views about a population based on its climate, international affluence and the sophistication of its medical services can be misleading. Both the United States and the Soviet Union trail behind most industrialized countries in such indicators as infant mortality and life expectancy at birth despite their affluence and the extraordinary sophistication and huge staffing of their health care industries. The importation of high technology and the staff to use it into an underdeveloped country will not prevent infants dying from diarrhoea in distant rural areas. Safe water newly provided for that village will do little to improve health until the population learns to use it freely in hygienically preparing foods and in caring for infants. By contrast countries which are very poor in terms of international banking, like Sri Lanka and Costa Rica, may enjoy better health than their equally poor neighbours. Their advantage appears to lie in their better level of primary schooling and the resulting favourable literacy levels. It has been argued that to educate young females to the point where they can usefully read and then teach each other should come before the provision of health care services, other than basic hygiene and immunization programs.

Health related indicators can be constructed for any population even without any of the information contained in Table 10.1. Simply by observing the answers to the questions suggested at different stages of the journey undertaken in chapter 9 a surprisingly accurate picture of a community and of its probable needs can be drawn. The following categories of observation are suggested.

1. The country, region or district

Define as far as possible its geographic features concentrating upon.
(a) assets — ease of terrain, soil fertility, opportunity for agricultural expansion, good and continuous water supply, easy communications within and to outside the area, natural resources able to feed population expansion.
(b) potential hazards — inhospitable climate, difficult access, poor communications, barren or misused land, no obvious sources of wealth creation.

2. The environment

(a) assets — geologically stable, even climate, healthy farm and wild animals, good game reserves and fish stocks, well drained soil, hygienic living practices.
(b) potential hazards — polluted rivers, air pollution from industrial effluent, extreme climatic variations, potential for periodic floods, earthquakes, crop failures, monsoon failures, potential disease vectors and breeding places, pollution of housing areas and water supplies with human wastes.

3. The economy

(a) assets — productive and well cared for fields, good crop storage, cash producing employment and spendable family income above basic necessities, goods available and at reasonable costs, net cash inflow from trade, reliable food and power sources, adequate and well maintained agricultural equipment.

(b) potential hazards — neglected fields, insecure food stores, derelict industrial buildings and equipment, rising trade debt, high proportion of unemployed family heads, little or no public transport, evident poverty and apathy.

4. The stage of development

(a) assets — appropriately dispersed primary health care centres with easy access to secondary referal, adequate primary schools for both sexes, school attendance well maintained, well kept public buildings, voluntarily restrained society, access to mass communications such as radios.
(b) potential hazards — poor quality housing (actual structure dependent upon culture, climate and migratory nature of the population), poor ventilation, overcrowded especially in wet or cold season, lack of basic domestic assets for food storage, cooking and hygiene, mixing of animals and people, repressive law and order or chaos and indiscipline, development of shanty towns.

5. The population

(a) numbers distribution and accessibility
(b) demography — evidence of any unusual sex or age ratio, frequency of conception, proportion of dependents in the average family.
(c) ethnic make up and evidence of minorities and their respective position in the society and its economy.
(d) language commonly understood or evidence of barriers to communication.
(e) tribal and family patterns and their stability — evidence of urbanization.
(f) nutritional appearance especially of pre-school children and including physical and mental alertness and activity.
(g) potentially restrictive cultural patterns, taboos, religious beliefs or ceremonial mutilations.
(h) presence of disabled, crippled or beggars, skin scars or blind persons.
(i) evidence of alcohol, tobacco or drug abuse.
(j) evidence of population fear of crime or uncontrolled adolescent street aggression.
(k) attitudes — cheerful relaxed, adaptable versus truculent, rigid, hostile, threatening violence.
(l) presence of bizarre or bigotted, conflicting religious groups.
(m) prosperity as evidenced by clothing, transport, property upkeep.

Observation alone, not accompanied by close enquiries and cross questionning of what is related can of course be misleading. An evidently prosperous well fed population may be experiencing the painful consequences of industrialization with breakdown in traditional, secure family patterns, an increase in single parent families and increasing disputes over authority within families and over property between families. In order to earn wages family heads may be absent from home for long periods. The outside observer will see little evidence of frequent after dark adolescent violence or alcohol related road accidents. It will take patient enquiry to reveal the potential hazards from new occupations especially as they are not evident at early stages of development when the work force is young and healthy.

In many ways the indicators of population well being or population stress summarized above are more useful than a passive analysis of such health data as may already exist or can be obtained. In the preceeding chapter caution was suggested in interpreting the significance of hospital inpatient or clinic outpatient records. If the morbidity and mortality do truly represent what is going on in the population they will be good indicators of need. Unfortunately that is not usually the case.

The measurement or quantifying of health resources, per head of population, suggests what could be attempted rather than what is actually achieved. Shere attendance numbers at outpatient services mean little unless the reasons for attending, who comes and how frequently, can be analysed. What the District Health Officer will need to know is the following.

1. what proportion of pregnancies result in both a healthy mother and a healthy infant.
2. what is the mean interval between pregnancies and the mean number of live infant-producing pregnancies per female in the childbearing age groups.
3. what proportion of infants is born with evidence of birth injury or congenital abnormality
4. what proportion of live born infants survives to school age
5. what are the strengths and potential dangers of traditional healing services especially in relation to childbirth.
6. what are the prevailing attitudes and beliefs in regard both to infant rearing and to the care of the elderly
7. what is the frequency of growth retarding sickness in childhood
8. what proportion of children, at different ages, fail to achieve or to maintain normal growth and development.
9. what proportion of school entrants survives to become work productive
10. what proportions of female and male children remain illiterate at the end of the primary school age.
11. how adequate is the diet available to young families in the lowest social class or income group
12. what proportion of mothers with young children are aware of and practice reasonable hygiene especially in the preparation of food.
13. what proportion of work age adults is unable to earn a living through physical or mental disability and what is the distribution of the causes of this disability.

14. what proportions of mature females and males are illiterate.
15. how frequently are working age adults acutely or chronically reduced in their capacity to work by ill health or disability.
16. what proportions of physically and mentally fit adults are underemployed or totally unemployed.
17. what is the mean family income for wage earners or what is the range of spendable income in excess of subsistence level at local commodity prices.
18. with what frequency do single or widowed parents of either sex head young families.
19. what is the level of knowledge about the means to preserve health in the average adult in the community.
20. in what proportion of family homes are the food preparation and storage areas within the general living area.
21. with what frequency and in what sections of the population do preventible diseases or those which are curable but not cured occur
22. in what quantities and by who are consumed potentially harmful substances such as alcohol, tobacco or drugs and from where do they come
23. with what frequency and in what sections of the population do serious domestic, occupational or civil disorder type episodes of injury occur.
24. what attitudes or criteria does the average individual use in deciding what is or is not 'normal' in her or his own health
25. at what age does a significant proportion of the population loose most of the teeth, suffer deteriorating eyesight or experience difficulty in performing hard labour.
26. what proportion of families have access to 'safe' water and in what proportion is this water available on tap in the home in unlimited quantity.
27. what proportion of family homes possess a 'safe' system of human waste disposal and what proportion of those use it regularly.
28. what proportion of the 'at risk' population is fully protected against the immunizable infections.
29. what is the activity and independence level of elderly persons in the community.
30. what disabling or independence threatening conditions of adults could be relatively easily corrected or prevented.

From the above and other similar measurements or estimates can be constructed health related indicators for any particular community. These will weave a pattern of now observed need in the population. They may also delineate a pattern of desire or 'wanting' in the population which will not necessarily coincide with what health personnel judge to be high priority needs. Many of the needs, perceived or otherwise, though indicating fairly the health of the population are not always best met by simply providing more health care or preventive services.

The District Health Officer may be unable to rehouse the population, persuade it to house its domestic animals apart or overnight change the attitudes of village midwives. Perhaps all that can be done at first is to assess the magnitude of the local health problems and to determine who is principally affected. Action to solve them will likely be a very slow process.

The nearness of existing health resources, their adequacy, accessibility, effectiveness and appropriateness are not health related indicators. They are not necessarily even related to need. There is no obvious correlation between medical resource development and established need. This is especially true in a free enterprise system where supply side economics dictate what actually will be made available to consumers. When need is examined in relation to measurable variations from normal health it is mental health which is most starved of resources in most societies.

Presumably what most agrarian peoples fear most is that their young families should be made motherless or should loose the principal breadwinner, that they will fail to raise sufficient children to maintain the parents in old age or that some large disaster, possibly divinely imposed, will disrupt their society and force them off their land. The ownership of land or the right to farm it is the most valued asset in all societies. A health service will be most valued to the extent that it is seen to be mitigating these dangers. Many well meaning programs based on Western standards of hygiene and infant survival fail to excite support from indigenous populations because they do not appear to address this first priority for survival of the agrarian family unit. The extent to which services, if any, are offered to the most difficult to reach sections of the population provides a useful measure of a program but not of the needs, perceived or otherwise, of the population itself.

TERMINOLOGY

Gross national product. The sum of the value of all industrial and agricultural production and of all services within the country upon which value can be placed. When expressed as 'per capita' the gross sum is divided not by the number of persons producing this wealth but by the total number of persons in the population. By thus correcting for differences in the numbers in different populations they can be compared together as though saying this particular country produces this much wealth for every person in it per year. To some extent the measurement exagerates the differences between the rich industrial and the poor agrarian ones as the GNP takes little account of home produced and consumed products.

Maternal Mortality Rate. The exact definition varies from country to country but it is meant to express in a rate the likelihood of pregnancy either terminating prematurely in the death of the woman or in causing such damage that death occurs fairly soon after the birth, miscarriage or abortion. The frequency indirectly indicates the effectiveness of the local obstetric services. Most commonly expressed by the formula.

Maternal mortality rate =

$$\frac{\text{deaths from pregnancy in a year} \times 1000}{\text{number of live births in the same year}}$$

Perinatal Mortality Rate By making no distinction between late fetal deaths and early infant deaths this rate measures the total risk to the child associated with the end of pregnancy and birth and indirectly the effectiveness of the obstetric and early post partum services. Expressed by the formula
  Perinatal mortality rate =

$$\frac{\text{Fetal deaths after 28 weeks of pregnancy} + \text{infant deaths under seven days} \times 1000}{\text{Total live births} + \text{late fetal deaths in the same year}}$$

REFERENCES

Swaroop S 1960 Introduction to health statistics. Livingstone, London.
WHO 1976. Applications of systems analysis to health management: report of a WHO expert committee. WHO Geneva.
WHO 1979. Measurement of levels of health. WHO Copenhagen.

Applying research techniques at community level

Four types of research are conducted at community level. It is as well from the onset to be clear which of these motivates the researcher.

1. To construct a 'profile' of the health of the individuals who collectively constitute that population. Usually the purpose is to identify the general burden of sickness; the needs for health protection and the ways in which the available resources can be spent. Much of this has been discussed in the preceding chapters.

2. To measure the endemicity of a particular disease; how many individuals are affected by it and why? What proportions of those affected are at the different stages of illness or incapacity? What proportion can be expected to die and at what age? What measures will be necessary to interrupt transmission or to remove other persons from risk and what measures of treatment will be required for those already affected? Such single problem research can also be adapted to measure the effect or outcome upon the community of a specific event or particular environmental conditions. The event may be an epidemic or a less well defined general deterioration in health. It might be man made or a natural disaster. The research will identify the cost in terms of lives shortened or made harder; resources lost and burdens of increased dependency forced upon the survivors.

3. To assess the effectiveness of specific modules of health care or entire health related programs. These might have been completed or be ongoing and might be designed to reduce a hazard or to alleviate its consequences. The investigation would reveal to what degree the original objectives of the program have been met. Equally well the outcome being studied could be the health consequences of changing the environment in some way, such as building a dam.

4. To test new drugs or techniques. This will generally involve comparisons of existing treatment or preventive methods with new ones to determine which is safest; which is most easily acceptable to the subjects and which, if there is a choice, is the cheapest.

Research type 1 is often identified as 'descriptive', type 2 is into 'causality', costs and control alternatives, type 3 is of 'cost benefit' or 'intervention outcome' and type 4 research would likely be an 'experimental trial'.

In practice and under field conditions many community research programs are a mixture of two or more of the above. Full accounts of the principles which must be considered in planning each of the above types of research program will be found in standard textbooks of epidemiology. Sufficient here to concentrate on the practical issues most likely to be of interest to the District or Regional Health Officer in a developing country.

THE POPULATION HEALTH PROFILE

The preceding chapters have dealt with the possible sources of health information about a particular population and need not be repeated. Assessments of community health based on periodic sampling of the population are also conducted in some affluent countries. Occasional single sample assessments, generally funded by overseas reaseach institutions, are also made in developing countries. Some caution is required in extrapolating the findings of such specially observed and specially treated groups to the general population. *Multiphasic* screening is also sometimes performed but it is clumsy and expensive even for affluent societies. In general it is probably just as useful to measure a few health related indicators in a population as described in the last chapter as to weigh the actual total burden of sickness.

SPECIFIC DISEASE PROBLEMS

Here there are three distinct aspects to consider
(a) Prevalence
(b) Causal relationships
(c) Costs and remedies.

Prevalence

The prevalence of a particular disease in a population can be calculated if the disease usually terminates in death and if the mean time between first onset and termination can be reasonably certainly calculated. The researcher need then only ascertain how many persons die of the disease in the community in order to calculate how many others are now affected but not yet dead. Such calculations could be made for a disease with a slowly progressive tendency like breast cancer or with a dramatic onset, like a stroke. Such events tend to be noticed and remembered and, with encouragement, will be reported. Greater difficulty is encountered in determining the prevalence of such a condition as rheumatic heart disease or lymphatic filariasis. For such health hazard in which many affected individuals will go unnoticed a special early disease detection program will probably have to be set up. Diseases can be detected at any one of five different stages.
   1. The earliest stage. Detection may be primarily immunological or may

depend upon the noting of a physiological reading beyond the 'normal' range. There is no sickness.

2. The stage when illness has begun but before any irreversible effects have occurred. Early enough treatment will bring about a complete cure.

3. The stage when damage has occurred to the individual but treatment will either prevent further transmission to others or will limit the effects of the damage on the original cases so that independence is maintained or restored.

4. The carrier state. An apparently well individual is able to transmit the disease.

5. The damaged, dependent or dying individual but who is not necessarily beyond hope of some alleviation of suffering.

Before embarking upon any disease detection program in a developing country it is essential that the researcher consider the following questions.

1. At what point does a detectable departure from perfect health become unacceptable?
2. What will be the cost benefit of detection to the individual or to the community?
3. Will the screening program itself change the expectations of those screened?
4. Is the condition sought reversible and are there facilities available to treat it?
5. What proportion of the health program manpower will be consumed by the disease detection program?
6. Will the survey commit future health teams to continuing a possibly unacceptable drain of resources to a constantly growing caseload of patients?
7. What quantity of follow up will be required to confirm the 'abnormal' screening findings and finally to categorise the 'borderlines'?
8. Will there be possible damage resulting from the labelling of 'abnormals'?
9. How wide should screening be in the population?
10. What should be the manner of the screening — single surveys, periodic bursts or low profile ongoing surveillance?

Even when these questions are satisfied the researcher will still need to bear in mind the following constraints.

(a) screening test results are commonly only *presumptive* in character and merely indicate that the positively identified individual should now go on to further diagnostic tests.

(b) The tests must be cheap, especially in developing countries, and must be acceptable to the population.

(c) The ethical consequences of what is being proposed must be carefully considered. Especially the procedure must not offer false hopes, must not shatter otherwise contented lives with bad news, must not turn respected individuals into objects of scorn or pity.

Next decide at which group in the population the screening program is aimed. Decide too whether the purpose is to establish a data base, to identify individuals who should be brought into surveillance because of the high risks they run or is to identify new cases requiring treatment. In a leishmaniasis control program the first objective would be achieved by fluorescent antibody screening, the second by using the leishmanin skin test, the third by diagnostically examining all persons with a large spleen. For the actual screening process itself the following technical considerations apply:

1. Normality

In practice relatively few physical, physiological or serological tests give, in the first instance, a clear distinction between what is abnormal and what is not. It is not even sufficient to use as a parameter the mean values of a healthy population, and then to assume that every individual value is abnormal if it falls outside the 95 per cent of readings lying nearest to the mean value for the whole population (that is two Standard Deviations in statistical language). As an example the 'normal' haemoglobin level for healthy adolescents in Hongkong will probably not apply to acceptably vigorous adolescents in a holoendemic malaria area of Africa. Similarly the normal values for the malaria affected population would probably be inappropriately high for a central American community with marginal nutrition and much hookworm (Haller 1980). Much unnecessary anxiety has been occasioned in developing countries by attempting to apply the 'normal' values obtained from measuring abnormally privileged sub groups.

2. Reliability of the proposed test

Will it give consistently similar results when applied again to the same subjects under similar circumstances? This question has as much to do with variations in the observers as with the laboratory procedures which might be involved. For example, the Mass Miniature Radiography (MMR) formerly used in screening for pulmonary tuberculosis could yield reasonably consistent radiographs of the chest but the readers of the films could neither agree with each other on what they meant nor consistently reproduce their own original interpretations when shown the same films again (Farer 1979).

3. Sensitivity

How nearly does the test detect ALL 'abnormals'? It might be dreadful to miss treatable disease and to reassure falsely those who in fact need treatment. Little reliance can be placed on negative results, for example in the searching of faeces to detect typhoid carriers where the detection of bacilli is highly satisfying to the observer but the absence of bacilli proves nothing. By contrast an oversensitive test will produce far more possible than real positives causing much anxiety and possibly overloading follow-up services.

4. Specificity

How well does the screening test distinguish ONLY the particular disease being sought? Many screening tests yield a range of variations from the 'normal' which may mean little or much such as the Weil Felix reaction and are further compromised by cross sensitisation produced by unrelated infection.

5. Yield

Will all the cost and effort produce a worthwhile crop of treatable disease? Moreover will those discovered to be in need of treatment actually stick to it? The lower the yield and interest in a population and the higher is the cost of finding each willing, treatable case. Conversely a high, cheap yield and worried screenees may overwhelm the curative services.

In practice most screening programs are run as a series of compromises especially in the attempt to balance the competing needs for sensitivity and specificity. As immunologic tests similar to the ELISA become more widely applicable to screening these problems will be somewhat reduced.

Too many screening programs have used a mindless approach to the subjects. A wide range of tests, unrelated to any evident needs of the individual, has aimed to discover any abnormality which might by chance be there. Hospital based personnel have been particularly guilty of such expensive practices and a whole cult of 'defensive medicine' has been built up to justify it. Regular 'health' examinations, which have become a cherished privilege of senior industrial executives in many countries rely on a battery of such tests often termed multiphasic. They have not been proved to be useful in prolonging life.

Causal relationships

The exact identification of the cause or combinations of causes or circumstances which lead to a particular damaging incident is the basis of investigative epidemiology. To identify accurately the circumstances is to provide a tool which, hopefully, will prevent the same problem occurring again. Nature occasionally provides an experimental situation. For example a measles epidemic will swing through a population only partly immunised against the disease. The opportunity to study the effectiveness of the vaccine will come through measuring attack rates in the vaccinated and unvaccinated — appropriately corrected for any differences there might otherwise be between the two groups in this 'natural experiment'.

In such circumstances a mere correction of age and social class differences may not suffice to avoid bias. Children may not have had a particular vaccine because they already had natural protection through early infection or their parents may have refused permission for them to have it. Families with strong views cannot be compared health wise with those who are quiescent. Unfortunately such comparisons of the outcome of tests using such unlike groups for subjects and controls have led to much confusion in the past.

The observer too needs to be very careful in weighing the evidence that there is a *direct relationship* between, say, the distance of an Ethiopian village from a colony of rock hyrax and the frequency of leishmaniasis in those villagers (Bray 1974). The true direct relationship might be with goat herding practices or, more fancifully, villagers already burdened with leishmaniasis might be ousted from more fertile valley land by stronger healthier competitors. In such cases the apparent direct relationship between where the sick lived and their degree of sickness would be described as an artefact or a *spurious relationship*.

In some instances what appears to be a true relationship between two factors or variables exists because both are related, though coincidentally, to a third factor or variable. It appears, for example, that persons who consume moderate amounts of alcohol also suffer less frequently from arteriosclerotic heart disease. There is, however, a third factor operating, good physical and emotional health. The fortunate individual possessing this will be, on average, physically active, well disciplined and a good but not over-dependent socialiser. This is also a description of the moderate drinker and coincidentally a description of those persons least likely to suffer coronary disease. Persons in poor health may have no opportunity for moderate social drinking while persons with good physical health but self indulgent will both tend to drink unwisely and lead a coronary prone unhealthy life. In fact (Petersson et al 1982) once the biasing differences between individuals are removed alcohol in *any* quantity is damaging and the damage rises progressively with consumption.

In real life many chance factors contribute to the likelihood of a particular individual's acquisition of a particular disease. What is called the '*web of causation*' will take a particular traveller in central South America to a particular remote valley, will oblige the traveller unexpectedly to spend the night at the poorest class of village inn with mud walls and unshuttered window through which the kerosene lamp has attracted a reduviid bug which earlier fed on an infected dog and which defaecates as it feeds, as the traveller scratches in his restless sleep and so introduces trypanosomes into his tissues. The web of causation is not quite finished with him for it will depend upon the state of his immune system on that particular day whether or not the infection proceeds. If he has been recently fatigued or has been drinking too much alcohol during his journey he may eventually die of Chagas' disease.

It was the biologist Koch, working at that time with tubercle bacilli, who first laid down the rules of proof that a particular infecting agent was the 'cause' of a particular disease. He postulated that the organism to be the cause must always be present in the appropriate lesion or clinical stage, must not be found in other diseases and, when isolated and cultured in the laboratory through several generations, must be capable of causing the original disease in whatever experimental animal is susceptible.

Costs and remedies

In chapter five reference has already been made to the way in which the amount of life disease steals from those it affects can be measured. Lives lost, families disrupted, industrial production dissipated, harvests left ungathered can all be quantified whatever the cause. Once a hazard is identified the costs of controlling or correcting it can also be measured. For example, potentially damaging chlorampenicol will protect a party of land surveyors from scrub typhus in the jungles of Indonesia. The intervention cost includes both the price of the drug and the potential costs of the bone marrow damage which may occur, if rarely. These are set against the costs of treating the scrub typhus including the evacuation of the occasionally very ill patients and the possible compensation for death, if rarely. Of course the epidemiologist comparing such alternate courses of action cannot promise either that disaster is inevitable if no intervention occurs or that there will never be damage from the intervention. In affluent societies parallel comparisons have been made to support the need for a legal requirement that drivers and passengers in road vehicles wear seat belts.

ASSESSMENT OF PROGRAM EFFECTIVENESS

In the next chapter are given some examples of the way in which a survey may be designed to measure the cost benefit derived from a particular form of intervention into the health of a community. Reference has already been made to the models which epidemiologist-planners use in order to forecast the probable cost benefits of several different kinds of program even before they are put into operation. In theory at least any application for the funding of a control or treatment program whose benefit is yet unproved should include a component to measure the benefit or long term outcome. These intervention analyses are not solely concerned with new techniques but periodically should also be with long accepted ones.

Some interventions are relatively easy to assess. An established vaccine or chemotherapeutic agent either does or does not work in particular circumstances.

Other interventions are much more difficult to measure. For example, how can it be shown that the health of a village was improved by setting up a primary health care program? Such care programs are customarily measured by the quantity of service which they provide. This says nothing about whether the villages derived any actual benefit from that service. Measurement of the proportion of pre school children with completed immunisations (not at all the same thing as the number of immunisations given), or of the proportion of women coming to labour already protected by tetanus vaccine tell little. The crucial tests are the numbers of individuals dying of diphtheria or tetanus before and after the program in the community.

Even more difficulty is encountered in attempting to measure the outcome or the benefits of such an intervention as, say, providing a pit latrine for every household in a small town. The base line information needed, the morbidity and mortality levels before the pit latrine program was instituted, are not usually available. The difficulty in measuring the effect of any intervention is greatly increased when several 'risk' factors or variables are contributing independently or synergistically. Such is the case in attempting to measure the effectiveness of programs to reduce the hazards of coronary artery disease (Hjermann et al 1981, Multiple Risk Factor Intervention Trial 1982).

Some, though inexact, measurements of benefit can be obtained through population surveys. In one type the population will be screened to discover previously untreated disease. In the second type the members of the community will be asked what value they put on a program that has been provided for them. The survey should also ask what alternate services they might still prefer to use. Such a survey conducted in Turkey (Hohmann 1982) revealed that most families in a rural community still preferred to use the private physicians in a distant town rather than the local free government clinics. This greatly reduced the benefit of providing the clinics for the community. Similar paradoxical situations can be found throughout the developing countries where inconvenient and costly services are often more highly valued that the free local government programs.

The basic technological requirement to any objective measurement of program effectiveness is that there must be some way in which the different effects of doing or failing to do something can be compared, some agreed way in which the outcome can be judged. Occasionally several entire communities can be compared though it requires great care to ensure that the population groups are reasonably alike socially, economically and educationally. It was in this way that the effects of high versus low fluoride levels in drinking water were demonstrated by measurements of the number of missing or decayed teeth and comparing like age groups. The most ecologically favoured communities, most likely to keep their teeth, were those with moderate fluoride concentrations in their drinking water.

Unfortunately the consequences of deliberate programs or natural occurrences cannot always be so easily measured as the simple counting of teeth. Moreover the effects of deliberate interventions or chance occurrences are not equally dispersed among all the individuals who go to make up a community. There are profound differences in the susceptibility of different individuals to different challenges. It is also useless to measure the effect of putting iodine into the cooking salt in New Guinea or to provide ear protectors for automobile workers in Sao Paulo unless most of the Papuans actually consume the salt or the Brazilian workers actually wear the protectors over their ears even when management is not watching.

In order to avoid the problems inherent in any comparisons between whole communities most research is done, if practicable, upon two or more groups of individuals specially selected to receive or not to receive a particular service. Selection may also be based on particular previous experiences, because certain individuals have lived or worked in a particular environment or because of a particular mode of behaviour. The differences between the groups will then be monitored until the assessment period is at an end. It is of course important to ensure that the factor being measured does not change during the assessment period. It would be useless, for example, to assess the health effects of chewing or not chewing betel nut over a ten year period if half the chewers cease and half the non chewers begin to do so during the study period.

To avoid the problems which would inevitably occur if two groups of individuals being measured and compared were not similar in all respects except the factor being measured epidemiologists use a system of *controls*. It is not only in the familiar characteristics of age, sex and social class that differences must be avoided. As an example the allocation by chance of middle aged men who have suffered a coronary episode to three different treatment groups would compare the long term outcome, as judged by the proportion in each group who survive. One group will be treated at home, one in any local hospital ward, the third by intensive care in a special unit in the university teaching hospital. If the groups are sufficiently large and if the temptation to treat those most ill in some special way can be resisted by the researchers the results are almost certain to show that the group admitted to the teaching hospital has the greatest proportion of survivors while those treated at home has the least. This will be so regardless of the relative appropriateness or the efficiency of the care given. Middle aged men who have suffered an acute coronary episode are most likely to die in the first hours and are likely to be at home when struck down. In the little time it takes to get group two to the local hospital some of the near dying are lost and are eliminated from the program. By the time the average group three patient has reached the teaching hospital alive several hours may have elapsed and those who are most likely to die in that group have already been eliminated. The variable being tested here is not the different forms of treatment but the time taken to get to it.

The following are the different kinds of 'controls' used in outcome studies.

1. Paired

For every individual being studied another is chosen at random and the study will compare the collective effects of treatment on the study group with no treatment in the control group.

2. Matched

Here an additional step is taken. The controls are now deliberately chosen so that for each study subject there is also a control subject as alike as possible in age, sex and background. Collectively the two groups differ only in the variable being tested.

In all comparative research properly matched controls are the most desirable. In practice providing there are sufficiently large numbers in the compared groups researchers will usually be satisfied if the mean, say for age, of the two groups is the same. It is not necessary to pick over a huge group of controls to find an individual exactly like each test subject. It is, however, particularly important to select proper matching controls in retrospective studies of the outcome of a program or environmental difference. In retrospective studies the researcher cannot exercise any discipline over the way in which test and control subjects behave or the degree of hazard to which they expose themselves — these events have already occurred. In prospective studies which will proceed as the program is implemented, it is usually easier to control the conditions under which the intervention takes place so that perfect matching is not so important. For example the progress of the first 100 babies born in village A can be compared with 100 babies born at the same time in village B in which a new Primary Health Clinic has been established. It is not essential even to attempt to match the groups individual to individual, presuming that the two villages are basically similar. Each group of babies is a 'cohort'. The comparing of the two cohorts as their lives proceed in all respects similar except for some factor, such as primary health care, is a basic epidemiologic tool.

In conducting prospective studies in any human population there is an additional danger to objectivity. That is the positive or negative attitudes of the subjects to what is happening to them plus the enthusiasm or disbelief of the observer in what is being investigated. For example, comparisons of disease levels in two similar groups of young male army conscripts, one assigned to a high plague risk area of rural Thailand the other to a low risk suburb of Bangkok, can be expected to produce more complaints of lymphadenopathy in the rural group which is scared of plague regardless of any actual infection. Similarly the trained observer noting episodes of diarrhoea in two groups of school children one in a school with a safe water supply the other highly suspect will expect more sickness in the second group. Unintentionally the observer is likely to discount sickness in the low risk group which is not frankly diarrhoeal.

To get over these and similar problems both the subject and the observer are 'blind'. That is the subject does not know what she or he is being treated with or observed for or even what the risk being investigated is. The observer reporting on the condition of the subjects is also kept in ignorance of which are the test and which the control subjects or if different therapies are being compared of what those drugs actually are. When both subject and observer are kept in ignorance this is called a 'double blind' trial. Once the measurements are completed the epidemiologist-researcher calculates the relative benefit or relative risk experienced collectively in the different test and control groups.

THE EXPERIMENTAL COMMUNITY TRIAL

The investigator working in the community must avoid two principal types of error. Either, if not carefully eliminated beforehand, will ruin the value of the observations and discredit the investigator. Far too many epidemiologic and research program planners simply neglect the details which are necessary to collect both accurate and unbiased data (Gordis 1979). In the first instance the researcher may use the wrong instruments for measurements, or may use the right instruments incorrectly or the instruments may be at fault. Questionnaires are a form of instrument and the questions and answers may be wrongly translated by an interpreter. Scales to weigh infants may give consistently erroneous or eccentric readings with the same child. Laboratory sera may be inactive or the technician wrongly trained to interpret microscopic preparations. All such errors once the data is collected are usually uncorrectable. Worse still if undetected the erroneous conclusions will mislead other researchers in the future. A 'bias' has been introduced as a consequence of these 'systematic errors'. It takes a brave researcher to admit to such a bias even though it would, of course, always be assumed that the bias had been introduced accidentally with no prior intention to mislead. Bias is particularly likely to occur in trials which do not use the double blind techniques.

The second type of error which the investigator must avoid is that which occurs by chance. In non jargon language that might be 'bad luck' but the epidemiologist prefers the term 'random error'.

In such a case the population may have been carefully chosen, there may be matched experimental and control groups of subjects, the measurements are all free of bias but the results are still erroneous. For some reason, hidden from the investigator, either the groups being compared are not truly comparable or the measurement is being made upon a section of the population which is not truly representative of the whole. Such chance errors are most likely to occur when the numbers being tested or measured are small. They can also occur in animal experiments. For example a batch of test animals after exposure to a pathogenic virus will be used to measure the protective effects of a new antibiotic. Unknown to the investigator the animals have already been exposed to the infection, perhaps through being housed close to other test animals and have already developed some natural immunity. Often the actual reasons why a test group of any kind fails to react as would the rest of the population remain obscure. It may only be a long time after the research has been completed that other investigators unable to repeat the experiments on an identical population, will question the validity of what was done earlier.

For the field researcher, once the instruments of measurement have been found reliable, the possible sources of systematic error eliminated from the procedures, attention will next fall on the selection of a truly representative sample group or groups from the population. Whenever possible, if unintentional bias is to be avoided, the samples should be chosen by 'random selection'.

Selection of a sample

(a) Individual versus family

There are several distinct methods by which to obtain a representative sample of any population. First though, in many developing countries, the investigator must decide whether to select individuals to study or whether instead to operate on the basis of families. In the highly literate community, with births and addresses well documented and with good communications most selections will be on the basis of individuals. The advantages of selecting individuals include direct one-to-one contact subject-to-observer, reduction of the errors introduced by intermediaries and the easy maintenance of confidentiality.

In practice in many developing societies the smallest unit which can be readily identified is the family — and even this is likely to be a broad grouping of several generations. There are some undoubted advantages in using whole families rather than individuals. Once the interest of the most influential member of the family has been aroused the cooperativeness of the rest is assured. One family member can provide information on several others. Family homes are obviously easier to map and to relocate than are individuals. In some societies even the family as a distinct unit is not demacrated and in these instances the sampling unit must be the entire village or commune.

(b) Size of the sample

This is usually a compromise between what is cheapest and easiest, the smallest possible number, and what is ideal, the whole population. There is no exact number of subjects which should be used in any trial or survey. It is the resources and time available which, more than anything else, dictate sample sizes. If, however, resources, are too limited to obtain a reasonable sample size the results may be meaningless and the investigator should consider whether or not to go ahead. By contrast there comes a point when riches of resources and an infinity of time used to vastly increase sample size improve accuracy so little as to be wasteful.

The minimum sample size to be aimed at is easily calculated if the information sought is itself simple. For example in a community survey designed to detect thoracic skin depigmentation or ulnar nerve thickening due to leprosy the observations will be positive or negative with no real variations inbetween. In such events the 'confidence limit' indicates the range on either side of the figures for the sample and within which the 'true value' for the whole population will itself lie. On being consulted the statistician will probably first ask the researcher to what degree of certainty she or he wishes to work. Is it good enough, for example, to report that the true leprosy prevalence in a community lies somewhere between 28 per cent and 36 per cent or must the answer be more specifically between 31.5 per cent and 32.5 per cent. To get to the latter degree of specificity a lot more subjects must be examined though perhaps the overall impression of the importance of leprosy in this population is not much changed.

On the assumption that a one in twenty or 95 per cent probability of being right is good enough (from minus 2 Standard Deviations to plus 2 Standard Deviations on a Normal curve) the confidence limit can be expressed as:

$$2 \times \sqrt{\frac{\% \text{ positive} \times \% \text{ negative}}{\text{number in the sample}}}$$

Following are four calculations differing only in the size of the population sampled. In each case the sample population contains 30 per cent with signs of leprosy.

Sample Size	Number +ve	Formula applied =	Confidence Limit
10	3	$2 \times\sqrt{\dfrac{30 \times 70}{10}}$	29.98
100	30	$2 \times\sqrt{\dfrac{30 \times 70}{100}}$	9.17
1000	300	$2 \times\sqrt{\dfrac{30 \times 70}{1000}}$	2.90
10 000	3000	$2 \times\sqrt{\dfrac{30 \times 70}{10\ 000}}$	0.92

In the case of the small sample of 10 the confidence limit of 28.98 suggests that the 'true value' for the entire population will lie somewhere between (30–28.98) per cent and (30 + 28.98) per cent that is from 1.02 per cent to 58.98 per cent. Such a huge range hardly indicates whether leprosy is a minor or a serious problem in this population. By contrast the sample of 1000 individuals indicates that the prevalence of leprosy in the population lies somewhere between (30–2.90) per cent and (30 + 2.90) per cent, that is 27.10 per cent to 32.90 per cent. This is an agreeably small and useful range and accurate enough for most researchers.

Frequently of course the yield on sampling will be much smaller than 30 per cent. If it were to be 3 per cent the confidence limit in a 1000 sample would be 1.08 so that we are now relatively less sure than we were before of where the actual figure lies. The sample size would have to be increased to regain sensitivity.

Research, whether in the laboratory or the community, is often so funded that the investigator has little control over sample sizes. Or in a retrospective study there are limited numbers of records available. In such cases it can be particularly helpful to use a 'nomogram' type of tool which permits the investigator to forecast the likely degree of significance when two samples are compared and where the effect of using different sample sizes can be directly read off (Altman 1980). This relatively simple procedure avoids having to make the alternate calculation of the '*Standard error of the mean*' otherwise necessary when the factor being tested is a continuously variable one, for example, haemoglobin levels in a population. Particular care must be exercised, and the statistician must certainly be consulted beforehand, when the investigation is in the nature of a trial which at best will have only a relatively small effect on the study population. An example might be an increase in weight expected in a child study population given nutritional supplements. Unless the sample sizes compared are sufficiently large real effects of the nutritional supplementation will actually appear not to be statistically significant (Freiman 1978).

(c) Sampling methods.

The so-called 'paired' and 'matched' samples have already been described. Others include the following:

1. Systematic sampling. Each of the smallest units which can be identified, individuals, families or village clusters, is allocated a number or the investigator can use any existing number in a register from an official record. If, for example, a sample size of 250 infants is desired and there are 2000 registered births it will be sufficient to take every eighth record to spread the sample over the whole available population. This is a frequently used method of selecting a sample. Care is needed to ensure that some bureaucratic procedure does not coincidentally use each eighth record for, say, unmarried mothers or that some chance arrangement of family homes in groups of eight does not result in an unrepresentative sample being chosen.

2. Random sampling. This provides an alternative method of extracting individuals from, for example, the above group of 2000 registered births. The numbers by which the infants are registered are again used but they are not selected in any particular sequence but from lists of random numbers published precisely for this purpose (Fisher 1963). The possible source of bias introduced by the systematic method is eliminated. No selection method is, however, foolproof. By chance the random numbers used to select villages, for example, from a larger rural population could select mostly those of one type. The investigator must not hesitate to reselect the sample if such a chance mishap occurs. Also in both systematic and random sampling individuals or families will be chosen for study who for one reason or another cannot cooperate. Unless such losses are very frequent it is better to explain them as losses together with any background information indicating whether they are or are not similar to those who were actually used in the investigation. If the loss is numerically serious the reasons for it must be explained and it is permissible to seek more subjects as replacement but only by the same random method as the original subjects were chosen. Do not be tempted to take on the next cooperative individual or family as replacements.

3. Stratified sampling. This is designed to economise on resources while at the same time being careful not to introduce a random error by selecting an unrepresentative population. At its simplest the method would, for example, only select families for investigation of possible complications to whooping cough immunisation where it was known that there was a child under five in the household. The cost benefit of surveying households with no pre school children would be rather low. At a more complex level the technique could be used deliberately to select low risk households or individuals when it was desired to calculate accurate data about prevalence in different risk groups. For example in a survey to count the number of persons with sickle cell disease (homozygotes) in Jamaica it would require relatively few infants to be screened to be able accurately to estimate the prevalence in that age group. As with rising age the disease, by death, becomes much less common the sample size chosen, if the estimate of prevalence is to be accurate, must be increased.

4. Cluster sampling. Transport is costly in developing countries and travel wastes precious staff time. A correctly randomised study in a scattered rural population can be very costly to conduct. Much easier in these circumstances to allocate numbers to whole villages and then randomly select villages and study the whole of their populations.

5. Grid sampling. A reasonably accurate map of the area is required. Upon this is superimposed a drawn grid of squares. The smaller the size of the squares, the more there are of them and the less likely is there to be a selection error. One kilometre squares are commonly employed in rural areas. The squares are numbered in the order they appear, that is sequentially, and they are not numbered unless at least half of the area covered by the square is in the study area. Squares are then selected for the study of their populations by the use of the random number tables. Again it is common sense to look at what has been selected and to start again if a chance bias seems to have been introduced. Mean values calculated for the population of each individual grid square must not be used to calculate

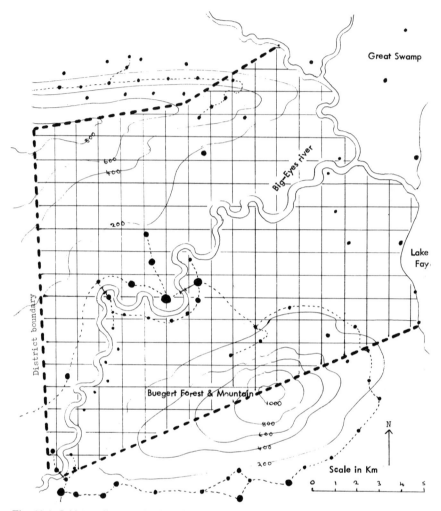

Fig. 11.1 Grid sampling — selection of map squares.

overall means for the total population as this would bias the results towards the values of the more sparsely populated squares.

6. *Multistage sampling.* In practice it is often convenient to combine several forms of population sampling in selecting individuals or families to be studied. As an example, groups of individuals will be chosen by grid or cluster sampling. Further random selection will now occur within each of the chosen squares or clusters. It is necessary to ensure that the same proportion, not the same actual number, of subjects is drawn from each grid square or cluster. Otherwise the rural populations will be unfairly represented in any final population mean.

Having finally decided upon the criteria to be used for producing the information required, having eliminated all probabilities of bias and system-

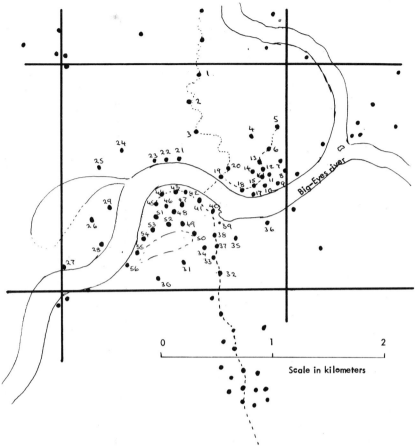

Fig. 11.2 Multistage sampling — Selected grid square for random sampling of nuclear families.

atic error and having chosen the sample population, or the test and control groups, three aspects remain to be considered. First, is the procedure proposed ethically or morally justifiable and will it not involve those studied in any extra risks? Second, will the confidentiality of the information sought be protected even against established authority? Third, are all individuals who will be involved completely educated to the point that they can give an informed and willing consent to the procedures and to their involvement in any extra risks however remote these appear to be? Once these points have been dealt with the immediate organisation of the investigation can begin.

TERMINOLOGY

Controls. Individuals or laboratory animals as much alike as possible to the test subjects and who will be investigated exactly like the test subjects except that they will not be subject to the variable which is being studied.

Direct relationship. An increase in the amount of one factor or variable is followed by an increase in the second factor. An *inverse direct* relationship can also exist when two factors are tied together, for example, vaccination cover and disease incidence, but an increase in one is automatically followed by a decline in the other.

Multiphasic. Used to describe a battery of tests, often unrelated to each other, performed as a group to screen for any possible abnormality rather than for purposeful diagnosis. Originally coined to fit in with the potential for doing several tests at once, regardless of their usefulness, on the same sample of blood in an autoanalyser.

Presumptive. When used to describe the result of a screening test means that there exists a suggestion of abnormality but this will require further tests to make sure.

Spurious relationship. By chance two factors appear to have a direct or inverse relationship but in fact this is because of some third factor to which both are actually related. For example poverty and child growth appear to be inversely related but the real relationship with both is with nutrition.

Standard error of the mean. In practice can be expressed as

$$\frac{\text{Standard deviation of values in a sample}^2}{\text{Number in the sample}}$$

Web of causation. An extension of what had been originally described as the 'epidemic triangle' the web further emphasised that much more than the simple coming together of infecting or toxic agent and Man was essential to the development of disease. Before that several chance or manipulable conditions or variables, such as the appropriate environment, would also have to be just right for transmission to occur. Today the emphasis is on the immune responsiveness of potential victims. Another way of emphasising this multiple causation was to describe Man as at the centre of a 'wheel of causation'.

REFERENCES

Altman D G 1980 Statistics and ethics in medical research iii How large a sample? British Medical Journal 281: 1336–1338

Bray R S 1974 Epidemiology of leishmaniasis: some reflections on causations. From Trypanosomiasis and Leishmaniasis with special reference to Chagas' disease. Associated Scientific Publishers. Amsterdam. pages 87–100

Farer L S 1979 Tuberculosis control for developing countries. US Department of Health and Human Services. Center for Disease Control, Atlanta

Fisher R A, Yates F 1963 Random numbers in statistical tables for biological, agricultural and medical research. Longmans. London. 6th edition. pages 134–143

Freiman J A, Chalmers T C, Smith H, Kuebler R R 1978 The importance of beta, the type 11 error and sample size in the design and interpretation of the randomised control trial. New England Journal of Medicine 299: 690–694

Gordis L 1979 Assessing the quality of questionnaire data in epidemiologic research. American Journal of Epidemiology 109: 21–24

Haller L, Lauber E 1980 Health of schoolchildren in the Ivory Coast. Acta Tropica. Vol 37. Supplementum 11

Hohmann H 1982 Health for rural Turkey. Dissertation submitted to Liverpool School of Tropical Medicine in part requirement for the degree of Master of International Community Health

Hjermann I, Byre K V, Holme I, Leren P 1981 Effect of diet and smoking intervention on the incidence of coronary heart disease. Report from the Oslo Study Group of a Randomised Trial in Healthy Men. Lancet ii: 1303–1310

Multiple Risk Factor Intervention Trial. 1982 Risk factor changes and mortality results. Journal of the American Medical Association 248: 1465–1477

Petersson B, Trell E, Kristenson H 1982 Alcohol abstention and premature mortality in middle-aged men. British Medical Journal 285: 1457–1459

Organization of community investigations

There are, it is suggested, seven stages in the planning of any type of investigation which involves the community. First it must be decided what final data will be required, second what measurements must be made to produce it, third what communications will be needed between investigator and community, fourth what personnel and materièl will be required, fifth how will the survey subjects be chosen, sixth how will the raw data be recorded and processed, seventh what form will the confrontation take between investigator and subject.

What follows is not an exhaustive account of how to plan any kind of survey or test. It is, however, intended to point out some of the avoidable pitfalls and some of the proven ways to success in gathering useful information.

STAGE 1: THE FINAL DATA REQUIRED

In the previous chapter were described the four basic types of investigation in which a District Health Officer might become involved. Briefly these are 1. Descriptive, 2. Causality, Costs and Controls, 3. Cost Benefit and Intervention Outcome, 4. Experimental trials. The kinds of concluding data each type requires have also been summarized.

Sufficient here to emphasise the essential nature of that first exercise in planning an investigation. That is to project the mind forward to sketch out the final report, its means, ranges, standardised ratios, tabulations and cross comparisons which will be used in supporting its observations, arguments and conclusions. Might further investigations be required on the same test population? What possible criticisms might be directed at the investigation especially over omitted or incomplete measurements?

Although deceptively simple it is probably in the descriptive type of survey that faults are most likely to be built in from the beginning. This is because many investigators have no clear idea what they wish to know. The investigation is founded upon such generic questions as 'What is the most important sickness in your village?' or 'What kind of health care does your community need?'. Such *open ended* questions, and those requiring a considered comparison with a non existent standard, pose insuperable challenges to the community spokesmen and yield at best uncertain answers.

In determinations of causal relationship, outcome and cost benefit as well as in trials the measurement must serve the purpose of what it is hoped to measure. In testing the effectiveness of a new virus vaccine it would be of little value to conduct a prospective survey of matched immunized and unimmunized groups in a community already heavily infected with the disease. The vaccine would be better tested on two previously unexposed groups but in whom subsequent high exposure could be expected. In real life this is hard to manage. The consequence is that some techniques, such as BCG vaccination, can be shown to be effective in a low risk test population but prove less useful when applied to a population in which the dose of pathogens is overhelming. A better indication of likely effectiveness came from the trials of the inactivated hepatitis B vaccine which was tested in homosexuals drawn from low risk populations but now behaviourally transferring themselves to a high risk status (Szmuness et al 1980).

STAGE 2: THE MEASUREMENTS

The raw measurements must entirely serve the purpose of the required final data. They should be specific and should be recorded in such standard units as skin fold thickness for assessing nutrition, modified E card testing for visual acuity, hemoglobin levels for anemia. In this regard bench-type laboratory research is inherently simpler than that involving subjects in the community.

Questions must be clear and appropriate to the subject's comprehension and life style. Whenever possible the investigator will already have prepared graded answers from which the subject will choose the most appropriate. For example, work ability can range from maximum sustained physical vigour down to an inability to do anything but watch and comment on the work of others. The young labourer and the elderly overseer will each claim that they 'work'.

In a group of individuals long infected with untreated leprosy, or for that matter degenerative arthritis, the investigator might explain that the information required was about the level of effort which could be sustained over a full work day. This might vary from:
'giving advice to workers returning from the fields'
'giving advice in the fields'
'supervising each worker in the fields'
'distributing and collecting equipment to individual workers'
'weeding and hoeing'
'planting by machine'
'harvesting by machine'
'planting by hand'
'harvesting by hand'

'clearing drainage ditches'

'ploughing with animals'

'heavy lifting, digging and carrying'

In this type of *structured question* the rating of the possible answers is sufficiently wide to accommodate a wide range of responses even if they do not exactly fit the description of what the worker actually does. It can be helpful if the answers are presented in turn to the subject so that the appropriate one will be selected once it is reached. Bias is minimised if rating scales begin with the least acceptable alternative answer. In a rating scale to find out how often a mother punishes her child the first suggestion offered might be 'Do you beat your child at least 20 times per day?' Hopefully no mother would agree to this horrendous suggestion but the succeeding answers offered, being less and less accusatory, the mother is glad to be able to go as far as some far more agreeable alternative such as 'Do you beat your child when he is particularly naughty about once a day?' The inference is nothing like so damaging and it may even be near the truth. If on the other hand the rating scale had begun from the kindly, socially acceptable end of the scale the mother would never have dared allow herself to be dragged too far into less respectable responses and would have given a hopelessly unrealistic answer. It must never be assumed that respondents are unaware of the direction and implications of the investigator's question.

Many errors stem from using what appear in the field to be convenient but unequal intervals, say of age, weight or parasite load. The problem is compounded if findings on the edge of a range are recorded, for example, as 'over six years of age'. Where lies the mean of such a group which can now never be more than a dustbin of subjects whose measurements are meaningless?

In actual field conditions it is faster and more convenient to record measurements within categories, such as '8.5 kilos to 9.4 kilos'. This reduces the necessity for much slower, accurate measurements except for those children near to the edge of a range. It also avoids the topping up or down which many field staff are tempted to do when for example 'the child was almost 9 kilos'. There is a final bonus to the use of such categories as in the above example the mean weight in the 8.5 to 9.4 kilo group will be exactly 9 kilos. Using a more conventional category of 9.0 to 9.9 kilos yields a mean of 9.5 kilos, somewhat more awkward.

Measurements sometimes have to be made by inference rather than through a scientific instrument. It can be embarassing to ask a mother how frequently her child has an event like diarrhoea especially as in the normal course of events it may not provoke much interest. It is easier for the mother to relate to a question which asks how often the child is unable to go to school because of the diarrhoea. Bias is always a danger as the person providing the information gets more remote from the subject being investigated. Surveys of infant feeding practices are all too often misled by seeking data from health personnel, clinic records or even from mothers attending a maternal and child health clinic. Even a random sample of houses may not be good enough in such a survey. A better way, if it is practicable, is to select a random sample of infants from the birth records and then, if necessary, go out into the fields to question the mother of each infant selected.

It has already been emphasised that, whenever possible, answers as well as questions should be constructed so that they cannot be misconstrued. The open ended question is a fine basis for confusion in processing data. In, for example, questionning adults about their attitude toward a local clinic use a pilot study to suggest the range of dislikes which may discourage attendance. Such a range might be 'too far away — have to wait too long — too crowded — afraid of baby catching sickness from others — ashamed of own clothes — ashamed of baby's poor development — staff not interested — staff aggressive or rude — staff from another tribe — staff not well trained — husband discourages my attendance — mother-in-law forbids me to go — other women tell tales'.

The technology which will be required to produce the data, for example laboratory tests, is mapped out and costed at this stage. Included is the degree of expertise which will be required of staff in making and interpreting the tests as well as educating the subjects and bringing them back if further tests, or follow up treatment, are required.

STAGE 3: COMMUNICATIONS

The first decision to be taken is on who will speak with the actual subjects. This is particularly important when there is a language barrier between the investigator and the community. Frequently, in developing countries, a third person will be required to act as the go-between or translator. The investigator must then test, using a second translator the reliability, understanding of what is being attempted and consistancy in translation of questions and answers. At village level volunteers, unpaid health auxillaries and even local officials may be neither trusted by the subjects nor reliable in transmitting the information which they are given. Local gossips and busybodies are only too eager to become involved in information gathering among their neighbours. Depending upon the nature of the investigation local health personnel may have too much personal interest in the outcome to be entrusted either with the selection of subjects or with the interpretation of their responses. Unless themselves of local origin they may not be trusted by the subjects.

The employment of literate, disinterested outsiders has a great deal to recommend it but it may introduce new problems, especially in conditions of inter tribal rivalry. Well educated outsiders, though native to the region, may be quite unable to understand the local dialect. Or their elitist attitude, especially on the Indian subcontinent, may antagonise the subjects.

Finally in the employment of personnel to assist in any survey program rates of pay must be agreed in advance including travel expenses and an agreement on who provides such items as pencils or blank paper sheets. It is wise to ensure that remuneration is sufficiently high to motivate temporary employees to be available exactly when required and the rates paid to different personnel must be seen to be comparable. A little extra reward to health care staff already full time employees but willing to help out with the community investigation will not be wasted.

Next the investigator must decide on how best to inform the community about what is proposed. House by house visits are too costly. Even village meetings can prove time consuming and can be the catalyst for a ground swell of complaints and objections with very little to do with the proposed survey itself. Religious and political meetings are good venues for announcements but the association with such pressure groups is not always beneficial. It might produce more hostility than cooperation in the intended subjects observing it.

Wallposters are useful and cheap but there must be a reasonable number of literate individuals in each community to read and explain them. Loudhalers can be used in market places or at race tracks and fairs but getting across a complex message is very difficult. Local newspapers will reach only a select literate audience, though a valuable one nevertheless. Radio and television are the most powerful of the communications media providing that they are accessible to the investigator and also reach the local populace.

Now the investigator must identify reliable local informants or influential individuals who can open the doors to those persons who hold the information desired. It is of utmost importance that local government authorities should feel involved, at the very least informed. They must never be made to loose face through not knowing what is going on in their district. Their advice, for example on communications and security can be invaluable but they should never be yielded the right of veto.

Discrete enquiries are advisable beforehand. Tribal or village leaders must inevitably be used, at the very least consulted, though their self interests may highly colour the information which they pass on. Religious and political leaders are not often very useful as direct informants but are more useful in both identifying sources of information and in encouraging those sources to be cooperative. In practice it is more important to ensure that they are not opposed to any program as their negative influence can be devastating. The education and experience of school teachers, civil servants and policemen makes them good observors. As minor but visible members of the establishment they transmit their respectability to the investigating team. In many developing and developed countries a tacit association with the police can be highly protective for the investigating team.

Consider always the degree to which local rivalries, customs and taboos will limit the operation of the investigating team. A local elite can be remarkably insensitive to the views and needs of the population. Minority group leaders must be dealt with very carefully if the researcher, who needs anyway to overcome deep suspicions in minority group members over any government associated program, is not to become entangled in minority political demands and agitations. The most delicate situations are to be found in countries and regions fired by pre-revolutionary ferment. If a survey must be completed under such conditions it may prove relatively easy to allay the suspicion of the revolutionary leaders but the investigators are in greatest danger from minor leaders especially in rural areas where communications may be poor and fright and hostility can occur with all too sudden violence.

Even the apparently compliant attitude of a population itself can be misleading. Many so-called primitive peoples are in reality highly sensitive. They may cover feelings of dislike or distrust with no more than a polite but otherwise unaccountable failure to cooperate. Beware especially of the community which has been offended by earlier contact with a failed clinic service or by contact with a survey team which appeared to offer promises of assistance which never materialised.

Finally at this stage the investigator must decide whether or not the proposed survey or trial may cause damage to the subjects. A break of confidentiality is one obvious hurt. Subjects may also be unintentionally damaged by having some previously undiscovered abnormality, such as rheumatic heart disease, placed on a register. The unhappy individual is forever labelled as disabled or at risk. Anxiety will be engendered if pathology is brought to light but no treatment is offered. Some discoveries, such as the presence of tubercle bacilli in the sputum, may result in legal sanctions being imposed on the unfortunate sufferer. Such events are not likely to inspire the trust of the community.

STAGE 4: PERSONNEL AND MATERIEL

As this is the stage of planning at which likely costs can be quantified the investigator may be hurried into it especially in preparing a budget for fund applications. Errors made now will have a negative effect upon the researcher's reputation. It is certainly wise not to apply for funds until the main points of the suggested earlier stages have been considered. Be sure of what is being attempted and what information will be sought, from whom and where. Otherwise the proposed investigators will find that the survey subsequently has to be fitted not to what is actually needed but to the resources which have been granted.

Consider first what quantity of personnel and supplies will be needed. The costing of them can come later. The nature of the country, of its population and the quality and fitness of the members of the investigating team will dictate what can be achieved with a given unit of resources. In general the following examples can be taken as the very best that can be expected under reasonable circumstances in warm climate conditions.

(a) a strong young man can carry 20 to 30 kilos on his back for 15 kilometers over flat dry ground in a day but over very much shorter distances if the ground is soft or steep. By contrast a well trained health assistant may perform 120 modules of a relatively simple, repetative task, such as taking venous blood samples, in the same period.

(b) A very simple, rapid wrist circumference measurement, up to 500 by a health assistant in a day, will indicate preschool age nutrition levels in a community. By contrast a child development survey will require much more time consuming weight and height measurements and age estimations.

(c) A skin depigmentation survey for leprosy in good light takes two minutes per unclothed subject and little training of personnel. By contrast though a dental survey can be completed almost in the same time it will require at least five years of training for the personnel.

(d) In a market crowd as many as 50 persons can give a range of answers to ten questions to a single language-fluent investigator in half a day. By contrast to search for and interview 50 subjects randomly selected in their own homes will take the investigator at least 10 working days.

The quantity of work which can reasonably be expected of available personnel will vary considerably by work ethic and by the training and morale of the individuals involved. Adding survey tasks, such as even simple measurements, will greatly reduce speed. The 50 persons questioned in the market place would be reduced in number to 20 if the investigator were also to take a rough measurement of their visual acuity. Speed is radically slowed, even in captive populations such as clinic attenders, if the reasons for the questions and measurements have to be explained separately to each subject. Transport, climate and translation difficulties will further slow surveys within the community itself. In many community research programs the investigator is obliged to be content with completing two family contacts, randomly selected, per half working day. If the family can be reached only at the evening meal only one may be reached each day (Lutz 1981). The number of subjects to be included in the survey or trial will have been determined either by the criteria set out in the previous chapter or will have been dictated by the resources and time available. The kind of information sought greatly influences what minimal size must be aimed at from an entire population, if the expectation of life is to be calculated, down to as few as ten for a pilot study. Figure 12.1 illustrates these differences.

The training the field staff will require is all too often underestimated. Modules of training, for example, to weigh a baby, to prepare a blood film for malaria parasite microscopy, are not difficult. The proper training in the completion of questionnaires takes much more time. In this case the staff must know exactly what the questions mean and must be able to comprehend the nuance of the responses by the subjects and their relation to the information being sought. It is not strictly necessary for field staff using a questionnaire to be literate. They can be taught to memorise the positions of the questions and if very skillful can even check the answers onto a

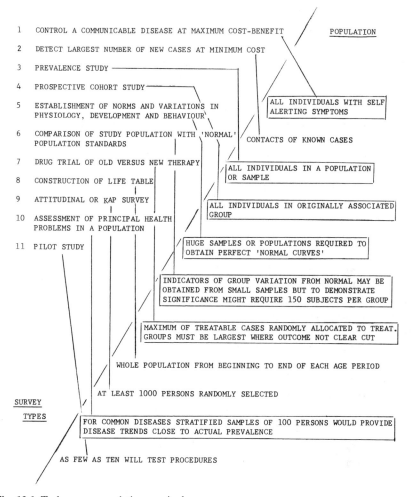

Fig. 12.1 Task versus population required

precoded answer sheet. It is well to remember that in some developing countries the value given to prompt timing and systematic order may be very different from that in the investigator's own country. It may also be difficult to instill a sympathetic approach to subjects in those societies in which respect for the rights of individuals, especially if they are poor, is somewhat limited.

Field service staff need to know not only what the research program is about but also about the importance of acting and reporting objectively. Their responses must not be designed to please the investigators. They must never be given the impression that this or that type of response or measurement is what the investigator is hoping to find. It is helpful though if field staff can visualise some possible benefit for the community emerging as a result of the study. Confidentially of the data and protection of the sources of information cannot be overemphasized.

STAGE 5: THE SURVEY SUBJECTS

The methods of selection of subjects and controls have already been outlined in chapter 11. Still earlier it was suggested that no community survey should be attempted until the area had been mapped geographically and the situations of the populations and its resources had been identified. The potential sources of information about where individuals or families are, for example birth registration, post office lists, taxation records, land and house registrations and health centre listings were outlined in chapter nine. A warning was also delivered about the potential biases inherent in such information sources. It is especially wise to be wary of outpatient or clinic listings as these tend to be loaded with nearby families and self selected individuals.

STAGE 6: THE RECORDING OF DATA

This is not an appropriate place to discuss in detail the processing of data. Many field surveys will produce at last a mean of one value or another, or a range of values within a population possibly stratified by age and sex. Reports are made more useful as well as more interesting when a *dependent variable* is plotted against an *independent variable* so allowing the relationship between two events or population variables to be quantified. Tests of significance will show whether the findings or the suggested associations between two apparently independant factors are real or merely chance departures from the normal.

It is more appropriate to consider here how to record the information as it is elicited or created. If it is not properly recorded from the outset no subsequent processing, however sophisticated, is likely to rescue the results. Space here is sufficient only to remind the the District Health Officer planning a research program of the principal points which should be considered to protect the data and preserve its usefulness.

First consider the advantages of permanently identifying the subjects and the controls who take part. Occasionally, such as when it concerns venereal infections, the information may be too sensitive to expect subjects to comply except on a basis of anonymity. In some screening programs it is both convenient and reassuring to the subjects to record their findings under a code number. It is reassuring to the investigator if a separate and well guarded sheet tallies names with those code numbers. Some form of identification is desirable in the event further information may be needed. Or it may later be advisable to bring the subjects in for treatment. Identification will also be necessary if records held elsewhere, such as in a district hospital, are to be used as verifying information. Addresses of subjects may also be useful but time can be wasted being too assiduous in this regard.

Additional personal information, such as marital status, religion, education or occupation can be useful not so much to identify the subject as to help in understanding what variables are at play in the population. Why do certain events occur to some individuals or families and not to their relatives or neighbours. Though it is often difficult to be precise about it in developing countries age is the most commonly used personal variable. Partly because of the imprecision to be expected age, unless it can be copied directly from a reliable record, is best recorded in small ranges such as 20 to 24, 25 to 29, 30 to 34 and so on. As in the example of weight recounted earlier some extra care is needed in assigning persons on the borders of two age groups to the correct one. In adults age can often be calculated from the memory of well remembered events. In the elderly, however, factors such as age can be greatly exagerated by adopting the memories, told as tales, of earlier generations (Robinson 1975, Doll 1983).

In questionnaire type surveys it is essential that the form of the questions should not betray the preferences of the investigator. Perjorative type questions which betray themselves include apparently simple enquiries like 'Do you breast feed your baby?', 'Did you take the medicine the doctor ordered?', 'Can you read?'. Each of these questions must be recast to avoid either an irrelevant excuse or an honest answer which would likely cause shame or embarassment to the subject. It is no accident that the structured answers discussed earlier also lend themselves especially well to precoding. They can be recorded as the information is provided simply as numbers on a sheet, not necessarily the original questionnaire. Needless to add that columns of numbers, one column for each subject, are also subsequently easier to process than piles of questionnaires.

Apart from the tactical mistake of asking open ended questions the most frequent regrets when it is too late are the consequences of asking too many. Ten questions, each with graded and coded answers, are sufficient for most purposes. Otherwise both subjects and field staff become wearied. Many more answers and the investigator will find the mass of data unusable.

The quantity mass of unused data mistakenly gathered by many past surveys was an error of judgement looking for an excuse. The computer has become that excuse. The computer has enabled a great many poorly planned research and survey programs to assume a false air of respectability. Sadly the accuracy of all processed data can never be greater than the efficiency of the most inept of those field personnel who provide the raw information. By contrast the discipline required in the coding of research measurements and answers to questions, as would be required anyway to make proper use of the computer, is an excellent one. Whether or not they are to be recorded on a computer, on simple punch cards for manual sorting or on even simpler cross tabulations of coded answers by hand, all data should be planned as a disciplined collection even before the facts are gathered.

What the computer does is to trace and to reproduce the information stored in it much more rapidly than could any human extract the same information from a ledger system and far far faster than could the same human sort through and extract from individual files and case notes.

The computer acts also as a rapid and accurate calculating machine. It can analyse the association, if any, between two or more different measurements on the same subjects and can then test these associations statistically. The investigator still has to interpret and explain the findings. The author's law of data chaos suggests that 'work related to the processing of survey report sheets or questionnaires can be expressed as the square of the number of questions, times the mean number of possible responses per question to the power of the number of sheets of answers used per survey subject'.

STAGE 7: THE CONFRONTATION

The investigator and subject must now be brought into contact and without threat to either. Traditionally in warm climate countries there has been much dependence upon safari-like expeditions, the team customarily led by a medical officer. In practice the present day District Health Officer may be obliged to rely upon spot surveys using air or jeep-type transport. Few programs these days can afford the special research medical teams which were stationed for long periods in specially chosen villages and whose sole purpose was to collect information.

There are acceptable alternatives. Simple surveys can be performed by much lower cost teams and without the constant presence of expensive health professionals once field staff have been adequately trained. Traditional health workers and local healers could, in theory, also be trained for this information gathering but the problems in making this actually work are formidable. Educated local personnel, such as school teachers can, by contrast, prove valued and effective field workers especially if there is some profit in it. Mobile and migratory populations can be surveyed as they periodically pass a certain geographic point, such as a water source.

At the opposite end of the scale, in countries where communications technology is widely spread questionnaire type surveys, occasionally even direct measurements, can be obtained through postal or telephone contacts. Simple periodic measurements, such as for blood pressure or glycosuria can be performed by the subject trained to do it. With some additional equipment in the subject's home it is already practicable to monitor through public telephone lines such readings as fetal heart rate (Dalton et al 1983). Local cell, commune, collective or cooperative leaders, once trained, can also be assigned such tasks where the system of government is appropriate.

The security of the field staff must be ensured. Some easily recognisable form of identification must be carried. It must be sufficiently convincing to be accepted by an illiterate tribesman, soldier or policeman who has never heard of the survey team. Government backed identification documents are invaluable in dealing with local authority but discretion is required in using such documents to avoid it appearing that the survey program is serving government interests. An official document describing what is being sought may avoid an allegation of spying. It should certainly never be assumed that a field research team will be accorded the status of friends or even of neutrals during times of local political disturbance.

Weapons or noise makers will scare off animals but if anything will tend to attract aggressive humans. Flares and emergency signals are useful only if there is regular observation and an evacuation plan. Certainly field staff chosen must be circumspect in behavior and will seek to avoid giving offence to the proposed subjects and their families. Care will be needed to avoid sparking off religious conflict. The advantages of using female staff must be weighed against the additional security problems this may engender in a society which has never heard of sex equality. Except where they are already known to the local population field staff should not work alone. Though the consequent possible biasing of any data based on personal verbal responses can be worrying any offers of the local army commander or police chief to provide an escort should not be lightly rejected.

Investigators can appear to be threatening even when attempting to reassure subjects. A statement such as 'I have the approval of your government in asking you these questions' is likely to be the opposite of reassuring. With the best of intentions investigators have sent home school children with letters to their parents saying in effect 'unless I hear to the contrary I assume that you agree to my giving your child a new vaccine which the experts hope will help the child avoid catching disease X'. The sensible parents object leaving children of the illiterate or uncaring to be tested with misleading results. Enthusiasm can lead a clinic clerk to remark that 'you must give me your parents address so that I can send you a reminder of when you are due to come back to the venereal disease clinic'.

Persuasion is important and must be subtle. The investigator in the first example should have said 'I am not doing this for the government but their experts agree that it will be a good thing for your village when I have all the information I am seeking'. The letter about the vaccine should have described why it was being used and emphasised the good fortune of this community in obtaining supplies early. Moreover it should have taken both agreeing and disagreeing responses with a community worker following up on the non responders. The clinic clerk might have obtained better cooperation by remarking 'I shall send you reminders of when you need to come back here but I shall arrange that the messages appear to come from a friend of yours'.

Never force a subject with no opinion to give an answer. Always in the range of possible answers include a 'Don't know' 'No opinion' or 'Not applicable'. Avoid if possible asking very personal questions in front of close relatives or even of staff who may be friends of the subject's family. If postal questionnaires are to be returned or subjects are requested to come in for examination do not expect the subjects to do this at their own expense.

The decisions on what to seek and how and from whom and when have been made. Approval has been obtained from the authorities, the community has been fully informed about what will take place and why, the field personnel have been trained and the subjects to be used have been identified. The necessary equipment has been obtained and tested.

At this stage, it is suggested, a pilot study under field conditions will measure the appropriateness of the plans and the feasibility of actually achieving what is being attempted. It will reveal any hitherto hidden blocks or an inherent weakness in any one of the modules of the program. There is still time to correct mistakes or to fill gaps or to make any adjustments_ in the way the information will be collected or measurements and laboratory procedures completed. If no major adjustments are necessary the information obtained in the pilot study can be incorporated into the main data base. If a radical redesign should be necessary the pilot study, far from being a waste, may have protected the main program from disaster.

When the objective of the pilot study is merely to demonstrate that the method of collecting data is a reasonable one the size of the sub sample can be very small. As few as ten subjects will show the investigators where any major problems are likely to occur. The pilot study needs to be larger if its objective is to test the original hypothesis and thus demonstrate whether or not there is possibly significant data to be uncovered. For the District Health Officer it is in the former more modest application, the testing of a survey method, that a pilot study is most likely to be used. Once this is completed satisfactorily the main investigation can begin.

TERMINOLOGY

Dependent variable. Any measurable response resulting from a graded change in some other factor which may either be subject to external manipulation, such as a change in drug dosage, or which may be an inherent difference between the tested subjects, such as age.

Independent variable. Any factor which on being measurably changed results in changes in some other dependent variable, such as different dosages of drug having measurably different reactions, or age which as it increases also increases the risk of death.

Open ended question. One which permits the subject to make his or her own interpretation of what the investigator is actually seeking and which provides no guidance on the limit or range of the response.

Structured question. One which specifies more exactly what response is sought usually through providing a range of possible answers together with 'escape' responses for the subject who cannot or does not wish to respond or for whom the question or responses suggested are inappropriate. An open ended 'other' response may overcome the objections that the range of suggested answers may bias the subject who attempts, perhaps inappropriately, to fit his or her experience into the limited format. Depends very much on the sagacity and experience of the investigators in considering all likely responses and pretesting or a pilot survey is very helpful here. The structured question and its limited range of responses is superbly easier than the open ended question to process the resulting data. It also lends itself to precoding, essentially giving each possible answer a number, and hence to recording and storage with economy of effort and space. Of course it is also ideally suited for computer processing and to the testing of association between one graded measured factor and another.

REFERENCES

Dalton K J, Dawson A J, Gough N A J 1983 Long distance telemetry of foetal heart rate from patients' homes using public telephone network. British Medical Journal 286: 1545
Doll R 1983 Prospects for prevention. British Medical Journal 286: 445–453
Lutz W 1981 Planning and organizing a health survey. International Epidemiological Association and WHO. Geneva
Robinson D 1975 Some complications of Methuselahism. New England Journal of Medicine 292: 357
Szmuness et al 1980 Hepatitis B vaccine: demonstration of efficacy in a controlled clinical trial in a high risk population in the United States. New England Journal of Medicine 303: 833–841

Acute respiratory infections

INTRODUCTION

Acute respiratory infections, together with diarrhoeal diseases, are the major causes of morbidity and mortality in children in warm countries. The term 'acute respiratory infections' (ARI) includes diseases and conditions such as the common cold, nasopharyngitis (including coryza), sinusitis, rhinitis, pharyngitis, tonsillitis, laryngitis, tracheitis, acute bronchitis, pneumonia and bronchopneumonia and bronchiolitis, as well as acute otitis media, measles, whooping cough, diphtheria and influenza. Some of these diseases, dealt with separately in this book, will not be referred to in this chapter.

The term ARI in its present broad sense is widely used only recently, following the World Health Organization's decision (WHO, 1976) to launch a specific programme of control of this group of diseases in children in developing countries. In view of the currently available means of controls, the first objective of the programme is to reduce mortality from acute lower respiratory tract infections by means of effective diagnosis and appropriate treatment, i.e., chemotherapy in some very well defined syndromes and supportive measures in all cases. Also included must be family and community education on the critical symptoms of these infections, as many children die without having been taken to the health services.

THE DISEASES

Acute respiratory diseases are often divided into two subgroups; the upper respiratory infection affecting the respiratory tract above the epiglottis such as rhinitis, pharyngitis, tonsillitis, otitis media, sinusitis; the lower respiratory infections, with pneumonia and bronchiolitis as examples of the most serious clinical infections. Most often, however, the infection affects several structures of the respiratory tract, either simultaneously or in sequence and it is more appropriate to describe it as nasopharyngitis, pharyngotonsillitis, laryngotracheobronchitis (croup) et cetera.

The vast majority of episodes of ARI are mild and self-limiting, requiring general supportive measures and/or symptomatic treatment in the form of aspirin and cough mixture. On the other hand, many deaths caused by ARI are due to the fact that children are brought to the attention of the qualified health worker too late, when they are already too sick to respond to treatment. The reason for this is often lack of adequate information on the part of mothers, as well as on the part of some less qualified primary health care workers, who are not aware of the significance of the key symptoms of the common infections and particularly the more severe infections of the lower respiratory tract.

The ability of primary health care workers and of mothers to discriminate mild and severe ARI is particularly relevant to warm climate countries, the majority of which belong to the group of least developed and developing countries. Only a few of the more common ARI will be discussed here, with emphasis on severe lower respiratory tract infections.

Common cold (Coryza)

Children under five years of age usually have four to six colds each year. The main symptoms are sneezing, nasal discharge and mild fever. For the first day or two the discharge is watery, then it becomes thick and yellow. The infected mucosa swells and obstructs a child's nose, so that he is obliged to breathe through the mouth. This is not important in older children, but may prevent babies from sucking. Postnasal discharge may produce coughing. Sometimes infection spreads below the larynx and causes laryngitis, bronchitis or pneumonia. A common complication is acute otitis media.

There is no specific treatment for the common cold, and antibiotics should not be given. A danger with nasal drops is that they will run down into the lower respiratory tract and may produce a secondary bacterial infection there.

Some children have an increased incidence of colds, tonsillitis and acute otitis media. The symptoms of recurrent cough without sneezing, often called a recurrent bronchitis, is most common during the second half of the first year of life and up to five years. The exact pathology of the condition is unknown, most of these children are not severely ill and symptoms gradually subside within a few days even without treatment. In a few of them however, by the age of 4–5 years, the characteristic features of bronchial asthma may develop.

Pneumonia

Pneumonia is an acute septic infection of the lung alveoli. It can be caused by a bacterial, viral or a mycoplasma infection, the latter affecting mainly older children in the form of so-called atypical pneumonia In bronchopneumonia, the infection is spread throughout the bronchial tree whereas in segmental pneumonia it is confined to the alveoli in one segment or lobe.

The major clinical signs of pneumonia include cough, dyspnea, tachypnea and often fever. Flaring of the *alae nasi* are almost always present and there may be reduced breath sounds over the affected area as well as crepitations. A raised respiratory rate at rest distinguishes pneumonia from acute bronchitis.

Pneumonias are usually preceded by several days of a cough and rhinitis — an upper respiratory tract infection. Typically, the child with a mild rhinitis suddenly becomes anorexic, listless and sometimes febrile. The loss of desire for food or liquid in a small child with a cold is a danger signal. The cough becomes dry and painful. The pain may be referred to the abdomen and can simulate appendicitis. Small children often suffer vomiting or mild diarrhoea, while in infants convulsions may occur at the onset. The normal respiratory rate of 20–25 increases to 50 and more per minute. Respiration which is often rapid and shallow, is frequently accompanied by an expiratory grunt. The pulse rate often doubles.

In addition to antibiotics, treatment includes bed rest, increased fluid intake and increased humidity. The child may be given antibiotics, analgesics and a cough medicine. In severely ill children (in hospitals) postural drainage, intravenous fluids and oxygen treatment are often necessary.

Bronchiolitis

Bronchiolitis, a viral infection of the lower respiratory tract, results from inflammatory destruction of the small airways, the bronchioles, causing necrosis of the cells lining the airways. It occurs most often during the winter and early spring months and affects infants under six months of age, with the peak incidence between two and five months of age.

Bronchiolitis, as pneumonia, is usually preceded by an upper respiratory infection for several days. The child has been sneezing, has a nasal discharge, loss of appetite, is difficult to feed, has a hacking, harsh cough, low-grade fever and wheezing with activity through the obstructed airways. The infant's respirations are laboured — rapid, shallow, often 60 breaths per minute, with nasal flaring and mild to severe intercostal and subcostal retractions at rest. All these signs are exaggerated by crying, feeding and any activity. The child is able to take in sufficient air, but has difficulty in expelling all the air from the lungs. This interferes with normal exchange of gases in the lungs, and hypoxemia as well as hypercapnia may develop. The most critical phase of the disease is the first 24 to 72 hours. Treatment is supportive only and includes oxygen and hydration, plus bed rest, increased humidity and neutral environmental temperature.

Laryngotracheobronchitis (croup)

The croup is a major cause of acute upper airways obstruction of viral origin in children. The disease most commonly occurs during the winter months and as is true of many respiratory infections, it starts with a history of cold for one to two days. Then a harsh, barky cough, hoarse voice, low grade fever and stridor develop. Stridor is a harsh sound caused by increased velocity and turbulence of airflow in the larynx or trachea. It is predominantly inspiratory. The child at rest may not demonstrate stridor. The age range affected is generally from three months to three years, with the peak incidence between nine and 18 months.

Treatment is essentially supportive. The basic measures include minimizing the child's anxiety, use of mist and adequate intake of fluids. In cases with severe obstruction, intubation may be mandatory.

THE AGENTS

There is widespread agreement that the principal initiators of ARI are viruses, and that bacteria may either super-infect the virus-damaged respiratory tract or cause a clinical infection on its own. The number of respiratory viruses that are pathogenic for man is enormous. They fall taxonomically into five viral families, represented by seven genera containing more than 200 serologically distinct viruses. The number of pathogenic bacteria is also enormous.

As far as severe ARI are concerned, the predominant viral pathogens appear to be respiratory syncytial virus (RSV), the parainfluenza viruses, the influenza virus and the adenoviruses. The predominant bacterial pathogens in severe ARI appear to be *Streptococcus pneumoniae*, *Haemophilus influenzae*, *Klebsiella pneumoniae* and *Staphylococcus aureus*. (the list of pathogens involved in ARI is given in tables 13.1 and 13.2.

EPIDEMIOLOGY

There is very little sound information on morbidity due to ARI, and data on mortality are far from complete and reliable. In a global review of the problem of ARI based on data from 88 countries in five continents with a total population of nearly 1200 million, Bulla and Hitze (1978) showed that in 1972 deaths due to ARI amounted to 666 000 and this figure represented 6.3 per cent of deaths from all cases. On the crude assumption that the same mortality rates might also be valid for non-reporting countries, one may estimate that about 2.2 million deaths due to ARI occur throughout the world every year. These estimates might well be too conservative, as the mortality from ARI in the non-reporting countries might conceivably be of greater magnitude than in the reporting countries. Mortality from ARI is highest in infants in pre-school children and old people, and considerable differences exist both between and within continents.

Bacterial and viral pneumonia are by far the most important causes of death, together accounting for 75· per cent of all deaths from ARI. If all causes of death reported in the world are taken into account, pneumonia accounts for about 5 per cent.

Table 13.1 Aetiology and clinical syndromes of acute viral respiratory disease*

Viruses associated with syndrome	SYNDROME					
	Coryza	Influenzae & febrile catarrh	Viral sore throat	Infantile croup	Infantile acute bronchiolitis	Non bacterial (atypical) pneumoniae
Influenzae A		+++	±	±	±	+
Influenzae B	+	++	+			±
Influenzae C	±	±				
Parainfluenzae	+			+++	+	+
Respiratory Syncytial	+				+++	
Rhinoviruses	+++					
Echo	+	+	±	+		
Coxackie	+	+	+			
Adenoviruses	±	+	+++			+
Mycoplasma	±	±			±	++

+++ to ± indicates relative frequency of virus in each clinical syndrome.
* Hobson D. (1972)

Table 13.2 Aetiology and clinical syndrome of bacterial ARI in children

Bacteria associated with Syndrome		Sinusitis	Pharyngitis	SYNDROME Epyglottitis, Laryngitis & Laryngotracheal bronchitis	Pneumonia*	Necrotizing pneumoniae
Haemophilus influenzae		++++		++±+	++++	
Streptococcus pneumoniae		++++		+++	++++	
Staphylococcus aureus		++++			++	
Streptococcus pyogenes	Group A	+++	++++			
	Groups B & C		+++			
Klebsiella pneumoniae					+++	
Bordetella pertussis				++++		
B. parapertussis				++++		

Table 13.2 cont.

Bacteria associated with Syndrome	Sinusitis	Pharyngitis	SYNDROME Epyglottitis, Laryngitis & Laryngotracheal bronchitis	Pneumonia*	Necrotizing pneumoniae
Corynebacterium diphtheriae		++**			
Neisseria meningitidis				+++	
Escherichia coli				+++	
other Enterobacteriaceae				++	
Pseudomonas aeruginosa				++	
Yersinia pestis				+	
Francisella tularensis				+	
Legionella pneumophila				+	
Anaerobic bacterial species					+
Chlamydia trachomatis				±	

* rickettsial pneumonias are not included.
** in a non-immunized population.
+++ to ± indicates the relative importance of bacteria in each clinical symdrome.
++++ the most important ± the least important.

There are many warm climate countries where death rates from ARI in 0–4 year old children are as much as 30–70 times higher than for children in developed temperate climate countries, although morbidity is similar. It does seem that bacterial pneumonia is relatively more important in warm climate countries than in developing countries of temperate zones and this may explain the very high mortality rate there.

A few community-based longitudinal studies on frequency of ARI have been conducted in warm climate countries. Frey and Wall (1977), James (1972) and Datta et al (1969) in three independent surveys conducted in Ethiopia, Costa Rica and India report that on average a child in an urban area has from five to eight annual episodes of ARI. Studies from Ethiopia and Guatemala by Dodge and Deneke (1970) and Gordon et al (1968) indicate that children in rural areas have on average one to three episodes of ARI per year.

Little is known about the relative importance of the different pathogens causing ARI as well as about other factors, environmental and personal, which influence susceptibility to ARI and its spread in different population groups and communities. Relevant factors which may affect the susceptibility to ARI as well as the distribution of pathogens are the tropical climate, high prevalence of parasitic diseases and nutritional deficiencies.

In the past 10 years it has become increasingly evident that the parasitic infections induced by protozoa (as in malaria and trypanosomiasis) or by helminths (as in schistosomiasis and filariasis) not only have a direct deleterious effect on the host, but also affect the host's immune system by impairing the immune response to other infections. Williamson and Greenwood (1978) observed that the immune response to vaccination with bacterial vaccines (e.g., tetanus toxoid, meningococcal vaccine, et cetera), was depressed in children with acute malaria. It has also been suggested that repeated episodes of malaria induced immunodepressions may contribute to the high incidence of bacterial infections among children in the tropics. Studies carried out in countries of Africa showed that patients homozygous for sickle-cell disease are at an increased risk of severe pneumococcal infection. Watkins et al (1979) reported that the incidence of bronchitis and pneumonia in breast-fed infants was significantly less common than in those who were bottle-fed only. Infant feeding and also parental smoking are examples of modifiable social factors, a change in which could produce desirable effects in a relatively short time, while other social and environmental changes to prevent the spread of infection and to enhance resistance to disease, such as improvement in living standards and control of air pollution, are examples of long term efforts to be undertaken. For the majority of warm climate countries at present, however, the single most important factor affecting the mortality rate from ARI seems to be an adequate, i.e., accessible and effective health care system for all children with symptoms of acute lower respiratory infections.

LABORATORY INVESTIGATION

Laboratory investigation for identification of etiological agents in acute respiratory diseases should be carried out for epidemiological purposes, rather than for the benefit of patients. The epidemiological data are of considerable importance, particularly for surveillance and for making decisions on appropriate preventive measures to control acute respiratory diseases.

To obtain laboratory data, it is essential to have a large enough sample of cases in all the main clinical categories over a long period of time and over a wide enough area. The requirement is for a laboratory adequately supplied with staff and material together with an appropriate system for the collection and transporting of the specimens.

For the diagnosis of viral pathogens three diagnostic approaches are considered: serology, virus isolation and demonstration of viral antigens in respiratory secretions by immunological methods. Serological tests are often unrealistic and less accurate. They require specimens from both acute and convalescent (2–3 weeks later) stages of the disease. Such specimens are usually difficult to obtain, particularly from infants. Furthermore, the antibody response to RS virus infections, that are observed mostly in infants and toddlers and are frequently associated with severe lower respiratory tract symptoms may not always be detectable in the first 3–5 months of life. (Cruickshank 1975) This is the consequence of the immaturity of the infants immune system and the presence of maternal antibodies.

Laboratory procedures for the isolation and identification of respiratory viruses are complicated and expensive. In addition, RS virus and parainfluenza viruses are very labile and require immediate inoculation into appropriate tissue culture. The appearance of local antibody may prevent isolation of viruses from patients investigated at an advanced stage of the disease.

Immunofluorescence has been shown to be a sensitive method to detect viral antigens in cells from respiratory (naso-pharyngeal) secretions and to give accurate and reliable diagnostic results, provided that standardized reagents that have acceptable levels of sensitivity and specificity are available. Other diagnostic methods such as the enzyme techniques and radioimmunoassay are still under development.

For the diagnosis of bacterial pathogens routine serology is not recommended for the same reason as in the viral diagnosis. Conventional microscopy and culture technique are the method of choice, provided that no antibacterial drugs have been taken before the bacteriological work was started. However, there are certain limiting factors when the specimens for diagnosis are selected. Throat swabs only yield a causative agent in about 15 per cent of cases. Naso-pharyngeal secretions are also unsatisfactory. Cough swabs give rather better results but can be distressing and dangerous if there is an upper airway obstruction. Bronchial aspiration is difficult to perform and disturbing and the specimen may be easily contaminated.

Tracheal aspiration can yield a high percentage of positive isolation of lower respiratory tract organisms but is technically difficult, particularly in children and unacceptable to mothers. Aspiration of a pleural fluid will yield a pathogen in about 40 per cent of cases. Blood culture yields the causative agent of pneumonia in about one third of cases and the negative results will not always exclude the presence of bacterial pathogens. Lung puncture and aspiration can give a very high proportion of positive results but to be effective and safe it should be performed by a skilled and experienced person under radiological control. There are, however, certain contraindications, particularly hyperinflation of the lungs, a haemorrhagic tendency and presence of cysts of any size in the lung or of a pleural effusion. The newly developed techniques of antigen detection in body fluids, (such as coagglutination, counterimmuno-electrophoresis, latex agglutination, ELISA, et cetera), can increase the number of positive findings if done in parallel with conventional bacteriology.

SURVEILLANCE

In all warm climate countries, ARI stands as a leading cause of hospitalization and of death. Although this is a widely acknowledged fact, there is still lack of adequate information both epidemiological and clinical. The surveillance mechanism should be developed on either a national or a regional basis to monitor mortality and morbidity attributable to ARI in defined populations, to monitor the prevailing pathogens, to define population groups at special risk, as well as to investigate host factors determining susceptibility and environmental conditions that influence the incidence and severity of ARI, and to monitor and evaluate control measures. Four principal types of data need to be collected and analysed:

(a) population identification data, including information on social and environmental characteristics of the individuals; (b) clinical data, including history of illness and examination results; (c) intervention data, including clinical management and outcome, as well as community oriented activities such as immunization programmes or social or environmental change; (d) laboratory data, including data on prevailing pathogens in ARI as well as serological surveys on healthy people, to provide background information.

CONTROL OF ARI

Many deaths caused by acute respiratory infections in warm climate countries are due to the fact that children are brought to the attention of the health worker too late, when they are already too sick to respond to treatment. There is a great need for education of mothers and other persons providing care to children about danger symptoms such as rapid breathing, indrawing of chest and cyanosis.

Mothers should also be informed about general supportive care of the sick child. They may not be aware of the importance of providing sufficient fluid (tea, fruit juice, etc.) and with a neutral environmental temperature.

The most important problem facing warm climate countries is the clinical management of severe acute lower respiratory infections at the peripheral level of health care delivery systems and the first decision by the primary health care worker is whether the child's illness is mild or severe.

For purpose of clinical management at the primary care level and for notification of epidemiological surveillance simplified clinical categories of acute respiratory diseases, based on symptomatology and applicable by relatively inexperienced health workers, have been outlined (WHO, 1980; Fig. 13.1). It has the advantage that it can be elaborated to a more precise diagnosis by more highly trained clinicians for their own needs.

In a WHO memorandum (1981) a very simplified flowchart for the clinical management of severe ARI (mainly pneumonia) in children under five years of age which has been developed in Papua New Guinea after several years of experimental trials, has been presented (Fig. 13.2). Only five clinical signs were found to be essential for selecting appropriate therapeutic or referral actions for children with a cough, namely:
— rapid breathing
— chest indrawing
— cyanosis
— heart failure
— too sick to feed

In other places, such as Brazil (see figure 13.3) fever was included together with cough and dyspnea, as a key symptom.

The choice of antibiotics for routine clinical management varies from one country to another depending on local drug supplies and on information about the susceptibility of bacteria to drugs. Among the antimicrobials, penicillin, sulfonamides, chloramphenicol and co-trimoxazole are relatively inexpensive and could be considered effective against many bacterial respiratory pathogens. Of these, penicillin administered parenterally, is the drug chosen for the initial treatment of pneumonia.

Antibiotics are given according to the chart when these key symptoms are present, provided there is no skin rash (for example, indicating measles) in which case antibiotics are only given if fever persists for longer than five days.

In table 13.3, other main antibacterial drugs for treatment of pneumonia are listed. It should be remembered, however, that it is difficult to make a rational choice of drug regimens when the common pathogens causing pneumonia, and their drug sensitivities, are unknown. A programme of antibiotic therapy should of course be associated with one of supportive therapy at all levels of health care delivery systems. As many severe ARI are caused by viruses and since so far the use of antiviral drugs against acute respiratory diseases has been limited owing to their relative ineffectiveness, occasional

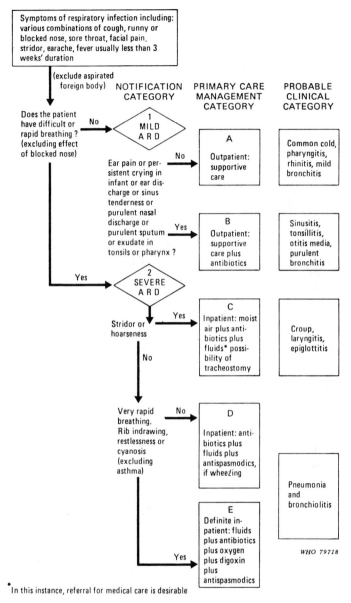

Symptoms of respiratory infection including: various combinations of cough, runny or blocked nose, sore throat, facial pain, stridor, earache, fever usually less than 3 weeks' duration

(exclude aspirated foreign body)

NOTIFICATION CATEGORY

PRIMARY CARE MANAGEMENT CATEGORY

PROBABLE CLINICAL CATEGORY

Does the patient have difficult or rapid breathing? (excluding effect of blocked nose)

No

1 MILD ARD

A
Outpatient: supportive care

Common cold, pharyngitis, rhinitis, mild bronchitis

No

Ear pain or persistent crying in infant or ear discharge or sinus tenderness or purulent nasal discharge or purulent sputum or exudate in tonsils or pharynx?

Yes

B
Outpatient: supportive care plus antibiotics

Sinusitis, tonsillitis, otitis media, purulent bronchitis

Yes

2 SEVERE ARD

Stridor or hoarseness

Yes

C
Inpatient: moist air plus antibiotics plus fluids* possibility of tracheostomy

Croup, laryngitis, epiglottitis

No

Very rapid breathing. Rib indrawing, restlessness or cyanosis (excluding asthma)

No

D
Inpatient: antibiotics plus fluids plus antispasmodics, if wheezing

Pneumonia and bronchiolitis

Yes

E
Definite inpatient: fluids plus antibiotics plus oxygen plus digoxin plus antispasmodics

WHO 79718

*In this instance, referral for medical care is desirable

Fig. 13.1 Simplified categories of acute respiratory disease

toxicity and high cost, supportive treatment in the form of extra fluids, administration of moist air, provision of a neutral environmental temperature, the administration of oxygen and, in the case of heart failure, of digoxin, may be life saving. Obviously, good nursing care and an adequate well-balanced diet including appropriate vitamins and mineral supplements, are the basic requirements.

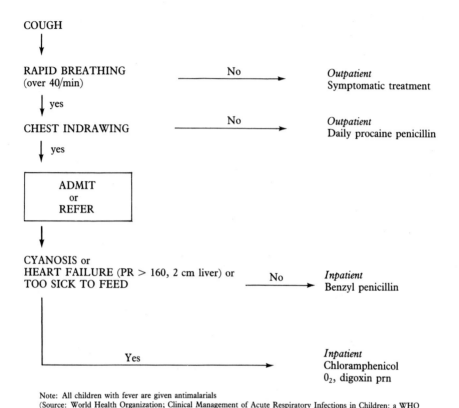

Note: All children with fever are given antimalarials
(Source: World Health Organization; Clinical Management of Acute Respiratory Infections in Children: a WHO memorandum; Bulletin of the World Health Organization (1981), 59(5), p. 710).

Fig. 13.2 Clinical management of ARI in child < 5 in Papua New Guinea

PREVENTION

Specific preventive measures against ARI are rather limited at present. Potent and safe vaccines against measles, pertussis and diphtheria are available and mass immunization in infancy, within the WHO expanded programme on immunization, should ensure a high coverage. In the majority of warm climate countries at present, however, the proportion of children vaccinated is still relatively low. Furthermore, the overall effect of these vaccines in reducing general ARI morbidity and mortality is as yet not known. *Pneumococcus* and *haemophilus influenzae* polysaccharide vaccines are also available but their effectiveness in children under the age of 18 months, those most susceptible to severe ARI, is limited, as they do not mount a good antibody response to polysaccharide challenge. Furthermore, the results of distribution of pneumococcal serotypes in countries of Africa showed that some of the types causing pneumococcal infections were not included in the 14 valent vaccines. (Greenwood et al 1980). They have been shown in clinical trials however, to prevent otitis media in chil-

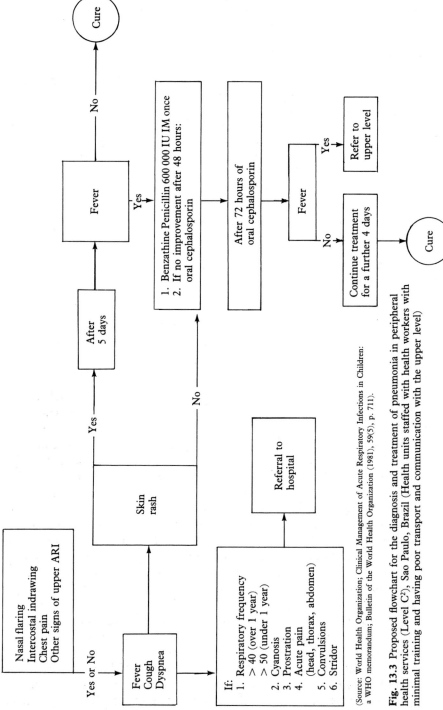

Fig. 13.3 Proposed flowchart for the diagnosis and treatment of pneumonia in peripheral health services (Level C²), São Paulo, Brazil (Health units staffed with health workers with minimal training and having poor transport and communication with the upper level)

(Source: World Health Organization; Clinical Management of Acute Respiratory Infections in Children: a WHO memorandum; Bulletin of the World Health Organization (1981), 59(5), p. 711).

Table 13.3 Main antibacterial drugs for treatment of pneumonia

Penicillin Ampicillin	Streptococcus pneumoniae
Ampicillin Chloramphenicol	Haemophilus influenzae
Oxacillin Flucloxacillin	Staphylococcus aureus penicillin-resistant
Gentamicin	Klebsiella pneumoniae Other Gram (−) agents
Erythromycin	Mycoplasma pneumoniae Chlamydia psittaci Legionella pneumophila
Metronidazole	Anaerobic agents

New broad spectrum antimicrobials		
*CEPHALOSPORINS:	First generation:	Cephalotin Cephaloridine Cephalexin
	Second generation:	Cefamandole
CO-TRIMOXAZOLE:	Trimethoprim + sulfamethoxazole	

NOTE: Tetracyclines should not be used in children
    a. they stain developing teeth and possibly interfere with dental development
    b. there are now a relatively large number of tetracycline-resistant bacteria causing respiratory infections.
    (Source: WHO (1981)).
* Recently cephalosporins of third generation have also been used for second line treatment of ARI. There will in future be new developments in the diagnosis, prevention and treatment of ARI which should be taken into consideration by clinicians.

dren. So far no available respiratory virus vaccine, with the possible exception of measles, has proved to be of practical value in preventing or modifying ARI in children. Mass immunization with currently available influenza vaccine, which in theory could prevent epidemics or halt their spread, is extremely difficult to achieve. Furthermore, the continuous process of the gradual alterations in the antigenic constitution of a viral strain (drift) and the occasional appearance of a 'new' strain with surface antigens serologically unrelated to previously circulating viruses (shift) make it necessary to constantly incorporate currently circulating viruses into the vaccine. So far, influenzae vaccines have been used primarily in certain selected population groups (industry, public service) and also in certain high risk groups (elderly and individuals in any age group, chronic and debilitating disease), in order to prevent severe complications and even fatal infections in such persons.

The development of vaccines against other viral infections (Parainfluenzae, RSV, Adenorivus, Rhinovirus) has been underway for some years. Nevertheless, this is a rapidly advancing area.

As far as nonspecific preventive measures against ARI are concerned, the improvement in nutritional status of children in warm climate countries seems to be essential. Because of the complex nature of ARI, it is probable that social and environmental improvements, in the long run, will produce a major decline in ARI mortality.

REFERENCES

Bulla A, Hitze K L 1978 Acute respiratory infections. A review Bulletin of the World Health Organization, 56(3), 481–498
Cruickshank R 1975 Respiratory infections in Epidemiology and Community Health in Warm Climate Countries p 57–62. Churchill-Livingstone. Edinburgh.
Datta B N D, Krishna R, Mane S I S, Raj L 1969 A longitudinal study of morbidity and mortality pattern in children under the age of five years in an urban community, Indian Journal of Medical Research, 57, 5: 948–957
Dodge R E, Demeke T 1970 The Epidemiology of infant malnutrition in Dabat. Ethiopian Medical Journal 82: 53–72
Frey L, Wall S 1977 Exploring Child Health and its Ecology — The Kirkos study in Addis Ababa. An evaluation of procedures in the measurement of acute morbidity and a search for causal structure. Acta Paediatrica Scandinavica Supl. 267. Almqvist and Wiksell periodical company, Stockholm, Sweden
Gordon J E, Ascol W, Mata L J, Guzman M A, Scrimshaw N S 1968 Nutritional and infection field study in Guatemalian villages (1959–1964) Archives of Environmental Health 16: 424–437
Greenwood B M et al. 1980 Pneumococcal serotypes in West Africa. Lancet. 1: 360
Hobson D 1972 Acute Respiratory Virus Infections. British Medical Journal 2: 229–231
James J W 1972 Longitudinal study of the morbidity of diarrhoeal and respiratory infections in malnourished children. American Journal of Clinical Nutrition. 25: 690–694
Watkins C J, Leeder S R, Corkhill R T 1979 The relationship between breast and bottle feeding and respiratory illness in the first year of life. Journal of Epidemiology and Community Health, 33, 3: 180–182
Williamson W A, Creenwood B M 1978 Impairment of the immune response to vaccination after acute malaria. Lancet 1: 1328–9
Viral Respiratory Diseases 1980 Report of a WHO Scientific Group WHO TRS 642
World Health Organization 1976 Sixth General Program of Work covering a specific period (1978–1983); WHO Official Records, No. 233, Annex 7, p 94
World Health Organization 1981 Clinical management of acute respiratory infections in children: a WHO memorandum, Bulletin of the World Health Organization, 59(5): 707–716

Streptococcal infections and their sequelae

INTRODUCTION

Streptococci pathogenic for man prevail in all the climatic zones. Available data on the incidence of streptococcal infections indicate that they belong among the most frequent bacterial diseases in the temperate zone and are common in the warm and hot regions. Although considerable improvement in the diagnosis, therapy and to some extent prevention of streptococcal diseases has been achieved over the last few decades, morbidity from streptococcal infections continues to be relatively high. Streptococcal diseases thus represent a world-wide health and economic problem.

THE DISEASES

Pathogenic streptococci produce diverse clinical patterns of disease.

Group A streptococcus (*Streptococcus pyogenes*) is the most significant streptococcal pathogen in man, causing acute upper-respiratory tract diseases including scarlet fever and a variety of septic lesions. The major clinical symptoms and signs of streptococcal pharyngitis or tonsillitis are a sudden onset of sore throat, fever, headache, pain on swallowing, malaise, exudate on the tonsils or posterior oropharynx and enlarged cervical lymph nodes. Characteristic of scarlet fever is the typical skin rash; desquamation of the skin occurs at a later stage of the disease.

In respiratory tract infection the streptococci can invade neighbouring tissues or other organs and provoke adenitis, otitis media, or osteomyelitis, or produce septicaemia. The most important streptococcal affections of the skin are erysipelas and impetigo.

A group A streptococcal infection of the throat may be followed by acute rheumatic fever, rheumatic heart disease and/or acute glomerulonephritis.

Rheumatic fever is a delayed sequela of acute streptococcal throat infection. After a latent period of usually 2 or 3 weeks, the disease starts with arthralgia, fever, pallor, tachycardia, often muffled heart sounds, accompanied by electro-cardiographic evidence of carditis (mostly, transitory prolongation of the P-Q interval). Tender, red and swollen joints are part of the typical clinical picture, but are less frequent than described in classical textbooks. Sometimes chorea* is the leading symptom. Subcutaneous nodules may be detected if carefully looked for. Erythema marginatum, mentioned in textbooks, is very rare.

The main laboratory signs are a high erythrocyte sedimentation rate (ESD), and a rise in some or all of the following antibodies: antistreptolysin O, anti-deoxyribonuclease B, antistreptokinase and antihyaluronidase. The most important characteristic of rheumatic fever is, however, its tendency for repeated recurrences following streptococcal reinfections.

Rheumatic heart disease in the acute phase involves the heart muscle and the endocardium, sometimes the pericardium as well. The myocardial and pericardial lesions are usually reversible, but the endocardial lesions as a rule lead to deformation of the heart valves, resulting in chronic rheumatic heart disease which becomes increasingly severe with each subsequent recurrence. Unless the recurrent attacks are prevented, chronic valvular heart disease evolves during childhood and adolescence into a crippling condition characterized by severe heart failure, usually leading to death in young adulthood. Valvular surgery and prostheses are palliative interventions.

Acute glomerulonephritis (AGN) is another important sequela of streptococcal infection. The disease occurs sporadically, sometimes in epidemic form, particularly in areas where the disease is considered to be endemic. (Potter et al 1968, Rodriguez et al 1977)

Clinical features of AGN in warm climatic countries do not differ remarkably from those in other parts of the world. The nephritic syndrome is characterized by oedema, dark urine, oliguria, haematuria, proteinuria, hypertension and azotemia. Asymptomatic cases of AGN were reported to be much more common than cases with symptoms (Seggie 1981, Simpson et al 1980).

Although AGN is now a much less common disease in many developed countries, (Mehta et al 1980) its occurrence has been shown to be relatively frequent in warm-climate countries. Sporadic cases and epidemics of AGN have been reported from countries of the African, Asian and American continents. (Anphaichitr et al 1976, Anthony et al 1969, Gallagher and Miller 1967, Hayes et al 1975, Nicholson 1977, Poon-King et al 1973, Rodriguez et al 1981) The throat or a skin lesion (pyoderma) may be the site of infection. Association of AGN with skin infection has been long recognized (Anthony et al 1967, Cruickshank et al 1975, Kaplan et al 1970, Parker 1969). It was also shown that persons most prone to the disease were children under 10 years of age and that there is a definite tendency for young children to have streptococcal skin infection rather than pharyngitis, which

---

* A neurologic disorder characterized by emotional lability, muscular weakness and rapid uncoordinated involuntary purposeless movements, which are most notable in the face, hands and feet.

is more common in early school years. The attack rate of AGN following skin infection varies in different countries and is between 3 to 20 per cent (Koshi 1972, Wannamaker 1970).

The causative agents of poststreptococcal AGN are nephritogenic group A streptococci belonging to particular types, e.g. M type 12, 49, 1, 3, 4, 25, and the types above 50.

The connection between AGN and the streptococcal infections has been proved in only a proportion of cases. Moreover, the ratio of streptococcal to non-streptococcal nephritis may vary locally and is virtually unknown. It is felt nevertheless, considering the public health importance of the streptococcal infection problem in warm-climate countries, that there is a need to develop an overall programme for the surveillance and control of streptococcal diseases and their sequelae, of which control of AGN should be an integral part.

Other streptococci

Group B streptococci (*Streptococcus agalactiae*) sporadically produce septic generalized infections of newborns, quite often with fatal outcome. In adults they can exceptionally cause systemic or localized pathogenic processes (meningitis, sepsis, pneumonia, etc.) (Anthony et al 1978, Bayer et al 1976, Parker 1979).

Streptococci of groups C, G and F occasionally act as agents of respiratory tract infections, which, however, are never followed by rheumatic fever or glomerulonephritis (Bannatyne and Randall 1977, Bouza et al 1978, Davies et al 1981, Mohr et al 1979). These streptococci can also cause localized sepsis.

Group D streptococci (this group includes enterococci) are responsible for low-grade sepsis. A particular species (S. bovis) may produce bacterial endocarditis (Bavikatte et al 1979, Fikar and Levy 1979).

Among usually non-groupable streptococci the most important species are *Streptococcus milleri*, *Streptococcus salivarius* and *Streptococcus sanguis*, which can cause localized sepsis or systemic infection (Blair and Nartin 1978, Lütticken et al 1978).

With a few exceptions there are no clinical features specific to the infections caused by most of the streptococcus species indicated above. To identify the etiological agent, bacteriological or serological examination is essential. It is advisable to test antibiotic sensitivity in pathogenic streptococci other than the invariably penicillin-sensitive group A streptococci.

THE AGENTS

Streptococci are Gram-positive organisms, spherical or oval in shape, which usually grow in short or long chains. They are aerobic, although they usually grow better in an atmosphere with a reduced oxygen content.

Group A streptococcus is by far the most significant streptococcal pathogen in man and the best known streptococcus as regards biological characteristics. The outermost part of its cell surface is a capsule composed of hyaluronic acid. Beneath the capsule is the cell wall, covered by fimbriae. One fimbrial determinant is lipoteichoic acid which enables the microorganism to adhere to the epithelial cells of the human oral mucosa (Beachey 1975, Klesius et al 1974, Maxted et al 1973, Rudzynski and Jackson, 1978, Selinger et al 1978). Another determinant is the M protein, which is a virulence factor responsible for resistence to phagocytosis and also the type-specific substance on the basis of which some seventy types of group A streptococci have been distinguished so far (Fischetti et al 1977, Fox 1974, Manjula and Fischetti 1980, Widdowson et al 1975). It is the antibody to the M protein that confers immunity to group A streptococcus infection; the immunity is therefore type-specific. Other cell-wall constituents are the T, R and MAP antigens and the SOF component, which have some additional importance for classification (Havlíček 1978, Johnson 1975, Johnson and Vosti 1977, Ludwicka 1976, Rijn 1980). The polysaccharide of the cell wall is the group-specific substance (Coligan et al 1975 and 1978) while peptidoglycan is the basic structure ensuring the rigidity of the cell wall (Rotta 1975, Rotta and Bednář 1969). Among the extracellular products of group A streptococcus the most important are the erythrogenic (or scarlet fever) toxin, streptolysin O and S, deoxyribonuclease B and some other substances (Bernheimer 1972, Wannamaker 1980).

Important facts have been brought to light about the structure and further biological characteristics of some other streptococcal species, viz. streptococci of groups B, C and D, S. sanguis and others (Russell et al 1980, Wilkinson 1972).

Diagnosis of acute throat and skin streptococcal infections based on clinical features always requires microbiological verification. In acute rheumatic fever and acute glomerulonephritis, identification of a preceding streptococcal infection by isolation of a group A streptococcus and/or by detection of an immunological response to it in the host is of basic importance for diagnosis. The prerequisites for obtaining a reliable answer from the microbiological laboratory are adequate sample collection, appropriate transport of the material to the laboratory, use of standard laboratory identification techniques and correct interpretation of the laboratory findings.

The bacteriological methods (Moody 1972, Rotta 1972, Rotta and Facklam 1980) for the recognition of streptococci include the following procedures: appropriate collection of throat, nose and skin swabs; transfer of the swabs to the laboratory within three hours. If this is not feasible for technical reasons, any of the following devices should be used for transport: filter-paper strips, the commercial silica gel transport system or the Stuart transport medium.

In the laboratory the material should be inoculated on a blood agar plate or plates, incubated aerobically at 37°C overnight, and the streptococci iden-

identified on the basis of their colony shape, haemolysis, and possibly microscopic appearance. A rough assessment of the growth in terms of colony count should be recorded.

All beta-haemolytic streptococci should be grouped, at least using sera for the identification of groups A, B, C, D, F and G. Serological grouping methods are preferable to physiological tests, viz. the bacitracin and CAMP tests. For serological grouping, the precipitation reaction using formamide or HCl extract of cells and group-specific serum is recommended. The coagglutination method, recently developed, also gives fully satisfactory results in routine practice and has the advantage of simplicity. Non-groupable streptococci should be classified by using physiological tests. The typing of group A streptococci, (Maxted et al 1974, Rotta et al 1971) and possibly also of group B (Cropp et al 1974, Stringer 1980) and D (Hérmán and Hoch 1971) streptococci, are specialized methods not required at the peripheral or district laboratory level.

Although a variety of laboratory tests have been developed for the titration of streptococcal antibodies, two especially should be used in routine diagnostic practice, viz. the tests for antistreptolysin O and antideoxyribonuclease B. They are of value as a means of confirming clinical diagnosis in patients suspected of streptococcal infection progressing with atypical features or without symptoms and in patients suffering from sequelae of streptococcal infections.

EPIDEMIOLOGY

The most significant pathogenic streptococci in man are those of group A. As has already been stated, group A streptococci cause diseases of the upper respiratory tract and skin, and these infections may lead to rheumatic fever or acute glomerulonephritis. Infections caused by other serological groups, the most important of which are B, C, D and G, or by the non-groupable species, are much less frequent (Kaplan 1972).

The rates for carrier status of haemolytic streptococci show considerable fluctuation at different times. Prospective studies on carrier status have disclosed that in temperate climatic regions even 30 or more per cent of individuals may be harbouring haemolytic streptococci in some situations. Data reported in recent years from tropical and subtropical countries indicate that the carrier rate is frequently no lower there.

The incidence of streptococcal acute upper respiratory tract disease in the temperate zone amounts to 5–15 cases per 100 individuals per year. Data on scarlet fever show an incidence variation from some 50 to 250 or more cases per 100 000 population per year in some geographic areas. In hot climatic regions streptococci tend to produce rather mild respiratory disorders, the frequency of which has not been yet adequately estimated by forecasts. Scarlet fever is very rarely seen in many of these areas. However, skin infections due to haemolytic streptococci (Dajani et al 1974, Selinger et al

1978) are very common there and their prevalence can even reach 20 per cent or more of the child population during particular seasons. The incidence of rheumatic fever has dramatically declined in the economically advanced countries and seems to have stabilized at some five cases per 100 000 inhabitants per year. In the developing countries of the tropical and subtropical regions rheumatic fever and rheumatic heart disease represent a health problem roughly of the same magnitude as they formerly were in Europe and the United States several decades ago (Rotta 1980, WHO 1980).

Group A streptococci spread among the population by the respiratory route, which implies close contact between individuals. The streptococci are conveyed by relatively large droplets up to a distance of about 3 metres. The symptoms of respiratory disease usually develop within 2 to 3 days. Acquisition rates are highest on exposure to acute infection; they decrease considerably with the length of the carrier state. Patients harbouring streptococci in the nose are particularly likely to transmit streptococcal infection. The microbe can also be dispersed in the air and on the surfaces of fomites by carriers, but these streptococci are not a source of respiratory infection as a rule.

Laboratory and clinical investigations have demonstrated that the microorganism must possess certain biological characteristics in order to cause disease. The most essential of these characteristics are the ability to adhere to epithelial cells and their virulence. These depend mainly on the presence of lipoteichoic acid and M protein, respectively, on the surface of the cell. In the process of infection transfer, the quantity of the harboured streptococci is an important factor in addition to their biological properties (Stollerman 1971).

The susceptibility of the host is obviously determined by a number of factors, of which, besides age, the best known and the most important one is the lack of type-specific immunity (Sramek et al 1968, Widdowson et al 1974).

Various health conditions which are characteristic of warm-climate countries, may also enhance a susceptibility to streptococcal infections; for instance, patients with thalassemia/haemoglobin E disease as well as splenoctomized patients have been shown to be unusually susceptible to streptococcal infections (Bhamarpravats 1967, Econonidou and Constandoulakis 1971, Sucroogreung and Wasi 1972, Wasi 1971). Based on this fact, some investigations claimed that these patients could have a higher incidence of rheumatic fever and AGN than the normal population. Others, however, do not confirm these observations (Anphaichitr et al 1976).

Human reservoirs are the only important source of microorganisms in respiratory streptococcal infection.

The density and magnitude of crowding is the decisive environmental factor in the spread of infection. Climate and the socio-economic status play an indirect role only. Secondary reservoirs (e.g. streptococci in the air, in the dust or on fomites) have no bearing on the epidemiology of respiratory infection, but these streptococci can cause skin infections or post-operative complications.

Hot and humid weather, when the skin is more apt to be exposed to minor trauma, as well as mosquito bites have been considered to be important predisposing factors for skin infections (Dillon 1967 and 1974). Of particular importance is scabies, which is common in warm-climate countries and may occur sometimes in epidemic forms. Evidence of a scabies epidemic producing an epidemic of AGN has periodically been reported (Fish et al 1970, Herch 1967, Poon-King et al 1967, Whittle et al 1973). Factors such as housing and nutrition, overcrowding and unhygienic conditions both at home and school, dust and dirt, infestation by head lice, the habit of sharing combs and clothing, as well as contact with cattle and fowl in the same dwelling may also contribute to the occurrence of skin infection. The higher prevalence of pyoderma in urban children reported in some warm-climate countries (Koshi and Benjamin 1977) may be due to overcrowding in classrooms with less open-air facilities than in rural schools.

The epidemiology of rheumatic fever and acute glomerulonephritis displays all the major characteristics of the epidemiology of acute infection (Stollerman 1964). Both sequelae may only develop in those cases in which the antecedent acute streptococcal infection has not been identified and therefore has not been treated or the treatment has not been adequate as regards the type of antibiotic given or the duration of the antibiotic therapy. The latent period preceding a rheumatic fever attack is usually 2 or 3 weeks, but it can vary from 5 to 45 days. In acute glomerulonephritis the latent period may very from 1 to 4 weeks.

It was shown that sequelae occur, in particular, during epidemics of streptococcal infections in those individuals where the disease has led to a greater immune response and possibly to prolonged convalescent throat carriage. In acute glomerulonephritis so-called nephritogenic types are known (e.g. types 12, 49, the types above 50 and some others). (Noble and Vosti 1973, Potter et al 1971). After infection by these types the incidence rates for acute glomerulonephritis are higher than after infection by other types. The existence of rheumatogenic streptococci has not been conclusively demonstrated. While both sequelae can develop after acute streptococcal respiratory infection, skin infection never leads to rheumatic fever.

In contrast to group A infections, which can occur either sporadically or in epidemics, the infections caused by other streptococci are almost always sporadic. This fact co-determines the different epidemiological character of these infections.

SURVEILLANCE

Assessment of the magnitude of the streptococcus problem in a particular geographical area or country is a prerequisite for launching control measures on a peripheral or central level. This goal can best be achieved through surveillance of streptococcal infections by means of epidemiological and microbiological surveys. These studies should be focused on the most important points. They should be developed gradually and their aim should be the introduction of new or improved methods for the diagnosis, therapy and prevention of streptococcal diseases and their sequelae.

Information on streptococcal infection can be collected either by (1) analysing morbidity notification data or (2) prospective studies on streptococcal infections in population samples.

Morbidity data are in practise available only for scarlet fever, but notification of this disease is at present obligatory in fewer countries that it used to be in the past. Consequently the major portion of reliable information, if not the only one, can be obtained though forecasts conducted either on samples of the general population or in selected communities such as schools, military units, etcetera.

The objectives of the studies are to learn: (a) the occurrence of particular groups of haemolytic streptococci; (b) carrier rates for haemolytic streptococci; (c) the incidence of (i) streptococcal diseases of the upper respiratory tract, including scarlet fever, and (ii) streptococcal skin lesions; (d) the incidence of rheumatic fever, acute glomerulonephritis and the prevalence of rheumatic heart disease (if the protocol of the study makes it possible to pursue this objective as well).

The surveillance programme should embody as many objectives as feasible. Attention would simultaneously have to be paid to the epidemiological and micro biological aspects of streptococcal infections.

The protocol of the studies must pay heed to the fact that there is frequently considerable fluctuation in the incidence as a result of many factors, such as the biological properties of the streptococcus in circulation, host characteristics of the study group, season of the year etc.

The implementation of the surveillance programme presupposes selection of a suitable study area, provision for clinical cooperation, setting up of an epidemiological group and the establishment of adequate laboratory facilities.

The studies require team-work between the epidemiologist, microbiologist and clinician. These specialists draw up the protocol of the study, carry out the study, analyze the results and recommend counter-measures to be introduced into practice by the public health services.

CONTROL

At present, the only approach to effective control of streptococcal infections is through early diagnosis, confirmed by microbiological examination, and followed by appropriate antibiotic treatment. The sequelae are reliably prevented, whenever the infection has been diagnosed early and properly treated (Report of a WHO Expert Committee 1966). The drug of choice for treatment is penicillin. The following doses are recommended: intramuscularly, benzathine penicillin G, 1.2 mil. I.U. (0.6–0.9 mil. I.U. for children), in a single injection or a combination of crystalline penicillin G, procaine penicillin and benzathine penicillin in a dose of 1.2 mil. I.U. (0.6–0.9 mil. I.U. for children), in a single injection; orally, penicillin G, 0.2 mil. I.U. three or four times a day for 7–10 days, or penicillin V, 100–125 mg four times a day for 7–10 days. In individuals with penicillin allergy, erythromycin is used in a dose of 250 mg four times a day for 7–10 days (40 mg/kg body weight/day in children). Tetracycline or sulphonamides should never be used for the treatment (Matsen and Coghlan 1972).

Early treatment of the acute streptococcal infection is thus a primary preventive measure against the sequelae of infection, in particular rheumatic fever and rheumatic heart disease, and should be the primary goal of streptococcal disease control. However, streptococcal throat infections often occur without major symptoms and, even if symptomatic, they may not be distinguished from a host of non-streptococcal sore throats, especially in tropical countries with developing health care systems and scarce resources.

The disease thus often escapes attention, is misdiagnosed or is not treated properly with penicillin, and so otherwise preventable heart damage may develop and may be recognized late, at an advanced stage, when it is already irreversible. Nevertheless, if at this stage systematic and long-term prophylaxis of streptococcal reinfections is established, further progression of the heart disease will be halted (secondary prevention) and the life expectation of the subject considerably improved. Long-term penicillin prophylaxis (1.2 mil benzathine penicillin in adults or 0.6 mil in children at three-week intervals) should be administered to all individuals who have experienced an attack of rheumatic fever or are suffering from rheumatic heart disease.

Secondary prevention by penicillin is recommended over a minimum period of five years after the attack (onset) of rheumatic fever. In young patients below 15 years, the prophylactic treatment should be continued until the age of 20.

Of particular importance is the prophylaxis in countries of tropical zones, particularly in developing countries where lifelong prophylaxis is recommended because of the risk of frequent exposure to reinfection. Lifelong prophylaxis is also recommended in some particular cases, for example for patients who have undergone heart valve surgery.

The main obstacles to successful secondary prevention of rheumatic heart disease are of an organizational and psychological nature. In some places benzathine penicillin may not be always available. Patients who need to receive repeated injections may forget or avoid the regular follow-up visits; (because of the painful injections) and left unprotected, they may become reinfected, and thus develop rheumatic fever recurrences, leading to increasingly severe valvular damage. Control at the community level therefore consists, in addition to surveillance and primary prevention (preferably organized through school health services), of organized, long-term secondary prevention in subjects with diagnosed rheumatic fever. Such programmes, shown to be feasible in developing countries even with limited resources, should include registration and active follow-up of the identified subjects. It has been demonstrated (Strasser 1978, Strasser et al 1981, WHO 1980) that such programmes are both feasible and cost-effective.

An AGN surveillance and control programme should aim at complete coverage of all cases in a community. Since the organizational pattern is very similar to that for rheumatic fever and rheumatic heart diseases, it is preferable to combine the AGN surveillance and control programme with that of rheumatic fever and rheumatic heart disease as concluded by an epidemiological study by Who (1971).

The questions to be elucidated by surveillance are: the incidence of streptococcal AGN, the epidemiological significance of various streptococcus strains and sites of infections and the frequency of transition from AGN to chronic glomerulonephritis (CGN). The last may be diagnosed either as a complication of a followed-up case of AGN or as being without a history of preceding AGN (since many a case of CGN is not preceded by clinically apparent AGN). Here it should also be mentioned that only a fraction of AGN cases evolve into CGN. Investigation of immunological features of the disease could also give useful information.

The frequency and world-wide occurrence of streptococcal infections calls for the elaboration and implementation of improved defense measures. One possibility would be an immunological approach, streptococcal vaccination (Polly et al 1975, Wittener et al 1979). The research in this direction is at the laboratory stage so far and the prospect of a vaccine becoming available is still rather distant.

REFERENCES

Anphiachitr P, Petchclai B, Bhanchet P, Hathurat P 1976
   Thalassaemic diseases and acute post-streptococcal glomerulonephritis. Lancet ii, p 861–
Anthony B F, Kaplan E L, Wannamaker L W, Briese F W, Champman S S 1969 Attack rates of acute nephritis after type 49 streptococcal infection of the skin and of respiratory tract. Journal of Clinical Investigation 48: 1697–1704
Anthony B F, Okada D M, Hobel C J 1978 Epidemiology of group B streptococcus: Longitudinal observations during pregnancy. The Journal of Infectious Disease 137: 524–530
Anthony B F, Perlman L V, Wannamaker L W 1967 Skin infections and acute nephritis in American Indian Children. Pediatrics 39: 263–279
Bannatyne R M, Randall C 1977 Ecology of 350 isolates of group F streptococcus. American Journal of Clinical Pathology 67: 184–186
Bayer A S, Chow A W, Anthony B F, Guze L B 1976 Serious infections in adults due to group B streptococci. The American Journal of Medicine 61: 498–502
Bavikatte K, Schreiner R L, Lemons J A, Gresham E L 1979 Group D streptococcal septicemia in the neonate. American Journal of Diseases of Children 133: 493–495
Beachey H B 1975 Binding of group A streptococci to human oral mucosal cells by lipoteichoic acid. Transactions of American Physicians 138: 285–291
Bernheimer A W 1972 Hemolysins of streptococci. In: Wannamaker L W, Matsen J M (ed) Streptococci and streptococcal diseases. Academic Press, New York and London. h 2, p 19
Bhamarpravats, N, Na-Nikorn S, Wasi P, Tuchinda S 1967 American Journal of Clinical Pathology 47: 745–

Blair D C, Nartin D B 1978 Beta hemolytic streptococcal endocarditis: predominance of non-group A organism. The American Journal of the Medical Sciences 276: 269–277

Bouza E, Meyer R D, Busch D F 1978 Group G streptococcal endocarditis. American Journal of Clinical Pathology 70: 108–110

Coligan J E, Schnute W C, Kindt T J 1975 Immunochemical and chemical studies on streptococcal group-specific carbohydrates. The Journal of Immunology 114: 1654–1658

Coligan J E, Kindt T J, Krause R M 1978 Structure of the streptococcal groups A A variant and C carbohydrates. Immunochemistry 15: 755–759

Cropp C B, Zimmermann R A, Jelinková J, Auerheimer A H, Bolin R A, Wyrick B C 1974 Serotyping of group B streptococci by slide agglutination, fluorescence microscopy and immunodiffusion. Journal of Laboratory and Clinical Medicine 84: 594–603

Cruickshank R, Duguid J P, Marmion B P, Swain R H A 1975 In: Medical Microbiology Vol II, 12 rd. Churchill Livingstone

Dajani A S, Ferrieri P, Chapman S S, Wannamaker L W 1974 Spread and persistence of cutaneous streptococcci and staphylococci. In: Haverkorn M J (ed) Streptococcal Disease and the Community Excerpta Medica, Amsterdam. ch p 243

Davies M K, Ireland M A, Clarke D B 1981 Infective endocarditis from group C streptococci causing stenosis of both the aortic and mitral valves. Thorax 36: 69–71

Dillon H C 1967 Pyoderma and Nephritis. Ann Rev. Med. 18: 207–

Dillon H C 1974 Streptococcal infections of the skin and their complications: impetigo and nephritis. In: Wannamaker L W, Matson J M (ed) Streptococci and Streptococcal Diseases. Academic Press, New York and London. ch 34 p 572–586

Economidou J, Constandoulakis M 1971 Streptococcal infection in thalassemia. Lancet ii: 1160–

Epidemiological study and control of streptococcal infections. Rheumatic fever and glomerulonephritis proposal for an international cooperative study 1971 CVD/70.5. WHO. Geneva

Fikar Ch R, Levy J 1979 Streptococcus bovis meningitis in neonate. The American Journal of Diseases of Children 133: 1149–1150

Fish A J, Herdman R C, Michael A F, Pickering R J, Good R A 1970 Epidemic acute glomerulonephritis associated with type 49 streptococcal pyoderma II correlative study of light. Immunoflurenscent and electron microscopic findings. American Journal of Medicine 48: 28–39

Fischetti V A, Gotschlich E C, Sivigkia G, Zabriskie J B 1977 Streptococcal M. protein: An antiphagocytic molecule assembled on the cell wall. The Journal of Infectious Diseases 136: S222–S233

Fox E N 1974 M proteins of group A streptococci. Bacteriological Reviews 38: 57–86

Gallagher B H and Miller C G 1967 Acute glomerulonephritis in Jamaican Children. West Indian Medical Journal 16(1): 17–32

Hayes J S, Persaud M P, Omess P J 1975 Post-streptococcal glomerulonephritis in North Trinidad. Tropial and Geographical Medicine 27: 253–256

Havliček J 1978 Occurrence of Fc-reacting factor in acid extracts of streptococcus pyogenes and its relationship to M protein. Experimental Cell Biology 46: 146–151

Herch C 1967 Acute glomerulonephritis due to skin disease with special reference to scabies. South African Medical Journal 41: 29–34

Hérmán G, Hoch V 1971 Phage typing of group D streptococci II. Isolation of supplementary phages for classification enterococci untypable with roumanian phages. Acta Microbiologica Academiae Scientiarum Hungaricae 18: 101–104

Johnson R H 1975 Characterization of group A streptococcal R-28 antigen purified by hydroxyapatite column chromatography. Infection and Immunity 12: 901–909

Johnson R H, Vosti K L 1977 Purification and characterization of group A streptococcal T-1 antigen. Infection and Immunity 16: 867–875

Kaplan E L 1972 Unresolved problem in diagnosis and epidemiology of streptococcal infection. In: Wannamaker L W, Matsen J M (ed) Streptococci and streptococcal diseases. Academic Press, New York and London. Ch 33 p 558–570

Kaplan E L, Anthony B F, Chapman S S, Wannamaker L W 1970 Epidemic acute glomerulonephritis associated with type 49 streptococcal pyoderma clinical and laboratory findings. American Journal of Medicine 48: 9–27

Klesius P H, Zimmerman R A, Mathes J H, Auernheimer A H 1974 Human antibody

response to group A streptococcal teichoic acid. Canadian Journal of Microbiology
20: 853–859

Koshi G 1972 The epidemiology of streptococcal infections with particular reference to the study in Vellore Ann IAMS. 8: 23–27

Koshi G, Benjamin V 1977 Surveillance of streptococcal infections in children in a South Indian community—A pilot survey. Indian Journal of Medical Research 66. 3: 379–388

Ludwicka A 1976 T. antigen of streptococcus pyogenes: isolation and purification. Infection and Immunity 13: 993–994

Lütticken R, Wendorff U, Lütticken D, Johnson E A, Wannamaker L W 1978 Studies on streptococci resembling streptococcus milleri and on an associated surface-protein antigen. Journal of Medical Microbiology 11: 419–431

Manjula B N, Fischetti V A 1980 Studies on group A streptococcal M-proteins: purification of type 5 M protein and comparison of its amino terminal sequence with two immunologically unrelated M protein molecules. The Journal of Immunology 124: 261–267

Matsen J M, Coghlan Ch R 1972 Antibiotic testing and susceptibility patterns of streptococci. In: Wannamaker L W, Matsen J M (ed) Streptococci and streptococcal diseases. Academic Press, New York and London. ch 12 p 189–203

Maxted W R, Widdowson J P, Fraser C A M, Ball L, Bassett D C J 1974 Streptococcal typing by means of the serum opacity reaction. In: Haverkorn M J (ed) Streptococcal Disease and the Community Excerpta Medica, Amsterdam. ch 1 p 48

Maxted W R, Widdowson J P, Fraser Ch A M 1973 Antibody to streptococcal opacity factor in human sera. Journal of Hygiene 71: 35–42

Mehta G, Prakash K, Sharma K B 1980 Streptococcal pyoderma and acute glomerulonephritis in children. Indian Journal of Medical Research 71: 692–700

Mohr D N, Feist D J, Washington J A, Hermans P E 1979 Infections due to group C streptococci in man. American Journal of Medicine 66: 450–455

Moody M D 1972 Old and new techniques for rapid identification of group A streptococci. In: Wannamaker L W, Matsen J M (ed) Streptococci and streptococcal diseases. Academic Press, New York and London. ch 11 p 178–187

Nicholson G D 1977 Post-streptococcal glomerulonephritis in adult Jamaicans with and without sickle-cell anaemia. West Indian Medical Journal 26(2): 78–84

Noble R C, Vosti K L 1973 Biologic and immunologic comparison of nephritogenic and non-nephritogenic strains of group A, M-type 12 streptococcus. The Journal of Infectious Diseases 128: 761–767

Parker M T 1969 Streptococcal skin infection and acute glomerulonephritis. British Journal of Dermatology 81. Suppl. 1: 37–46

Parker M T 1979 Infections with group B streptococci. Journal of Antimicrobial Chemotherapy 5: 27–37

Polly S M, Waldman R H, High P, Wittner M K, Dorfman A, Fox E N 1975 Protective studies with group A streptococcal M protein vaccine. II. Challenge of volunteers after local immunization in the upper respiratory tract. The Journal of Infectious Diseases 131: 217–223

Poon-King T, Mohammed I, Cox R, Potter E V, Simon N M, Siegal A C, Earle D P 1967 Recurrent Epidemic Nephritis in South Trinidad. New England Journal of Medicine 277(13): 728–733

Poon-King T, Svastman M, Mohammed I, Potter E V, Achong J, Cox R, Earle D P 1973 Epidemic acute nephritis with reappearance of M type 55 streptococci in Trinidad. Lancet 1: 475–479

Potter E V, Oritz J S, Sharratt A R 1971 Changing types of nephritogenic streptococci in Trinidad. Journal of Clinical Investigation 50: 1197–1205

Potter E V, Siegal A C, Simon N M, McAninch J, Earle D P, Poon-King T, Mohammed I, Adibh S 1968 Streptococcal infections and epidemic acute glomerulonephrits in South Trinidad. Journal of Pediatrics 72: 871–84

Report of a WHO Expert Committee 1966 Prevention of rheumatic fever. World Health Organization Technical Report Series 342: 5–27

Rijn van de I 1980 Structure and immunochemistry of the group A streptococcal membrane. In: Read S E, Zabirskie J B (ed) Streptococcal disease and the immune response. Academic Press, New York and London. p 161

Rodriguez, Iturbe B, Garcia R, Rubio L 1977 Post-streptococcal glomerulonephritis. Controversial aspects of recent investigations. The disease in Venezuela. Acta Cientif. Venezuela 28: 245–248

Rodriguez, Iturbe B, Rubio L, Garcia R 1981 Attack rate of post-streptococcal nephritis in families. A prospective study. Lancet 1: 401–403

Rotta J 1972 Prospects for improved approaches to and reagents for identification of streptococci. In: Wannamaker L W, Matsen J M (ed) Streptococci and streptococcal diseases. Academic Press, New York and London. ch 16 p 268–279

Rotta J 1980 The rheumatic fever problem in some areas of the world. In: Read S E, Zabriskie J B (ed) Streptococcal disease and the immune response. Academic Press, New York and London. p 751

Rotta J, 1975 Endotoxin-like properties of the peptidoglycan. Zeitschrift für Immunitätforschung 149: 230–244

Rotta J, Bednář B 1969 Biological properties of cell wall mucopeptide of hemolytic streptococci. The Journal of Experimental Medicine 130: 31–47

Rotta J, Facklam R 1980 Manual of microbiological diagnostic methods for streptococcal infections and their sequelae. World Health Organization p 3–69

Rotta J, Krause R M, Lancefield R C, Everly E, Lackland H 1971 New approaches for the laboratory recognition of M types of group A streptococci. The Journal of Experimental Medicine 134: 1298–1315

Rudzynski A B, Jackson R W 1978 The properties of a lipoteichoic acid antigen from streptococcus pyogenes. Immunochemistry 15: 83–91

Russell M W, Bergmeier L A, Zanders E D, Lehner T 1980 Protein antigens of streptococcus mutans: purification and properties of a double antigen and its protease resistant component. Infection and Immunity 28: 486–493

Seggie J 1981 Glomerulonephritis in Zimbabwe. Experience of Harare Hospital during 1978. Central African Journal of Medicine 27. 5: 77–84

Selinger D S, Julie N, Reed W Q, Williams R C 1978 Adherence of group A streptococci to pharyngeal cells: a role in the pathogenesis of rheumatic fever. Science 201: 455–457

Simpson W A, Ofek I, Sarasohn, Mirrison J C, Beachey E H 1980 Characteristics of the binding of streptococcal lipoteichoic acid to human oral epithelial cells. The Journal of Infectious Diseases 141: 457–461

Stollerman G H 1964 The epidemiology of primary and secondary rheumatic fever. In: Uhr J W (ed) The Streptococcus, Rheumatic Fever and Glomerulonephritis. The Williams & Wilkins Company, Baltimore. p 311

Stollerman G H 1971 Rheumatogenic and nephritogenic streptococci. Circulation 43: 915–921

Strasser T 1978 Rheumatic fever and rheumatic heart disease in the 1970s. WHO Chronicle 32: 18–25

Strasser T et al 1981 The community control of rheumatic fever and rheumatic heart disease: report of a WHO international cooperative project. Bulletin of the World Health Organization 59: 285–294

Stringer J 1980 The development of a phage-typing system for group B streptococci. The Journal of Medical Microbiology 13: 133–143

Sramek J, Baculard A, Gerbeaux J, Mozziconacci P 1968 Acquisition of type-specific immunity by group A streptococcus carriers. In: Caravano R (ed) Current Research on Group A Streptococcus. Excerpta Medica, Amsterdam, p 253

Sucroogreung S, Wasi P 1972 Antistreptolysin O titres in thalassaemic diseases and the effect of splenoctomy. Journal of the Medical Association of Thailand 55: 287–293

Wannamaker L W 1970 Medical Progress. Differences between streptococcal infections of the thorat and the skin. New England Journal of Medicine 282: 78–85

Wannamaker L W 1980 The extracellular products of group A streptococci. In: Read S E, Zabriskie J B (ed) Streptococcal Disease and the Immune Response. Academic Press, New York and London. p 177

Wasi P 1971 Streptococcal infection leading to cardiac and renal involvement in thalassemia. Lancet i: 949–950

Whittle H C, Abdullah M T, Fakulle F, Parry E H O, Rajkovic A D 1973 Scabies Pyoderma and Nephritis in Zaria, Nigeria A clinical and Epidemiological study. Transactions of the Royal Society of Tropical Medicine and Hygiene 67: 349–363

Widdowson J P, Maxted W R, Notley C M, Pinney A M 1974 The antibody responses in man to infection with different serotypes of group A streptococci. The Journal of Medical Microbiology 7: 483–495

Widdowson J P, Maxted W R, Pineey A M 1975 Immunological heterogenity among the M protein antigens of group A streptococci. The Journal of Medical Microbiology 9: 73–87

Wilkinson H W 1972 Comparison of streptococcal R antigens. Applied Microbiology 24: 669–670

Wittner M K et al 1979 Protective studies with group A streptococcal M protein vaccines. In: Parker M T (ed) Pathogenic Streptococci, Reedbooks, London. p 33

WHO, Community control of rheumatic heart diseases in developing countries 1. WHO Chronicle 1980 34 334–345

WHO, Community control of rheumatic heart diseases in developing countries 1. WHO Chronicle 1980 34: 389–395

Measles and whooping cough

INTRODUCTION

Those specific infections which all children are likely to develop and which are usually easily recogizable, have been called the 'immunizing diseases' of childhood. Among these immunizing diseases, measles and whooping cough are the most import. Both diseases show a high fatality rate in tropical countries, but for different reasons: measles because of the interaction with malnutrition, and whooping cough because it develops at a very early age. In warm climate countries, health data depends heavily on clinical experience in hospital. As a result both of these diseases have been under-reported, in measles due to local beliefs, and in whooping cough due partly to the high case fatality in the early months of life. A further, but largely theoretical reason why both diseases may be more severe in developing countries is the evidence that in each, though for different reasons, the infecting dose may be heavier than in more developed countries. Both diseases may be prevented by active immunization but in each infection epidemiological ignorance has led to squandering of immunization resources.

MEASLES

Measles is the outstanding example of the interaction of malnutrition and infection. The association of nutritional deficiency as a cause of death has been well documented. A PAHO study (Paffer and Serrano 1973) produced further evidence and nutritional deficiency was found as a contributory cause in around 80 per cent of children in two areas of Bolivia, and in 70 per cent in the north-east of Brazil.

Measles is more severe in the malnourished child. In no other common disease is there so much difference in the course and outcome of measles between children living in a satisfactory socio-economic environment and those from less privileged situations. The difference in fatality rate for measles between European and African communities has been estimated to be at least four hundred-fold, and the PAHO study found differences of a similar order among children living in good and poor environments. This difference in fatality rates can be most easily explained on two grounds: (1) measles develops at an earlier age in the developing countries, and (2) the children living there are less well nourished. The child's age, and his poor nutritional state, are also inter-linked. Because the child develops measles at a period of maximum growth, when malnutrition is most likely to be present, the disease is more severe than it might be in an older child.

Severity and infecting dose of the virus

Although the importance of under-nutrition is now widely accepted, a further cause for the severity of measles is now becoming apparent from work in Guinea Bissau and Indonesia. Studies have shown considerable differences in the mortality from measles between families in which only one index child is involved compared with families in which there are multiple cases. There are a number of possible reasons why the mortality is higher where there are multiple cases and so far these have not been adequately researched. First of all, more than one severely sick child in a family may be more than the adults can cope with. Another possibility is that where there is more than one child, the possibility of a secondary infection might be greater, particularly due to a virus such as herpes simplex, which is now known to be very serious in measles. Another and interesting possibility is that, in the case of the index child, the infecting dose is likely to be fairly small when that child was in contact with another child secreting measles virus. Where, however, there are multiple cases within a family, it is likely that the child infecting the other children will have been in close contact with them; perhaps even sleeping in the same bed for a considerable period. For this reason the infecting dose of the virus may be much greater.

If, as seems possible, the last of these suppositions is true then it does suggest that where measles cases are occurring a new emphasis is required in health education. Experience has shown that infection cannot be avoided by isolation of cases. It is, however, possible that the severity of the disease in other children may be reduced by separating infective cases, particularly early in the disease, from children who have yet to experience it.

Historical and geographical variations in severity of measles

Historically there is evidence of catastrophic attacks of measles in such areas as Fiji, the Hudson Bay region, South America, and Terra del Fuego. In some of these epidemics, a considerable fraction, at times possibly over a quarter of the population, died. The circumstances in these areas were, however, different from those that exist at the present time anywhere in the world. In these isolated communities when measles struck, whole families would be infected at the same time. No one was well enough to undertake the routine work of bringing water and food necessary to the nutrition and life of the family. For this reason, there is little doubt that in these areas there was acute starvation which would follow in the wake of the disease. This was described in the Lancet in 1875 in the Fijian outbreak of that year '. . . the great mortality has been in large measure due to the fact that sick were exposed to the most unfavourable conditions. Unprotected from exposure, untended and untreated chiefly because of their unhappy prejudices . . .'

In many of these areas, measles was a recent arrival and the greater severity of the disease was ascribed to the lack of herd immunity. This is unlikely to be the case in countries in Africa and Asia. Here there is evidence that measles has been present for thousands of years, with exceptional outbreaks in which fatality rates between 15 per cent and 30 per cent of all children in a village have been recorded.

In Europe, measles has a peak incidence in the winter months, and in each area there tend to be epidemic waves in alternate years. From experience in Africa, the suggestion was made that the nearer the community lies to the equator, the less evidence there is of a seasonal increase. In detailed records of the disease in Nigeria, the start of the epidemic occurred in the driest and often the hottest season of the year. This finding was related to the fact that at this season the ground was too hard for tilling and the people crowded together for celebrations. The epidemic decreased when, with the onset of the rains, the people dispersed to their farms.

In Nigeria the prevalence of the disease in young infants (Fig. 15.1) has been related to the custom of carrying the child on the back, so that the infant attends with the mother in the market and at all functions, and is in close proximity to other children of a similar age. Also, the extended family, with several young children from different parents all living in close prox-

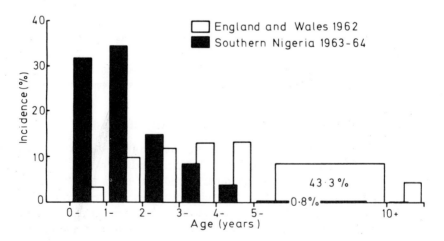

Fig. 15.1 Measles, in common with other droplet diseases, is more common in the first years of life in developing countries

imity, offers additional opportunities for the spread of droplet infections, all of which occur at an early age in such societies.

Severe measles: clinical manifestations of the disease in the malnourished child

Differences in the rash and subsequent changes in the skin have been described over the last 20 years in the malnourished child: reference to the older literature from Europe and America in the last century reveals a similar appearance in those countries at that time. The appearence of Koplik's spots in the early stages of the disease is similar, but in a proportion of the children the rash darkens to a deep red and violet colour and desquamation ensues. A mild branny desquamation is seen in all children after measles, but in the malnourished child in whom the rash has taken on a darker colour, this desquamation may become very marked indeed. If this marked difference in the rash is seen on the skin, it is perhaps not surprising that a similar change should be occurring on other epithelial surfaces, such as mucous membranes in the respiratory and intestinal tracts, as suggested in Fig. 15.2. The difference in the outcome of the infection on these other surfaces may well do much to explain the difference in the disease. The difference in the type of rash was recognised in antiquity, and Rhazes in the year A.D. 850 wrote 'Measles which are of a deep red and violet colour are a bad and fatal kind'. The equivalent pathological changes

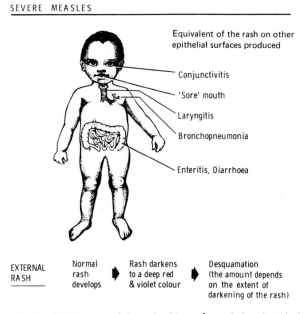

SEVERE MEASLES

Equivalent of the rash on other epithelial surfaces produced

Conjunctivitis

'Sore' mouth

Laryngitis

Bronchopneumonia

Enteritis, Diarrhoea

| EXTERNAL RASH | Normal rash develops | ▶ | Rash darkens to a deep red & violet colour | ▶ | Desquamation (the amount depends on the extent of darkening of the rash) |

Fig. 15.2 Stages in the development of the rash of 'severe measles' and equivalent changes on other surfaces

in the mouth are responsible for the extreme soreness of the mouth recorded in some areas, and the dreaded condition of cancrum oris is most frequently related to a recent attack of measles. Laryngitis which may require tracheotomy in many developing countries, is further evidence of epithelial changes. In the respiratory tract, the frequency of bronchopneumonia, and in the bowel the association with diarrhoea, are all well documented. Diarrhoea in West Africa was first noted as a severe complication of measles in 1850 and it is now recognized as a major cause for the severity of the disease in areas where it is so dangerous.

Studies in East Africa and elsewhere suggest some explanation for 'severe measles'. In the well nourished child multi-nucleate giant cells may be identified in the saliva or in scrapings from the oropharynx, but they disappear within 48 hours of the appearance of the rash. In the malnourished child they have been shown to persist for three weeks or longer. During this period it is possible that these children may still be infective. The persistence of these cells suggests that the production of lymphocytes competent to destroy cells infected with measles virus is delayed. As a result the virus multiplies for a longer period and most cells are infected. When sufficient competent lymphocytes are produced there is greater destruction of the epithelium, as seen on the skin and suggested by the blood-stained diarrhoea (Forbes and Sheifele 1972).

The frequency of encephalitis in the severe measles of poorly-nourished children in developing countries has not yet been fully documented, but convulsions and coma in children with measles are common.

Other reasons for measles being more severe

The view that severe measles is related to the poor nutrition of a child has only recently been developed, and consideration must be given to other arguments for a more severe variety of the disease. In particular, the suggestion has been made that there may be variation in the virulence of the virus. Yet in these days of rapid mass transport, there seems no reason for a virus to remain isolated to various areas of the world. There are now good studies of measles varying in severity within one community, being very much more severe in the less favoured socio-economic group.

One of the most revealing studies of the ravages of measles as a social disease was that undertaken in Glasgow early in this century (Chalmers 1930) when the fatality rate of measles had a six-fold difference depending on the socio-economic condition of the parents. At that time, economic differences were measured by the number of rooms occupied by the family. The case fatality rate in families who shared one room was nearly 10 per cent, whereas in those with four rooms or more it was under two per cent (see Fig. 15.3).

The occurrence of higher mortality rates in measles in younger children has long been recognised. This relationship was well demonstrated in an

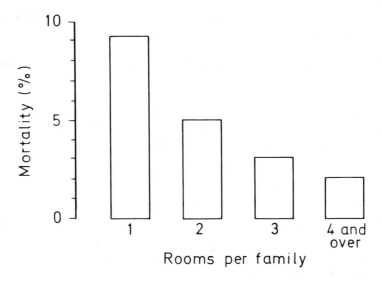

Fig. 15.3 Deaths from measles related to the socio-economic state of the family

American study (PAHO 1973). In Africa, where the case fatality rate has been studied, it is clear that infection is severe probably down to the age of nine months. An age-specific case fatality rate such as that found in the United Kingdom, if applied to the age structure of measles in a developing country, would explain only a part of a very much higher mortality in these areas. Evidence points, therefore, to other factors in the child's environment as being related to the type and severity of measles. Of these, as suggested already, the state of nutrition of the child and the size of the infecting dose

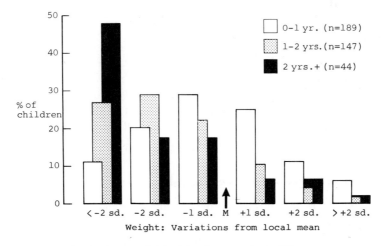

Fig. 15.4 Weight distribution of children dying from measles in different age groups/Manshande et al, *Lancet* 1981 (1) 779

are two possibilities. A recent study from Africa points to the possibility that in the older child of two to three years, nutrition is likely to be the important variable. (Fig. 15.4). By contrast, in the younger child it would seem that nutrition is not important as the distribution by weight of children dying in this age group is similar to that of the general local population. Perhaps this group of children suffers more severe measles because of higher infecting doses. They receive this higher infecting dose in part because of long contact over a period with the infecting child and also perhaps because, in the malnourished child, not only will the infecting period be longer, but the child may also secrete more virus.

Detrimental effect of measles on the nutritional state of the child

So far emphasis has been placed on measles as being more severe in the malnourished child, but of equal importance is the effect of measles on the child's nutrition. This was well brought out by a longitudinal study in Africa (see Table 15.1) when almost a quarter of the children with measles lost 10 per cent weight: further studies showed that full recovery could take up to three months. The place that measles plays in precipitating children into marasmus in infancy, and particularly kwashiorkor in toddler, is now well recognized in East and West Africa.

Table 15.1 Percentage of former weight lost during measles by 220 Imesi (Nigeria) village children

	None	Under 5%	5%	10%	20% 15%	and over
No. of children	24	71	72+	34	16	3
Percentage	11	32	32.7	15.5	7.3	1.5

To summarize the interaction of measles and poor nutrition on the child it may be concluded that the less well-nourished child has a more severe form of the disease, in which a darkening of the rash is followed by desquamation and that equivalent changes on other epithelial surfaces, for examples the respiratory and intestinal tracts, are probably responsible for the so-called complications of the disease, particularly brochopneumonia and diarrhoea. At the same time, the child's nutrition in these communities is likely to suffer a severe setback from the attack of measles, and as a result he or she may be precipitated into marasmus or kwashiorkor.

Geographical limitations of severe measles

Severe measles is now limited to the economically less privileged areas of the world, most of which lie in warm climate countries. Table 15.2 indicates that measles as it occurred more than 50 years ago in the U.K. was very similar to the disease as it now manifests in the developing countries.

Although in these areas measles is the most severe of the immunizing

Table 15.2 Features of measles in West Africa today, and in Great Britain today and before about 1920

	West Africa (today)	Great Britain (today)	Great Britain (before 1920)
Peak age incidence	17 months (Ilesha)	4 years	Under 3 years
Bronchopneumonia	Common and severe	Uncommon	Common and severe
Pharngitis	Common	Uncommon	Common
Diarrhoea	Frequent	Almost unknown	Frequent
Darkening of rash	Common	Unknown	Common
Desquamation	Common, may be severe	Practically unnoticed	Common
Effect on Child's Nutrition	Severe	Transient	Probably severe
Otitis media	? Uncommon	? Common	? Uncommon
Mortality	1:2	1:10 000	1:20(Glasgow 1908)

diseases of childhood, and is exceeded as a cause of death only by respiratory and diarrhoeal diseases, its importance has only recently been widely recognised; this is probably related to the strong beliefs about the disease that are found in almost every community. In rural India, measles is believed to be due to a goddess, Mata, and the child is often kept in the dark at the back of the house. Even the neighbours are unlikely to be informed of the illness, and the child is not usually seen by a doctor. In Africa, as in many other areas, the diet may be restricted, and fluid intake reduced, while treatment which includes injections is avoided. In South America, a very wide range of beliefs, depending on the origins of the people, are to be found.

In the industrialized countries of the world, measles used to be considered a 'natural' disease, through which all children must pass; this is still the case in many developing countries where on this account the disease is often not brought to the attention of health workers. Even when children die from measles and a death certificate is issued, the importance of this disease may not be appreciated as was illustrated in a study of the causes of death among children in different areas of South and Central America (Puffer and Serrano 1973). The assignment of deaths to measles among children less than five years of age was then compared with the causes stated on their death certificates; in only half of those considered to have died from measles was this the stated cause on the death certificate (Table 15.3).

Measles immunization

In terms of cost-effectiveness measles immunization is likely to be the most effective of all measures that an epidemiologist can persuade the health services to embark on. As so often in the present delivery of health services all over the world, those least in need of a service are the first to receive it. Measles vaccine is a live attenuated vaccine. It has been particularly successfully used in the United States, where an enegetic policy had led to virtual

Table 15.3 Final assignment for deaths of children under five to measles, compared with causes stated on death certificates (PAHO Report 1973)

Recorded on death certificate	Finally assigned to measles	
	No.	%
Measles	915	51.5
Pneumonia, influenza and other diseases of the respiratory tract	339	19.1
Diarrhoea	288	16.2
Other infections and other parasitic diseases	77	4.3
Nutritional deficiencies	79	4.4
All other cases	79	4.5
Total deaths	1777	100.0

eradication by the end of 1982. By that time, transmission in the U.S.A. had ceased, although cases will still be introduced from across the border which may lead to further cases amongst those who have escaped immunization. In the rest of the world and particularly Europe, measles vaccine has not been used so energetically. In the developing countries, however, thanks to the W.H.O. Expanded Program of Immunization (see Robinson, Chapter 4) levels are much improved on those of a few years ago, although the goal of universal immunization by the year 1990 will be difficult to achieve. This program has shown that the problems are largely logistic and that the expense of immunization is largely in the personnel and equipment rather than in the vaccine. Currently, in multi-dose ampules the vacine will cost between 10 to 20 U.S. cents per dose.

Vaccine is prepared from a live attenuated strain grown in chick-embryo fibroblasts. Recently, the vaccine in the dry form has been much improved in terms of theromolability. This has been achieved through using a variety of sugars, including sorbitol, in the drying process. With the modern vaccines, the reactions are minimal, although a small proportion will experience a rise in body temperature and perhaps one in a thousand children may have a convulsion. This is less than a tenth of what would be expected with natural measles and the convulsions in the natural disease are much more severe. Protection after measles vaccination persists for many years and probably for life.

A difficulty in developing countries is the age at which the vaccine should be given. In more developed countries the vaccine is usually given at around 14 months. If, however, vaccination is delayed to this age in developing countries a third or more of the children will have suffered from measles. After a number of trials and using mathematical models W.H.O. has come out with a strong recommendation that measles vaccine should be given at nine months or as soon as possible afterwards. Unfortunately even by nine months a considerable proportion, perhaps over 10 per cent of children, may have already had measles. Also as so often happens the child will not be available for vaccination at nine months so that a number of children are likely to develop measles before vaccination. A possible important new development is the use of measles vaccine through an aerosol. Sabin has shown that using this route, children between four and six months may be safely immunized. (Sabin et al 1983).

WHOOPING COUGH

Whooping cough is a disease that has declined in importance in industrialized countries, as shown in Fig. 15.5 for England and Wales. Thirty years ago it was a cause of many thousands of deaths, whereas in the last few years the number of deaths per annum has fallen below 50. This decline in morbidity and mortality has been reflected in a decline in the research and study undertaken on the disease. In the developing countries, the importance of this disease still remains an enigma, for although the evidence from epidemiological studies indicates that whooping cough causes many deaths, the evidence from clinical sources does not confirm this. The possible reasons for this discrepancy will be considered.

As indicated in discussing measles, 'droplet infections' in developing countries occur in early childhood and this factor, in conjunction with

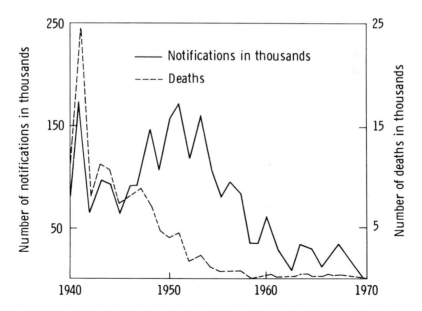

Fig. 15.5 The decline in whooping cough morbidity and mortality. The mortality was falling before immunization was introduced in the fifties

malnutrition, is a major reason why 97 per cent of all deaths among the under-five year olds now take place in the developing countries.

In measles, the high death rates in early life in developing countries are associated with the interaction between the disease and malnutrition. In whooping cough, the more important factor is the occurrence of this infection in the first months or years of life. The high case fatality rate in early infancy is a feature of whooping cough. This disease in the older child is well recognized by the community and by health workers. In the infant in the first six months of life, whooping cough is frequently unrecognized by the community and may not be diagnosed by health workers. Death from whooping cough in the early age group is sudden and unexpected and for this reason may not come to the notice of health personnel.

A failure of immunization in England during the '70s and early '80s has led to a fairly major epidemic of whooping cough. Unexpectedly, the mortality among small babies has remained relatively low. This may, in part, be due to the better management of these infants in severe respiratory stress. Another possibility is that unlike in developing countries, the population recognise the 'germ theory' of disease, and small babies are likely to be kept separate in most families from older children who have whooping cough even if this is only considered by the parents to be an ordinary respiratory illness. The same separation does not exist in less developed countries and, here again, as in measles the young infant may receive a massive infecting dose leading to a more severe infection.

Age incidence of whooping cough

Figures from a number of developing countries in Africa are compared with England and North America and given in Table 15.4. From this it will be seen that whooping cough is common in the first two years of life in these countries, whereas in England and North America it was more common around the fourth and fifty years of life. The importance of this age incidence is brought out in Fig. 15.6, in which the mortality at different ages in children in the Ilesha hospital, West Africa, is compared with figures

Table 15.4 The medium age of whooping cough in developing countries compared with U.S. and U.K.

	Number of cases	Median age (months)
West Africa	2569	24.4
East Africa	2778	35.1
Congo and South Africa	860	23.6
Jordan	942	23.5
Lebanon and North Afriuca	954	35.6
England and Wales (1945)	92 266	45.6
Aberdeen (1890–1900)	15 094	38.4
Massachusetts (1945)	15 094	62.4

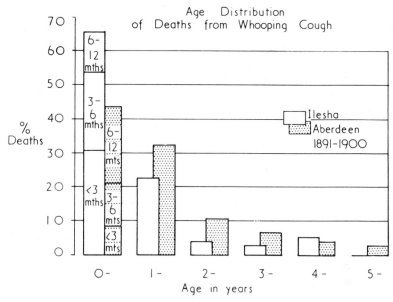

Fig. 15.6 These and many other studies have shown that the majority of deaths from whooping cough occur in the early years of life

from the city of Aberdeen in the last decade of the nineteenth century. These are confirmed by figures from North America and the U.K. in the last 20 years, in which deaths from whooping cough have occurred mainly in the first two years of life.

Although the clinical syndrome of whooping cough may rarely be caused by organisms and viruses other than *Bordetella pertussis*, the latter remains responsible for the majority of clinically diagnosed cases in both the developed and developing countries. Most cases will continue to be diagnosed on clinical features, so that an understanding of the march of synptoms, as described below, is essential if the disease is to be satisfactorily dignosed. A typical description of the development of the disease is as follows*

Whooping cough should be considered as an acute respiratory disease, beginning with a slight cough, usually accompanied by coryza; the cough then assumes a frequency which is out of proportion with the thin nasal discharge, and comes in bursts.

Unlike the child with bronchitis, the child with whooping cough does not take a breath in anticipation of the burst of coughing. At the end of the second week the coughing spasms increase in speed, rise in pitch, and the paroxysms become longer and more intense. The rapid spasmodic cough is at this stage generally associated with choking and vomiting, with the production of sticky, stringy sputum. In spite of the disturbing spasmodic cough, ausculatory signs may be absent from the lungs, and in the early stages the effect on the child's health may be surprisingly small.

To this may be added the fact that in developing countries where a degree of undernourishment is present, oedema of the eyelids is more common, and its presence is useful in aiding diagnosis. In those communities in which breast-feeding is well maintained, the mother has an intimate knowledge of the state of her child's mouth, and the presence of whooping cough may be indicated by the way she recognizes and picks out stringy sputum from the mouth.

The succession of events in the development of whooping cough in the older child is shown in Fig. 15.7. The stages of the disease are as follows. After an incubation period of one to two weeks there is a catarrhal stage, when cough and nasal discharge are present, sometimes with sneezing, and post-nasal swab cultures are usually positive. This syndrome, which cannot easily be differentiated from any other respiratory infection, is soon followed by the paroxysmal period, in which the spasmodic cough becomes more and more severe. The bursts of coughing are not preceded by inspiration; they may produce cyanosis, choking, vomiting and particularly in older children end with the typical whoop. The paroxysmal period may last for several weeks, and from this the child passes into convalescence. During this period of convalescence and for the subsequent year the child is in considerable danger of developing a recrudescene. In this period any mild upper respiratory infection may rapidly progress to a cough and pneumonia. Possibly the bronchioles becomes obstructed, causing persistent collapse in the lung, and within a few hours the child may be very ill with evidence of local atelectasis, and later bronchopneumonia.

In the younger child, as shown in Fig. 15.8, the disease may run a different course. It may develop within the first few weeks of life, and in

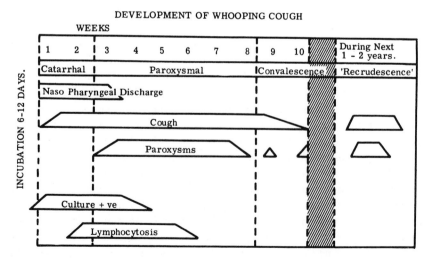

Fig. 15.7 The natural history of easily recognizable whooping cough in the older child

DEVELOPMENT OF WHOOPING COUGH IN BABIES UNDER 3 MONTHS

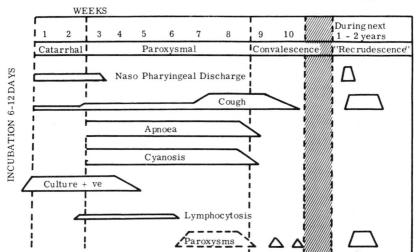

Fig. 15.8 Whooping cough in babies under 3 months. It is difficult to recognize in the early stages

all young infants it will create problems in diagnosis. The nasopharyngeal discharge may be scanty and is not followed by the development of a typical paroxysmal cough. Instead there may be apnoeic periods with intense cyanosis and sometimes convulsive episodes. Subconjunctival haemorrhages are common. The disease has a severe effect on the infant's nutrition, and frequently results in failure to gain weight over several months. In the first few months of life, fatality rates as high as 30 to 40 per cent have occurred, and whooping cough is one of the few diseases in which both incidence and case fatality are higher in girls than in boys.

The medical services of developing countries fail to make allowance for their large population of children, and any service that is effective will be swamped with children. Under these conditions the young infant arrives at a clinic or hospital in the early stages of whooping cough, is seen by the medical worker sleeping on his mother's knee with a chest free of physical signs of disease and does not gain admission to hospital. Such a child will receive scant attention compared with the child obviously ill, suffering from measles bronchopneumonia. This same infant may well die an acute and sudden death within an hour or so, on the way home with the mother. Recent evidence for this comes from the PAHO study, where in the city of Recife, Brazil, only three deaths from whooping cough were recorded on the certificates, whereas 28 were certified on final assignment. In the whole PAHO study, the assignment for infective diseases was low on death certificates, and as shown in Fig. 15.9 whooping cough was second only to measles in being under-diagnosed as a cause of death.

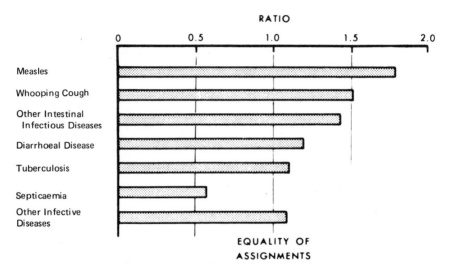

Fig. 15.9 The cause of death or death certificates was compared with that following full investigation. In this figure the ratio between death certification and final assignment shows that many cases of measles and whooping cough go unreported

Treatment and prevention

If epidemiological studies can awaken clinicians to the importance of whooping cough in the early months, then it is possible that a great many early infections can be aborted, and the lives of the children saved. In the author's West African clinics, all the nurses responsible for seeing children were taught that when a two- or three-year old was brought with whooping cough, their main responsibility was to enquire whether there were young infants in the household with coughs, and to explain to the mother the urgency of bringing such infants for treatment in the first few days of their symptoms. Such children can be treated with chloramphenicol or erythromycin and the infection, which results from their proximity to older children with the disease can be assumed to be whooping cough and may be satisfactorily aborted.

Immunization with pertussis vaccine contained in the DPT prophylactic has been the major reason for the decline in incidence of the disease in many developed countries. As with measles, the Expanded Program of Immunization is already reaching a quarter, or more, of children in some of the less developed countries, and in the majority there are programs to spread this immunization widely. As it is the small child who is so much in danger from whooping cough, immunization should be given early starting, if possible, at three months. The second and third doses should be at least a month apart and there are some advantages in having six weeks between injections. Where a child has not been brought for some months there is no need to restart the schedule. There is also concern that many children are not immunized due to other intercurrent infections or under-nutrition. The present policy is to give immunization to all children attending clinics unless they have a severe febrile infection. Immunization against illnesses such as whooping cough and measles should be available at every contact between child and health personnel. Only in this way can most of the infants be immunized as so many parents only bring their children for treatment when they are sick. Immunization is one of the key factors in the package of health measures available from an effective underfives clinic offering comprehensive care to all children brought to it.

REFERENCES

Chalmers A K 1930 The Health of Glasgow 1818–1925 p 343. Glasgow: Bell & Bain
Forbes C E, Scheifele D W 1973 The Management of Measles in Nairobi. E.Afr. Med.J. 50: 159
Krugman S, Ward R 5th Edition 1973 Infectious Diseases of Children. New York C V Mosby
Morley D C Paediatric Priorities in the Developing World 1973 London: Butterworths (This monograph contains many references on these diseases)
Puffer R R, Serrano C V 1973 Patterns of Mortality in Childhood. Pan American Health Organization Publication No 262
Sabin et al 1983 Measles Immunization by Aerosol. Journal of American Medical Association, 249: 2651–2662

Leprosy

INTRODUCTION

Leprosy is a chronic disease of man attributed to infection by *Mycobacterium leprae* and affecting primarily nerves, skin and the mucosa of the upper respiratory tract. It is also a social disease, associated with fear, stigma and social disruption in many communities. Though once found as far north as the Arctic Circle (Irgens, 1980), leprosy is largely restricted to the tropical and subtropical regions of the world today.

This chapter reviews current understanding of the natural history of leprosy, and discusses practical considerations of its control in endemic regions. For fuller treatment of these subjects, the reader is referred to specialised reviews and textbooks (Bryceson and Pfaltzgraff 1979; Canizares 1975; Fine 1982; Fitzpatrick 1979; World Health Organisation 1977, 1980, 1982).

THE DISEASE

Clinical leprosy manifests itself in a variety of forms, conventionally class-ified along a spectrum from tuberculoid through borderline to lepromatous. This spectrum coincides with important immunological, bacteriological and histopathological differences (Fig. 16.1). Several classification systems have been used to describe this spectrum, the most important being the 'Madrid' classification which is based upon clinical criteria and widely used in field-work (Committee on Classification 1953) and the 'Ridley-Jopling' classifi-cation which emphasises histopathological and immunological criteria, and is widely used in research (Ridley and Jopling 1966). An Indian classifi-cation, preferred in that country, is substantially similar (Association of Indian Leprologists 1982).

Pure or 'polar' tuberculoid leprosy is characterised by a single lesion showing anhidrosis and diminished sensitivity to light touch, which appears hypopigmented in dark skin and has a well-defined raised edge. The edge may be pebbled or slightly scaly. If the edge is not well defined, or if satellite lesions have appeared near the main lesion, containment is not complete and

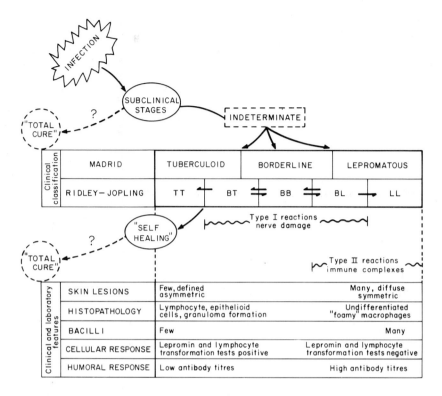

Fig. 16.1 The course of leprosy: infection and disease. Heavy solid arrows and compartments represent accepted pathways; dotted arrows and compartments denote controversial stages. 'Total cure' implies freedom of the host from bacilli. The clinical spectrum is described according to the Madrid and the Ridley-Jopling classification systems: TT = polar tuberculoid; BT = borderline tuberculoid; BB = borderline lepromatous; LL = polar lepromatous. The lower table summarises the basic clinical and laboratory features of leprosy at opposite ends of the spectrum. (Adapted from Fine 1982).

the disease is said to approach the middle or 'borderline' region of the range. Enlargement of and damage to nerves in tuberculoid leprosy is usually restricted to peripheral nerves near the skin lesions, though it is possible for nerve damage to occur without any skin lesion. In borderline-tuberculoid forms it is not uncommon for skin and nerve lesions to be unrelated. Tuberculoid leprosy is associated with few bacilli, granulomatous histology, low specific antibody titres and with strong specific cell-mediated immunity.

At the other end of the spectrum is pure lepromatous leprosy, which usually begins with widespread, ill-defined erythematous lesions. The macules, papules or nodules may be difficult to see. If the lesions are well defined and there are areas of normal skin between them the correct classification will be borderline lepromatous. At the lepromatous end of the spectrum nerve damage usually starts with the nerve endings in the skin leading to what is sometimes called 'high glove and stocking' anaesthesia (although palms and soles are typically spared until later stages in the disease process). Motor fibre damage is not initially a feature of lepromatous disease. Lepromatous leprosy is associated with masses of bacilli in globi within dermal histiocytes, often high titres of *M. Leprae*- specific antibodies and an apparent absence of specific cell-mediated immunity.

It is important to appreciate the temporal development of leprosy. The incubation period is long and variable. Though clinical lesions may appear during the first year of life in infants born to parents with the disease, infection in later life may not become manifest for many years. There is evidence that the incubation period preceding tuberculoid leprosy (2–5 year median) is shorter than that preceding lepromatous forms (8–12 years) (Brubaker et al 1969).

Many leprologists believe that the disease may go through an 'indeterminate' stage before becoming classifiable along the main tuberculoid-lepromatous spectrum. Indeterminate lesions are generally defined as flat and hypopigmented macules with or without signs of anaesthesia (Bryceson and Pfaltzgraff 1979). The definition of this type of leprosy is vague and unsatisfactory and there is bound to be some confusion with secondary hypopigmentation, particularly in dark skin, due to birthmarks, the application of 'local' medicine, fungous infections, infected insect bites, malnutrition and other stimuli.

A more important issue concerns the fate of established clinical lesions. Tuberculoid leprosy may self-heal, leaving little or no residual sign; or it may remain stationary for long periods of time; or it may gradually shift towards the borderline region. Alternatively, the disease process may shift suddenly towards the borderline or lepromatous region, associated with irreversible nerve damage and disabilities (Type-1, 'downgrading' reaction). The opposite shift may also occur, from borderline towards tuberculoid disease, particularly in patients under treatment. This shift may be associated with an acute or subacute clinical episode, often with nerve damage (Type-1, 'reversal' or 'upgrading' reaction). Polar lepromatous leprosy usually progresses relentlessly, leaving its victim with severe disabilities unless the process is halted by treatment. Approximately 50 per cent of treated lepromatous patients suffer at least one acute reactional episode involving immune complexes — erythema nodosum leprosum (ENL, Type-2 reaction) — generally within 18 months of commencing chemotherapy.

Clinical diagnosis of tuberculoid or borderline leprosy is often based on the appearance of skin lesions, but should include a systematic examination of peripheral nerves for enlargement, asymmetry and tenderness, together with testing for loss of sensation and muscle power. Slit skin smears (see below) should be performed if there is any indication of borderline or lepromatous disease. A positive smear is necessary for the diagnosis of early lepromatous disease. Reliance upon clinical criteria for diagnosis is often unsatisfactory, but unavoidable unless facilities are available to take and examine biopsies.

Treatment

Since 1950, dapsone monotherapy has been conventional treatment in most areas of the world. 100 mg daily for adults has been the preferred dose in recent years, but much lower doses were used widely before 1970. It has generally been recommended that tuberculoid cases should continue such treatment for at least two years after their lesions have become inactive, but that patients near the lepromatous end of the spectrum should continue treatment for life. Multiple drug regimens combining clofazimine or rifampicin with dapsone have been recommended increasingly for patients with multibacillary disease in order to hasten the disappearance of viable bacilli and to impede the appearance of dapsone resistance.

Dapsone monotherapy and poor compliance have encouraged the emergence of dapsone resistance worldwide. This has led to radically new recommendations for short course multiple drug therapy for all leprosy patients, by a WHO Study Group on Chemotherapy of Leprosy Control Programmes (1982). Their basic recommendation is as follows:

— for multibacillary leprosy (adult dosages)
    Rifampicin   — 600 mg once monthly, supervised
    Dapsone   — 100 mg daily, self-administered
    Clofazimine   — 300 mg once monthly, supervised, and 50 mg daily
        self-administered

(This regimen should be given for at least two years, and be continued wherever possible up to smear negativity).

— for paucibacillary leprosy (adult dosages)
    Rifampicin   — 600 mg once monthly, supervised
    Dapsone   — 100 mg daily, self-administered

(This combined treatment should be given for six months only).

Type-1 reactions should be treated as early as possible with corticosteroids. The treatment of Type-2 reactions is less uniform and depends upon the severity of the reaction and its response to treatment (Jolliffe 1977).

Untreated lepromatous patients may be a source of infection for the community but are rendered non-infectious within 3–4 months on dapsone alone, and within 3–7 days on rifampicin (Shepard et al 1964; WHO 1982). They may be treated at home in the same manner as tuberculoid cases. Institutionalisation is no longer recommended in most countries, and is now discouraged as the practice increases popular fear of the disease and makes control programmes more difficult.

THE AGENT

Clinical leprosy is a response to infection with the leprosy bacillus, *Mycobacterium leprae*, discovered by Armauer Hansen in 1873. Though the bacilli are scanty and found with difficulty in tuberculoid patients, they are found in abundance in biopsies, slit skin smears and frequently also the nasal discharge of active lepromatous patients (Davey and Rees 1974; Shepard 1962). They are acid-fast rods, 2–3 μ long, often seen as intracellular clumps or globi.

The skin slit smear is the classical technique for identifying leprosy bacilli in patients. Using a sterile scalpel, a small incision is made into the upper part of the dermis, without drawing blood. A small amount of tissue fluid is obtained by scraping the base and sides of the incision with the blade. This fluid is smeared on a slide, heat fixed and stained for acid-fast bacilli (Bryceson and Pfaltzgraff 1979). The number of M. leprae in skin slit smears is conventionally expressed on a logarithmic scale as the 'Bacillary Index' or 'BI' (Ridley 1958).

	Number of M. leprae seen
BI	per oil immersion (1000X) microscope field
1	1–9 per 100 fields
2	1–9 per 10 fields
3	1–9 per field
4	10–99 per field
5	100–999 per field
6	⩾1000 per field

A BI of 6 implies that there are between 10^9 and 10^{13} organisms in the patient's body. In addition to the simple BI count, the percentage of solidly staining M. leprae, as distinct from fragments and granules, is often determined and expressed as the 'Morphological Index' (MI). It is generally believed that the MI reflects the proportion of viable bacilli in the patient (Rees and Valentine 1962). Other indices have been suggested and are in use (e.g. Ridley 1971).

Skin slit smears should be taken from the earlobes and from skin lesions of all suspected borderline or lepromatous cases, from relapsed cases, and from all cases before release from control. Results may differ markedly between sites, in particular during relapses and also during reactions, and should be reported separately. For district hospitals and smaller institutions a simple grading of skin slit smear results from negative to highly positive, without a morphological index, will probably have to suffice unless the laboratory technician can be specially trained and has considerable practice in the procedure.

Though M. leprae has not yet been grown in vitro, it grows in the mouse foot pad (Shepard 1960), nine banded armadillo (Kirchheimer and Storrs 1971), and in nude mice (Hastings et al 1981). This has allowed detailed bacteriological characterisation and drug sensitivity studies. Animal inoculation experiments have revealed that M. leprae remains viable outside the human body for several days, in particular under humid conditions (Davey and Rees 1974).

EPIDEMIOLOGY

Time and place

It is estimated that there are approximately 10.5 million clinical cases of leprosy in the world today (Sansarricq 1981). On the basis of broad geographic patterns and secular trends of leprosy the world may be divided into 7 zones (Fine 1982):

1. The Old World tropical and subtropical belt: this area is considered the ancestral home of leprosy. Approximately 90 per cent of the world's leprosy patients live in subsaharan Africa or southern Asia. A third of them live in India.

2. Mediterranean Basin: prevalence is low (below 0.0001 in the general population), focal, and probably decreasing.

3. Northern Europe: it is believed that leprosy was widespread in Northern Europe a thousand years ago but that it started to decline after the thirteenth century. The last known endemic case in the British Isles was recorded in 1798. In Norway approximately 8000 leprosy patients were registered in the latter half of the nineteenth century and the last recorded endemic case had onset in 1950. The disappearance of leprosy from Northern Europe remains a major puzzle, and has been attributed to a variety of influences, such as: decreased importation of cases after the last Crusade; high mortality of the susceptible population from plague; cross protection by tuberculosis infections; improved nutrition; improved living standards (decreased crowding, improved hygiene, better clothing), and/or isolation of infectious leprosy patients from the community (Chaussinand 1948).

4. Northern Asia: leprosy is present in parts of Russia and China, but there is little published information on its prevalence and distribution.

5. South and Central America, including southern United States: it is thought that *M. leprae* was introduced into this region from Southern Europe and Africa. It has remained endemic at a low level ever since, except in Chile, which appears to have remained free of transmission.

6. Northern United States and Eastern Canada: leprosy was introduced by French, German and Norwegian immigrants. It persisted in several well-defined foci and within certain families for several generations and then disappeared.

7. Pacific Islands and Australia: leprosy was introduced into a number of islands and into Australia during the past two centuries. The best known example is that of the island of Nauru (1°S, 167°E), where a single case was introduced into a population of approximately 1300 people in 1912, resulting in an epidemic which is reported to have affected some 30 per cent of the population over the next 20 years. In Australia leprosy still persists among aborigines in the Northern regions of that continent.

The clinical type distribution varies between different regions of the world. In general the proportion of lepromatous cases among newly diagnosed patients (the 'lepromatous rate') is highest (above 20 per cent) in Europe and the Americas, intermediate (5–20 per cent) in Asia, and lowest in subsaharan Africa (below 5 per cent).

A prominent feature of leprosy in endemic areas is clustering within certain families, villages or areas. This has been widely discussed and is an important reason for the view that genetics plays an important part in leprosy. But it is in general difficult to assess to what extent the clustering of leprosy may be real, reflecting focal incidence patterns or shared susceptibility, or else an artifact, reflecting social forces tending to segregate cases or ascertainment bias (non-homogenous case detection). A clear explanation of the roles played by these several factors would represent a major advance in our understanding of leprosy.

There is evidence that leprosy is more rural than urban in its distribution in many areas of the world. On the other hand, a tendency for rural incidence may be counteracted by the movement of cases towards urban centres to seek medical attention or to beg, leading to an accumulation of cases in cities (Fine 1982).

Age and sex

Routinely available statistics generally reflect prevalence, i.e. case loads on registers or treatment programmes. Such data are strongly affected by local policies of case ascertainment (e.g. whether or not school surveys or household contact surveys are performed) and registry maintenance (e.g. policies for updating ages and for deleting cured, lost or dead cases), and generally

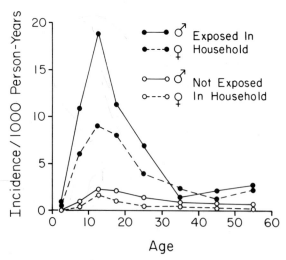

Fig. 16.2 Incidence rates of clinical leprosy in Cordova and Talisay municipalities, Cebu, Philippines, by age, sex, and whether exposed in household. Data refer to the first third of the 20th century. (From Doull et al 1942).

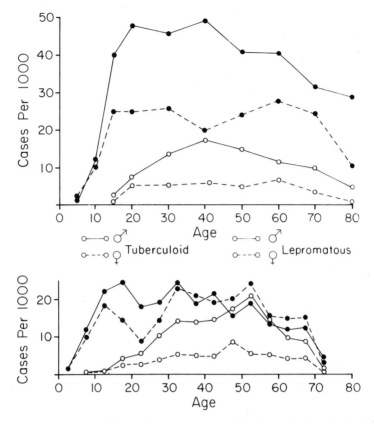

Fig. 16.3 Prevalence rates of leprosy by age, sex, and clinical type (Madrid classification). A: data for BCG trial area in northern Burma (Bechelli et al 1973). B: data from Gudiyatham Taluk in Tamil Nadu, South India (Rao et al 1972a). In both populations the prevalence of borderline disease was lower than that for either tuberculoid or lepromatous types.

are very poor reflections of the actual leprosy distribution in a community. Our only reliable data come from a few systematic surveys of populations, in particular those associated with BCG trials (Bechelli et al 1973; Dominguez et al 1980; Doull et al 1942; Rao et al 1972a 1972b). These studies allow several generalisations (see Figs. 16.2, 16.3). Clinical leprosy is rare among children under the age of 5 years. In most areas incidence rates rise to a peak between age 10–25 and then fall, and are consistently higher for those in household contact with leprosy cases than for the general population. Incidence rates of lepromatous disease are lower, and rise at a later age, than those for tuberculoid disease. The latter observation may reflect the longer incubation period preceding lepromatous disease. There is little difference in leprosy incidence between the sexes among children, but higher incidence rates have frequently been observed among male than among female adults, in particular for lepromatous disease.

Prevalence patterns reflect the accumulation of past incidence, recoveries, cures and deaths. Prevalence rates generally rise to a plateau between 30–50 years of age and then decline. The longer incubation period and duration of lepromatous disease mean that the lepromatous rate generally increases with age, though this may be counteracted among the very old by an elevated mortality rate among lepromatous patients (Smith and Guinto 1978). A male excess is generally observed among adults, in particular among lepromatous cases, though exceptions to this rule of male excess are reported in some African populations (Bechelli et al 1966).

Sources and modes of infection

The transmission of *M. leprae* remains one of the major riddles in leprosy. It is generally presumed that *M. leprae* is maintained by direct human-to-human transmission. Though there has long been discussion of possible environmental sources of infection, the only confirmed extra human resorvoir is in armadillos of the southern United States (Walsh et al 1981). This appears to be an example of 'reverse zoonosis' (*M. leprae* having been introduced into the new world armadillos by man) and there is no evidence that it is an important source of human infection.

The problem thus probably resolves to identifying the human sources of infection in the community and how transmission occurs. Patients towards the lepromatous end of the spectrum would seem the most obvious sources of bacilli, as it has been demonstrated that they may shed very large numbers of viable bacilli (up to 10^7 per day) in their nasal discharge (Davey and Rees 1974). They may thus be analagous to open pulmonary cases of tuberculosis as sources of infection in the community. On the other hand, many workers have argued that tuberculoid cases are also infectious. Though it is conceded that tuberculoid cases are individually far less important than individual lepromatous cases, the fact that the great majority of cases are tuberculoid might mean that they are in fact responsible for most of the transmission in a community (e.g. Guinto 1978). The argument is further complicated by the varying importance which different workers would place upon subclinical cases or cases in reaction as sources of bacilli.

The view that the upper respiratory tract of lepromatous cases is the predominant source of infection in the community has bacteriological support. It has proved difficult to identify leprosy bacilli on the skin of lepromatous cases, or from any portal of exit of tuberculoid cases (Pedley 1978). The major arguments against it concern the rarity of known lepromatous cases in most endemic communities, in particular in Africa, and an inability to elicit a history of contact between most incident cases and known lepromatous patients. This paradox may just reflect the difficulties of tracing contacts years after the event. Similarly, the fact that household contacts of tuberculoid cases are found to have an elevated risk of developing clinical leprosy may just reflect the fact that such individuals are more likely to have had contact with extra familial lepromatous cases than are individuals with no known household contact with any leprosy.

Some workers have suggested that insects might serve as vectors of *M. leprae* (Kirchheimer 1976). While there is evidence that culicine mosquitoes or bedbugs can pick up viable bacilli from lepromatous patients, there is no compelling evidence that this mechanism is important in nature.

The argument favouring lepromatous cases as the predominant sources of infection in communities has several important implications. First, it contradicts the traditional view that prolonged or intimate contact is necessary for transmission of *M. leprae*. Second, it suggests that *M. leprae* infection is far more widespread in endemic communities than is clinical disease. If only transient contact with lepromatous cases is sufficient for transmission of infection, then almost all individuals in daily contact with such cases are likely to be infected, though most of them never develop clinical disease. Third, as a consequence of the above, it means that the distribution of clinical leprosy in communities is not just a reflection of the distribution of infection *per se*, but is influenced to an important degree by the distribution of factors regulating the response to infection in the human host.

The inference that *M. leprae* infection is far more widespread in endemic communities than is clinical disease is now supported by a growing body of bacteriological and immunological evidence. Several surveys in India have revealed *M. leprae*-like bacilli in the skin of up to five per cent of healthy persons in endemic areas (Chatterjee et al 1976). And surveys with lymphocyte transformation tests (Godal and Negassi 1973), skin tests with soluble *M. leprae* antigens (Convit et al 1975) and fluorescent antibody tests (Abe et al 1980) have all suggested a high prevalence of *M. leprae* infection or at least of sensitisation to *M. leprae* antigens. None of these tests is ideal in terms of sensitivity and specificity; but nonetheless the accumulating evidence is consistent in indicating widespread subclinical *M. leprae* infection in endemic communities.

Factors determining clinical expression of infection

Despite the increasing evidence that factors affecting the host response to infection determine the distribution of disease in communities, we are still unclear as to the nature and relative importance of these factors. Many have been suggested and studied: e.g. host genetics, route and dose of infection, immunological interactions between responses to different infections, or physiological factors such as nutrition and pregnancy.

The apparent family clustering of leprosy has engendered a long tradition of considering genetical factors. Twin studies have found higher concordance rates for leprosy among monozygote than dizygote pairs, but biases in ascertainment and diagnosis have weakened the strength of these studies. More convincing evidence has come from studies of the segregation of the

HLA types within families with multiple cases of leprosy (Fine 1981). These investigations suggest that an HLA-linked allele, perhaps HLA-DR2, acts in a recessive manner and predisposes to tuberculoid leprosy. Though these and related studies indicate that host genes do have some influence on the type of clinical response, it is apparent that they act in a complicated fashion and are by no means the only determinants involved.

Evidence that dose or route of infection might be important in determining clinical outcome has come largely from animal studies. It has been suggested that exposure to large doses might overwhelm the host's immune response and predispose towards lepromatous disease. Such a mechanism would predict that the risk of lepromatous disease should correlate to closeness of contact with lepromatous cases — but there is little or no evidence for such clustering. The argument for route of infection being important is based upon evidence in animal studies that an oral route may predispose to T cell suppression (and lepromatous disease) whereas skin or upper respiratory tract entry may lead to involvement of dermal Langerhans cells and strong cellular immunity (tuberculoid type disease). There is very little evidence bearing upon actual routes of infection in human communities (Fine 1982).

There is strong evidence that prior immunological experience can effect a host's response to *M. leprae* infection. BCG vaccination has been shown to provide approximately 80 per cent protection in Uganda (Stanley et al 1981), 45 per cent protection in New Guinea (Scott et al 1976), 30 per cent protection in South India (Tripathy, personal communication, 1982) and 20–30 per cent protection in Burma (Bechelli et al 1974). This evidence for varying protection efficacy is similar to the situation with tuberculosis. It has been argued that this variation may be due to the prevalence of infection with different environmental mycobacteria in the several study areas. Consistent with this view is the observation that natural tuberculin sensitivity was associated with protection against leprosy among unvaccinated persons in Uganda, though not in Burma (Stanley et al 1981).

With regard to physiological influences on host response, there is widespread belief and limited data that pregnancy and lactation may increase the risk of clinical onset or reaction among women (Duncan et al 1981). Similarly, there is widespread belief but almost no data supporting an association between malnutrition and leprosy (Edelman 1979; Rees 1981). As leprosy is associated with poverty in most endemic areas its relationship to the many factors of the poverty complex — crowding, poor hygiene, malnutrition and intercurrent infection — is difficult to untangle.

SURVEILLANCE

The combination of low prevalence, clustering, stigma and difficult diagnosis makes it difficult to obtain reliable estimates of prevalence or incidence of leprosy in any given area. Passive case detection and reporting are liable to give a low and distorted picture. Routine statistics are further affected by differences and changes in policies of maintaining case registers. School surveys provide one method for population screening, and are routine in some areas. Such surveys may not give an accurate assessment of leprosy in the community, in particular if school attendance rates are low and if there is the possibility that attendance is selectively low from families with leprosy. On the other hand, repeated school surveys may provide an indication of incidence trends in a population.

The optimal approach to assessing the extent and distribution of leprosy in a region is thus by household surveys either throughout the population or in a random sample of villages or townships. Such surveys are expensive in time and personnel and require careful planning, organisation and field supervision. Though it may not be possible to carry out such surveys on a routine basis, even a single survey can be valuable in providing a baseline against which to assess information obtained from routine sources.

CONTROL

In theory the objectives of a control programme are to reduce the incidence and prevalence of disease in the community. While it is reasonable to suppose that effective ascertainment and treatment of infectious cases should lead to reduced incidence rates of leprosy, there is little hard evidence that this has ever been achieved (Fine 1982). This may reflect our ignorance of the natural history of leprosy, or it may indicate inadequate assessment of control programmes. On the other hand it may lead us to argue that the primary goal of leprosy control programmes today should be the prevention of disabilities rather than reduction in incidence of disease *per se*. Given that nerve damage during reactions is a major cause of disability, it is particularly important that staff be able to recognise and treat patients in reaction.

Case finding procedures should be optimised within the constraints of the funds and staff available, with due consideration to the relative priority of leprosy in an area. In most areas there are insufficient resources for active case finding activities, but the examination of household and neighbourhood contacts of newly discovered lepromatous cases should be carried out routinely if at all feasible.

Integration of a leprosy control programme into the general health services, though desirable for the sake of reducing the stigma of the disease, can be difficult for a number of reasons. Health services in the third world are in general neither organised nor equipped for the treatment of the chronically ill — whether they be patients with hypertension, mental illness or leprosy. Furthermore, the relative rarity of leprosy means that few staff will see sufficient cases to gain the experience necessary to diagnose early leprosy, at a stage when there are yet no disabilities, and also to recognise and to treat reactions competently. Often the distance to the health centre will discourage patients from attending at all. And even more discouraging than distance are disinterested and unsympathetic staff.

It is possible for treatment to be given by village health workers, or primary health care workers; but it is particularly important that they be trained to recognise symptoms, reactions or allergies and to refer such patients to a supervisor. Some beds should be made available for the admission and treatment of leprosy patients in reaction and with other complications such as severe allergy against dapsone (Stevens-Johnson syndrome).

Regardless of whether a leprosy control programme is integrated into the general health services, or whether it is a separate vertical programme, it may be worthwhile to link it to existing tuberculosis services. Laboratory requirements are very similar for both services. And both patient groups require intensive encouragement and follow-up in order to achieve high attendance and success rates.

In any case, leprosy treatment should be on an out-patient or home-treatment basis. Enforced hospitalisation and segregation of patients are likely to be counter productive in that they will discourage patients from reporting early to the health services. Wherever possible the treatment should be based upon multiple drug short term regimens (see WHO recommendations above) rather than traditional dapsone monotherapy. Low compliance is a universal problem in leprosy control (Ellard 1981) and every effort should be made to ensure that the prescribed drug regimen is taken in full. The 1982 WHO recommendations require a minimum of monthly patient contact in order to supervise rifampicin administration. More frequent contact between health workers and patients, and appropriate discrimination in the handling of patients, should improve both compliance and case finding and should minimise the development of disabilities during treatment.

A leprosy control programme which continues to rely upon dapsone monotherapy will have to face the problem of secondary dapsone resistance in lepromatous patients and eventually also primary resistance in both tuberculoid and lepromatous patients. Clinically, secondary resistance becomes apparent when a lepromatous patient who has been treated for some years, and who is still on treatment, develops new lesions — for example nodules or papules — which are positive for solid M. leprae on skin slit smear. These new lesions do not disappear under supervised dapsone intake. Where feasible the resistance can be confirmed by sensitivity assays in the mouse footpad. In contrast, if someone has been infected de novo with dapsone resistant organisms there will be no — or hardly any — initial improvement with dapsone treatment. This is called primary resistance. The proportion of patients with dapsone resistance is now approximately five per cent in many areas of the world (Levy et al 1982). Resistance to the more powerful drugs, rifampicin or clofazimine, is still very rare.

The success of a leprosy control programme is extrememly difficult to evaluate within the usual financial and staffing constraints. Usually it will only be possible to monitor the functioning of the programme. Helpful parameters for such assessment include attendance rates, regularity of re-examination of patients ('reviews'), regularity of skin slit smears taken from multi-bacillary patients, and the percentage of patients discharged after review rather than 'lost' from follow-up. The proportion of incident cases with disabilities, and the average severity of disabilities, should decrease over time if a programme has been effective.

IMPROVED DEFENSE (PREVENTION)

Primary prevention of leprosy (reduction in incidence of new disease) can in principle be achieved either by removing the source of bacilli from the community (isolation or treatment of infectious cases) by impeding trans-mission (environmental changes) or by protecting potential recipients (chemoprophylaxis or immunisation).

Physical isolation of leprosy patients has been carried out in many soci-eties, but it is arguable whether it has had any impact on incidence (Irgens 1980). Given that modern drugs render patients non-infectious within a short period of time, there is no longer any rationale for isolation, in particular because the practice encourages fear and stigma of the disease. Chemical isolation of cases by effective drug therapy should lead to a reduc-tion of transmission in the community. Though sound in principle, this relationship has been difficult to demonstrate in practice (see above), and thus chemotherapy must still be considered of unproved efficacy as a method of primary prevention.

There is considerable circumstantial evidence that environmental changes and improvements in living standards may lead to reductions in leprosy risk. The mechanism of this relationship is not understood, but may function by improving host defenses (e.g. nutrition, changes in patterns of infection) as well as by reducing infection *per se* (e.g. by reducing crowding and improving hygiene). While this may provide some long range optimism, it provides little immediate comfort to those responsible for leprosy control today.

Chemoprophylaxis with long-acting injectable dapsone (DADDS) has been found effective in reducing incidence of clinical leprosy among high risk groups in several studies (Noordeen and Neelan 1978). But there is considerable cost and logistic complexity to this approach, and thus it has not been routinely recommended as a part of leprosy control.

BCG vaccination is probably the most effective preventive measure against leprosy being carried out in the world today. Protection afforded by the vaccine appears to vary between 30 and 80 per cent in different regions of the world. However, BCG vaccines are now being used on a large scale in many leprosy endemic areas, and are undoubtedly preventing many thou-sands of leprosy cases. It may be that this intervention has been more effective in controlling leprosy than in controlling tuberculosis! It is arguable whether BCG vaccination is sufficiently cost-effective to be recommended for leprosy control alone; however, given that it is being used, we must recognise that it is probably making an important contribution to leprosy control today.

CONSEQUENCES

Leprosy is a cause of severe physical and social disability. Physical disfigurement is largely the result of nerve involvement leading to paralysis, anaesthesia, ulcers, distortion and resorption of digits. Social problems arise from the stigma attached to the disease in many communities. Though originally a cultural response to the progressive disfigurement of the leprosy sufferers, this stigma has been inadvertently encouraged by certain Biblical and linguistic references to the disease, and in particular by the widespread practice of segregating patients and their families in leprosy 'colonies'. Rehabilitation of leprosy sufferers should thus be included in any community approach to the disease. Though elaborate surgical procedures and prosthetic devices have been developed for correction of many of the physical effects of leprosy, they are expensive, and available to relatively few of those who need them. Better by far is to prevent the disabilities by early case finding and careful management of the disease in its early stages.

REFERENCES

Abe M, Minagawa F, Yoshino Y, Ozawa T, Saikawa K, Saito T 1980 Fluorescent antibody absorption (FLA-ABS) test for detecting subclinical infection with Mycobacterium leprae. International Journal of Leprosy 48: 109–119

Bechelli L M, Dominguez V M, Patwary K M 1966 WHO epidemiological random sample surveys of leprosy in Northern Nigeria (Katsina), Cameroon and Thailand (Khon Kaen). International Journal of Leprosy 34: 223–243

Bechelli L M et al 1973 Some epidemiological data on leprosy collected in a mass survey in Burma. World Health Organisation Bulletin 48: 335–344

Bechelli et al 1974 BCG vaccination of children against leprosy: nine year findings of the controlled WHO trial in Burma. World Health Organisation Bulletin 51: 93–99

Brubaker M L, Binford C H, Trautman J R 1969 Occurrence of leprosy in U.S. veterans after service in endemic areas abroad. Public Health Reports 84: 1051–1058

Bryceson A, Pfaltzgraff R E 1979 Leprosy. 2nd edn. Churchill Livingstone London

Canizares O 1975 Clinical Tropical Dermatology. Ed Canizares O. Blackwell Scientific Publishers. Oxford

Chatterjee B R, Taylor C E, Thomas J, Naidu G N 1976. Acid-fast bacillary positivity in asymptomatic individuals in leprosy endemic villages around Jhalda in West Bengal. Leprosy in India 48: 119–131

Chaussinand R 1948 Tuberculose et lèpre, maladies antacomques. Eviction de la lèpre par la tuberculose. International Journal of Leprosy 16: 431–438

Committee on Classification 1953 Technical resolutions: Classification. International Journal of Leprosy 21: 504–510

Convit J et al 1975 Tests with three antigens in leprosy-endemic and non-endemic areas. World Health Organisation Bulletin 52: 193–198

Davey T F, Rees R J W 1974 The nasal discharge in leprosy: Clinical and bacteriological aspects. Leprosy Review 45: 121–134

Dominguez V M et al 1980 Epidemiological information on leprosy in the Singu area of Upper Burma. World Health Organisation Bulletin 58: 81–89

Doull S A, Guinto R S, Rodriguez J N, Bancroft H 1942 The incidence of leprosy in Cordova and Talisay, Cebo, Philippines. International Journal of Leprosy 10: 107–131

Duncan M E, Melsom R, Pearson J M H, Ridley D S 1981 The association of pregnancy and leprosy I. New cases, relapse of cured patients and deterioration in patients on treatment during pregnancy and lactation — results of a prospective study of 154 pregnancies in 147 Ethiopian women. Leprosy Review 52: 245–262

Edelman R 1979 Malnutrition and leprosy — an analytical review. Leprosy in India 51: 376–388

Ellard G A 1981 Drug compliance in the treatment of leprosy. Leprosy Review 52: 201–213

Fine P E M 1981 Immunogenetics of susceptibility to leprosy, tuberculosis and leishmaniasis: an epidemiological perspective. International Journal of Leprosy 49: 387–454

Fine P E M 1982 Leprosy — the epidemiology of a slow bacterium. Epidemiological Reviews 4: 161–188

Fitzpatrick T B 1979 Dermatology in General Medicine. 2nd edn. Eds Fitzpatrick T B, Eisen A Z, Wolff K, Freedberg I M, Austen K F. McGraw-Hill Book Company. New York

Godal T, Negassi K 1973 Subclinical infection in leprosy. British Medical Journal III: 557–559

Guinto R S 1978 Epidemiology of leprosy; current news, concepts and problems. In: Chatterjee B R (ed) A Window on Leprosy, Gandhi Memorial Leprosy Foundation, pp 36–53

Hastings R C, Chehl S K, Black G, Morales M J, Shannon E J, Kirchheimer W F 1981 Growth of M. leprae in nude (athymic) mice. In Humber D P (ed) Immunological aspects of Leprosy, Tuberculosis and Leishmaniasis. Excerpta Medica, Amsterdam, Princeton, pp 166–176

Indian Association of Leprologists 1982 The concensus classification approved by the Indian Association of Leprologists. Leprosy in India 54: 17–25

Irgens L M 1980 Leprosy in Norway — an epidemiological study based on a national patient registry. Leprosy Review 51: Suppl 1, 1–130

Jolliffe D S 1977 Leprosy reactional states and their treatment. British Journal of Dermatology 97: 345–

Kirchheimer W F 1976 The role of arthropods in the transmission of leprosy. International Journal of Leprosy 44: 104–107

Kirchheimer W F, Storrs E H 1971 Attempts to establish the armadillo (Dasypus novemcinctus Linn.) as a model for the study of leprosy I. Report of lepromatoid leprosy in an infected armadillo. International Journal of Leprosy 39: 693–702

Levy L, Noordeen S K, Sansarricq H 1982 Increase in prevalence of leprosy caused by dapsone-resistant Mycobacterium leprae. Morbidity and Mortality Weekly Report 30: 637–638

Noordeen S K, Neelan P N 1978 Extended studies on chemoprophylaxis against leprosy. Indian Journal of Medical Research 67: 515–527

Pedley J C 1978 Transmission of leprosy. In: Chatterjee B R (ed) A Window on Leprosy, Gandhi Memorial Leprosy Foundation, pp 54–58

Rao P S S, Karat A B A, Kaliaperumal V G, Karat S 1972a Prevalence of leprosy in Gudiyatham Taluk, South India. Part I. Specific rates with reference to age, sex and type. International Journal of Leprosy 40: 157–163

Rao P S S, Karat A B A, Kaliaperumal V G and Karat S 1972b Incidence of leprosy in Gudiyatham Taluk, South India. Indian Journal of Medical Research 60: 97–105

Rees R J W 1981 Non-specific factors that influence susceptibility to leprosy. Leprosy Review 52: Suppl, 137–146

Rees R J W, Valentine R C 1962 The appearance of dead leprosy bacilli by light and electron microscopy. International Journal of Leprosy 30: 1–9

Ridley D S 1958 Therapeutic trials in leprosy using serial biopsies. Leprosy Review 29: 45–52

Ridley D S 1971 The SGF (Solid, Fragmented, Granular) index for bacterial morphology. Leprosy Review 42: 96–97

Ridley D S, Jopling W H 1966 Classification of leprosy according to immunity. A five group system. International Journal of Leprosy 34: 255–273

Sansarricq H 1981 Leprosy in the world today. Leprosy Review 52: Suppl, 15–31

Scott G C, Russell D A, Boughton C R, Vincin D R 1976 Untreated leprosy. Probability for shifts in Ridley-Jopling classification. Development of 'flares', or disappearance of clinically apparent disease. International Journal of Leprosy 44: 110–122

Shepard C C 1960 The experimental disease that follows the injection of human leprosy bacilli into footpads of mice. Journal of Experimental Medicine 112: 445–454

Shepard C C 1962 The nasal excretion of Mycobacterium leprae in leprosy. International Journal of Leprosy 30: 10–18

Shepard C C. Levy L, Fasal P 1974 Further experience with the rapid bacteriological effect of rifampin in Myocobacterium leprae. American Journal of Tropical Medicine and Hygiene 23: 1120–1124

Smith D G, Guinto R S 1978 The association between age of onset and mortality in lepromatous leprosy. International Journal of Leprosy 46: 25–29

Walsh G P, Meyers W M, Binford C H, Gerone P J, Wolf R H, Leininger J R 1981 Leprosy — a zoonosis. Leprosy Review 52: Suppl 1, 77–83

World Health Organisation 1977 Expert committee on leprosy — fifth report. World Health Organisation Technical Report Series 607

World Health Organisation 1980 A guide to leprosy control. World Health Organisation: Geneva

World Health Organisation 1982 Chemotherapy of leprosy for control programs Technical Report Series 675

Tuberculosis

INTRODUCTION

Tuberculosis is a conglomerate of diseases resulting from several distinct *Mycobacteria*. The worldwide distribution, its slow, diverse, inexorable but unpredictable course among high and low, rich and poor alike attracted, to the pulmonary forms especially, a profusion of studies unmatched by any other disease group.

The universality of the pulmonary forms has led to the misleading custom of using the term 'tuberculosis' as synonymous with 'pulmonary tuberculosis'. The special curative services also developed to deal primarily with the pulmonary forms.

The syndrome of emaciation, cough and hemoptysis was recognised in China about 5000 years ago. Extra pulmonary disease is evident in the mummified corpses from the early dynastic period in Egypt (Keers 1978). Apparently by 700 BC the disease was being quite logically treated in India with good hygiene, a healthy balanced diet, high altitudes and gentle horse riding. The genetic susceptibility to the disease seems to have been recognised by the prohibition of Brahmins from marrying into affected families.

With the establishment of the Alexandrian school the science of autopsy produced the 'tubercle' the nodule in the tissues. About 320 BC Aristotle hypothesized that the infective agent was exhaled. Further progress was halted when the Middle Ages stifled scientific thought and precipitated European Man into ignorance and superstition. It was not until 1867, when Budd reported on the way tuberculosis spread among African seamen that the contagious nature of the disease was accepted by British physicians. European scientific progress initiated by Sylvius in Leyden had been faster but attempts to control the disease, by for example, notification of cases and dissinfection in Napoleonic Europe, were frustrated by the costs. Too many individuals were affected.

After description of the organism in 1882 by Koch progress, at least epidemiologically, was rapid. Clinicians once more resorted to the healthy diet and high altitudes. For the affluent the private sanatorium in the picturesque mountains became not only the hope of eventual cure but the symbol of a leisured and disciplined but healthy life in communities upon which their patients came ultimately to depend. For the less affluent there were also later to be public sanatoria as anxious tax payers became eager to remove all possible sources of infection whatever the cost. Real progress, with diminution of the disease irrespective of sanatorium availability, had to await the coincidental improvements in housing and nutrition which were to be the eventual reward of the industrial revolution in Europe and north America.

Whether or not BCG, first developed in the 1920s, and specific therapy, beginning with Streptomycin in 1948, contributed all that much to the decline of the disease in industrial countries is controversial. Much more dramatic, though now often forgotten, were the measures to eliminate the crippling non pulmonary forms of the disease, principally through the pasteurization of milk. Resistance to this basic public health measure continues in conservative communities even into the present time.

THE AGENT

Three *Mycobacteria* are responsible for most of the cases of infection included within the rubric 'tuberculosis'. They are *M. tuberculosis*, *M. bovis* and *M. africanum*. Several other *Mycobacteria* including *M. avium* (or *intracellulare*), *M. kansasii* and *M. xenopi* also give rise to tuberculosis type disease (Communicable Disease Reports 1979). The first is usually found in the swollen lymph glands of children, the second and third are particularly associated with drug resistant pulmonary disease in ageing alcoholics with a previous history of bronchitis. These so called 'atypical' infections are currently a problem in the technologically developed societies. They form a residue of resistant and difficult disease though their epidemiologic importance is not clear. It is characteristic of their opportunistic nature that atypical mycobacterial infections should now be cropping up in persons with the acquired immune deficiency syndrome (AIDS) (Fainstein et al 1982). This is not to say that the atypical infections are not also found in developing countries. Their potential for causing confusion in the interpretation of the unspecific 'tuberculin test' is confirmed by specific antigen screening (Wells and Rao 1982). Additional evidence from Lagos (Ogummekan 1980) suggests that children are particularly likely to be infected early in life by atypical or opportunistic mycobacteria producing an indecisive reaction to the tuberculin test. How far such atypical infections affect immunity to the typical tubercle bacilli is not clear. Once the tuberculin test is frankly positive it seems that the infecting agent causing it is likely to be one of the full blown variety.

The possibility of an 'atypical' organism should always be considered once a patient's disease fails to respond to normal therapy. Research in Africa has demonstrated that even in the common *M. africanum* 30 per cent of strains isolated may be resistant to at least some of the antituberculosis drugs (WHO 1979).

There are also a number of fungal type organisms, including Coccidioidomycosis, North American Blastomycosis, Cryptococcosis and Histoplasmosis which can not only give rise to tuberculosis-like disease but also cause epidemiologic confusion by converting tuberculin negative individuals to tuberculin positive. An examination of the sputum is required to distinguish these infecting agents. There are also some *Mycobacteria* which can produce only limited disease in Man, for example *M. ulcerans* and *M. balnei* which cause local skin effects reflecting the lupus forms of the major infective agents. The *Mycobacteria* are seen microscopically as slightly curved rods not forming chains or capsules. There are several distinctive characteristics which account for the epidemiology and pathogenicity of them as infective agents, not excepting *M. leprae* (See Fine and Ponnighaus chapter 16).

1. They thrive only in high oxygen conditions
2. The single bacilli are about one micron long
3. They can successfully invade new host tissues as a single organism but usually multiply only slowly
4. They evade the antibody mechanism under control of the body's B cells but in time can be combatted by a fairly effective T lymphocyte mechanism
5. They can mutate to produce resistant types to whatever drug they are exposed
6. They can apparently retreat into a dormant stage within animal tissue and may emerge again and invade aggressively after long periods, often many years
7. They cause the formation of granulation tissue as the host body attempts to heal the damage to its own cells
8. They are highly susceptible to drying and to sunlight
9. They can pass out in milk from the breast of an infected female
10. They are antigenically similar and are relatively simple organisms
11. They are not highly selective on the animal species they parasitize
12. They are known as 'acid fast bacilli' because when stained they retain the dye even when washed with acid-alcohol solutions. The dye most commonly used is the Ziehl-Neelson stain.

In consequence of the above the *Mycobacteria* in general might be expected to cause disease on the body surfaces, the lungs and skin, or in well blood supplied tissues such as the brain, kidneys and epiphyseal lines of growing bones. They will also be slowly invasive and at any stage of disease might be eliminated by the host but at a cost of tissue scarring or deformation especially damaging to long bones or to the spine. They will be especially well able to penetrate by air spread to the terminal alveolus of the lungs evading the mucus surfaces and ciliated epithelium which keeps out most infectious or irritating agents. As contaminants of food of animal origin, especially dairy products, they will also invade the gastrointestinal tract.

The development of immunity, regardless of infection site, will be slow and will not be passed on to an infant from its mother in the form of immune globulins. The immune system, having learned to deal with one mycobacterial invasion will deal far more effectively with any later mycobacteria. They will be unpredictable infections, sometimes reactivating in the victim long after the body had apparently overcome either clinically apparent or covert disease.

The common 'tuberculosis' types will spread indescriminately between different animal species but only usually after a long and intimate contact between reservoir host and victim. Skin forms excepted, they will not usually be transmitted via inanimate objects and the bacilli will soon perish even in room dust.

Newborn infants of infected mothers, and young animals in general, will be susceptible because of high dose on an immature immune system. Though easily transmitted by food they are easily eliminated from it by heating. In animal tissues and secretions they will be relatively easily identified though the existance of many non pathogenic bacilli which are also acid-fast makes this a helpful rather than certain diagnostic technique.

THE DISEASE

As chronic respiratory tract tuberculosis is the most dangerous of the sources of infection it follows that detection, diagnosis and treatment of individual cases forms an essential corner stone of any tuberculosis control program. At some time or other, sooner rather than later, virtually every human is exposed to tuberculosis type mycobacterial organisms. The first successful bacillus which by chance penetrates the body's outer defences finds macrophage cells eager to eliminate it, as a foreign particle, but not always capable of killing it. As no useful antibody is produced any bacilli which survive the initial clumsy cellular attack enjoy a period, of up to six weeks, in which to divide and spread in the host tissues. During this time bacilli may reach the blood stream and be widely disseminated to cause miliary disease.

Normally in the immunologically mature human the sluggish mycobacterial invasion spreads only slowly, if at all, so that the T lymphocytes have sufficient time to learn to recognise the foreign antigen before any real disease has resulted. The T lymphocytes now influence the macrophages to produce the tuberculous granuloma and the giant multinucleated cells typical of a host tissue beginning successfully to respond to a mycobacterial invasion (Unanue 1980). The activated macrophages now destroy any extra-cellular mycobacteria and the host is said to be 'sensitive'. Any subsequent invasions will be dealt with quickly by macrophage cells under the influence of T lymphocytes cloned from those with the 'memory' of the original mycobacterial antigen. It is the relative failure or success of the original invasion which usually determines whether or not a new host develops disease. Most individuals will completely overcome this infection but for some years after, often for life, will remain sensitive to any mycobacterial antigens. This sensitivity is the basis of the tuberculin test.

In other, less immunologically competent individuals, the initial invasion will progress to some extent. The old 'primary lesion' in the middle lobe of the right lung is a typical limited episode. Usually there is ultimate resolution and healing but with scar tissue which, at least in the case of the lung, may be detected radiologically. Similar primary foci in the gastro-intestinal tract and kidneys would only be detectable on autopsy.

In the days before milk began to be pasteurized the primary lesion in children in Europe tended to be in the cervical lymph glands which became swollen in active disease and hard and nodular as healing was completed. Typically even this relatively localised form could continue to progress with abscess formation and consequent chronically suppurating sinus to the skin of the neck. Extra pulmonary disease, such as cervical adenitis, is still important in the warm climate countries. In Singapore it is reported to be particularly a problem for women (Epidemiological Record 1978).

Unfortunately in some individuals and despite antigen sensitization the disease not only progresses locally but leaps via the blood stream to distant sites. Even at this stage the rather unspecific complaints of the victims, or the observation that a child is simply failing to thrive and appears to have a slight fever, are unlikely to lead to a suspicion of tuberculosis.

The upper part of the human lung is the most important of the final sites for disease to progress though the damage produced there is not as immediately dangerous as, say, in the brain. It is though from the lung site that progressive invasion may break through into a bronchus resulting in the coughing of an aerosol spray of bacilli to new victims. A chronic, radiologically detectable cavity part filled with air will be the late consequence. The patient is now said to have 'open' cavitary tuberculosis.

At this stage most patients will know that they are sick. The screening of any population for those individuals feeling chronically unwell, with a mild sweaty fever especially at night and with a troublesome cough will produce most of the infectious cases (Meijer 1971). The ultimate fate of the untreated tuberculosis patient is always unpredictable. Healing can occur at any stage though tissue damage and subsequent slow healing with scar formation is an especially destructive process in the genitourinary tract and bones. The bones of the leg and spine are particularly vulnerable. Like leprosy tuberculosis produces most long term damage in those individuals with a reasonably but not quite sufficiently good resistance to the disease. The patient survives but at great cost to affected tissues and to general health.

For the immune deficient progress can be very rapid with tissue invasion and destruction far outstripping healing until death occurs through miliary infection or through damage of vital centers. The more bizarre patterns of disease are found especially in those victims in whom earlier apparent cure has left some dormant forms of the organism. Dramatic recurrences occur as immunity wanes especially in old age or when nutritional status declines. A glacially slow erosion of an artery in the lung terminates in the sudden rush of blood, the hemoptysis, in an apparently well individual.

Diagnosis of the disease, at least of the common pulmonary forms, is relatively easy. Paradoxically delay in diagnosis is most likely in those societies in which tuberculosis has become uncommon and especially in cold climate countries with much chronic respiratory infection of non tuberculous origin. Any history of close contact with a previously known or suspected case would be prime presumptive evidence which should always be solicited.

The tuberculin test is not diagnostically useful except in the uncommon case of an individual known quite recently to have been tuberculin negative. It may not become positive until six weeks after the primary infection. It may remain negative in individuals who are immune deficient. Chest radiography is not much more helpful though the location of infiltrates, especially at the apices of the lungs, and their character may encourage a suspicion of tuberculosis. So also will the finding of a typical part-filled or empty cavity but negative findings on a full sized postero-anterior X-ray film do not exclude the possibility of there being active disease.

Immunodiagnostic tests such as the enzyme linked immunoabsorbent assay (ELISA) can radically sharpen diagnostic confidence but in practice, especially at District Health Center level suspected pulmonary tuberculosis is best confirmed bacteriologically. The reliance placed on the finding of acid-fast bacilli in sputum from case suspects must from time to time lead to misdiagnosis. To be certain of diagnosis culture is mandatory (Farer 1979) though in many developing countries it is not practicable. Simple acid-fast identification is rapid and can be performed efficiently by properly trained auxillary health personnel cautioned on the dangers of handling potentially infectious materials. Not all experts agree that even this procedure is appropriate at a District Health Center. They argue that efficiency can only be maintained when there is a large volume of the same kind of work (Fox 1976).

Not all infectious patients excrete bacilli in such quantities or so consistently as to be picked up in a single sputum microscopy. Culture is certainly helpful in these cases but, like the decision on whether or not to treat soley on the presumptive evidence of acid-fast bacilli, depends upon the extent of local resources. In those priviliged conditions in which laboratory resources are almost unlimited clinicians sometimes prefer to prescribe therapy under guidance of culture sensitivity tests (Wilcocks and Manson-Bahr 1972). These assume real value when faced with patients who have failed to respond to a normal course of therapy, where relapse has occurred after apparent cure or where the relapse has occurred after apparent cure or where the patient has repeatedly reneged on treatment (Glassroth et al 1980). Any tuberculosis control program needs to pay special attention to patients who come from an area where a poorly conducted service has led to INH resistant disease (Pichenik et al 1982). Trials are currently under way to test the suitability of techniques promising a quick detection of drug insensitivity in particular cases.

As the treatment of most forms of tuberculosis is medically simple, at least in the essentials of eliminating a source of further infection, it can usually be undertaken on an outpatient basis. Inpatient care is for the complex cases, for the acutely ill, for those living far away from any primary health care service and for those highly infectious individuals for whom temporary separation from susceptibles in their families is desirable. Institutional, sanatorium care is seldom required. It is useful only for the persistantly uncooperative patient, for the homeless, for those too damaged or too old to return to society or for those cases of atypical infection for which current schedules of therapy may be ineffective. Inpatient and institutional care merely divert resources from where they should be spent, in providing care for ambulatory infectious patients in the community.

The continued disagreement between proponents of this or that regimen suggests that properly controlled, randomized studies of the long term outcome of different schedules of treatment are either too few or too inconclusive in their findings. There are many different roads to the therapeutic cure of tuberculosis. The fastest and most reliable ones require that at least three drugs be used simultaneously, one of them being INH, depending upon what is locally available. To be effective therapy must be regular, though not necessarily daily, and must be maintained in the patient who is obviously responding for at least six months.

Recently even four and a half months has been reported as sufficient providing that four drugs are given simultaneously (Abeles et al 1982). Relapse rates in US Public Health Service trials have, however, been as high as nine per cent only six months after completion even in six months treatment schedules (Glassroth et al 1980). This contrasts with the more optimistic reports from British trials in East Africa (Second East African/British Medical Research Council study 1974). Treatment beyond 12 months is considered to be of little or no value (WHO 1974). Some physicians with a wide variety of drugs available to them prefer periodically to change the constituents of the triple or quadruple therapy though INH usually remains constant. What is really important is that treatment should not lapse otherwise drug resistant mutants have a chance to become dominant with all the problems and epidemiologic hazards that produces.

The difficulty in actually treating the disease is in keeping up therapy which may be somewhat unpleasant and at best inconvenient in a patient who quite soon begins to feel well again. Case finding and treatment programs are best not begun unless community follow up of patients can ensure that all prescribed treatment is completed. For this reason community nursing personnel are far more important than are clinicians in curing tuberculosis. To provide casual, walk in services for the obviously sick may be satisfying to clinic personnel but it may be of little long term benefit to the community, may actually constitute a menace unless all suspect cases are thoroughly treated. A minimal additional service should be the examination of all close contacts, especially children and young people, of the infectious cases. It is from these contacts that the next generation of infectious cases will originate.

Once fully treated, clinically well and with no signs or symptoms of active disease the patient is discharged from care. Though inevitably a small proportion of properly treated patients will relapse, perhaps many years later, there is no evidence that keeping all cured patients under surveillance serves any useful purpose — and it unnecessarily stigmatizes the former patients. Those who are discharged, or a responsible member of their family, should be advised to return to the health center should there be any return of symptoms.

EPIDEMIOLOGY

Distribution

Pulmonary tuberculosis is found in every society and is not influenced in its distribution by climate or vectors. It is commonest where poverty is greatest and where people, or animals, are crowded together for whatever reason. It presents as a more acute problem with rapidly progressive disease in those populations only recently exposed to infection, such as Amerindians and Pacific Islanders. It tends to be a more chronic disease in populations long experienced, such as India, China and the eastern Mediterranean. It has been characteristically devastating in relatively isolated communities at the edges of major population groups, such in Europe as the Irish and Scandinavians, in Asia the Tibetans. Gastrointestinal forms of the disease will obviously be commonest in populations heavily dependant for food on animals, especially milk products. Skin infections will be commonest in persons handling infected animals or animal products. The extra pulmonary forms of tuberculosis are actually likely to increase in frequency as populations move from a poverty associated vegetarian diet to the consumption of more animal products which come with affluence.

Although it is relatively easy in a population to estimate the number of individuals with active pulmonary disease the larger number of those who have been infected will be at some stage of quiescence or natural cure. Currently used case finding methods identify only those individuals with the most highly infectious pulmonary disease. Except in the most sophisticated societies little reliance can be placed upon disease notification figures. In a high proportion of persons whose death is hastened by tuberculosis or whose health and vitality are undermined the disease is never actually identified.

The important human cases are those who are potentially infectious to others usually with pulmonary disease and it is estimated that there are about seven million of those in the world. Three quarters of those individuals live in the warm climate countries. Each year, it is estimated, about 3.5 million new infections occur and half a million persons die of the disease, four hundred thousand of those in the warm climate countries of Africa, Asia and Latin America.

The incidence of new disease varies widely from the lowest levels of 20 or fewer per 100 000 population in most of the cold climate industrialized countries, through about 100 per 100 000 in rapidly developing countries, levels of 200 per 100 000 in Africa to an extraordinary high of 500 per 100 000 population in some crowded parts of South East Asia.

Incidence figures of course relate to new cases. These as they occur are added to the pool of sickening, dying or gradually recovering earlier cases. In terms of prevalence in the maximally infected population as many as 4.5 per cent of individuals may at any one time have infectious pulmonary disease. Any serious social disruption will soon eliminate the old and sick but even in those who survived to become refugees in IndoChina examination revealed a prevalence of 926 active tuberculosis cases per 100 000 population (Morbidity and Mortality Weekly Reports 1979).

As current medical technology could either prevent or treat most of this disease and relatively cheaply it is hardly surprising that in many warm climate countries more attention is given to tuberculosis control than to programs for the more traditional or exotic tropical diseases. In the technologically advanced countries extra pulmonary tuberculosis has been almost eradicated while pulmonary disease, though relatively infrequent, tends to linger on as the principal death-causing infectious disease.

More reliance can be placed on case notification of tuberculosis where it is mandatory, where the government funds and controls the diagnostic laboratories, provides treatment free and where prevalence is fairly low. The incidence figure of new infections in low risk countries like Sweden or the United States is also influenced by strict diagnostic criteria, such as the requirement that to be counted as a case of tuberculosis there must be a positive culture. Inside even the favoured countries there are pockets of much more prevalent infection. These more commonly occur in the big cities and in the under priviliged minorities within those cities (US. DHHS. 1979).

Outbreak characteristics

The long period of time between the original primary infection and the subsequent symptomatic disease, in all but the most immunologically deficient individuals, militates against the occurrence of epidemics of tuberculosis. Nevertheless primary infection in the lung can cause a mild but recognisable sickness especially in young people. The term 'epidemic' has been applied to a group of such infections resulting from a single source exposure, say to an infectious schoolteacher (Rao et al 1980) or barman (Hill and Stevenson 1983).

The ease with which *M. tuberculosis* can spread by air also puts previously uninfected persons at particular risk when they are gathered into new communities. Examples include army recruits, the inpatients of mental institutions and prisons, or in air enclosed and air ducted environments such as hospitals and ships (Riley 1961). As such incidents can only occur in groups of previously uninfected, that is tuberculin negative, individuals they would be unlikely to occur in societies in which exposure to tuberculosis occurs universally at an early age. In these societies tuberculosis can be thought of as a family infection; a relatively rapid spread of tuberculin sensitivity occurs once one member of the family becomes infectious. This is followed by new cases of sickness at irregular and generally long intervals of time. In Western societies the disease has changed from being one which affects primarily the young to one in which most newly recognised, infectious illness is recorded in the long infected elderly. Part of the change in age distribution is due to the very effective control of extra pulmonary tuberculosis which previously affected the milk consuming young population.

Sources of infection

Once zoonotic, food borne infection is controlled human victims with pulmonary disease become virtually the sole reservoir of infection. Contact with infectious animals will produce occasional human cases. Inanimate objects, even those handled by infectious humans seems not to be epidemiologically important though some of the mycobacterial skin infections may be transmitted through, for example, the grazing of bare skin in a well used swimming pool.

Transmission

Between humans by far the greater part of infection by *M. tuberculosis* and *M. africanum* occurs via air spread from the infected lungs of the host to the lungs or upper respiratory tract of an individual who has not yet learned to deal with mycobacterial antigens. An impressive aerosol of organisms can be expelled in the cough or sneeze of an individual with open cavitary disease. The larynx when infected produces clouds of organisms especially especially when the voice is used. In a study in Tanzania it was found that the larynx was involved in 27 per cent of previously untreated cases of tuberculosis (Manni 1982).

The largest particles of saliva-wet aerosol fall relatively harmlessly to the ground or far more harmfully onto the face and conjunctiva of the lap held child. Large salivary particles inhaled by potential victims are usually safely dealt with by the mucus blanket of the oropharynx and trachea or by the ciliated epithelium of the bronchial tree. They are eventually spat out, or somewhat less safely swallowed. The small salivary particles, less than ten microns in diameter, are the most dangerous as they float in air currents and if inhaled are quite likely to reach the terminal alveoli of the unprotected lung where any contained bacillus may begin a new infection. In theory tuberculosis could be transmitted over considerable distances by air currents. In practice only the moist, comforting darkness of air conditioning systems found in closed environments such as ships, schools, government buildings and hospitals provide the *Mycobacteria* with a good chance of spreading far beyond the source (Houk 1980).

The natural disease regulators of sunshine; drying or simply being lost in the infinity of the atmosphere which limit air spread transmissions do not apply when the source is food. Consequently *M. bovis*, usually derived from a domestic animal source, can be very widely spread along the food distribution lines. Providing that it is unheated the organism can survive very well in the interior of such foods as butter and cheese. The danger from infected meat, especially from infected lymph glands, is somewhat less as such foods are not customarily consumed uncooked though diseased flesh might well be mixed in with other minced preparations which might be eaten cold. Farmers and handlers of infected animals and carcases are at the same risk as though they were exposed to infected humans.

Individual susceptibility

Three principal factors determine which individuals are likely to develop actual tuberculous disease of whatever form.

1. The dose

The more frequently does a previously uninfected individual come into contact with tubercle bacilli the more likely is primary infection to occur. The higher the dosage of bacilli in the community and the more likely is this primary infection to occur in early life. Not surprisingly those persons living in crowded conditions and for long periods are at high risk of tuberculosis and the more infectious cases there are in that community the more likely is infection to occur. Dose/Time relationships thus determine that tuberculosis will be a greater problem among the less affluent among whom the resevoir of disease is more likely to be maintained because of the poorer diagnostic, therapeutic and follow-up services which they are obliged to tolerate. As resistance aquired from the primary infection is not absolute it follows that even immunologically competent individuals may eventually be overcome if the dose of mycobacteria is sufficiently high and persists for very long.

2. Inate immunologic competence

Though apparently susceptible populations have been identified epidemiologically for some time it is only recently that laboratory tests have become available which reveal, for example, an eight times likelihood of developing severe disease in certain individuals of African origin (Al-Arif et al 1979). Within any population will be families whose members are more likely, it would appear, to develop secondary or adult type disease. Although some of this familial susceptibility could be ascribed to contact, and hence to dose, the findings of Kellman and Reisner (1943) did suggest that there is a genetically determined susceptibility with, for example, the heterozygote twin of a case having a 25.6 per cent chance of also developing the disease. This compares with the near certainty of 87.3 per cent that a monozygote or identical twin will also fall victim.

3. Immunologic damage

The competence of an individual who would normally be resistant to mycobacterial invasion may apparently be undermined by several stresses. Among these is malnutrition. In wartime Europe it was observed that the advance and retreat of tuberculosis prevalence was inversely related to the decline and recovery of protein levels in the food of those populations (Heaf 1957).

Chronic alcoholism is an adverse factor though at least some of the risk of aquiring tuberculosis is probably secondary to the notoriously poor diets of many chronic alcoholics as well as the company they keep. The apparently adverse influence of cold damp climates, noticed long ago in ancient Greece, is probably a consequence of the crowding indoors which is encouraged by inclement conditions and which increases contacts and dosages of bacilli. Exposure to dusty conditions, usually a consequence of occupation, also appears to undermine individual resistance. As was confirmed in Zimbabwe (Girwood 1962) susceptibility to tuberculosis is greatly increased when the dust is silicon dioxide (SiO_2) which causes the pneumoconiosis of coal miners and the silicosis of stone workers.

Immunologic competenence also appears to be stressed by pregnancy, especially at its termination, by old age and by certain medical conditions such as diabetes, blood dyscrasias or through the prolonged administration of steroid-like compounds. Stress in a psychological sense, as would occur in disasters, in refugees, in wartime or internecine conflicts, is commonly followed by an increase in the amount of tuberculosis in that particular community. Any disruption to social life, however, also predicates an increase in the exposure to bacilli and a worsening of nutrition so that the influence of stress alone is not measurable. University students in developing countries, removed from the certainties of village life to what appears as a far away and alien environment, become highly susceptible to tuberculosis (Wigley 1980).

SURVEILLANCE

Screening for tuberculosis is deceptively simple. Injected intradermally as in the Mantoux test, five units of purified protein derived from tuberculin and stabilized against its precipitation onto the glass wall of the vial (PPD-T) will reliably cause a tissue reaction in those individuals who have been sensitized by an initial invasion of mycobacteria. Unfortunately the test is not specific to tuberculosis and indicates nothing about when the initial infection occured or if it is still active. Read 48 to 72 hours later a positive reaction is constituted by 10 mm or more of tissue induration around the injection site — not redness. Where the objective is simply to obtain prevalence data rather than to provide service for individuals it may be justifiable to use one of the simpler tuberculin tests such as the Tine. In these speed and subject acceptance outweigh problems of sensitivity. The relative inaccuracy of these simple adaptations of the Mantoux test does greatly limit their usefulness (Lunn and Johnson 1978).

Used as a population disease screening technique the tuberculin test provides a gauge of previous infectivity in that community and little more. It would, of course be useless in a population vaccinated with BCG. As a screening measure in special highly susceptible groups, the contacts of cases or such as school leavers going into industrial employment screening might be justified on the grounds that the early convertors, those individuals earliest infected, are also those most likely to develop actual disease (American Thoracic Society 1974). In the first years following infection the risk of developing actual disease has been calculated as about four per cent per year.

Unfortunately the translation of this knowledge into a useful program implies that all young people found to be tuberculin positive should either be brought under surveillance for many years or should be treated by INH chemoprophylaxis. Pediatricians have used INH for this purpose in many affluent countries but it is doubtful if such a program could or should be supported under conditions of most warm climate countries. An exception might be a young person, recently converted to tuberculin positive in consequence of exposure to an open case in the family. In any case INH is a potentially hepatotoxic drug and should not be scattered around too freely (Comstock and Edwards 1975). More recently Rifampicin has been used for the same preventive purpose.

Screening for actual disease in any community, whether based on seeking individuals with the triad of symptoms or on the presence of acid-fast bacilli, or both, can be justified on the grounds that it discovers the infectious resevoir. When, however, a reasonably efficient tubberculosis treatment program has been operating for some time, and where the population is not too scattered to benefit by easy access to those services, screening will probably uncover relatively few new infectious cases. The District Health Officer planning programs for a previously untreated population faces a dilemma.

If few new cases are produced the screening will have wasted valuable resources; if many new cases are found the existing treatment and follow-up resources may be unable to cope.

Limited screening for active disease is sometimes defended on the grounds that in some sensitive situations such individuals would pose a special threat. School teachers are those most often screened as a routine both before and periodically during their employment. Inevitably the rationale that any profession which brings close contact with the public, especially young people, should be screened for tuberculosis casts suspicion at school bus drivers, hairdressers, restaurant employees and shop assistants but it is doubtful if such enthusiasm is cost effective. The justification for screening immigrants into an area or country is based not so much on the risk they pose as a group but on their relative inability or unwillingness, should an individual be sick with tuberculosis-like symptoms, either to use the existing services or to refer themselves if illness should be noticed later. The District Health Officer will not, of course, forget that health personnel should be screened for tuberculosis both on being first recruited and at later regular intervals.

The use of Mass Miniature Radiography as a case finding technique is no longer advocated (Toman 1976).

CONTROL

Eradication of the zoonotic and food-borne types of tuberculosis are entirely feasible, at least for the general public. The sterilization or pasteurization of milk or milk products produces a dramatic fall in $M.$ $bovis$ type new cases (See Abdussalam Chapter 39). A modern meat inspection and meat condemnation program and the culling of tuberculin positive animal reactors from domestic herds are late but necessary steps in control. They can only be effective if allied with a fair scheme for the compensation of owners of destroyed animals. Some spill over from wild animal sources is bound to occur occasionally and cattle can be infected by infectious humans. Each such incident is not in itself an epidemiologic disaster but its possibility makes it necessary to continue tuberculosis surveillance in agricultural animals indefinitely.

Much more difficult to eradicate is the commonest form, pulmonary tuberculosis, and this despite the fact that Man is the only important reservoir. Eradication of this source of infection can only come through the seeking out and treatment of every single pulmonary case including those who have relapsed or never completed treatment. A community rendered free of tuberculosis would either from then on have to artificially raise immunity levels in all susceptibles, especially the newborn, or would have to surround itself with a sanitary cordon with entrance restricted to those proved uninfected or totally immune.

Variations on these methods have indeed been tried. Unfortunately there is as yet no completely effective, safe, immunity raising agent and the sanitory cordon is irksome or impossible to enforce except in small specialised, self contained communities. For some time to come it appears likely that we shall have to be content to reduce pulmonary tuberculosis case incidence slowly to a reasonable level in the developing countries. This will be done in the knowledge that in the affluent societies it has been economic and social progress rather than active medical intervention which have reduced the incidence of tuberculosis to its present low levels. It is to largely similar improvements in living standards that the decline in mortality from tuberculosis in China has been attributed (Peking Tuberculosis Institute 1977).

Unfortunately in many poorer warm climate countries the existing resources could not bear the cost in manpower and drugs necessary for a careful tuberculosis case finding program. Even in more fortunate societies it is essential to make sure that continuity of treatment once begun can be guaranteed, including all drugs and follow-up for the drop-outs, before any case finding is begun. The attitudes and understanding of the community and of its constituent family units are crucial to success. It might even be as well not to tackle the general problem of pulmonary tuberculosis in a high endemic society until the later stages of economic and social development.

Initially then a District Health Officer would be wise to concentrate upon treating known or symptomatic cases, encouraging their contacts to be screened for the disease and spreading the message in the community about the clinical symptoms which suggest tuberculosis. Understanding needs to be increased about the ways in which airborne infections occur and may be reduced by home ventilation, safe coughing and disposal of sputum and about the special dangers to which infants and young children may unwittingly be exposed within the family circle.

Beyond the most passive program, gradual progress toward the control of pulmonary tuberculosis will depend very largely on the development of laboratory capabilities, upon the stocking of supplies of drugs and upon a health infrastructure which keeps diagnosed cases within care until treatment is completed. Only when local services can deal with the flow of obvious cases with acid-fast bacilli in the sputum should there be any question of expanding diagnostic capability into culture of the bacilli and still later into testing those bacilli found for their sensitivity to the drugs being used. Culture of tubercle bacilli is not difficult but it is slow. It requires not only a well trained staff but also sophisticated protection against these hazardous procedures (Harrington and Shannon 1976). Such techniques are anyway probably best performed in regional or national central laboratories which become the quality control, reference and training centers for the entire tuberculosis program (Farer 1979).

Most of the diagnosis and treatment, especially of the epidemiologically important infectious cases, should take place in District Centers where all but the most uncooperative or therapeutically resistant cases can be dealt with adequately. Neither radiologic facilities nor the constant supervision of a physician are essential to diagnosis and treatment. Whoever is directing care does need to ensure that staff understand the tranmission pathways of the disease and the conditions which might lead to chemotherapeutic resistance. The success of any tuberculosis control program depends more than any other factor on the strength and continuity of the relationship between local health care staff and the patients and the latters' immediate contacts. Farer (1979) has also suggested that a system of evaluating progress should be built into any tuberculosis control effort. In most tuberculosis control programs the principal weakness lies in failure of patients to comply with treatment (Fox 1983).

PREVENTION

It has already been emphasized that a reduction in the sickness due to pulmonary tuberculosis comes principally through economic and social development. As far as it is possible to see, the two crucial factors in reducing the risk of pulmonary disease are good housing and nutrition. To these must be added the understanding and the will of the community to overcome the hazards of tuberculosis and this without authoritarian measures being taken against those already infected.

Prevention of food-borne disease, though not technically difficult, is expensive and requires, if anything, an even higher degree of societal cooperation. Safe food is inevitably more expensive and health standard requirements are sometimes inimical to the peasant farmer. Unlike pulmonary tuberculosis reduction in food-borne transmission does not come automatically as living standards increase.

It was hoped that the vaccine derived from that first developed by Calmette and Guerin in 1921 would provide just that boost to the immune state of most members of heavily infected communities which simply cannot afford to await the generations of investment and development from which the northern countries now benefit. BCG vaccination given at or soon after birth has seemed to be a cheap and safe way of decelerating the spread of tuberculosis especially in those communities in which there are too many sources to be able to isolate them from the susceptibles. As shown by tuberculin sensitivity BCG appears to alert the T lymphocytes, sensitises the body against further invasions of mycobacteria and in prospective trials in countries not overburdened with tuberculosis has seemed to reduce the chances of those vaccinated from being infected. The technique never found universal favour partly because of the unreliability of some of the vaccines and partly because to vaccinate was also to undermine the usefulness of the tuberculin test as an epidemiologic tool. The actual contribution made by BCG vaccination in reducing disease in countries like the United Kingdom in which the incidence of infection was falling anyway has also been questioned (Hart and Sutherland 1977).

The reports from India on long term outcome trials of BCG vaccination have thrown further doubt on its cost effectiveness, at least in those populations very heavily affected by the disease (Tuberculosis Prevention Trial, Madras 1979). Yet in 1984 BCG seems still able to prevent disease within moderate risk populations (Curtis, Leck and Bamford 1984). It will prove to be an irony if BCG vaccination, like so much else in the control of tuberculosis, has to wait to be truly effective until economic and social development have taken the population into conditions favorable to medical intervention. One way in which the District Health Officer might solve the dilemma posed by BCG is to provide a single mass program of vaccination. Thereafter the vaccine will be given only to those at special risk, like the newborn infants of infected mothers (Sutherland 1981). Even this policy would have an additional complication as if the mother were to be under treatment the infant would require an INH resistant form of BCG which is not generally available in developing countries.

It has already been noted that chemoprophylaxis designed to halt the progress of as yet incipient infection in tuberculin positive but healthy young people, though technically effective, is probably unjustifiable in terms of cost benefit in tuberculosis control in most developing countries. The District Health Officer will of course be faced most frequently with the desirability of interupting mycobacterial transmission not only within affected families but also within the wider context of the staff and other patients of clinics and hospitals in which care for the patient with open cavitary disease is provided. Appropriate multiple therapy renders the patient harmless within days (Gunnels et al 1974). Patients and their relatives should be instructed in the proper techniques of coughing to avoid wide air spread and on the safe disposal of sputum into a closed container. Some precautionary isolation of the more susceptible members of a family is common sense in the first few days of out-patient treatment. This is particularly important for the patient likely to prove unreliable in the taking of the prescribed drugs (Rouillon et al 1976). In the home increased air ventilation is probably useful. Draconian measures such as bannishing infected patients to isolated huts are probably no longer justifiable. Even if they work they are hardly likely to encourage other individuals with symptoms of infection to come forward for examination. In practice it is usually better to forfeit some safety in order to gain confidence and trust in the community.

Effort is best expended on ensuring that all close contacts with infectious patients are initially examined and consideration given, depending upon the local circumstances and resources, to continued surveillance, to BCG vaccination or, in a country where it is practised, to INH chemoprophylaxis.

Similar principles apply in the prevention of transmission in clinic or hospital. Forced ventilation of air by fans to the outside should be considered in any building area where high dose acid-fast bacilli producers are likely to be breathing the same air as other patients or staff. Particular problems are posed by some modern hospitals in warm climate countries with their air recirculating and conditioning systems. The use of ultra violet light as a mycobacteriacide is probably ineffective, especially in humid climates (Bagshawe et al 1978). In practice it may be better, when dealing with highly infectious patients, to block the air conditioner's extraction duct, to open a window and place there a fan which will draw air from the inside of the room and the corridor beyond and send it safely to the outside. Such actions are not popular with hospital designers and administrators.

Where some mixing of patients is inevitable it might be helful, or at least reassuring, to have the careless, highly infectious patient wear a surgical mask. No special precautions are necessary in handling inanimate objects such as books and barrier nursing is not indicated. The room occupied by an acutely infectious tuberculosis patient can be used again for others safely after all bedding has been normally laundered, the floor washed and the windows fully openned for half a day.

All hospital, clinic and laboratory staff on recruitment should be tuberculin tested and either given BCG if negative or additionally screened for disease if tuberculin positive. Regular six monthly surveillance should be conducted on all high risk staff though with care to avoid too many chest radiographs and to make sure that female staff are not pregnant. Tuberculin screening is safer where appropriate for younger staff but if performed too often can lead to sensitivity to the PPD-T itself and to a false positive result.

All health personnel should be taught to self recognise the symptoms of pulmonary tuberculosis. Very special care is needed in the disposal of laboratory materials especially of cultures. INH chemoprophylaxis might very well be considered for younger health personnel found to have converted to tuberculin positive but with no history of BCG vaccination. Health personnel found to have active disease should be treated as outpatients in the normal way and resume normal duties though preferably avoiding infant care, as soon as practicable and without waiting for treatment to be completed.

REFERENCES

Abeles H, Rodesco D, Williams M H 1982 Shortened chemotherapy for pulmonary tuberculosis. New England Journal of Medicine 307: 1527
Al-Arif L I, Goldstein R, Affronti L F, Jamicki B W, HLA-Bw 15 and tuberculosis in a North American black population. 1979 American Review of Respiratory Disease. 120: 1275–1278
American Thoracic Society. 1974. Preventive therapy of tuberculous infection. American Review of Respiratory Disease 110: 371–378
Bagshawe K D, Blowers R, Lidwell O M 1978 Isolating patients in hospital to control infection: Part II — Design and construction of isolation accommodation. British Medical Journal 2: 744–748
Comstock G W, Edwards P Q 1975 The competing risks of tuberculosis and hepatitis for adult tuberculin reactors. American Review of Respiraory Disease   : 573–577
Curtis H M, Leck I, Bamford F N 1984. Incidence of childhood tuberculosis after neonatal BCG vaccination. Lancet 1: 145–148

Fainstein V, Bolivar R. Mavligit G, Rios A, Luna M 1982. Disseminated infection due to Mycobacterium avium intracellulare in a homosexual man with Kaposi's syndrome. Journal of Infectious disease 145: 586

Farer L S 1979 Tuberculosis control for developing countries. US Department of Health and Human Services, Center for Disease control. Atlanta.

Fox W 1976 Tuberculosis control — a cost effective approach from Epidemiology and Community Health in Warm Climate Countries. ed Cruickshank R et al. Churchill Livingstone. Edinburgh pages 83–94

Fox W 1983 Compliance of patients and physicians: Experience and lessons from tuberculosis i. British Medical Journal 287: 33–35

Girdwood M I, Transactions of the sixth Commonwealth Health and Tuberculosis Conference 1962. Chest and Heart Association. London page 62

Glassroth J, Robins A G, Snider D E 1980 Tuberculosis in the 1980s. New England Journal of Medicne 302: 1441–1450

Gunnels J J, Bates J H, Swindell H 1974 Infectivity of sputum-positive tuberculosis patients on chemotherapy. American Review of Respiratory Disease 109: 323–330

Harrington J M, Shannon H S 1976 Incidence of tuberculosis, hepatitis, brucellosis and shigellosis in British medical laboratory workers. British Medical Journal 1: 759–762

Hart P D, Sutherland I 1977 BCG and vole bacillus vaccines in the prevention of tuberculosis in adolescence and early adult life. Final report to the Medical Research Council. British Medical Journal 2: 293–295

Heaf F R G 1957 Symposium of tuberculosis. Cassell. London. page 225

Hill J D, Stevenson D K 1983 Tuberculosis in unvaccinated children, adolescents and young adults: a city epidemic British Medical Journal 286: 1471–1473

Houk V N 1980 Spread of tuberculosis via recirculated air in a naval vessel: The Byrd study. Annals of the New York Academy of Science 353: 10–24

Kellman F J, Reisner D 1943 Twin studies on the significance of genetic factors in tuberculosis. American Review of Tuberculosis 47: 549

Keers R Y 1978 Pulmonary tuberculosis — a journey down the centuries. Baillière Tindall. London

Lunn J A, Johnson A J 1978 Comparison of the Tine and Mantoux tuberculin tests. Report of the Tuberculin Subcommittee of the Research Committee of the British Thoracic Association. British Medical Journal 1: 1451–1453

Manni J J 1982 The prevalence of tuberculous laryngitis in pulmonary tuberculosis in Tanzania. Tropical and Geographical Medicine 34/2: 159–162

Meijer J et al. 1971 in Tuberculosis Surveillance Research Unit of the International Union against Tuberculosis. The Hague. KNCV

Ogummekan D A 1980 Differential tuberculin testing in Lagos. African Journal of Medical Science 9: 21–26

Peking Tuberculosis Institute 1977 Tuberculosis control in New China. Chinese Medical Journal 3(4): 218–223

Pitchenik A E et al. 1982 The prevalence of tuberculosis and drug resistance among Haitians. New England Journal of Medicine 307: 162–165

Rao V R et al. 1980 Outbreak of tuberculosis after minimal exposure to infection. British Medical Journal 281: 187–189

Riley R L, O'Grady F 1961 Airborne infection: transmission and control. Macmillan. New York page 180

Rouillon A, Perdrozet S, Parrot R 1976 Transmission of tubercle bacilli: The effects of chemotherapy. Tubercle 57: 275–299

Second East African/British Medical Research Council Study 1974 Controlled clinical trial of four short-course (6-month) regimens of chemotherapy for treatment of pulmonary tuberculosis. Lancet 2: 1100–1106

Sutherland I 1981 The epidemiology of tuberculosis. Is prevention better than cure? Bulletin of the International Union against tuberculosis 56: 127–134

Tuberculosis prevention trial, Madras. 1979 Trial of BCG vaccines in south India for tuberculosis prevention. Indian Journal of Medical Research 70: 349–363

Toman K 1976 Mass radiography in tuberculosis control. WHO Chronicle 30: 51–57

UK, DHSS, Public Health Laboratory Service. 1979 Myobacterial infections, 1975–77: Part 2. Communicable Disease Reports. No 79

Unanue E R 1980 Cooperation between mononuclear phagocytes and lymphocytes in immunity. New England Journal of Medicine 303: 977–985

US, DHHS, Center for Disease Control. Tuberculosis in the United States, 1977, 1979, (DHEW publication no. (CDC)79–8322) Atlanta

US, DHHS, Center for Disease Control. 1980 Tuberculosis among Indochinese refugees. Morbidity and Mortality Weekly Reports. 29: 383–390

Well A V, Rao K R 1982 Dual intradermal testing of Barbadian children with tuberculin and Battey bacillus antigen. West Indian Medical Journal 31/4: 198–204

WHO Expert Committee on Tuberculosis. 1974 Ninth Report. Technical Report Series. WHO Geneva. page 552

WHO, 1978 Weekly Epidemiological Record No. 14 WHO Geneva page 101

WHO, 1979 Notes and news: Review of medical research activities in the African Region. WHO Chronicle 33: 391–392

Wigley S C 1980 Psychosomatics of tuberculosis. Papua New Guinea Medical Journal 23/1: 34–40

Wilcocks C, Manson-Bahr P E C, Manson's Tropical Diseases 1972 Williams and Wilkins. Baltimore. 17th Edition. page 450

18

B. Cvjetanović

Meningococcal meningitis

INTRODUCTION:

Meningococcal meningitis is an important public health problem in warm countries and in particular in the part of Africa and Latin America in areas such as is the so-called 'cerebrospinal meningitis belt' (Fig. 18.1) which lies north of the equator and south of the Sahara (Lapeyssonnie, 1963).

Large epidemics flare up from time to time in the Sahelian area as the

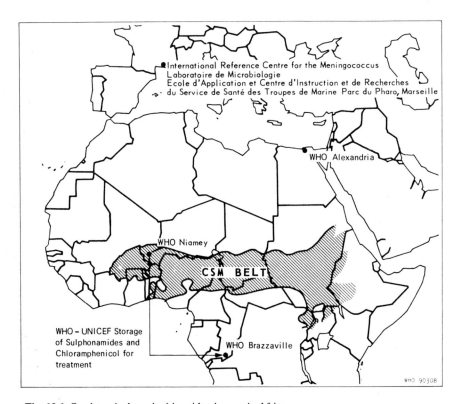

Fig. 18.1 Cerebrospinal meningitis epidemic zone in Africa

immunity of the population diminishes and favourable conditions for spread arrive in the dry season when, due to the cold nights, people crowd together in small dwellings. Sometimes, as in the case of famines or pilgrimages, mass migrations aggravate the situation.

In this area of Africa and in Brazil large outbreaks occur. Follow-up of the evolution of outbreaks and of the development of the resistance of meningococci is under way with the objective of making available effective drugs in case of possible outbreaks due to resistant micro-organisms. Stores of sulpha drugs and chloramphenicol are kept by the World Health Organization for immediate use in case of emergency. Vaccines are also kept ready to use if necessary.

THE DISEASE

Individuals become infected through colonisation of the nasopharynx. Some protective mechanism, which probably depends on circulating antibodies, is usually present and prevents the further spread and penetration of the meningococus into the blood stream. In some individuals whose serum does not have a highly bactericidal action on the meningococcus or who have lesions or a locus minoris resistentiae' in the nosopharyngeal membranes, the meningococci may penetrate into the blood stream. In such cases, bacteraemia and skin rash often result but meningeal symptoms are rarely provoked. Only in few individuals will the meningococci, which have a predilection for the serosal membranes in the central nervous system, pass through the blood-brain barrier and cause cerebrospinal meningitis. Purulent meningitis only occurs in one out of several hundreds of infected individuals. Incubation is 2–10 days, on average 3–4 days.

Clinical symptoms which have a sudden onset comprise: fever, intense headache, stiff neck and nausea. As the central nervous system is affected, delirium and coma may rapidly appear and later on the patients who survive may suffer from sequelae such as deafness or other defects due to the neurological lesions. Rapid treatment with sulphonamides, chloramphenicol or other antibiotics to which N. meningitidis is sensitive is important in order to save lives and prevent the sequelae.

THE AGENT

Neisseria meningitidis is divided into serogroups A,B,C,D,X and Y; there are also some untypable strains. The organism occurs in pairs or tetrades; it has the typical appearance of a diplococcus and is gram negative. It is easily recognized when stained on film preparations of meningeal exudate (CSF). Specimens for culturing and media must be kept warm until incubated. Growth is favored by incubating in an atmosphere with 10 per cent CO_2 at 37 °C. It is identified by biochemical tests and serological procedures. The antigenic differences, which are due to the different cell-wall polysaccharides that characterize each group, are of practical significance for the typing of strains and the preparation of group-specific polysaccharides for use as vaccine. The parasite is harboured in the nasopharynx of carriers usually for relatively long periods (10 months or so). Its survival time outside the body is very short as it is rather fragile, so that close contact is necessary for its transmission which occurs through air-borne droplets expelled by carriers and cases. During epidemics due to group A and C meningococci and especially towards their end, other groups and many atypical forms are observed. As the population, through the carrier state, becomes immune to the prevalent group other groups make their appearance. Prompt laboratory diagnosis of cases of meningitis is very important as it enables the early establishment of proper specific treatment (with drugs to which *N. meningitidis* is sensitive) and of control measures.

EPIDEMIOLOGY

Meningococcal meningitis appears in epidemic form when the relationships between parasite, host (man) and environment are favourable for the spread of infection. This, in the CSM zone in Africa, occurs every year in the dry winter months in one area or another, and ceases three to five months later with the rainy season. The three main epidemiological factors (parasite, man and environment) and their interplay deserve detailed consideration in each area and community as they differ in the various climatic areas and socio-economic conditions.

In temperate zones outbreaks of meningitis are usually limited to a relatively small number of cases among army recruits and other similar groups. In non epidemic areas, besides meningococcal infections, there are other microorganisms that cause meningitis, particularly infections due to pneumonococci and *H. influenzae*. The source of infection is a case or carrier. Transmission takes place when such a person is speaking, coughing or sneezing. Droplets bearing meningococci are expelled from the oropharynx into the air and then are inhaled into the respiratory tract of another person. Close contact such as in dormitories has often been shown to promote transmission of this airborne droplet infection.

It is probable that dust and dryness in the air which cause irritation of the mucous membranes of the nasopharynx facilitate infection.

The climate, in the 'meningitis belt' of Africa and elsewhere plays an important role. In Africa the semi-arid zone called the 'Sahel' is characterized ecologically by scarce vegetation with a typical dry climate in the winter months and a desert wind, the 'Harmatan'. This unusual climatic and ecological entity seems to facilitate the spread of meningitis because of a favorable microclimate in human habitations — small, closed, mud-walled houses in which there is practically no light or ventilation. The degree of crowding and of air pollution by oral airborne bacteria in these houses was observed to parallel the incidence of meningitis (Ghipponi et al, 1971; Fig. 18.2).

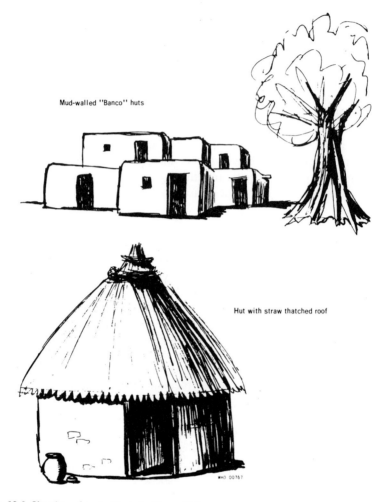

Mud-walled "Banco" huts

Hut with straw thatched roof

Fig. 18.2 Sketches of typical huts in Upper Volta

SURVEILLANCE

National laboratories and the WHO International Collaborating Laboratories for Meningococci are surveying the evolution of outbreaks and the development of the resistance of meningococci thus providing information for rational control. However, for early warning and timely implementation of control measures in the field a simple system of reporting clinical cases in sufficient.

CONTROL

Control measures to prevent the spread of infection are neither easy nor always effective. Consequently treatment should be made available to the population in all instances to save the lives and to prevent sequelae and deaths among those who develop illness.

Treatment with sulphonamides and antibiotics is effective if applied in the early stages of the disease. The earlier the treatment is begun the better the outcome will be. When treatment is delayed until the fifth day or later, the prognosis is poor.

The most practical method is a single injection of sulphamethoxypyridazine or sulphormetoxine, which will be enough to cure an uncomplicated case (Lapeyssonnie and Torres, 1962). The advantage of these drugs is that they are also available in tablet form and can easily be administered orally in the villages. In view of the ever-increasing use of antimicrobial drugs accompanied by an increasing resistance of *N. meningitidis* to sulphonamides, chloramphenicol and other antibiotics should be kept in reserve.

Early treatment of CSM is important in order to prevent invalidity from sequelae such as deafness. WHO, with UNICEF assistance, has made sulphonamides and chloramphenicol available to the countries in need.

It should be kept in mind that neither sulpha drugs nor chloramphenicol are harmless. When mass prophylaxis was carried out during an outbreak in Morocco, sulphormetoxine caused 11 deaths due to Stevens-Johnson syndrome (Bergoend et al, 1968).

Mass prophylaxis with sulphonamides is sometimes proposed and carried out with success. However, due consideration should be paid to the implications. In view of the increasing resistance of meningococci to sulphonamides, the sensitivity of the causative organism must first be proved and the risk of untoward reactions to the drug should be kept in mind. It is therefore considered that mass prophylaxis of general populations as a routine measure is contra-indicated. However, chemoprophylaxis can be used in closed communities (army units, boarding schools, etc.) where it can be applied under medical supervision, and possible mis-uses of the drugs are avoided.

IMMUNIZATION

Group A and C polysaccharides proved to be effective as vaccines in studies in Africa, and elsewhere but immunity is strictly serogroup specific (Gold, Artensten, 1971, Wahdan et al, 1973; Erwa et al, 1973). While the vaccines are effective there is still a problem of how, when and where to apply them in order to obtain the best results in the event of epidemics. The method used must be economically sound and acceptable for both the health authorities and the population.

ENVIRONMENTAL SANITATION

Since it is impossible to change any macroclimate, conducive to CSM outbreaks the obvious alternative is the modification of the microclimate in dwellings by building larger and better ventilated houses where epidemic waves recur. Unfortunately it is a formidable task in African and other countries to change housing conditions not only because of the limited financial resources but also because of the difficulty of persuading the population to change their traditional houses and way of life.

Disinfection of the air would be useless as it would not affect the spread of infection among close contacts. The cumulative cost of continuous disinfection of the air would probably turn out in the long run to be more expensive than the construction of new houses or the modification of existing ones.

Health education has its place during outbreaks in decreasing unnecessary contacts and gatherings.

CONSEQUENCES

Sequelae of which deafness is the most important represent a socio-economic problem. Detection of persons who have suffered damage of CNS after outbreaks is important in order to rehabilitate such persons as much as possible.

REFERENCE

Bergoend R et al 1968 Ann. Derm. Syph 95: 481–490
Erwa H H, Haseeb M A, Idris A A, Lapeyssonnie L, Sanborn W R, Sippel J E 1973 A serogroup A meningococcal polysaccharide vaccine Bulletin of the World Health Organization 49: 301–305
Ghipponi P, Darrigol J, Skalova R, Cvetanovic B 1971 Study of bacterial air pollution in an arid region of Africa affected by cerebrospinal meningitis. Bulletin of the World Health Organization 45: 95–101
Gold R, Artenstein M S 1971 Meningococcal infections. 2 Field trial of Group C meningococcal polysaccharide vaccine in 1969–70. Bulletin of the World Health Organization 45: 279–282
Lapeyssonnie L 1963 La Méningite cérébro-spinale en Afrique. Bulletin of the World Health Organization supplement to vol 28. 114 pages.
Lapeyssonie L, Torres F 1962 Presse med. 70: 2277–2279
Wahdan M H et al. A controlled field trial of a serogroup A meningococcal polysaccharide vaccine Bulletin of the World Health Organization 48: 667–673

Smallpox — Lessons from a successful eradication program

INTRODUCTION

On 8 May 1980, the World Health Assembly resolved 'that smallpox eradication has been achieved throughout the world ... and that there is no evidence that smallpox will return as an endemic disease.' The Assembly urged that smallpox vaccination be stopped except for investigators at special risk and that the requirement for international certificates of vaccination be terminated.

The last known endemic case of smallpox occurred in Merka, Somalia, on 26 October 1977. For more than two years, tens of thousands of health workers searched for cases, stimulated by a World Health Organization (WHO) reward of $1,000 to be given to anyone who discovered a case of smallpox. Countless rumors were investigated and thousands of specimens from cases with rash and fever were examined by WHO Reference Laboratories in Atlanta, USA, and Moscow. Except for two cases which occurred in 1978 in Birmingham, England, following a laboratory accident, no other cases of smallpox have been found. Smallpox virus is now believed to be confined to only two laboratories in the USA and the USSR.

Nevertheless, because the disease was so recently prevalent and geographically disperse, it has been difficult for some to accept that the virus itself might no longer exist in nature. As will be subsequently described, however, substantial evidence has been accumulated which documents this fact.

Since 1980 when smallpox was declared to have been eradicated, rumors and false reports of smallpox cases have continued to be received by WHO and each has been investigated. None has been smallpox. Many such reports have emanated from the news media who have mistakenly identified as smallpox epidemics of measles in which deaths have occurred. Some reports have been received from senior national and expatriate health personnel who have dealt with smallpox epidemics throughout their professional careers and assume, without evidence, that cases must still be present somewhere in the distant rural areas. Two diseases which clinically may resemble smallpox account for some of the reports and these are important to note. The causative agents of both diseases are virologically distinct from smallpox. Cases of severe chickenpox, especially in adults, occasionally may resemble smallpox and are mistakenly diagnosed as such. A second disease caused by the closely related monkeypox virus is clinically indistinguishable from smallpox but less than 100 cases have been identified. All have occurred in remote villages of the tropical rain forest in central and western Africa. Transmission of monkeypox from person to person rarely occurs and sustained human transmission has not been observed.

Accordingly, for health authorities everywhere, the occurrence of a single suspected case of smallpox continues to demand immediate and competent investigation by both clinical and laboratory means. Confirmation of a case as smallpox implies the possibility that the virus has escaped from a laboratory or that some other presently unforeseen event has occurred. The discovery of such a case thus represents a true public health emergency.

THE DISEASE

Smallpox was an acute exanthematous disease caused by variola virus. The incubation period varied from seven to 17 days, with most cases occurring 10 to 14 days after close contact with a previous case. The illness began with a high prodromal fever and mild to severe constitutional symptoms which resembled those of influenza. Between the second and fifth day, a rash developed. In the usual or 'ordinary' type of smallpox, the rash first appeared as macules on the face and upper part of the body and, within a day or two, on the lower part of the body and legs. Lesions frequently appeared on the hard and soft palate, cheeks and tongue as well as on the palms and soles. Over a three- to four-day period, the macules evolved into vesicles and then pustules. By the fifth day of rash, the appearance of the characteristic, deep-seated pustules, the similarity of all lesions on any given part of the body and the 'centrifugal' distribution of lesions on the face, arms and legs, characterized the illness as smallpox. The pustules began to be replaced by crusts about the tenth day of rash. These crusts separated over the following one to three weeks.

Although the ordinary type of smallpox accounted for 80 to 90 percent of cases, three other clinical types were recognized: (1) haemorrhagic, (2) flat, and (3) modified. In the uniformly fatal haemorrhagic type, the patient experienced a severely prostrating prodromal illness followed by the development of a dusky erythema and eventually petechiae and frank haemorrhages into the skin and mucous membranes. Death usually occurred by the fifth or sixth day after onset. In the frequently fatal 'flat' variety, the patient experienced prostrating constitutional symptoms. The lesions developed slowly and were essentially confluent. The skin took on the appearance of a fine-grained reddish-colored crepe rubber. Haemorrhages into the skin sometimes occurred. In the 'modified' variety which occurred in previously vaccinated persons, the patient experienced less severe symptoms, the lesions were fewer in number and matured more rapidly than in the ordinary case. Occasionally, they did not progress beyond the papular stage before resolving.

Case-fatality rates of 20 percent and greater were customary for smallpox caused by the pathogenic *variola major* strain. This strain of the virus, once prevalent throughout the world, was endemic only on the Indian subcontinent within the past two decades. A less pathogenic strain was prevalent in Indonesia and in most African countries with case-fatality rates of 5 to 15 percent. Least virulent was disease caused by the strain, *variola minor*, which was found most recently in South America, in southern Africa and in Ethiopia and Somalia on the eastern horn of Africa. Here, case-fatality rates of less than one percent were observed.

Cases of chickenpox most frequently presented problems in differential diagnosis. Such cases differ in several respects. Crops of lesions erupt over a period of many days and, on any part of the body, vesicles, pustules and scabs are found together. The lesions are superficial and a vesicle, when pricked, collapses. Moreover, the lesions are more densely concentrated on the trunk than on the extremities and, only rarely, are lesions found on the palms or soles. In contrast, smallpox lesions were more deep-seated in the skin and on each part of the body were all at a similar stage of development; the lesions were more densely concentrated on the extremities than on the trunk; and lesions were often found on the palms and soles.

THE AGENT

Variola virus is one of a group of orthopoxviruses which includes vaccinia, monkeypox, cowpox, buffalo pox, rabbit pox, camel pox, and ectromelia. The poxviruses are the largest viruses so recognized, having a diameter of about 200 mu. The genome consists of a single molecule of double-stranded DNA.

For virological diagnosis, vesicular or pustular fluid or scabs is examined under the electron microscope. This permits rapid identification of an orthopoxvirus if present. Differentiation as to which pox-virus might be causing illness requires that the virus be isolated on chick chorioallantoic membrane and its properties characterized by specific biological tests. WHO Reference Laboratories at the Centers for Disease Control, Atlanta, Georgia, and at the Institute for Virus Preparations, Moscow, continue to work with poxviruses and are prepared at any time to undertake necessary diagnostic studies. Shipment of specimens can be arranged through WHO. For patients who have recovered from their illnesses, diagnosis can be determined through the measurement of neutralizing, complement fixing and hemagglutinin-inhibiting antibody in serum specimens.

EPIDEMIOLOGY

Because smallpox has no known animal reservoir and because the virus persisted in man only during the three- to four-week period of illness, smallpox virus had to spread continually from person to person in order to survive. Since the recovered patient was effectively immune to subsequent infection, the persistence of smallpox required a population adequate in size to permit a sufficient number of new susceptibles to be infected each year. Only then could a continuing chain of virus transmission persist. Historians speculate that the disease could not have emerged until sometime after the first agricultural settlements, about 10 000 B.C., presumably as a result of a mutation of a related mammalian orthopoxvirus. The presence of the distinctive smallpox rash on the mummy of Pharaoh Ramses V documents its existence more than 3,000 years ago.

In ancient times, only a few populated areas, perhaps in India, China or Egypt, could have supported its continued transmission. If occasionally introduced into less populated areas, the virus would not long persist before dying out. As the world's population increased, smallpox progressively spread to infect all parts of the world.

Over the centuries, smallpox proved to be one of the most devastating diseases known to man. Its impact on history and human affairs was profound. Case-fatality rates of 20 percent or more were characteristic and where the disease became endemic, virtually all persons eventually contracted smallpox. Deities to smallpox were a part of the culture in India and a number of African countries. In Europe, at the end of the 18th century, it killed an estimated 400 000 persons each year and was responsible for one-third of all cases of blindness. In the Americas, within a few years after smallpox was introduced, more than 3.5 million Mexican Indians died and it was smallpox which was primarily responsible for the collapse of the Aztec and Incan empires. The devastation wrought by smallpox in Africa and Asia is less completely documented but appears to have been no less severe.

In 1796, Edward Jenner, an English physician, showed that smallpox could be prevented by inoculation into the skin of material taken from a lesion caused by cowpox. This technique he called 'vaccination.' Cowpox virus, which is related to but distinct from variola virus, was the world's first vaccine. Moreover, Jenner demonstrated that material taken from the cowpox lesion which had been induced by vaccination could be transferred from one person to another. The infection was mild, almost never fatal and was almost never transmitted naturally from person to person. Before Jenner's discovery, the only defense against smallpox had been to deliberately inoculate scabs or pustular material from smallpox patients into the skin of susceptibles. This procedure was called 'variolation.' The infection which resulted was usually less severe than infection acquired by the natural respiratory route of infection. Although case-fatality rates among those with induced infection were 'only' one to two percent, the variolated patients readily transmitted infection to others. Variolation gradually ceased as vaccination became known and available. However, in the more remote areas of Afghanistan, Pakistan and Africa, variolation persisted until the 1970s.

During the 19th century, vaccination was increasingly widely practised, especially in the more developed, temperate-climate countries. Its wider application was inhibited by the fact that the cowpox virus (later termed vaccinia virus) had to be successively transferred from one to another by arm to arm inoculation. Large scale vaccination was difficult and periodically the strain was lost when vaccinations proved unsuccessful. Late in the 19th century, vaccinia virus began to be propagated on the flank of a calf and this permitted large quantities to be produced. However, such virus remained viable for only a few days at ambient temperature. Finally, in the 1950s, a commercially feasible method was developed which permitted large-scale production of vaccine which was stable for a month or longer at temperatures of 37°C or greater.

In the industrialized countries, smallpox incidence steadily declined as vaccination became more widespread. However, not until after World War II did Europe and North America finally interrupt smallpox transmission. In the developing countries, vaccination was less widely practised and, in the tropical regions, vaccination with the available heat labile vaccine was frequently unsuccessful.

From its founding in 1948, the World Health Assembly had expressed concern about smallpox and had encouraged all member countries to take more vigorous control measures. Smallpox was a problem to all. Even those without disease feared importations and conducted vaccination programs to prevent epidemics should cases be imported. Finally, in 1959, the Assembly decided that a global eradication program should be undertaken. During the succeeding seven years, a number of countries undertook mass-vaccination campaigns but few succeeded in interrupting smallpox transmission. The few countries which were successful were plagued by repeated importations from neighbors. Surveillance for smallpox was poor and reporting was woefully incomplete. Vaccine donations were too limited to meet the needs and vaccine quality was generally poor. Serious setbacks in WHO's only other eradication program, the malaria program, caused the concept of eradication itself to be viewed with increasing skepticism.

However, in 1966, the Assembly decided that one further effort should be made to eradicate the disease. They voted to allot $US 2.5 million annually for an intensified eradication program. Although a modest sum to support programs which would need to be conducted in 50 countries, this represented five percent of WHO's budget that year. A 10-year goal was proposed. The intensified program commenced on January 1, 1967. Its objective was to eliminate smallpox from the world by December, 1976.

In 1967, smallpox was considered to be endemic in 33 countries; 14

additional countries reported cases that year which were attributed to importations. Although 131,000 cases were officially reported, later studies showed that only about one percent of all cases were notified. Thus, the true number of cases was about 10 to 15 million. Four geographic reservoirs of smallpox were identified: (1) virtually the whole of Africa south of the Sahara; (2) a band of southeast Asia countries extending from Bangladesh through India, Nepal, Pakistan and Afghanistan; (3) Indonesia; and (4) Brazil. The estimated population of these countries was more than 1.2 billion persons.

PROGRAM STRATEGY

WHO's program strategy initially called for each country to undertake an intensive, systematic program of vaccination with the objective of vaccinating at least 80 percent of the population during a two- to three-year period. During this time, it was expected that a reliable reporting system could be developed which would serve to identify the remaining foci of smallpox. These would be eliminated by isolation of patients and vaccination of contacts. The initial extensive vaccination campaign was believed necessary to increase population immunity and so reduce the number of smallpox cases to a level low enough to permit disease surveillance and containment activities to be effective.

Experience soon showed that the surveillance-containment component of the program could be developed more quickly and was more effective than had been thought. Its effective implementation proved to be the essential factor in the program's success. In part, this was due to the unique clinical and epidemiological characteristics of smallpox. An infected patient was able to transmit infection only from the time of first appearance of rash until the last scabs had separated. There were no chronic carriers nor individuals with latent infections. The rash was sufficiently characteristic to be diagnosed with a high degree of accuracy by clinicians and villagers alike. The presence or absence of smallpox in an area could thus be reliably determined without laboratory studies. Moreover, approximately two-thirds of all recovered patients in Asia and most parts of Africa had characteristic residual facial scars. Thus, it was possible, through survey, to determine not only the present status of smallpox but also its past history in an area.

To persist, smallpox virus had to be transmitted in a continuing chain of infection from patient to susceptible contact. By isolation of the patient and by vaccination of contacts, a barrier to transmission was created and the chain of infection interrupted. In small villages and in scattered populations, chains of transmission often terminated without intervention. Contrary to conventional wisdom, smallpox did not spread rapidly and then only to those in face-to-face contact. A given patient rarely infected more than two or three others and, even in infected households, three and sometimes four generations of cases occurred. Secondary cases were usually found among neighbors, relatives and friends — persons who had been in close personal contact with the patient. The cases tended to cluster within parts of a town or city and in localized areas within broader geographic regions. Because of the 10- to 14-day interval between generations of cases, outbreaks developed slowly. Because they developed slowly and the cases clustered geographically, early detection of cases followed by isolation of patients and intensive vaccination throughout the immediate community proved remarkably effective in stopping transmission, even when there was a comparatively low level of population immunity. These observations, made early in the program, resulted in a redirection of strategy to give priority to case reporting, surveillance and containment at the expense of mass vaccination programs.

VACCINE AND VACCINATION DEVICES

Smallpox vaccine which conferred durable immunity was an additional important factor in the program's success. Although it had been a common belief that effective levels of protection extended for no more than three to five years, studies during the program revealed vaccine-efficacy ratios of more than 90 percent after 20 years. Emphasis in program strategy was thus given to primary vaccination. Since the lyophilized vaccine retained its potency after incubation at 37°C for one month or longer, the logistics of vaccine storage and distribution were greatly simplified.

Unfortunately, when the program began, less than 10 percent of the vaccine then in use was found by WHO Collaborating Reference Centers to meet accepted standards. Through WHO assistance to laboratories and through a continuing program which monitored vaccine quality, standards improved. By 1970, all vaccine in use met stipulated requirements of potency and stability and, by 1973, 80 percent of the vaccine was being produced in the developing countries.

A new device for vaccination was introduced — the bifurcated needle, best described as a large sewing needle with part of the eye ground off to leave two small prongs. An invention of Wyeth Laboratories, the needle was dipped into the vaccine solution and just sufficient for inoculation adhered by capillarity between the prongs. The needle was held perpendicularly to the skin and 15 quick punctures were made. Only one-fourth as much vaccine was required as with the conventional scratch method; vaccinators could be trained within minutes, and take rates approached 100 percent. The needles could be repeatedly sterilized and reused 200 times or more.

A further simplification of vaccination technique was achieved by dispensing with solutions for cleansing the skin. Studies revealed that secondary infections of the vaccination site were the same whether or not acetone or soap was first applied. Vaccinators were ultimately instructed only to wipe away obvious caked dirt with a damp cloth.

With these changes in technique, a vaccinator needed only to carry the small 100-dose vials of dried vaccine and diluent and a supply of needles. A week's supply could be carried in a shirt pocket.

PROGRESS IN THE PROGRAM

By 1969, eradication programs were in progress in all of the infected and immediately adjacent countries except for Ethiopia, whose program began in 1971. A program manual set forth the strategy and provided overall guidance, but each country was encouraged to develop a reporting network, to evaluate its own epidemiological situation and to modify the program to best suit its own circumstances. WHO surveillance reports which documented program progress and recorded epidemiological observations, were issued every two to three weeks. Also distributed were technical papers describing scientific findings and field observations in different countries to facilitate a continuing interchange of experience.

By 1970, the number of endemic countries had decreased from 33 to 18. Eleven of the 15 which became smallpox-free were in western and central Africa where a regional program was assisted by the U.S. Center for Disease Control. Success in this region was an important stimulus to the global program because the health structures, as well as transport and communication systems, in many of these countries were among the least developed. Brazil registered its last case in 1971 and Indonesia and Afghanistan in 1972. By 1973, all of Africa had become smallpox-free except for Ethiopia whose program had only recently begun and Botswana, which was reinfected concident with the last cases in neighboring South Africa. In addition to Ethiopia and Botswana, there were only four other smallpox-endemic countries — India, Pakistan, Nepal and Bangladesh. However, the population of these four was over 700 million and the techniques of surveillance and containment which had been applied elsewhere were far less successful. Primarily, this could be attributed to the greater population density of these countries and the much more extensive movement of the population from place to place.

A new strategy for the Indian program was worked out during the summer of 1973 and implemented that autumn. It was decided that much more rapid case detection and more effective containment of outbreaks was needed. Accordingly, it was decided to mobilize for one week each month more than 100,000 health workers to search village-by-village, later house-by-house, to detect cases. Hundreds of special surveillance-containment teams were trained to contain the outbreaks which were found. In the period between the searches, the teams travelled throughout their assigned areas, stopping at markets and schools to question residents about rumors of cases. The number of reported cases rose sharply. More than 214,000 cases were recorded in 1974, the highest total notified in India in almost 20 years. Far more complete and more rapid reporting was being achieved, and the outbreaks more effectively contained. A similar strategy was soon adopted in the neighboring countries. During the summer of 1974, new cases declined rapidly in number and a cash reward began to be offered to anyone who reported a case and to the health worker who investigated it. As cases further declined, the reward was increased. In May, 1975, the last case was detected in India and on October 16, 1975, the last case in Asia.

The only remaining endemic country was Ethiopia. It posed an entirely different set of problems. Its 25 million people are scattered across a rugged mountainous plateau and desert area. More than half of its population lived more than a day's walk from any accessible road and its health structure was vestigial. With the end of smallpox in Asia, resources were shifted to Ethiopia and its 150-person smallpox program staff increased. Helicopters were added to facilitate transport. Intensive search for cases coupled with extensive vaccination programs interrupted transmission in August, 1976. Unfortunately, as the last outbreaks were being contained, the disease was introduced into neighboring Somalia. Cases were not promptly detected and the disease spread. Intensive surveillance and vaccination programs were immediately begun but not until October 26, 1977 was transmission finally stopped.

CONFIRMATION OF ERADICATION

Although eradication had apparently been achieved, it was important for scientists and policy makers alike to have confidence that this was fact. To foster that confidence, WHO established formal procedures for certification of eradication. The plan called for each country where smallpox had been endemic since 1967 and those at risk of importations to conduct a program of active search for cases for at least two years after the last known case. At the end of this period, a WHO-appointed International Commission visited each country, reviewed the record of work and conducted extensive field visits to confirm the results. In addition, the Commissions investigated special areas which were considered most likely to harbor cases of smallpox if present. Between 1973 and 1979, 21 different Commissions visited and certified eradication in 49 countries. The two-year period of search was confirmed in practise to be more than adequate. During the program, smallpox had not persisted without being detected for more than eight months in any country thought to be smallpox-free.

Finally, in 1978, the Director-General of WHO appointed a Global Commission for the Certification of Smallpox Eradication. The Commission, comprised of 21 scientists from 19 countries, reviewed reports submitted by each country and the findings of each of the International Commissions. Members of the Global Commission made special field visits and requested further information and studies from countries about which they had any question as to the status of smallpox. After satisfying itself that eradication had been achieved, the Global Commission reported its findings to the World Health Assembly. The Assembly considered the report and on May.

8, 1980, declared its agreement. It recommended that 'smallpox vaccination be discontinued in every country except for investigators at special risk' and advised that 'an international certificate of vaccination against smallpox should no longer be required of any traveller.'

POSSIBLE SOURCES FOR A RETURN OF SMALLPOX

As of June 1984, variola virus was known to exist only in two special laboratories, both of which had been inspected by WHO-appointed international teams to verify conditions of virus storage and laboratory safety. The risk of accidental escape from either was considered by the WHO Global Commission to be extremely small.

Extensive studies had been conducted since 1967 to discover a possible animal or other natural reservoir of the virus. None was found. The best evidence that such a reservoir does not exist derives from epidemiological observations that all smallpox outbreaks detected in otherwise smallpox-free areas during the past 12 years were able to be traced to other known human cases. If there were an animal reservoir or if the virus were able to persist in nature in crusts or other material, apparently 'spontaneous' outbreaks should have been discovered, but they were not.

Nearly 100 cases of a newly recognized disease which is clinically indistinguishable from smallpox but caused by the related monkey pox virus occurred in five central and west African countries between 1970 and 1983. All but two of the cases lived in small villages in the tropical rain forest. Person-to-person transmission may have occurred in six instances but it was apparent that the virus is transmitted only with difficulty even when many susceptibles are in close contact. Genome maps of this and other animal poxviruses reveal many differences between them and variola, suggesting that a mutation to variola virus would be highly unlikely.

The recurrence of smallpox due to a deliberate release of variola virus as an act of terrorism cannot, unhappily, be ruled out despite an International Convention which outlaws biological weapons in warfare. The potential harm of such an act will increase as population immunity wanes. However, the potential damage of such an act should not be exaggerated. As pointed out, smallpox does not spread rapidly, as does influenza or measles, and unless the public health services have completely broken down, an outbreak caused in this manner should be able to be contained within three to four weeks. Moreover, if someone were to decide to employ biological weapons, there are other agents whose virulence and characteristics of spread are superior to those of variola virus.

As insurance against presently unforeseen events, the WHO has established vaccine storage reserves containing some 200 million doses of vaccine. Additional stocks are being retained by a number of governments. Since vaccine has been shown to be potent after 17 years of storage at −20°C, it is believed these stocks can be retained indefinitely.

Barring unforeseen circumstances, a human case of smallpox will never again be seen. However, the problem of mistaken diagnosis is a real one. As noted by the WHO Global Commission: 'Experience in many countries indicates that reports of suspected cases of smallpox can be expected to be received from many sources for several years after the certification of eradication.' For this reason, WHO medical officers with expertise in diagnosis remain on call to investigate such rumors and an expertise in laboratory diagnoses will be maintained by WHO Diagnostic Reference Laboratories (Center for Disease Control, Atlanta, and the Institute for Virus Preparations, Moscow).

LESSONS FROM THE PROGRAM

Many lessons and observations may be drawn from the experience gained in the smallpox eradication program. I will discuss only three: (1) the importance of epidemiological surveillance to the program; (2) the potential for the mobilization of manpower; and (3) the prospects for eradication of other diseases.

In retrospect, it is clear that the most important decision in regard to the strategy of the program was the emphasis placed on the reporting of cases, the epidemiological evaluation of the occurrence and patterns of spread of smallpox and the continuing modification of the strategy and tactics of the program in response to these observations. Before 1967, program progress had been assessed primarily in terms of the numbers of persons vaccinated. The goal of the program then had been to achieve vaccination of 80 percent of the population, believing that when this proportion of the population had been rendered immune, smallpox transmission would cease. In fact, however, it was found that transmission could and did continue, especially in densely populated areas, when more than 90 percent of the population had been vaccinated. Conversely, transmission was interrupted in other densely populated areas when only half the population had been vaccinated. Whether smallpox transmission was interrupted or not depended on the prompt discovery of cases, their isolation and thorough vaccination of contacts and those living in the immediate vicinity. This was the essence of the "surveillance-containment" strategy.

Through surveillance, many observations were made which had practical program implications. The discovery that smallpox spread more slowly then was commonly thought resulted in more resources being diverted to the discovery of outbreaks and their containment. Many had believed that airborne transmission of the virus over long distances was common, but this was discovered to be erroneous. Containment procedures were modified accordingly. The finding that vaccine immunity was far more durable than had been believed resulted in a shift in emphasis from time-consuming systematic programs of revaccination to an emphasis on primary vaccination.

These are but a few illustrations of a multitude of important observations which altered program strategy.

Early in the program, the slogan, "Smallpox — Target Zero" was adopted. Progress was focused thereby, not in terms of numbers of persons vaccinated, but in terms of numbers of cases of smallpox. Inevitably, this sustained the focus of interest on the epidemiology of smallpox and this, in turn, directed changes in strategy and tactics.

No other disease has the same epidemiological characteristics as does smallpox and therefore the smallpox eradication program cannot serve as a template for any other disease control program. However, it would seem logical and desirable to incorporate as a basic element of strategy in any program, the principle of disease surveillance as the ultimate measure of progress or lack thereof and to utilize these findings in continuing modification of program strategy.

When the program began, many believed that a principal constraint in surveillance, as well as in the broader aspects of program implementation, would be the lack of clinics, health posts and hospitals which could report cases and of health personnel to undertake vaccination and containment activities. In some countries, this was indeed a constraint. However, in the majority, it was found that there were surprisingly large numbers of trained, well-motivated health personnel who had few or no supplies with which to work, no supervision and no defined program of activities. Health centers, dressers stations and other health units were surprisingly numerous in most countries but few had more than the most minimal resources. A small number of smallpox eradication program staff with transport to move from place to place distributed vaccines and vaccinostyles, trained health staff in reporting and containment activities and provided continuing supervision of activities. In many countries, they were the only health staff actively providing training and supervision in this manner. Given this type of support and encouragement, many health personnel responded with interest and enthusiasm and performed both competently and conscienciously. One cannot help but speculate about the existing potential for the delivery of other health services if objectives and procedures were better defined, if regular and effective field supervision of activities were provided and if effective distribution systems were established to provide the necessary vaccines, drugs, instruments, etc. I would guess that even today in most countries less than 20 percent of the capacity of the health services is utilized.

Finally, we must ask about the potential for the eradication of other diseases. Many factors were favorable for the eradication of smallpox. When the intensified program began in 1967, the practical feasibility of eradication had already been demonstrated. Disease transmission had been interrupted in all industralized countries *and* in many developing countries as well, including those in Central America and in North Africa, as well as Thailand, Philippines, Burma, Laos, Cambodia, Vietnam and others. The disease itself was feared by countries throughout the world and almost all were conducting vaccination programs of some type. The universal requirement that international certificates of vaccination be produced by travelers reflected this concern. Available to control the disease was an inexpensive, stable, highly protective vaccine which could be easily administered. The epidemiological characteristics of smallpox were exceptionally favorable — an easily diagnosed disease which spread slowly and whose chains of transmission could be interrupted in a comparatively straightforward manner. Despite these many favorable attributes and despite the previous demonstration of the practical feasibility of eradication in both developed and developing countries, global eradication was achieved only with the greatest of difficulty. Voluntary contributions to the program were meager and difficult to obtain, civil wars and political disturbances regularly interrupted progress and cooperation from many governments with endemic infection was grudging and reluctant.

Should we today consider embarking on the eradication of another disease given the available technology, the less favorable epidemiological characteristics of essentially all other diseases, the lesser concern about other diseases on the part of potential donor countries and the civil disorder extant throughout so much of the world? I think not. Moreover, to proclaim as an objective the eradication of a disease and to fail so substantially, as we did with malaria eradication, can only serve to discredit public health. Scientific and political wisdom points to disease control for the foreseeable future.

FURTHER READING

World Health Organization (1980) *The Global Eradication of Smallpox*, Final Report of the Global Commission for the Certification of Smallpox Eradication.

Joarder, A K, Tarantola, D, Tulloch, J. (1980) *The Eradication of Smallpox from Bangladesh*, World Health Organization, New Delhi.

Basu, R N, Jesek, Z. and Ward, N A (1979) *The Eradication of Smallpox from India*, World Health Organization, New Delhi.

Henderson, D A (1980) Smallpox, Maxcy-Rosenau *Preventive Medicine and Public Health*, edited by Last, J M. Appleton-Century-Crofts, New York.

Diarrhoeal infections

INTRODUCTION

Diarrhoea, the first or second most important cause of childhood death in the world, (Walsh, Warren, 1979) is in fact not a disease but a symptom complex of multiple aetiologies. Variously defined in terms of frequency and consistency of faecal passage, diarrhoea is ultimately identified by the liquid nature of the stool, loss of fluid is the most important cause of death. Infectious agents (bacteria, parasites, viruses) cause the vast majority of cases, and this chapter will concentrate on these.

In addition to claiming the lives of an estimated five million children per year, (Rohde, 1983) diarrhoea is a major contributor to malnutrition through a variety of mechanisms including anorexia, intestinal malabsorption and social practices depriving the patient of food. Prevention of diarrhoea requires vast, complex and expensive environmental improvements designed to reduce ingestion or contact with faecal organisms. Clean, protected water supplies and effective universal sanitation systems as well as the control of vectors and a high degree of personal hygiene must be widely available before a significant fall in the incidence of diarrhoea will occur. Even under sanitary circumstances prevailing in western nations, diarrhoea remains relatively high on the list of morbid conditions affecting children. The deaths and the morbid effects on nutrition can, however, be prevented by cheap and readily available oral rehydration and intensified attention to the nutritional needs of the sick and convalescing child. The universal understanding and use of home rehydration measures and effective back-up referral services should reduce deaths from diarrhoea by from 50–90 per cent, and may be the most effective intervention against malnutrition among the five hundred million children of the developing world.

The following is a brief review of the multitude of causative agents and the various pathogenic mechanisms (see Table 1). (Diarrhoea Dialogue, 1981)

Table 20.1

Complaint	Associated clinical features		Incubation period	Epidemiological features	Organisms	First line treatment	Percent of cases**	
	Common	Others					Child	Adult
Acute Watery Diarrhoea	• Vomiting • Fever	• Severe dehydration in some	24–72 hours	• Infants and young children • Common world-wide in all socioeconomic groups • Peak in colder seasons in temperate climates	Rotavirus	• Rehydration therapy	30–60	0–5
The stool takes the shape of the container	• Nausea • Vomiting • Abdominal pain	• Fever • Malaise • Severe dehydration	6–72 hours	• Infants and young children in developing countries • Travellers diarrhoea in adults	Enterotoxigenic *Escherichia coli* (ETEC)	• Rehydration therapy	5–25	10–30
	• Nausea • Vomiting • Fever • Chills • Abdominal pain	• Malaise	8–36 hours	• Children • Common world-wide • Food-borne outbreaks (animal products) • Warmer seasons	Non-typhoid Salmonellae	• Rehydration therapy	2–10	5–20

Table 20.1 cont.

| Complaint | Associated clinical features | | Incubation period | Epidemiological features | Organisms | First line treatment | Percent of cases** | |
	Common	Others					Child	Adult
Acute watery diarrhoea cont	• Abdominal pain • Fever • Malaise	• Chills • Blood and pus in the stools	3–5 days	• World-wide distribution • In developed countries may be food-borne (animal products) or transmitted by handling of animals	*Campylobacter*	• Rehydration therapy • Erythromycin in severe cases	2–15	5–15
	• Vomiting • Abdominal pain	• Severe dehydration • Circulatory collapse, 'shock'	1–3 days	• Children in endemic areas • Adults in newly affected areas • Not found in Latin America	*Vibrio cholerae*	• Rehydration therapy • Tetracycline	0–15	0–30
	• Nausea • Vomiting	• Fever	6–72 hours	• Nursery outbreaks in developed countries • Uncertain in developing countries	Enteropathogenic *Escherichia coli* (EPEC)	• Rehydration therapy	0–5	0

Table 20.1 cont.

Dysentery The stool is soft and watery with blood and/or pus	• Fever • Abdominal pain • Malaise • Vomiting • Urgency to defaecate • Painful spasm on defaecation	36–72 hours	• Children • Poor hygiene • Malnutrition • Institutions • Warmer seasons	Shigellae	• Rehydration therapy • Ampicillin or Trimethoprim Sulfamethoxazole	2–15	5–30
Prolonged Diarrhoea or dysentery	• Abdominal discomfort	2–6 weeks	• All age groups • World-wide distribution	Entamoeba* histolytica	• Metronidazole	0–3	0–10
For at least 7 days, stools have been more frequent or of softer consistency (with or without blood or pus)	• Abdominal distension • Flatulence • Anorexia • Nausea • Malbsorption • Frothy stools	1–3 weeks	• Young children • Some travellers • Poor hygiene • World-wide distribution	Giardia* lamblia	• Metronidazole	0–5	0–20

Can be identified on examination of the stools with a light microscope.
Blood and pus from Shigellae and Campylobacter can also be identified.
Produced in collaboration with the Ross Institute of the London School of Hygiene and Tropical Medicine and The Save the Children Fund
**Approximate percent of cases in reported series due to each agent. Table does not include non enteric infections which may account for 10–20% of cases in some series: measles, malaria, otitis media, meningitis. No etiologic diagnosis is found in 20–40% in most series.

THE AGENT

Bacteria

a. Toxins

Cholera is the most dramatic infective diarrhoea with massive isotonic fluid losses leading to fatal dehydration in a few hours. The study of cholera led to an understanding not only of the mechanisms of intestinal absorption but of all toxin induced diarrhoeas. *E. coli* and some shigella, which also produce toxins, account for far more cases of diarrhoea worldwide. The ability of an organism to produce toxin is genetically coded, and in some organisms is found on a plasmid (Finkelstein, 1973). Additionally, adherence factors on the cell surface of the bacterium are necessary for the organism both to colonise and to produce disease. Such factors, associated with the presence of pili or fimbriae, are known to be critical in the pathogenesis of animal diarrhoea (Dupont, 1980). Recently, similar colonisation factors have been identified in human *E. coli* pathogens (CFA — I and II) the absence of which renders non-pathogenic even toxin-producing organisms (Evans and Evans, 1978).

First, the bacterium adheres to the gut wall, then the toxin fixes to binding sites (gangliosides) on the cell wall. The toxin stimulates the cell mechanisms to produce cyclicnucleotides which in turn both decrease the absorption of sodium from gut lumen by the villous tips, and increase the secretion of sodium chloride and water from the blood to the lumen by the crypts (Field 1980). Cholera and related toxins of enterobacteriaceae such as the heat labile toxin (LT) of *E. coli* work through a cyclic AMP mechanism. This is characterised by a time lag in onset and subsequent continued effect for up to 48 hours with increase in crypt secretion as well as decreased villous absorption (Field, 1978). *E. coli* heat stable toxin (ST), on the other hand, activates guanyl cyclase to produce cyclic GMP almost immediately, an effect which can also be reversed by removal of the toxin. Decreased villous tip absorption results with no apparent effect on crypt mechanisms (Hughes et al, 1978). Intracellular mechanisms are mediated through or modulated by calcium and a variety of intracellular enzyme and transport systems susceptible to prostaglandins, cardiac glycosides and other pharmacologic agents. While the kinetics of these various mechanisms vary according to the toxins and particular cellular mechanism activated, it appears that the predominant mechanism of recovery from toxin diarrhoea is the replacement of the affected cells by the normal regeneration of the intestinal villus. (Pierce et al, 1971) Thus the diarrhoea is self-limited lasting for in most cases from two to five days.

b. Invasive diarrhoeas

Shigella is the classical agent. The organism elaborates a variety of products, many plasmid encoded, enabling it to penetrate the mucosa of the colon and to establish local inflammation, micro ulcers and resulting diarrhoea

(Keusch, 1979). Highly host specific a relatively few organisms, $10^1 - 10^2$, are required to produce disease. By contrast in cholera $10^5 - 10^7$ organisms, or in salmonella $10^6 - 10^9$ organisms, are needed to produce infections in a majority of cases (Keusch, 1981). The mechanism of other invasive diarrhoeas, campylobacter, *Vibrio parahemolyticus*, yersinia and salmonellas are apparently similar. Some of these, including shigella, may also produce entero-toxins that affect fluid absorption and secretion. The resulting diarrhoea is generally accompanied by fever and has mucus, pus and sometimes blood in the stool. Recovery occurs by removal of the organisms and repair of the damaged gut surface.

c. Enteric fevers

Classical typhoid fever may present with either diarrhoea, constipation, or indeed no intestinal symptoms. (See Robinson Chapter 23) Salmonella Typhi, a group D organism causes the most severe disease, which is best characterised as a reticuloendothelial systemic infection. From the intestinal Peyers patches, to the liver, spleen bone marrow and nodes, the organisms invade and proliferate in this system leading to severe septicaemia and endotoxigenic shock. Necrosis and breakdown of Peyers patches can lead to both bloody diarrhoea and intestinal perforation, both occurring some 10–14 days into the acute illness. A similar though generally more mild illness is caused by the paratyphoid organism.

More than 1700 serotypes comprise the rest of the salmonellae which are ubiquitous pathogens of higher animals. These cause a more mild usually afebrile enteritis that is readily transmitted through food or fomites. These are generally self limited non systemic infections.

Virus

For many years, although the epidemiology of childhood diarrhoea indicated an infectious origin, the incrimination of viruses was uncertain. In the last decade with the discovery of the Norwalk agent and rotavirus up to 80 per cent of diarrhoeal episodes in children can now be ascribed to specific aetiological agents. Norwalk and Norwalk-like agents account for about one-third of epidemic outbreaks in the U.S. (Kapikian et al, 1976; Greenberg et al, 1979) Worldwide, rotavirus is present in 30–40 per cent of diarrhoeas in children under age two years (Soenarto et al, 1981). Other viruses in the calicivirus, corona and adeno-virus groups have been identified and implicated both epidemiologically and pathologically in smaller studies. The consistent and continuing absence of aetiologic explanation in 20–40 per cent of diarrhoeal cases suggests that additional viral agents will be identified.

Intestinal viruses (rotavirus is the best studied) invade the enterocytes and cause a denuding of the villus columnar epithelium, resulting in diminished absorption of fluids electrolytes and monosaccharides (Davidson and Barnes, 1979). Recovery occurs when the mucosal surface regenerates.

Parasites

The most important parasites known to cause diarrhoea are *Giardia lamblia* and *Entamoeba histolytica*, although *Strongyloides* and occasionally *Trichuris* have also been implicated. There is no good evidence that ascaris or hookworm cause diarrhoea. The mechanism of amoebic dysentery is clearly invasion and microabscess formation the resulting diarrhoea tends to be chronic, painful, debilitating and associated with pus and blood (*See* McFadzean and Pugh Chapter 21).

Giardia attacks the upper intestine, usually the duodenum, and may be most reliably diagnosed by duodenal biopsy or the string test. The pathogenesis of the diarrhoea is unclear. It may produce toxins. While it can locally invade, it does not cause abscess formation. The symptoms of epigastric distress, foamy stools and foul smell suggest this diagnosis. While most diarrhoea associated with parasites tends to be chronic and not the acute dehydrating illness of the previous groups *Giardia* has occurred in epidemic proportions and can present with an explosive as well as a chronic onset (Craun, 1979).

Other mechanisms

Acute onset of vomiting and diarrhoea, is a hallmark of food poisoning, usually caused by ingestion of preformed toxins elaborated by *Staph aureus* or *B. cereus* in improperly preserved foods. Common source outbreaks of explosive onset are typical of such food poisoning. Ciguatera and other fish poisons and toxins of various mushrooms are distinguished not only by diarrhoea but also neurologic disturbances ranging from paresthesias to seizures, coma and death.

Diarrhoea commonly accompanies infections in other parts of the body. It has been associated with malaria, otitis media, pneumonias, streptococcal sore throat and a variety of other common conditions. It almost invariably accompanies measles and accounts for a substantial proportion of measles deaths. Those persons sick with intestinal tuberculosis and a variety of diseases of the liver including cirrhosis and biliary tract disease often have diarrhoea. Poisons and various toxins affecting the parasympathetic nervous system frequently cause acute diarrhoea.

Less frequently, especially in developing countries, a wide array of other aetiologic mechanisms exist. Food intolerance, for example lactose deficiency found predominantly in dark-skinned people, and food allergies, especially to foreign animal protein, can cause acute and chronic diarrhoea (Sunshine et al, 1977). Cow's milk formula provided early in life may lead to a high degree of sensitization to cow's milk proteins and other antigens, and result in lifelong sensitivity to these agents (Yadav, Iyngkaran, 1981). Granulomatous diseases of the gut and tumours elaborating gastrointestinal hormones are proven causes of severe diarrhoea. While these must be considered in the workup of chronic diarrhoea in Western countries, where 10 per cent or even 20 per cent of cases are related to such noninfectious causes, they account for a negligible part of the 500–1500 million diarrhoea episodes occurring in the world each year. In these infection is the cause of all but a small proportion.

THE DISEASE

Fluid and electrolytes

Diarrhoea of whatever aetiology precipitates acute Fluid and Electrolyte Malnutrition — FEM (Rohde and Northrup, 1976). The acute loss of fluid and body salts leads to dehydration and in some cases to death. Fluid losses in cholera can exceed 20 ml per kilogram per hour, rapidly leading to extreme hemoconcentration and shock. Usually fluid loss is slower. The composition of the lost fluid depends on the age of the patient, the rate of stool loss and the causative agent. Younger children tend to lose more potassium and less sodium in their stools. The higher the stool rate the more the sodium electrolyte level tends to approach serum level. This is probably a result of rapid passage through the colon where sodium-potassium exchange occurs. Cholera or *E. coli* stools contain sodium in concentration of 80–120 mg/litre while rotavirus stools have sodium consistently below 50 mg/litre.

Nutrition

Of all common childhood illnesses, diarrhoea has the most important nutritional effect (Rowland et al, 1980; Chen and Scrimshaw, 1982). This effect works through a variety of mechanisms including decreased intake due to sociologic factors as well as anorexia, decreased absorption of nutrients, increased catabolism through fever and activation of hormonal mechanisms. During an episode of diarrhoea, absorption of fats diminishes by as much as 50 per cent although the absorption of carbohydrates diminishes less than 20 per cent (Molla et al, 1982). Gastrointestinal protein loss has been documented in shigella, rotavirus and enterotoxigenic *E. coli* (not in cholera) (Rahaman and Wahed, 1982). Protein loss may be extreme in measles, accounting for its frequent association with the onset of kwashiorkor. In the marginally nourished child, diarrhoea of any aetiology may be the precipitating factor in the manifestation of florid malnutrition. Only in intestinal lymphagectasia is diarrhoea accompanied by a significant chronic loss of nutrients in the form of fats and body protein that can itself lead to severe growth retardation and even nutritional death.

Most toxin induced diarrhoeas are not accompanied by fever. The illness represents a derangement of intestinal luminal mechanisms rather than a systemic infection per se. Fever, however, does characterise many of the invasive diarrhoeas including rotavirus, especially in the early stages of infection (Steinhoff, 1980). The anorexia associated with diarrhoea seems to play a major role in inducing malnutrition. This comes as no surprise to mothers, as careful dietary measurements have now shown that a child will only eat 30–70 per cent of his normal intake during diarrhoea (Hoyle et al, 1980). The mechanisms for anorexia are unknown. Electrolyte imbalance, especially hypokalemia, as well as dehydration reduce appetite (Rowland et al, 1980). Various hormones are stimulated in response to diarrhoea, either as part of a general stress response (steroids) or specific gastrointestinal substances (VIP, secretin, prostaglandins). These contribute to the catabolic state. For example, the increased level of corticosteroids found during diarrhoea in Gambian children seems to contribute to development of marasmus in this population (Whitehead et al, 1977).

Altogether, because of the fluid and electrolyte secretion, the malabsorption and the lack of food intake, the child suffering from diarrhoea may lose from two to five grams per kilogram of body mass per day representing a deficit of some 20–50 grams in daily weight gain in the early years of life. Where normal monthly weight gain between ages one and five years is 170–200 grams, regression analysis of weight loss against days ill with diarrhoea shows a net loss of 500–700 grams per month ill (Rowland et al, 1980). The annual diarrhoea incidence in weanling children varies from two to twelve episodes, each lasting from three to seven days. As the point prevalence of diarrhoea ranges from 5–15 per cent this means that 20–60 days per year will be spent sick with diarrhoea for the average child in a developing country (Rohde, 1978). Consequently, the annual weight deficit associated with diarrhoea may be from 400–1500 grams or 25–75 per cent of expected normal growth. Compounded over the first five years of life, diarrhoea related nitritional deficits alone can leave a child in second or even third degree malnutrition.

Immune response

Immune mechanisms particularly related to the intestines involve antigen processing by lymphocytes in the lamina propria with formation of specific antibody, particularly of the IgA secretory class. Stimulated lymphocytes have been shown to travel centrally through the lymphatic system and to concentrate specifically in the Peyer's patches, salivary glands and mammary glands. Thus, a lactating mother secretes milk with both secretory antibodies and activated macrophages directed specifically against the antigens in her own intestine (Svennerholm et al, 1981). These appear to protect the nursing child. For example, nursing infants of mothers with cholera have a very low incidence of cholera (Gangarosa and Mosley, 1974). This offers the prospect of actively immunising mothers with oral immunogens to stimulate protective immune antibodies and cells in her milk against a wide range of potential pathogens. The role of intestinal immunity in protection from infection is, however, still largely unknown.

Systemic antibodies are formed against numerous agents. While these provide useful diagnostic tests, particularly where titre rises can be documented (rotavirus, Norwalk agent, cholera, amoebiasis) their role in recovery and subsequent protection is variable. Antibodies against cholera somatic antigens appear to protect, at least when in high titre (Levine et al, 1981); and volunteers infected with cholera are immune to repeat challenge. Protection is, however, not complete and in endemic regions, repeat cholera infection occurs with a frequency similar to index or first infection (Woodward, 1971). While duration of immune protection in cholera appears to be partial and shortlived, in rotavirus it may be lifelong. For infectious diarrhoeas, immune protection is intermediate, lasting from only a few months to several years.

Host response

Recovery from diarrhoea is related to elimination of the offending organism and to regeneration of damaged intestinal epithelial cells. In the case of simple infection with rotavirus or poisoning of cell mechanisms by toxins, this regeneration effectively takes only several days, thus accounting for the normal limitation seen in the duration of diarrhoea. A certain proportion of cases will, however, become chronic with associated food intolerance and a continued malabsorption of both nutrients and fluids. Antibiotics appear to favour development of abnormal gut flora and inhibit recolonisation by normal types and numbers of organisms. Withdrawal of food, even briefly, is associated with reduction of GI digestive enzymes and absorptive function, after which refeeding is associated with intolerance and indigestibility (Maclean et al, 1980). Thus chronic diarrhoea appears to be, in part, an iatrogenic complication of simple acute diarrhoea treated inappropriately with antibiotics and harmful dietary restrictions. In this small proportion of cases, careful continued feeding and replacement of lost fluids is essential.

EPIDEMIOLOGY

In field studies the incidence of diarrhoea varies widely and depends upon definition, sample size, duration of recall, intensity of surveillance as well as upon seasonal and other factors all affecting the accuracy of the results. From the United States to India, from South Africa to the Arctic, diarrhoea is common and the incidence is variously estimated from as few as one to as many as twelve or more episodes of diarrhoea per child per year (Gordon,

1971). Obviously the incidence varies with the environment as well as with the definition, perception and observation of illness. The WHO estimates 500–1500 million episodes of diarrhoea among the 600 million children under five years of age in the world each year (WHO 1980). The age specific incidence appears closely associated with the introduction of foods, peaking in the second year of life and diminishing constantly thereafter. Adults generally suffer fewer than one episode per year, an estimated rate rather than documented observation in most parts of the world.

Microbiological studies of weaning foods in the Gambia show a large innoculum of potentially pathogenic bacteria associated with feeding and a corresponding peak in diarrhoea incidence (Rowland et al, 1978). With the worsening crises in firewood for cooking, the poor in many countries prepare fewer daily meals. Bacterial overgrowth in unheated food and less frequent meals may contribute to rising rates of both diarrhoea and malnutrition.

Babies fed milk from bottles are exposed to large innocula of bacteria and in all reported studies have a much increased diarrhoea and death rate when compared to exclusively breast fed peers (Surjono et al, 1980; Jelliffe and Jelliffe, 1978) The earlier the bottle is introduced, the higher the risk. In an urban slum of Port-au-Prince, Haiti, children fed with a bottle during the first month of life had five times the risk of death in the next 17 months as peers exclusively breast fed in the first month (Berggren et al, 1981). The association of 'artificial feeding,' diarrhoea and death has been documented in detail by many authors in the United States, Europe and the developing world since the late 19th century (Wray, 1977).

Malnourished children have a higher incidence and suffer more severe disease than their better-nourished peers (Tomkins, 1981). They are more susceptible to a given challenge, most have greater exposure to environmental pathogens, and their intestinal function is reduced leading to more severe fluid and nutrient looses.

Using estimates for global protein-energy malnutrition (PEM) (See Eddy chapter 4) and relative risk of diarrhoea, the author has estimated that up to 30 per cent of diarrhoea cases are related to the increased incidence found in malnourished children (Rohde, 1978). On the other hand, the crude estimate of the nutritional impact of the 500–1500 million diarrhoea episodes in the world per year, with an average annual weight deficit of 400–1500 grammes in the first five years of life, shows the tremendous contribution to malnutrition made by diarrhoea. Thus, the commonly recognised interaction of diarrhoea and malnutrition, the FEM-PEM cycle (Rohde and Northrup, 1976) is an important part of the epidemiology of diarrhoea.

Infectious diarrhoea is transmitted by the ingestion of faecal organisms. Conditions encouraging contact or spread of faeces are invariably associated with higher incidence. Contaminated water supplies in closed resorts or cruise ships provide dramatic outbreaks in Western countries (Rosenberg et al, 1977), while in developing countries diarrhoea incidence is highest in crowded urban slums where filth and lack of clean water abound. In temperate climates diarrhoea tends to be associated with the warm summer months, probably related both to the viability of the organism in the environment, and to more frequent human contact such as in swimming pools, et cetera. Interestingly, rotavirus epidemiology shows distinct peaks in the colder and drier season, especially in temperate climates; this appears to be transmitted in patterns similar to streptococcus, measles, mumps, and other person-to-person contact and airborne diseases (Yolken et al, 1978). While studies continue to find little evidence for respiratory spread of this virus, it appears more related to direct contact than to water or food. *Yersinia enterocolitica*, which thrives and produces toxin only at sub-body temperatures (less than 30 C), also shows winter peaks (Marks et al, 1980).

The salmonellas are classically transmitted through foods, especially poultry and poultry products. Transmission of *S. Typhi* is usually by sewage contaminated water or food, but food handling by a chronic asymptomatic carrier has been a key epidemiologic factor leading in many countries to hygiene laws governing public food establishments. Shigellas and the amoebas appear to be more affected by personal hygiene than by water or food per se. Cholera is widely known as a waterborne disease since the day John Snow condemned the water of the Broad Street pump (Snow, 1965). However, the epidemic in Israel in the early 1970's and recent limited outbreaks in the United States and Europe have linked the transmission of cholera both to contaminated vegetables and to poorly cooked shellfish (Bain et al, 1974). Thus epidemiology varies extensively according to aetiologic agent. Where an organism is highly host-specific and requires a small mean innoculum size to infect (such as with Shigellas) person-to-person contact is important, and spread can be controlled through personal hygiene (Black et al, 1981). Where wide host ranges and higher innocula are required (such as for salmonella, E. coli, etc), the importance of food sources and water is even greater (WHO, 1980). In addition, host responsiveness changes with age. The rotaviruses are by far the major pathogen in children under two years (Banatvla, 1979), toxigenic *E. coli* are particularly important among travellers and adults in tropical areas (Traveller's Diarrhoea, 1982), and cholera affects all ages in epidemic virgin areas but predominantly attacks children in endemic areas (Gangarosa and Mosley, 1974).

The epidemiology of diarrhoea gives important clues to aetiology and defines risk groups, seasonality and environments where interventions are most likely to be effective. Because diarrhoea results from many different causes there are several different methods of control. They vary in their effectiveness depending on the cause of the diarrhoea. They include:

Prevention of contact with the infecting agent — hygiene, water supplies and sanitation,

Prevention of infection through the use of immunologic agents —
vaccines,
Breast milk protection,
Interference with the mechanisms of diarrhoea,
Antibiotics,
Replacement of losses — sodium, bicarbonate, potassium, substrate,
water,
Convalescent nutritional care.

PREVENTION

Prevention of contact with the infecting agent: Hygiene, Water Supplies and Sanitation

Interruption of the faecal-oral transmission of diarrhoea agents is accomplished through widespread introduction and proper use of effective clean water supplies, food hygiene and the elimination of vectors such as flies which can carry the infecting organism (Wolff et al, 1969). The effectiveness of environmental and public health measures have been proven more in historical perspective than in carefully controlled studies. That best known is the control of cholera in London due to improvement of public water supplies. Similar reduction in mortality from diarrhoeal diseases was seen in the United States in the early 20th century, and in a few documented studies in rural areas (WHO, 1980). In general, the impact of rural water and sanitation systems has been difficult to measure and often has not been apparent. Not only must water be provided in large quantities in the household, but also habits regarding personal hygiene must be developed to ensure interruption of faecal-oral transmission. A recent WHO review of the literature shows that abundant clean water supplies, or clean water provided very close to the home, are often associated with less diarrhoea. The most consistent positive results were, however, seen in communities in the United States and a few third world areas where demand for and use of water was affected by long cultural indoctrination on its proper use to avoid disease (WHO, 1980). Numerous attempts to reduce diarrhoea by improving water availability and quality have failed (Levine et al, 1976). Reasons are numerous and complex, and include technical inadequacies (broken pumps, leaking pipes, unprotected sources), improper use (storage of clean drinking water in unclean domestic containers), and deep cultural constraints (river water tastes better).

The impact of sanitary waste disposal is even more difficult to document. While a latrine program in an urban Philippine slum reduced the incidence of cholera, no impact was seen on acute non-cholera diarrhoea (Azurin and Alvero, 1974). These results are less surprising when one recalls that by far the major burden of diarrhoea is upon the very young, peaking around age two years. Children in this age group are generally not users of latrines or even clean water, and they are often the most exposed to the ground, the dirt, and the contaminants in the environment. Nothing short of an immaculate environment is likely to prevent this group from gaining access to the organisms causing diarrhoea.

Prevention of infection through the use of immunologic agents: Vaccines

While cholera vaccine does afford some protection, perhaps more than 50 per cent for a period up to six months, it is not effective in reducing transmission of the disease, nor does it alter the course of illness (Sommer et al, 1973). Cholera in patients with or without pre-existing antibodies is equally severe (Woodward et al, 1970). Vaccines for shigella and salmonella have been developed and tested, but none is yet effective enough to recommend for mass programs. Oral attenuated strains of shigella do offer partial protection. Newer typhoid vaccines offer high levels of protection for at least several years, but no vaccines for the 1500 or more known types of the common salmonellas are effective. With the identification of rotavirus as a major cause of fatal diarrhoea in young childhood, strong efforts have been made to produce a vaccine against this virus which appears to have only two or perhaps three serotypes (Blacklow and Cukor, 1981). The mapping of rotavirus DNA and hybridoma techniques of reproducing highly specific antigens now make vaccine production feasible within a few years. The highly limited age-specific attack rate of this virus suggests that immune mechanisms are indeed protective, and vaccines are a promising intervention.

In view of the wide range of aetiologic agents and the difficulty of eliciting effective immune protection for each, the likely impact of effective vaccination coverage against diarrhoea in developing countries is small. Nevertheless, if protection from specific diseases of high prevalence and importance, particularly rotavirus, the toxins of E. coli, cholera and shigella, could be provided simultaneously, perhaps through antibody to common colonisation factors, mass vaccination programs may become a reasonable, cost-effective intervention.

Breast milk protection

The remarkably high level of protection from diarrhoea enjoyed by the nursing infant is due to a myriad of factors which have been extensively reviewed (Berggren et al, 1981). An enteric antigen challenge to a lactating or pregnant mother leads to production of specific immune factors in the mother's milk. As protective antigens are discovered and produced through cloning a 'diarrhoea antigen cocktail' may be foreseen that will allow nursing mothers to produce natural protective passive immunity for the nursing infant. Not only do immune factors in mother's milk (macrophages, antibodies, lactoferrin) protect the child but, perhaps more importantly, the child is *not* exposed to the heavy contamination of the feeding bottle.

Unclean water, utensils and hands all contribute to the high bacterial count found in milk. Furthermore, the absence of refrigeration and the general need to save unused milk until a later feeding make bacterial proliferation inevitable in this ideal culture medium. The impact of breast milk on reducing diarrhoea among those most vulnerable make active promotion of lactation one of the essential interventions in the diarrhoea problems.

TREATMENT OF THE DIARRHOEA

Interference with the mechanisms of diarrhoea

In the face of infection by pathogenic organisms, interference with colonisation, with toxin production, with invasion, or with physiologic responses to the organism's presence offers mechanisms of intervention against diarrhoea. Breast milk may protect through denying bacteria nutrients such as iron which is effectively bound by lactoferrin. Cellular elements and antibodies may destroy or inactivate pathogens. Interference with adhesion of organisms to the intestinal mucosa through immunologic or chemical agents will render even toxigenic organisms ineffective. While no practical means are presently available, absorbents such as charcoal or gangliosides have been shown to reduce toxin effects in experimental situations (Fishman 1980). Drugs such as amphoterecin B or other membrane active drugs may alter permeability effects of toxin, thereby offsetting the loss of fluid and electrolytes (Chen et al, 1973). A number of anti-secretory drugs (aspirin, indomethacin, prostaglandins, chlorpromazine, loperamide) working through a variety of mechanisms in the mucosal cells have been shown to diminish or to reverse the secretory process, and therefore effectively to reduce loss of fluid and electrolytes (Powell and Field 1980). It is important to note, however that in no case has this reduction been clinically very significant, nor has it obviated the need to replace fluids and electrolytes lost before therapy. For cholera, chlorpromazine reduces fluid losses, but this reduction is no greater than that seen by the use of tetracycline, an antibiotic which effectively eliminates the organism from the gut (Rabbini et al, 1979).

The search for anti-diarrhoeal drugs has been confounded by the uncontrolled way in which most of the products have been introduced. Because diarrhoea is so often a brief and self-limited illness, numerous 'cures' have been used and accepted, ranging from exotic herbal concoctions to injected aminoglycosides. Anti-motility agents (opiates, Lomotil) may increase duration of secretion of fluid, prolong passage of pathogens, increase fever and related catabolism, and may decrease absorption of nutrients through statsis and pooling in the gut (Dupont and Hornick, 1973). Traditional wisdom notwithstanding, there is no evidence for an inverse relationship of gut transit time and nutrient absorption in acute diarrhoea. Anti-motility agents should not be used, except for control of severe cramps and tenesmus in children above infant ages.

Absorbents (Kaolin, charcoal) have no demonstrated effect on either duration or severity of diarrhoea. While not apparently harmful, they detract from more important therapy and should be avoided. It may be concluded while the pathophysiology of diarrhoea offers numerous potential intervention points, careful research and documentation of efficacy and safety are needed before any can be recommended.

Antibiotics ˙

Use of antibiotics has been shown in most studies of undifferentiated acute diarrhoea to be ineffective, and may in some cases lead to prolongation of the diarrhoea; non-use is the best general policy unless specific indications are present. In areas where cholera is endemic, or in the case of clinical dysentry, stool culture is critical for optimal management. While tetracycline is the drug of choice for cholera, the shigellas are notable for multiple drug resistance and locally determined recent antibiotic sensitivity patterns must be known in order to make proper therapeutic decisions. Erythromycin is the current drug of choice for campylobacter. Salmonellas, except for enteric fever, are best not treated, as antibiotics appear to prolong clinical illness as well as to increase the rate of chronic carriers.

With the possible exception of doxycycline, used to prevent travellers' diarrhoea (Sack et al, 1978) prophylactic antibiotics are contra-indicated and will only lead to the development of resistant organisms in the body. There is no evidence that the administration of tetracycline to a population at risk will reduce the incidence of cholera or other diarrhoeal diseases (Sack, 1979). A number of trials of low level non-absorbable antibiotics such as 'feed' antibiotics used in animal husbandry have not proved promising (Rosenberg et al, 1974). While diarrhoea incidence may be slightly reduced, potential complications in the form of resistant flora and logistical problems of assuring daily adherence to such prophylactic regimens make this tactic impractical.

Initial enthusiasm for the iodated chloroquine derivatives (Vioform) were not based on careful experimental evidence of efficacy. In fact, these agents appear to be of no value in any but amoebic diarrhoea, and even then are not the drugs of choice. Drug toxicity with retinal degeneration has proven a high risk for such an ineffective agent (Traveller's Warning, 1975).

Replacement of losses

By far the most effective intervention, reducing both deaths and nutritional morbidity, is through rapid replacement of fluid and electrolytes. Once viewed as a complex metabolic process to be carried out in a paediatric ward involving calculation of various body spaces and ion deficits, rehydration is now a simple procedure that, if started early in the home by mothers, can save lives for pennies. No doubt, initial intravenous rehydration with isotonic solutions containing a base (Ringers lactate is ideal) is critical for the severely dehydrated child, more so if unconscious or in shock. In such cases, ten per cent of body weight given rapidly over two hours will restore the child to a state where oral rehydration can take over. Hypertonic states are so uncommon in developing countries that they are virtually unrecognised, making the caution over speed and tonicity of rehydrating fluid far less a concern than in the wealthy northern nations. If bottle feeding continues, however, to make inroads into the poorer countries, hypertonic dehydration may well become one more 'imported' disease.

Extensive reviews have documented both the scientific basis and the efficacy of oral rehydration therapy (ORT) in acute diarrhoea (Parker et al, 1980; Baumslag et al, 1980). It is safe and more effective, as well as far cheaper, than intravenous fluid replacement (Santosham et al, 1982).

The WHO oral rehydration solution formula (ORS) (See Eddy, Chapter 45) has proven effective in millions of cases of diverse aetiologies throughout the world. To avoid excessive retention of sodium, especially in the younger infant, the WHO ORS should be diluted 2:1 with water, or extra water should be given to the child. For the youngest infant, lower sodium seems desirable but such a solution would be inadequate for cholera or severe toxigenic *E. coli* diarrhoea (Nalin el al, 1980). Bicarbonate can be replaced by other base (lactate, acetate, citrate) and some studies indicate that especially in malnourished children, potassium levels should be increased. Two per cent glucose stimulates absorption of the salt solution but higher concentrations may exacerbate diarrhoea due to osmotic load. Recent research confirms the value of hypoosmotic substrate sources such as cereal powders. Protein hydrolysates stimulate further fluid and salt absorption as well. Inclusion of more nutritious substrates absorbed by various non-competing pathways offers the prospect of a more efficacious and nutrient-dense rehydration solution. Exploitation of multiple absorptive mechanisms affords possible benefits in the form of:

a. increased and faster fluid and electrolyte absorption;

b. increased nutrient absorption, providing both energy and amino acids (absorbed by at least four independent or quasi-independent intestinal mechanisms);

c. decreased stool volume, thereby overcoming one of the greatest impediments to lay acceptance of oral rehydration solutions;

d. faster recovery due, first to shorter cell renewal time as a result of readily available basic nutrients for cell metabolism, and secondly, to better absorption of ORS;

e. better digestion of diet in recovery due to continued enzyme induction, offsetting the known effects of starvation in reducing enzymes.

Cereals, legumes, and other locally available simple foods may thus become, in proper quantities, the basis of a combined fluid-protein-energy oral therapy for diarrhoea, a single antidote for the FEM-PEM cycle.

While the literature abounds with arguments on the 'ideal' composition of ORS, the key factor to success on a global scale is the availability and acceptability of ORS and accessibility of the packets or materials to make it at home.

The best quality water available should be used to prepare ORS, but standards of purity that inhibit the use of ORT should be avoided. There is no evidence that ingestion of ORS prepared with normally consumed water is any more detrimental than the routine daily risk of the water alone (Shields et al, 1981).

While the efficacy of ORT is unquestioned, present efforts are focussed on developing the most efficient ways in which to deliver this treatment to each child early in the course of diarrhoea. The most successful programs have provided ORT at home, where high acceptance has led to the greatest fall in mortality. When ORT has been confined to medical facilities, or not used early or in adequate quantities, the impact has been less. Salt-sugar mixtures have been shown to be effective in treating dehydration, although when started late in the illness they will not correct acidosis. When distributed to households, salt-sugar packets were as effective as ORT in reducing diarrhoea deaths in one large Egyptian study (Mobarak, 1982). Carefully controlled large field trials of salt-sugar versus ORS are awaited, but most studies indicate that early replacement of losses is a key to effective impact, even if salt-sugar is the only solution available. Home mixtures made either with household implements or special plastic measures result in solutions of acceptable composition in most studies (Hendrata et al, 1980; Ellerbrock, 1981). Mixing errors appear no more likely with home mixtures than packaged ORT.

It appears from studies in the Philippines (WHO, 1977) Turkey, (Egeman and Bertan, 1980), Egypt (El-Sherbini et al, 1978) and Iran (Barzgar et al, 1980) as well as the earlier studies of Apaches (Hirschorn and Denny, 1975), that early rehydration leads to improved food intake and absorption resulting in a diminished negative nutritional impact of diarrhoea. In programs where oral rehydration is accompanied by strong nutritional advice, continued feeding of the child, and attention to food in early convalescence, improved nutritional status has been associated with the use of oral therapy. Thus ORT has provided both a dramatic reduction in mortality and a reduction of malnutrition.

Convalescent care

The nutritional care which follows a period of acute diarrhoea may be important in reducing the subsequent incidence of diarrhoea. Immediately following the cessation of diarrhoea there is an apparent rise in appetite, often to supra-normal levels, as shown by consumption studies in hospitalised patients. Molla has shown appetite recovery in acute rotavirus, ETEC (enterotoxigenic *Escherichia coli*), shigella and cholera diarrhoea occurring between the fourth and seventh days of illness, evidenced by spontaneous consumption of recommended dietary allowance (RDA) quantities or more of usual foods (Molla et al, 1982). Supra-normal appetite with intake exceeding 130 Kcal per kilogram of body weight has been documented in several hsopital studies.

While admittedly difficult to achieve in some patients, especially in the home setting, the accomplishment of supra-normal food intakes (25–50 per cent above RDA) for a period two times the duration of illness is an effective means to restore growth and obviate the nutritional effects of diarrhoea. Nutrition supplement programs highly targeted to this brief, but critical, period may be the most nutritionally effective intervention point in the diarrhoea-malnutrition cycle.

There is evidence that adequate feeding results, even before any significant gain in weight, in a reduced susceptibility to further episodes of diarrhoea, and thus to an improvement in the overall diarrhoea-malnutrition cycle (Wray, 1978). Increased emphasis on feeding during convalescence could lead to a reduction by up to 50 per cent in subsequent attack rates in these children. Nutrition interventions, targeted for brief periods in convalescing children, offer a greater nutritional impact both through rapid catch-up growth during the week or so after illness and through preventing future episodes of diarrhoea and resulting nutritional losses.

PROGRAM OPTIONS

There is no single superior method of dealing with diarrhoea in a community. All are operative and contribute to reduction in morbidity, mortality or both. Unit costs vary widely with actual programs, and for many, the estimate is at best a guess. Per capita cost of water varies from US$20 to $50 for capital investment with 10 per cent annual maintenance costs. Impact on diarrhoea depends upon aetiology, age groups, habits and the water system itself. Water supply has no effect on rotavirus, has very little effect on the youngest age groups, depends upon proper use for any effect at all and is useless when the supply fails. Water was piped throughout London in the mid-19th century, but diarrhoea death rates remained constantly high until the first decade of the 20th century (McKeown, 1976). In 1854 the Southwark and Vauxhall Company piped cholera into 10 per cent of London homes, enabling John Snow to prove once and forever the waterborne nature of cholera, held by most at that time to be a miasma (Snow, 1965). Clean, abundant, available water is a necessary prerequisite for sustained reduction in diarrhoea incidence, but its high cost and uncertain impact make it a long-range strategy at best.

Latrines have even less to recommend them as a means to control diarrhoea. Pit or water seal units cost US$5–$10 per capita initially and costs for more sanitary designs are higher. While they clearly contribute to the quality of the environment, sound evidence for their contribution to a reduction in diarrhoea is lacking. Only in the case of cholera is a good study available demonstrating an impact (Azurin and Alvero, 1974), and this same study showed no reduction in diarrhoea of other aetiologies.

Vaccines cost only US10 to 25 cents per dose but delivery, especially in rural areas, may cost $2 or more. Even this might be worthwhile if effective vaccines were available, but even cholera, the oldest bacterial vaccine in medicine, is so ineffective that treatment of cases is cheaper and more efficacious. No vaccines yet exist against the agents of 90–95 per cent of diarrhoea cases.

No one knows the price of encouraging breast feeding but its value is unquestioned. The economic value of breast milk to a developing country is itself a major reason to encourage lactation (Rohde, 1982). Where bottle feeding is prevalent, no other intervention offers such promise for saving lives and reducing malnutrition in the very young.

Antibiotics are of use only to short term travellers in tropical countries for protection from ETEC.

By far the best buy is oral rehydration. At a cost of 10 US. cents per litre of ORS, 20 cent per episode, the cost of materials to treat 500–1500 million cases annually is substantial: $100–300 million. Cost per life saved, assuming a 50 per cent effectiveness rate is $40–120 and this does not include the delivery cost of ORS packages which are undoubtedly five to ten times as much. For this reason, country programs are seeking strategies using homemade solutions to manage the majority of cases, while the more severe 10 per cent or so have access to ORS packets and to management by health personnel. The unit cost per death averted or per unit improvement in nutrition can thus be minimised. This is by far the most cost-effective strategy.

Convalescent nutritional care, the provision of additional food during the early recovery from diarrhoea, requires a hypothetical cost structure based on the known growth rates during recovery from illness. Normally, efficiency of conversion of food energy to lean body mass is about five kcal/gram tissue *above* basal metabolic needs (Spady et al, 1976). This efficiency may be raised in the malnourished, but is lowered by malabsorption or by factors which divert the food from the target child. Having estimated the nutritional cost of diarrhoea in preschool children in the developing world as 400–1500 grams per year (see p. 270), some 2000–7500 kcal of balanced diet are needed to replace this deficit. Provided as daily average, this is a negligible quantity of food: 5–20 kcal/day. Even if concentrated in convalescent periods, it is a small amount, costing perhaps only $1–2, depending on the diet. By avoiding the nutritional consequences of diarrhoea, subsequent attack rates could be reduced by up to 30 per cent (but a more likely reduction is 15–20 per cent). Thus, while such targeted feeding is likely to have the greatest nutritional impact at the least cost, its contribution to lowered diarrhoea incidence and death, though not negligible, would be small.

Coverage of the population at risk is a measure of key importance; all interventions must consider that total impact is a product of effectiveness times coverage. Even choices within an intervention strategy must consider this element. Compromises are needed that may well decrease program effectiveness but that will increase coverage to a large enough degree to give a greater overall impact. For example, in oral rehydration therapy it may be that homemade sugar-salt solutions increase the coverage to a large enough degree to offset any reduced effectiveness in comparison to packaged solutions. On the other hand, the cost of providing water which is pure may preclude delivery of that adequate volume which is essential to maximise health effects. Likewise the money spent on water and latrines for a small portion of a population could perhaps be better spent on providing nearly total coverage of an ORT and convalescent feeding program.

Cultural and social adaptation will have to be made by the community if the various prevention and control methods are to be accepted for wide and appropriate use in the target population. This applies to water systems, latrines, and vaccinations as well as to oral therapy and feeding. The credibility of any intervention, that is to say, its cultural acceptability and use by the population, will determine its overall impact to a large degree. Communication strategy supporting each intervention must be considered as an important part of extending the impact.

In the final analysis, intervention programs must consider the resources available and the impact to be expected from the mix of feasible alternative stategies. Cost-benefit analysis is not very helpful owing to the impossibility of pricing lives saved, illness averted or improved nutrition. A careful weighing of the relative effectiveness of various interventions at a given cost provides the best guide to both short and long term health planning.

SUMMARY AND CONCLUSION

Diarrhoea is a complex illness of multiple aetiologies accounting for a substantial number of deaths as well as significant disability in populations throughout the world. An understanding of the pathogenesis and epidemiology of this disease complex leads to a large spectrum of possible interventions. By far the most efficient and successful is the widespread use of oral rehydration and procedures designed to improve the nutritional intake of a child during and immediately following a diarrhoeal episode. Programs to introduce rehydration therapy into populationwide health systems must carefully consider social, cultural and practical factors to assure maximal coverage and acceptance of this proven effective modality. It is evident that the death rates and associated nutritional effects of diarrhoea can be reduced by as much as 80 or 90 per cent with effective introduction of this strategy.

REFERENCES

Azurin J A, Alvero M 1974 Field Evaluation of Environmental Sanitation Measures Against Cholera. Bull Wld Hlth Org 51: 19–26

Bain W B, Zampieri A M, Mazzotti M, Angioni G 1974 Epidemiology of Cholera in Italy in 1973. Lancet 2: 1370–1375

Bauatvala J E 1979 The Role of Viruses in Acute Diarrhoeal Disease. Clin Gastroenterol 8: 569–598

Barzgar M A, Ourshano S, Amini J N 1980 The Evaluation of the Effectiveness of Oral Rehydration in Acute Diarrhoea of Children Under Three Years of Age in West Azerbaijan, Iran. J. Trop Pedr 26: 217–222

Baumslag N, et al. 1980 (eds), Oral Rehydration Therapy: An Annotated Bibliography. Pan Am Hlth Org DC, pp 116

Berggren G, Ewbank D, Boulos C, Boulos L M, Mode F 1981 Baseline Survey of Nutritional Status of Mothers and Children in Cite Simone. USAID, Port-ou-Prince, Haiti

Black R E, Dykes A C 1981 Handwashing to Prevent Diarrhoea in Day-Care Centers. Am J Epid 113: 445–451

Blacklow N R, Cukor G 1981 Viral Gastroenteritis. New Eng J Med 304: 394–406

Chen L C, Scrimshaw N S 1983 (eds) Diarrhoea and Malnutrition: Interactions, Mechanisms and Interventions. Plenum, New York

Chen L C, Guerrant R L, Rohde J E, Casper A G 1973 Effect of Amphotericin B on Sodium and Water Movement Across Normal and Cholera Toxin-Challenged Canine Jejunum. Gastroenterology 65: 252–258

Craun G F 1979 Waterborne Giardiasis in the United States: A Review. Am J Publ Hlth 69: 817–819

Davidson G P, Barnes G I 1979 Structural and Functional Abnormalities of the Small Intestine in Infants and Young Children with Rotavirus Enteritis. Acta Paediatr Scand 68: 181–186

Diarrhoea Dialogue. 1981, 7: 6

Dupont H L 1980 Interactions of Enteric Pathogens with the Intestines. In: Field M, Fordtran J S Schultz S G (eds) Secretory Diarrhoea. American Physiol Soc, Bethesda: 61–65

Dupont H L, Hornick R B 1973 Adverse Effect of Lomotil Therapy in Chigellosis, JAMA 226: 1525–1528

Egeman A, Bertan M 1980 A Study of Oral Rehydration Therapy by Midwives in a Rural Area near Ankara. Bull Wrld Hlth Org 58: 333–338

Ellerbrock T V 1981 Oral Replacement Therapy in Rural Bangladesh with Home Ingredients. Trop Doctor 11: 179–183

El-Sherbini A F, Fahmy S F, Eid E E, Goda M Y, Eltantawy A S, El-Sayyed L 1978 The Use of Oral Rehydration in Infantile Diarrhoea. J Egyptian Publ Hlth Assn 53: (Suppl. 5–6): 82–104

Evans D G, Evans D J Jr 1978 New Surface — Associated Heat Labile Colonization Factor Antigen (CFA/II) Produced by Enterotoxigenic — Escherichia Coli of Serogroups: 06 and 08. Infect Immun 21: 638–647

Field M 1980 Regulation of Small Intestinal Ion Transport by Cyclic Nucleotides and Calcium. In: Field, M, Fordtran J S, Schultz S G (eds) Secretory Diarrhoea. American Physiology Society. Bethesda. 21–23

Field M 1978 Choleratoxin, Adenylate Cyclase and the Process of Active Secretion in the Small Intestine: The Pathogenesis of Diarrhoea in Cholera. In: Andreoli T E, Hoffman J F, Fansestil D D (eds) The Physiological Basis for Disorders of Biomembranes, New York Plenum: 788–899, 1978

Finkelstein R A 1973 Cholera. CRC Crit Rev Microbial 2: 553–623

Fishman P H 1980 Mechanism of Action of Cholera Toxin: Events on the Cell Surface. In: Field M, Fortran J S, Schultz S G (eds) Secretory Diarrhoea American Physiology Society. Bethesda. 85–106

Gangarosa E J, Mosley W H 1974 Epidemiology and Surveillance of Cholera. In: Barua D and Burrows W. Cholera. Saunders W B, Philadelphia, 381–403

Gordon J E 1971 Diarrhoeal Disease of Early Childhood — Worldwide Scope of the Problem. Am New York Acad Sci 176: 9–15,

Greenberg H B, et al 1979 Role of Norwalk Virus in Outbreaks of Nonbacterial Gastroenteritis. Infect Dis 139: 564–568

Hendrata L, Rohde J E, Idrus D 1980 Paed Indonesiana 20: 91–92

Hirschorn N 1980 The Treatment of Acute Diarrhea in Children — An Historical and

Physiological Perspective. Am J Clin Nutr 33: 637–663

Hirschorn N, Denny K M 1975 Oral Glucose-Electrolyte Therapy for Diarrhea: A means to Maintain or Improve Nutrition? Am J Clin Nutr 28: 198–192

Hoyle B, Yunus M, Chen L C 1980 Breast-Feeding and Food Intake Among Children with Acute Diarrheal Disease. Am J Clin Nutr 33: 2365–2371

Hughes J M, Murad F, Chang B, Guerrant R L 1978 Role of Cyclic GMP in the Action of Heat Stable Enterotoxin of Escherichia Coli. Nature London 271: 755–756

Jelliffe D B, Jelliffe E F P 1978 Human Milk in the Modern World. Oxford Univ Press, Oxford: pp 500

Kapikian A Z, et al 1976 Human Reovirus-like Agent as the Major Pathogen Associated with Winter Gastroenteritis in Hospitalized Infants and Young Children. N Engl J Med 294: 965–972

Keusch G T 1979 Shigella Infections. Clin Gastroenterol 8: 645–662

Keusch G T 1981 Ecological Control of the Bacterial Diarrheas: A Scientific Strategy. Am J Clin Nutr 31: 2208–2218

Levine M M, Black R E, Clements M L, Cisneros L, Nalin D R, Young C R 1981 Duration of Infection-Derived Immunity to Cholera. J Infect Dis 143: 818–820

Levine R J, Khan M R, Desouza S, Nalin D R 1976 Failure of Sanitary Wells to Protect Against Cholera and Other Diarrhoeas in Bangladesh. Lancet 2: 85–89

Maclean W C Jr, Lopez G, Massa E, Graham G G 1980 Nutritional Management of Chronic Diarrhea and Malnutrition: Primary Reliance on Oral Feeding. J Pediatr 97: 316–323

McKeown T 1976 The Role of Medicine: Dream, Mirage or Nemesis? Nuffield Provincial Hospitals Trust

Marks M I, Pai C H, Lafleur L, Lackman L, Hammerberg O 1980 Yersinia Enterocolitica Gastroenteritis: A Prospective Study of Clinical Bacteriologic and Epidemiologic Features. J Pediatr 96: 26–31

Mobarak A B 1982 Egypt: Mothers Cut Diarrheal Deaths in Half with Homemade Treatment. Salubritas (Am Publ Hlth Assn/Wash DC) 6: 1

Molla A, Molla A M, Sarkar S A, Khatoon M, Rahaman M M 1982 Effects of Diarrhea on Absorption of Macronutrients During Acute Stage and After Recovery. In: Chen L C, N S Scrimshaw, op cit

Molla A M, Molla M, Sakar S A, Rahaman M M 1982 Intake of Nutrients During and After Recovery from Diarrhea in Children. In: Chen L C and M S Scrimshaw, op cit

Nalin D R, et al 1980 Comparison of Low and High Sodium and Potassium Content in Oral Rehydration Solutions. J Pediatr 97: 848–853

Parker R L, Rinehart W, Piotrow P T, Doucette L 1980 Rehydration Therapy (ORT) for Childhood Diarrhea. Pop Reports 8: L41–L75

Pierce N F, Greenough W S, Carpenter C C J 1971 Vibrio Cholerae Enterotoxin and its Mode of Action. Bacterial Rev 35: 1–12

Powell D W, Field M 1980 Pharmacological Approaches to Treatment of Secretory Diarrhea. In: Field M. Fordtran J S. Schultz S G (eds) Secretory Diarrhea. American Physiology Society. Bethesda. 187–209

Rabbini C H, Greenough W B, Holmgren J, Lonnroth I 1979 Chlorpromazine Reduces Fluid Loss in Cholera. Lancet 1: 410–412

Rahaman M M, Wahed M A 1982 Direct Nutrient Loss and Diarrhea. In: Chen L C, Scrimshaw N S op cit

Rohde J E, Northrup R S 1976 Taking Science Where the Diarrhea Is. In: Acute Diarrhea in Childhood — Ciba Foundation Symposium 42, Elsevier Excepta Medica. North Holland: 339–366

Rohde J E 1978 Preparing for the Next Round: Convalescent Care After Acute Infections. Am J Clin Nutr 32: 2258–2272

Rohde J E 1982 Mother Milk and the Indonesian Economy. J Trop Ped 28: 166–174

Rohde J E 1983 Why the Other Half Dies: The Science and Politics of Child Mortality in the Third World. Assignment Children 61/62: 35–67

Rosenberg M L et al 1977 Epidemic Diarrhea at Crater Lake from Enterotoxigenic Escherichia Coli. A Large Waterborne Outbreak. Ann Intern Med 86: 714–718, 1977

Rosenberg I H, et al 1974 Infant and Child Enteritis-Malabsorption malnutrition: The Potential of Limited Studies with Low-dose Antibiotic Feeding. Am J Clin Nutr 27: 304–309

Rowland M G M, Cole T J, Whitehead R G 1980 A Quantitative Study Into the Role of Infection in Determining Nutritional Status in Gambian Village Children Brit J Nutr 37

Rowland M G, Barrell R A, Whitehead R G 1978 Bacterial Contamination in Traditional Gambian Weaning Foods. Lancet 1: 136–138

Sack D A, et al 1978 Prophylactic Deoxcycline for Traveller's Diarrhea. Results of a Double-Blind Study of Peace Corps Volunteers in Kenya. N Engl J Med 298: 758–763

Sack R B 1979 Prophylactic Antibiotics the Individual Versus the Community. (editorial) N Engl J Med 300: 1107–1108

Santosham M, et al 1982 Oral Rehydration Therapy in Infantile Diarrhea. A Controlled Study of Well-Nourished Children Hospitalized in the United States and Panama. N Engl J Med 306: 1071–1076

Shields D S, Naitons-Shields M, Hook E W, Araujo J G, De Souza M A, Gurrant R L 1981 Electrolyte/Glucose Concentration and Bacterial Contamination in Home-Prepared Oral Rehydration Solution: A Field Experience in Northeastern Brazil. J Pediatr 98: 839–841

Snow J 1965 Snow on Cholera. Hafner Publ Co, New York: p 191

Soenarto Y, et al 1981 Acute Diarrhea and Rotavirus Infection in Newborn Babies and Children in Yogyakarta, Indonesia. Clin Microbiol 14: 123–129

Sommer A, Khan M, Mosley W H 1973 Efficacy of Vaccination of Family Contacts of Cholera Cases. Lancet 1: 1230–1232

Spady D W, Payne P R, Picou D, Waterlow J C 1977 Energy Balance during Recovery from Malnutrition. Am J Clin Nutr 29: 1073–1078

Steinhoff M C 1980 Rotavirus: The First Five Years. J Pediatr 96: 611–622

Sunshine P, Sinatra F R, Mitchell C H 1977 Intractable Diarrhoea in Infancy. Clinics in Gastro 6: 445–461

Surjono D, Ismadi S D, Suwardji, Rohde J E 1980 Bacterial Contaminations and Dilution of Milk in Infant Feeding Bottles J Trop Pedr 26: 58–61, 1980

Svennerholm A M, et al 1981 Antibody Response to Live and Killed Poliovirus Vaccines in the Milk of Pakistani and Swedish Women. J Infect Dis 143: 707–711

Tomkins A 1981 Nutritional Status and Severity of Diarrhoea Among Pre-School Children in Rural Nigeria. Lancet 1: 860–862

Traveller's Diarrhoea 1982 (editorial) Lancet 1: 777–778

Traveller's Warning 1975. Entero-Vioform Abroad. Med Lett Drugs Ther 17: 105–106

Walsh J A, Warren K S 1979 Selective Primary Health Care: An Interim Strategy for Disease Control in Developing Countries. N Engl J Med 301: 967–974

Whitehead R G, Coward W A, Lunn P G, Ruteshauser I H E 1977 A Comparison of the Pathogenesis of Protein-Energy Malnutrition in Uganda and the Gambia. Trans Royal Soc Trop Med Hyg 71: 189–195

WHO. A Manual for the Treatment of Acute Diarrhea. WHO/CDD/SER/80.2

WHO. Scientific Working Group 1980. Environmental Health and Diarrhoeal Disease Prevention. World Health Organization. WHO/DDC/80.5: pp 33

WHO International Study Group. 1977 A Positive Effect of the Nutrition of Philippine Children of an Oral Glucose-Electrolyte Solution Given at Home for the Treatment of Diarrhoea: Report of a Field Trial. Bull Wld Hlth Org 55: 87–94

Wolff H L, Van Zijl W J, Roy M 1969 The Availability of Water and Diarrhoeal Diseases. Bull Wld Hlth Org 41: 952–959

Woodward W E 1971 Cholera Reinfection in Man. J Infect Dis 123: 61–66

Woodward W E, Mosley. W H, McCormack W M 1970 The Spectrum of Cholera in Rural East Pakistan. 1-Correlation of Bacteriologic and Serologic Results. J Infect Dis 121: (Suppl) 510–516

Wray J D 1977 Maternal Nutrition, Breast Feeding and Infant Survival. In: Mosley W H, (ed), Nutrition and Human Reproduction. Plenum, New York: 197–229

Wray J D 1978 Direct Nutrition Intervention and the Control of Diarrheal Diseases in Preschool Children. Am J Clin Nutr 31: 2073–2082

Yadav M, Iyngkaran N 1981 Immunological Studies in Cows' Milk Protein-Sensitive Enteropathy. Arch Dis Chldhd 56: 24–30

Yolken R H, et al 1978 Epidemiology of Human Rotavirus Types 1 and 2 as Studied by Enzyme-linked Immunosorbent Assay. N Engl J Med 299: 1156–1161

Amoebiasis

INTRODUCTION

Amoebiasis is defined as 'the condition of harbouring *Entamoeba histolytica* with or without clinical manifestations' (WHO Expert Committee, Tech. Rep. Ser. No. 421, 1969), and occurs throughout the world in some 10 per cent of the world's population. There are a number of ameobae which inhabit the large intestine of man but *Entamoeba histolytica* is the only species known to be pathogenic.

With a few rare exceptions man can become infected only by ingesting the mature cysts of the parasite, and these can only derive from the faeces of an individual who is harbouring the parasite. The transmission of the cysts from the faeces of one person to their ingestion by another, can take place in a variety of ways, e.g., by faecal contamination of drinking water.

THE DISEASE

Clinical

Asymptomatic infections

Many individuals harbour *E. histolytica* in their colons without any signs or symptoms, and they may be quite unaware of being infected until the parasite is found on a stool examination. However, at any time and for reasons unknown, the host tissue may be invaded by the amoebae to produce any of the clinical manifestations described below.

Amoebic dysentery

Dysentery can occur within one to two weeks of ingesting cysts or can develop at any time in a person with an asymptomatic infection. The main presenting feature is diarrhoea, six to eight stools per day which are usually blood-stained and contain mucus. The degree of systemic upset is variable, but commonly this is minimal with little fever or toxaemia. The attack may last from a few days to several weeks, and is followed by periods if intermittent diarrhoea and remissions. Fulminating attacks even with perforation of the intestine can occur, and these are often precipitated by other factors such as malnutrition, another infection or by pregnancy.

Liver abscess

The amoebae may pass from the colon via the portal viens to the liver, where they can produce an abscess. Rarely does the patient present with a liver abscess during an attack of dysentery, and it can be that no history of dysentery is given. There is often a long latent period between the patient being infected and the appearance of a liver abscess.

A painful, tender, enlarged liver should be regarded as suggestive of amoebic liver abscess in an area where amoebiasis is endemic or in a person who at some time has been to such an area. Obviously, depending on the size of the abscess and the duration of the condition, a patient can present with few symptoms and signs, or on the other hand can be moribund. An intermittent pyrexia is common. The abscess may subsequently rupture usually into the abdominal cavity or into the thoracic cavity.

Some five to 15 per cent of patients with amoebic dysentery who are not treated or are inadequately treated, develop liver abscesses.

Other lesions

Abscesses may occur at other sites in the body, e.g., in the brain, and depending on the location, so will depend the presenting feature. However, abscesses at other sites are much less common than liver abscesses.

Amoebae can invade the integuments and due to tissue response, tumour masses (amoebomata) may develop.

PATHOLOGY

In the colon

In amoebic dysentery the amoebae invade the gut wall and produce necrosis, resulting in ulceration of the mucosa and submucosa. This may occur anywhere along the large intestine, but it is most common in the caecum and rectum. Ulceration can vary in degree from a minute ulcer to almost complete sloughing of the lining of the colon.

In the liver

An amoebic liver abscess is bacteriologically sterile and the lesion is one of an area of necrotic liver tissue surrounded by an area in which the amoebae are penetrating further into the liver tissue. Rarely is there any fibrotic reaction round the abscess.

DIAGNOSIS

As in all conditions caused by a parasite, the diagnosis is made by isolating the parasite from the patient and identifying it correctly. However, the finding of amoebae or cysts in a patient's stool has often resulted in a wide variety of clinical conditions being unjustly attributed to the amoebae. Therefore, the finding of the parasite must be taken in conjunction with the presenting clinical features. A useful aid in attributing the patient's illness to the amoeba is the finding of a positive serological test. The subject of serological tests is dealt with later

Treatment

It has been stressed that the patient with amoebic dysentery is not a source of infection to others but becomes such when in remission. It is important therefore that individual patients with amoebiasis be treated adequately with chemotherapeutic agents to ensure complete elimination of the parasite from the gut.

A number of therapeutic agents is available. Over the last 15 years metronidazole has become the treatment of choice using various dose regimes, but the best results have been obtained with 800 mg t.d.s. for five to 10 days, for all forms of amoebiasis. Other nitroimidazoles are being evaluated. Diloxanide furoate, 500 mg t.d.s. for 10 days can be used in addition as a lumenal amoebicide.

THE AGENT

Life cycle of E. histolytica.

Stage I: The mature four-nucleated cysts, derived from the formed stool of a person harbouring the parasite, are ingested, via contaminated food or water.

Stage II: In the distal part of the small intestine, four-nucleated amoebae hatch from the cysts and divide in the large intestine to prodice uninucleate amoebae. These amoebae reproduce by binary fission and may remain within the lumen of the large intestine or may invade the mucosa.

When no invasion occurs

Stage III: The amoebae continue to multiply without invading the mucosa of the intestine and the rate of passage of the colonic contents, being normal, allows time for the amoebae to encyst as follows:

As the luminar contents become drier the trophozoites become smaller, gradually round off and secrete a cyst wall. Two nuclear divisions take place in the maturation of the cysts to produce a four-nucleated (infectious) cyst which is excreted in the faeces. Cysts containing only one or two nuclei are also excreted. This completes the cycle.

When invasion occurs

Stage IV: Invasion of the gut wall can take place from Stages II or III causing ulceration. This results in rapid passage of the intestinal contents, and the amoebae do not encyst. Trophozoites are therefore excreted in the fluid stools and die rapidly.

During remissions the situation changes to Stage III

Stage V: The amoebae are disseminated from the gut wall via the portal veins to other sites, most frequently the liver, where abscesses may be produced.

Isolation and identification

Asymptomatic amoebiasis

The great majority of individuals with asymptomatic amoebiasis will be passing formed stools and the diagnosis will often be made by chance as a result of examining the stool for other parasites, or during the conduct of a survey. The formed stools will contain the cysts of *E. histolytica*, and it is important to be able to differentiate these from the cysts of non-pathogenic amoebae which commonly occur in man, often in association with *E. histolytica*.

The most efficient method of examining a formed stool for cysts, is the formal-water concentration technique as described by Allen and Ridley. This concentrates the number of cysts by factor of 20 to 30. Cysts and ova of other parasites such as helminth eggs and cysts of *Giardia lamblia* are also concentrated by this method. this fairly simple procedure is as follows:

Reagents

10 per cent formalin (one volume of 40 per cent formaldehyde diluted with nine volumes of distilled water).
Ether.

Apparatus

Centrifuge; conical centrifuge tubes of approximately 15 ml capacity; swab sticks; wire gauze, mesh 40 to the inch (15 per cm) (any other mesh is unsuitable); evaporating dish.

Procedure

(1) Into seven mls of 10 per cent formalin in a centrifuge tube, emulsify a specimen of faeces about the size of a pea taken on the end of a swab stick.

(2) Sieve by pouring whole contents of tube through wire gauze into an evaporating dish. Wash out the tube.

(3) Return the fluid in the evaporating dish to the centrifuge tube. Add three ml of ether. Shake vigorously for a full 30 seconds.

(4) Place tubes into centrifuge. Immediately set the regulator of the centrifuge to a mark corresponding to 3000 rpm and switch off exactly 60 seconds after starting. If the centrifuge is only capable of a speed of 2000 rpm spin for one and a half minutes.

(5) A layer of debris will have accumulated at the interphase between the two liquids. Loosen it by passing a swab stick gently round the circumference of the tube. Pour the contents of the tube down the sink, allowing only the last one or two drops to return to the bottom, where there will be a small deposit.

(6) Shake up the deposit. If the inside of the tube is dirty, wipe with cottonwool, and transfer the deposit to the slide with a Pasteur pipette.

Add a drop of Lugol's iodine and examine under a cover glass, with a × 40 objective. A calibrated micrometer scale should always be kept in one ocular of the microscope.

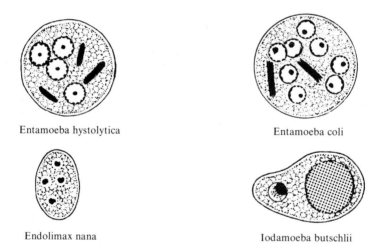

Entamoeba hystolytica

Entamoeba coli

Endolimax nana

Iodamoeba butschlii

Fig. 21.1 Diagrammatic representations of the common amoebic cysts of man.

Figure 21.1 represents, diagrammatically, the appearance of the cysts of *E. histolytica* and of the non-pathogenic amoebae commonly found in the faeces of man and the main distinguishing features are tabulated below.

For more detailed descriptions of the cysts and for staining techniques, which demonstrate nuclear structures in greater detail, reference should be made to standard parasitological works on the subject, such as The Color Atlas of Intestinal Parasites by Spencer and Monroe, published by C. C. Thomas, Illinois.

Table 1

Features	E. histolytica	E. hartmanii	E. coli	End. nana	Iod. butschlii
Shape	Spherical	As E. hist.	Spherical	Often oval	Irregular
Size	>10μ	<10μ	10–25μ	5–15μ	5–20μ
Karyosome	Often central	As E. hist.	Usually eccentric	–	–
Nuclei	1–4	As E. hist.	Up to 8	1–4 Usually indistinct	1
Other	Chromidial bars have rounded ends	As E. hist.	Chromidial bars have splintered ends	–	Large glycogen vacuole

Amoebic dysentery

With unformed stools a simple wet smear should be made, as trophozoites are destroyed by the concentration technique. The stool must be freshly passed as the amoebae soon round off and die and become unrecognizable. A drop of saline is placed on a slide and a portion of an abnormal part of the stool, e.g., mucus, is mixed with the saline, using a swab stick. The finding of motile amoebae with ingested red cells is diagnostic. The amoebae are from $10-40\mu$ in diameter and in fresh faeces they are very active and push out finger-like pseudopodia. The cytoplasm is granular and contains ingested red blood cells. The single nucleus is not clearly visible unless the specimen is stained.

It has been stated above that patients with asymptomatic amoebiasis usually passed formed stools. However, if the individual develops diarrhoea due to another agent, e.g., a bacterium or a virus, trophozoites will be found in the stools. These trophozoites will not contain ingested red cells as occurs in amoebic dysentery. Care must therefore be taken to avoid diagnosing amoebic dysentery solely on the presence of vegetative amoebae in the faeces.

Prevalence

Amoebiasis occurs throughout the world but accurate figures for prevalence are rare. Many areas have not been surveyed for amoebiasis and some surveys are unreliable due to the fact that the amoebic cysts are excreted intermittently and a large number of specimens requires to be examined from each individual in order to obtain accurate figures. However, where relatively low or high figures have been reported, these can serve as a general indication of prevalence.

The major factors responsible for a high prevalence are conditions of poor hygiene and sanitation. Climate per se has no direct influence, as amoebiasis has been reported from Arctic regions, but the highest prevalence figures are associated with warm countries where there tend to be poorer standards of hygiene and sanitation. Other factors must be involved, as where there are apparently identical conditions of hygiene and sanitation, whether good or bad, the prevalence figures are not necessarily identical. Amoebiasis in epidemic form has been recorded usually as a result of gross contamination of a water supply.

The prevalence of the parasite does not necessarily parallel the occurrence of symptomatic amoebiasis. A good example of this is the high prevalence of *E. histolytica* in hospitals for subnormality in the U.K., where invasive amoebiasis has not been recorded. The reasons for the wide variation in morbidity in different parts of the world are by no means clear. Various factors have been considered such as the virulence of the parasite, the diet, nutritional and immune state of the host, other disease conditions present, and variations in the gut flora, but no satisfactory explanation has yet been produced.

The race, age and sex of the host appear to be of little significance in the morbidity of the infection.

Transmission and sources of infection

The cyst and not the trophozoite is the infectious stage of the parasite. Virtually the only source of the cyst is the formed stool passed by individuals who have amoebiasis, either asymptomatic or those who are in a remission stage of amoebic dysentery. Thus man can be infected only through contamination by human faeces of food, drink or other objects placed in the mouth.

Faecal contamination may take place by any of the following methods.

Direct contamination of food and water by infected individuals

The importance, in the transmission of amoebiasis, of food handlers whose hands become contaminated after defaecation and who subsequently do not wash their hands properly, is still open to question. Cysts can remain viable for five minutes on the skin or for 45 minutes under the fingernails. Cysts die rapidly on dry food but not in liquids. From these data it would be quite wrong to ignore food handlers as a potential source of transmission, but their relative importance is still in doubt.

Sewage contamination of water

This is probably the most important factor in the transmission of amoebiasis for the following reasons.
(1) Contamination of water can occur easily and at several points in its distribution.
(2) The bulk of water is drunk "uncooked".

(3) A contaminated water supply will be widely distributed.
(4) Cysts can survive in water for a period of several weeks.
(5) The normal level of chlorine, if added, has no effect on the cysts.
(6) Even a satisfactory water supply can be contaminated by accident.

Night soil

Night soil apart from contamination of a water supply is now believed not to be an important factor in transmission of amoebiasis, except where it is applied directly to the crop in a vegetable farm shortly before harvesting. Washing vegetables, which are to be eaten raw, in water contaminated with night soil, is a likely way in which fresh vegetables can become contaminated.

Insects

Flies and cockroaches can harbour viable cysts and subsequently contaminate food with their vomitus or excreta.

Animal Reservoirs

A source of cysts other than man are animals which are infected with *E. histolytica*, particularly monkeys, but they are believed at present to be of little importance.

SURVEILLANCE

The frequency of the occurrence of the clinical pictures described above and correctly diagnosed, will indicate the magnitude of the problem in a population, particularly where the data have been recorded reliably over a period of years. Thus, hospital records when available, can be of great assistance. In the absence of reliable medical records, there are two principal ways in which to assess the situation, namely by a parasitological survey of stools as described above which will give a measure of the prevalence of the parasite, and, by undertaking a serological survey. Positive serological tests indicate the presence of invasive amoebiasis either currently or in the recent past. These are a number of serological tests but these are sophisticated and require complex equipment.

Unfortunately a reliable skin test is not yet universally available.

Control

Mass treatment and prophylaxis

The widerspread use of efficient chemotherapy in an attempt to eradicate

E. histolytica, followed by maintenance chemoprophylaxis is an attractive proposition. There are a number of reports in the literature, one being a study in an Indian reservation in northern Canada using metronidazole for a period of 12 months. Once monthly dosage for three months followed by bi-monthly treatment with single doses of 1.5 g to 2 g was used. This resulted in a seven-fold reduction in the number of cases of amoebic disease. However, further work requires to be done in this field and at present such a approach can be advocated only in acute situations.

PUBLIC HEALTH AND HYGIENE

The most important approach is to control the transmission of the parasite and all of the measures involved are based on preventing excreted cysts from being ingested by others. Hence, the proper disposal of faeces, the provision of an adequate water supply, health education and correct personal hygiene and the control of insects are all involved.

Disposal of faeces

The disposal of faeces so that cysts are not ingested by others is of paramount importance. This can be achieved by sophisticated or by simple methods either of which may be satisfactory if correctly designed and maintained. Details of techniques for the disposal of faeces and sewage are available in reference volumes. It is vital to avoid contamination of the drinking water supply whatever method of disposal is used.

Water supply

Proper filtration should be instituted wherever possible; as has been stated above, normal chlorination has no effect on the cysts of *E. histolytica*. A system for regular inspection and proper maintenance of the supply must be instituted.

Education and personal hygiene

Any measures which can be taken to educate the population on the association of faeces with the disease will be of value. The stressing of good personal hygiene, showing the population how to wash their hands properly, how to prepare and to protect food against insects are all of importance.

Control of insects

This embraces all aspects of insect control and includes the correct disposal of refuse by burning or burying, and the disposal of animal excreta. The use of insecticides should also be considered.

Typhoid

INTRODUCTION

The typhoid and paratyphoid infections together cause the enteric fevers. They are epidemiologically, diagnostically and therapeutically distinct from the diarrhoeal infections dealt with by Rohde in Chapter 20. The enteric fevers are primarily toxemias. Only in the cases of *Salmonella paratyphi A* and *B* can irritation of the gut be found with reasonable consistancy.

In earlier times there was a confusion with typhus fevers. It was not until the mid nineteenth century that typhoid became recognised as a specific disease (Budd 1873). Typhoid appears to be an exception to several epidemiologic expectations partly because it may be in the process of establishing a comfortable commensal relationship with man. Already it causes relatively few of those it infects to become sick. It cleverly continues to live and multiply especially in the gall bladders of carriers whose health it obligingly does not affect. Both urine and feces are transmission vehicles.

Though an infection transmitted by both food and water typhoid does not necessarily manifest itself through gastrointestinal symptoms. As it is primarily an infection of the reticuloendothelial system it does not respond, as would most gastrointestinal infections, to the rehydration of the patient. Though a single source in the community may infect many persons simultaneously the relatively few unlucky ones who actually become sick may become ill at widely different intervals.

Though part of the Salmonella family there is no important zoonotic element for the enteric fevers. The potentially most dangerous reservoirs are human carriers who have not suffered apparent disease.

Enteric fever is worldwide in distribution but has become particularly associated with social dislocation. Probably large proportions of cases, including those causing death, are never properly diagnosed and in areas where malaria is prevalent symptomatic differentation is not always easy. Both can cause chills, splenomegaly and neutropenia. Death may occur suddenly in a patient whose enteric fever has resolved and whose convalescence has begun. The single, reliable, presenting sign is a progressively rising and sustained fever.

THE AGENT

The enteric group consists of the four salmonellae *S. typhi.*, *S. paratyphi A.*, *S. paratyphi B.* and *S. paratyphi C.* They are Gram negative bacilli and in liquid media move about rapidly with the aid of flagellae. They are up to four microns in length. They are fairly fragile organisms soon killed by dessication, chlorine disinfection or heat. They remain alive in heavily polluted water for several weeks. Though they are easily cultivated in the laboratory it is not always possible to grow them from the feces of those who are sick. In typhoid itself the bacilli are most likely to be isolated in the second and third weeks of illness. Blood culture or aspiration of bone marrow are more reliable especially in the early stages of sickness. The continuation of bacilli in the blood stream after the first week of illness is an indicator of severity of the toxemia (Christie 1980).

A series of elegant laboratory procedures has evolved over the years. These distinguish not only between the different members of the enteric group but, by phage typing are able to distinguish as many as 80 different strains of *S. typhi*, many more still of the paratyphi. This phage typing, in effect the vulnerability of the bacilli to certain viruses, is sometimes epidemiologically useful as an indicator of the probable source of infection in a community: or if the phage type of suspect and cases is different it indicates that the correct source is yet to be discovered.

The so-called Widal reaction is an attempt to use the rising titers of IgG and IgM agglutinating antibodies (the H and O agglutinins) to make an early diagnosis where the disease is suspected. Previous typhoid vaccination complicates the interpretation especially of the H agglutinins. A third antigen, the Vi, plays an obscure part in the protection of the bacillus from O antibodies but its use as a detector of continuing *S. typhi* excretors, the carriers, is not reliable.

None of the bacterial isolation or serologic techniques can be relied upon diagnostically. They must often be repeated or, as in the case of the agglutination tests are only useful in a series of readings. A rising O agglutinin level most certainly indicates new typhoid infection. At the primary health care center in a developing country such tests have very limited applicability. The initial diagnosis must be made, and treatment begun on reasonable suspicion. In any case the likely many sources of infection in the community not only cloud the antigen picture in suspects but also render local eradication attempts impracticable. When enteric fever occurs in epidemics it is said that a single Widal reaction can prove useful as a means of screening out those sick who are actually infected with one of the enteric organisms (Shehabi 1981). Other antigen detection tests are also being reported (Sivadasan, Kurien and John 1984).

THE DISEASE

In general the paratyphoid infections cause the milder variations of enteric fever. Even in typhoid itself, however, there is a wide range of effects on different individuals from completely inapparent but antigenically stimulating infection to fulminating, septicemic toxemia and early death. The variably long incubation period, it can be up to four weeks, poses an additional problem in retrospectively pinpointing the source of any infection. Especially in typhoid itself the onset of the actual illness tends to be insidiously slow and there is considerable variation in virulence in the different strains. Initial complaints will be unspecific apart from the headache related to fever. Diarrhoea sometimes occurs as the disease develops and even in the paradoxically constipated patient there may be some abdominal discomfort, For the full range of presenting signs the reader should consult a clinical textbook.

Sometimes the only indication that a sickness is likely to be enteric fever is the step by step progressively upward fever in a step by step progressively prostrated patient. The strange feature which may alert the observor is the failure of the pulse rate to match the increases in the fever. Some typhoid fever sufferers may be brought to the District Health Center on the supposition that they are suffering from an acute psychiatric disturbance. Especially in children the history may be of little more than a short, sharp fever with a cough. If the child is severely anemic even the fever may be missed.

The fever resolves by gradual spikey lysis after the third week in untreated sufferers who are going to recover. Even so in the pretreatment days dangerous relapse of the fever and deaths, still later, from cardiac failure were not infrequent. In fact the heart appears to be involved in a substantial proportion of cases. In an Indian study electrocardiographic changes were found in 11.9 per cent of the patients (Khosla 1981). The degree of abnormality was related to the severity of the illness and to the ultimate prognosis.

The palpable spleen and the transient rose spots rash are of little or no diagnostic value in the populations of most warm climate countries. Nowadays the commonest complications are intestinal perforation or bleeding requiring respectively surgery or blood transfusion. Of the late complications the most important epidemiologically is cholecystitis because this is one of the commonest reasons for the recovered patient to become a carrier.

The treatment of typhoid, unlike the typical diarrhoeal infections, depends soley upon the use of antibiotics. Chloramphenicol was the earliest to be effective but it must be given in an adequately large dose and therapy must be continued for at least two weeks if either relapse or an increased likelihood of the carrier state are to be avoided. Unfortunately resistance of S. typhi to chloramphenicol soon became evident. In Peru it was reported that as few as 30 per cent of cases remained sensitive (WHO 1978i) though sensitivity to ampicillin remained.

Since then several drugs, as well as ampicillin, have been used as alternatives but with greater relapse rates and with the same problems emerging of resistant strains. Recently co-trimoxazole has been recommended as the drug of choice when chloramphenicol is proving to be ineffective (Herzog 1980). Most District Health Officers will in practice find themselves limited to using chloramphenicol for some time to come as it is cheap, relatively safe and easy to adminster.

The finding of identical phage types in victims with severe drug resistant disease underlines the danger if such cases become carriers able to transmit their drug resistant organisms within the community. High dosages of ampicillin or co-trimoxazole often still fail to sterilize the unlucky hosts. If the gall bladder is suspected as the source of the bacilli its removal may offer the only chance of eradicating a source of infection to others. Such heroic measures may not only be out of the range of options available in the health centers of many developing countries but would also be diluted in their effect by the inevitable persistance of many other sources of infection within the same community. Even given all the treatments available for typhoid the mortality rate can still be expected to be at least one per cent. It will be higher at the extremes of age or in the undernourished. The case fatality rate in the untreated has been found during disease outbreaks to be within the range of 10 to 15 per cent (Gorbach 1979). Corticosteroids may reduce case fatality in the most gravely ill (Hoffman et al 1984).

EPIDEMIOLOGY

1 Distribution

The disease is found world-wide but as one of the fecal-oral group of bacilli its prevalence will be determined largely by hygienic standards. Its prevalence has indeed been used as an indicator of the level of community hygiene. Even the best hygiene practices can of course be overcome by the importation of infected foodstuffs or by the moving of carriers into a community especially if they become involved in food preparation for the public. The fecal-oral spread within the family and village is probably the common pattern within most warm climate societies. In the industrialized countries outbreaks are usually traced to contamination of a water supply by a carrier. This contaminated water may be consumed directly or may itself contaminate foods, especially salads and canned foods. Contaminated water will also ensure that other fluids, such as milk and milk products act as vehicles of infection. As enteric salmonellae withstand cold temperatures very well neither refrigeration nor freezing reduce the risk from such consumables as ice cream or other fluids to which ice may be added.

In populations in which enteric infections occur fairly regularly children appear most frequently to be the victims. In communities long priviliged with good hygiene, and almost certainly less frequent disease, the age preference is lost. In India, it is suggested that about one child in every hundred between the ages of one and 15 years is newly infected each year (Cruickshank 1976). It is reasonable to suppose that as defects in basic hygiene and in the safety of the water supply are being corrected in a community the familiar endemic pattern of enteric fevers will be replaced by occasional epidemics. How widespread such epidemics would be would depend upon which part of the water or food distribution system was breached as well as upon the immunity level of the population. Though official reports suggest that there are about half a million cases of typhoid each year with about 25 000 deaths the true picture is clouded by the unspecific nature of much of the sickness while the milder diarrhoeal paratyphoid infections are likely to be ascribed to dysenteric-like infections.

2. Outbreak characteristics

The enteric fevers are typically family, closed community or village affairs. It is mainly because of the improved hygiene of the industrialized societies that typhoid became notorious as an explosive epidemic disease. The salmonella organisms are well adapted to Man's changing environment by their ability to multiply in such excellent culture media as dairy cream and meat based soups held at room temperature. A carrier handling food may only occasionally infect others depending upon the suitability of the food being handled and the susceptibility of those who consume it.

Of all the group of the enteric fevers only *S. typhi* itself seems well able to cause disease from apparently clean water. This is not because it survives well or multiplies away from its favourite medium, human sewage, but because of its ability to infect through relatively small doses of bacilli. Even after considerable dilution of sewage with clean water the bacilli may remain in sufficient concentration to cause invasive disease. Chance dictates that large outbreaks of enteric infection are more likely to be attributable to contaminated water than to food. As the epidemiologic generation time of *S. typhi* can be up to five weeks a single point source of infection in an immunologically innocent population will cause a typical outburst of disease but at a leisurely pace of new cases. The primary outburst can then be expected to subside completely with a secondary wave of new cases several weeks later as the families of the first cases develop the disease. In seasonal climates the greatest danger has been typically toward the end of a long period of hot weather.

3. Sources of infection

In practice Man is the only source and anything which Man can contaminate, including his own hands, will act as the vehicle of infection. Dairy products become less of a problem once milk pasteurization is enforced though clean milk can still be contaminated by dirty water. Vegetables fertilized with human feces will transmit enteric fever if the soil is not washed off with clean water or if the vegetables are not cooked before eating. Of course any liquid or solid food can be contaminated by a carrier after heating. Cold cooked meat dishes have always been a particular problem. An uncontaminated food can be contaminated by the dirty knife which cuts it into portions for tthe table or the dirty fingers which serve it out. Egg products have proved repeatedly to be an excellent vehicle for *S. paratyphi B*.

Canned foods are not foolproof against *S. typhi* which is particularly adept at entering cans being cooled after processing through minute defects in the metal. Contaminated cans are usually expected to 'blow' owing to the presence of gas producing organisms. In the case of the enteric fevers this is not a foolproof sign.

Shellfish are a particular danger as human food owing to their propensity for concentraing the bacilli just as they do the saxatoxin produced by the marine dinoflagellate *Gonyaulux tamarensis* (Red Tide). Sea water itself when ingested does not appear to be especially dangerous even though often heavily contaminated with human sewage. Shellfish though should never be eaten raw unless they come from an unimpeachable source or have been maintained for some days in clean, dilute salt water in which they will purge themselves of earlier contaminants.

Though enteric type bacilli are commonly found in such various human pets as tortoises and dogs the part these play in the infection of humans is unknown. Similarly though house flies could, by alternately landing on human sewage and food or by resting on the lips of infants, transmit bacilli their true importance as carriers is unknown. In any event there are many obvious transmission routes in communities whose hygiene is deficient. For laboratory workers an additional hazard is posed by fecal and urinary specimens and especially by culture plates. Bacilli from such sources have been transmitted in aerosols (Holmes et al 1980). In practice cross infection in hospitals is quite rare. Indeed it does not seem to require all that advanced a state of family hygiene greatly to slow down transmission within a community.

4. Transmission

As has already been suggested any drinkable fluid or edible solid handled by Man, or for that matter any contaminated object entering the mouth of a previously uninfected individual, may initiate infection. The nature of the intestinal pathology dictates that most new infections come from either convalescent recent cases or from carriers. Transmission can be greatly delayed by the ability of *S. typhi* to remain alive in well oxygenated sewage almost indefinitely. In dairy products such as cheese the bacilli remain alive for at least two months while in apparently clean water they will stay viable for at least four weeks. The increasing technological sophistication of the food distribution system also ensures that cases can occur separated by thousands of miles from the source.

5. Inidividual susceptibility

Quite a large dose of enteric organisms is required to ensure that a reasonable proportion of potential victims exposed actually become sick. The dose is smallest for *S. typhi* but other than prefering the immunologically immature or stressed, the young, the old and the malnourished, the enteric fevers have few prejudices in their selection of victims. Whether or not an individual becomes sick is largely a function of dose. In their remarkable experiments with volunteers Hornick et al (1970) demonstrated that more than 100 *S. typhi* bacilli must be swallowed for there to be any chance of infection. Indeed to cause typhoid fever in 95 per cent of those at risk required for each potential victim 10^9 (1 000 000 000) live bacilli.

SURVEILLANCE

No practicable system exists either to screen for or reliably to record new infections as they occur in large populations. In some countries handlers of food for public consumption are required to produce periodic stool samples which must be negative for *S. typhi* if they are to retain their jobs. Unfortunately even notorious carriers are not consistant bacilli excretors and so might easily be missed in such screening. The severity of the toxemia and fever in typhoid itself, if not in paratyphoid, will probably bring any multiple case outbreak to attention even when the number of cases is small. Antibody testing is probably too unreliable and too difficult to interpret for all but the serial surveillance of individuals already known to have been recently exposed. By contrast the registration and regular surveillance of known carriers has proved useful in those societies in which the disease has ceased to be a common fecal-oral family infection.

At the intermediate stage of development when public hygiene is also reasonably secure and typhoid should be, but too often is not, controlled it is worth remembering that individuals with chronic gall bladder disease are especially likely to be carriers. In Chile 3.8 per cent of such patients were found to carry *S. typhi* with a further 3.5 per cent carrying paratyphoid bacilli (Ristori et al 1982).

Some of the European socialist countries are especially eager to ensure that their citizens returning from work or vacation in typhoid endemic areas should be screened for infection, or at least advised to seek medical care should fever occur after returning home. Western industrial countries have been somewhat less concerned partly because of the logistics of coping with the huge numbers of international travellers. In consequence cases of typhoid are imported from time to time though the general standards of hygiene predicate against there being any wide spread of infection within the victim's community. In the period 1974 to 1978 45 different phage types were detected in West Germany in returning travellers (Brandis et al 1980).

CONTROL

In the western industrialized societies the reduction in typhoid from being an endemic to a now very sporadic disease can be ascribed to improvements in family and public hygiene, regulation of the food preparation and distribution system and especially to the ready availability of clean water for washing. This is not entirely comforting for the District Health Officer faced with a constantly recurring problem of enteric fever in a population with little education and few resources. Even the provision of a bacteriologically safe water supply will probably have little effect on enteric disease prevalence unless the water is convenient enough and liked enough for the washing of hands in the home to break the fecal-oral cycle of infection. The salmonellae are certainly sensitive enough to a simple soap and water washing of the hands of carriers (Pether and Scott 1982).

Controls are more easily applied and are better accepted when there is a major epidemic in a community especially when preliminary investigation points to a single source such as a particular well or food. In such conditions effective treatment is also more likely to reduce the chance of subsequent carriers than in sporadic unnoticed events.

In an area where the danger of enteric fever is high large stocks of chloramphenicol should be maintained. While bearing in mind the dangers of aplastic anemia a special effort to bring therapy to all those with possible enteric fever may reduce the community load of bacilli. Pasteurization of dairy products and chlorination of drinking water supplies will help in some populations. Until, however, the District Health Officer has begun to identify the likely carriers, and has some laboratory capability permitting repeated examination of the stools of suspects, controls will be rather hit or miss. The difficulty in limiting actual outbreaks is not all that great but finding the carrier sources can be most frustrating. Even in a relatively small, relatively closed island community like Dominica attempts to find the carrier(s) from outbreaks beginning in 1977 have still been inconclusive (Fortune 1981). In such circumstances further explosive outbreaks seem inevitable. Once they have been identified carriers should either be bacteriologically sterilized or kept well away from preparation of food for public consumption and from public water supplies. Pether and Scott (1981) have argued that effort is really better spent on improving hygiene practices in all food handlers than in chasing after individual carriers.

PREVENTION

Though given confidently for many years the actual effectiveness of the traditional enteric fever vaccines has never been irrefutably demonstrated. Part of the difficulty lies in the absence of an entirely satisfactory laboratory animal. The antigen which, if given as a vaccine, might produce active resistance is still to be identified. Even typhoid fever itself may not protect the victim against subsequent reinfection. Certainly it appears that immunization campaigns against typhoid in disaster situations or in conditions of upheaval such as a refugee camp are a waste of time (Bollag 1980). The results of the massive WHO trials have never been encouraging (WHO 1962) though WHO has not given up hope that a typhoid vaccine of known potency would prove useful in areas where surveillance suggests a continuing high risk or in situations where a limited outbreak stems from a single but continuing source (WHO 1978ii).

The problem with the dead vaccines may lie in their failure to stimulate specific T lymphocytes rather than in the production of antibodies which was the original objective. The old vaccines appeared to be effective in protecting against small dose water borne infections but proved useless when the dose of *S. typhi* was large as is often the case in food contamination.

New live vaccines given by mouth and using a mutant strain of *S. typhi* have produced promising results. The mutant invades, alerts T lymphocytes but causes no sickness. In Egypt this vaccine was found to be effective for at least a year in a large field trial (Wahdan et al 1980). Such a vaccine would indeed be analagous to that against poliomyelitis and would also be expected to work best in those communities in which rapid fecal-oral spread would ensure widespread infection but this time by the immunizing vaccine.

REFERENCES

Bollag U 1980 Practical evaluation of a pilot immunization campaign against typhoid fever in a Cambodian refugee camp. International Journal of Epidemiology 9/2: 121–122

Brandis H, Lenk V, Wuershing F 1980 Results of phage typing of Salmonella typhi and Salmonella paratyphi-B in the years 1974–1978 Federal Republic og Germany including Berlin (West). Zentralbl. Bacteriol. Microbiol. Hyg. 274: 440–459

Budd W 1873 Typhoid fever. Its nature, mode of spreading and prevention. Longmans, London

Christie A B 1980 Infectious diseases. Epidemiology and clinical practice, 3rd edn. Churchill-Livingstone, Edinburg, P 47–102

Cruickshank R 1976 Enteric infections: Gastroenteritis, dysentery, typhoid, cholera. from Epidemiology and community health in warm climate countries. Cruickshank (ed). p 111. Churchill-Livingstone, Edinburgh

Gorbach S L 1979 Typhoid fever. In Cecil textbook of medicine, 15th edn. Saunders, Philadelphia, P 446–449

Herzog Ch 1980 New trends in the chemotherapy of typhoid fever. Acta tropica 37: 275–280

Hoffman S L et al 1984 Reduction of mortality in chloramphenicol-treated severe typhoid fever by high-dose dexamethasone. New England Journal of Medicine 310: 82–88

Holmes M B et al 1980 Acquisition of typhoid fever from proficiency testing specimens. New England Journal of Medicine 303: 519–521

Hornick R B et al 1970 Typhoid fever pathogenesis and immunologic control. New England Journal of Medicine 283: 686–691

Khosla S N 1981 The heart in enteric (typhoid) fever. Journal of Tropical Medicine and Hygiene 84: 125–131

Pether J V S, Scott R J D 1982 Salmonella carriers; are they dangerous? A study to identify finger contamination with Salmonellae by convalescent carriers. Journal of Infection 5/1: 81–88

Ristori C et al 1982 Investigation of the Salmonella typhi — paratyphi carrier state in cases of surgical intervention for gallbladder disease. Bulletin of the Pan American Health Organization 16/2: 161–171

Shehabi A A 1981 The value of a single Widal test in the diagnosis of acute typhoid fever. Tropical and Geographical Medicine 33/2: 113–116

Sivadasan K, Kurien B, John T J 1984 Rapid diagnosis of typhoid fever by antigen detection. Lancet 1: 134–135

Wahdan M H et al 1980 A controlled field trial of live oral typhoid vaccine. Bulletin of the World Health Organization 58/3: 469–474

WHO Yugoslav typhoid commission 1962. A controlled field trial of the effectiveness of phenol and alcohol typhoid vaccines. Bulletin of the World Health Organization 26: 357

WHOi 1978 Surveillance for the prevention and control of health hazards due to antibiotic resistant enterobacteria. Technical Report Series No 624. Geneva

WHOii 1978 Control of diarrhoeal disease: WHO's programme takes shape. WHO Chronicle 32: 369–372

Enterovirus infections: Poliomyelitis

INTRODUCTION

The regular use of poliovirus vaccines on a large scale during the last two decades has resulted in almost complete elimination of poliomyelitis in those economically developed countries where this disease had formerly been a serious public health problem. During this time poliomyelitis received little attention in developing warm climate countries owing to an assumption that it occurred relatively infrequently. This assumption was based on formal morbidity reports and on certain accepted dogmas about the epidemiology of poliomyelitis.

Though it had been apparent for some years that considerable discrepancies existed between the reported and the real incidence rates (Dömök, 1972) and that there were indications of a changing pattern of the disease (Sabin, 1963; Cockburn and Drozdov, 1970), the validity of the aforementioned assumption came into question only most recently owing to the results of the lameness surveys which have been carried out in a number of warm climate countries since the original publication of Nicholas et al (1977). These surveys unanimously indicated that in these countries the mean annual incidence rate of poliomyelitis even under endemic circumstances had been as high as, or even higher than, in temperate climate countries during epidemic periods. These findings as well as some other considerations (Nathanson and Martin, 1979) led to the recognition that some accepted concepts on poliomyelitis needed revision, and that poliomyelitis was a major public health problem in warm climate countries.

This chapter will focus mainly on poliomyelitis with special regard to the above mentioned developments in theory and practice. Since, however, the nosocomial entity of poliomyelitis as a disease caused by polio viruses is now debated (Sabin, 1981a,b) owing to the similarity of clinical features elicited by non-polio enteroviruses and the similarities in other ways of the enteroviruses, certain topics will cover a broadened field for a clear understanding of pertaining questions.

THE DISEASES AND THE PATHOGENETIC PROCESSES

By classical definition paralytic poliomyelitis is the most serious clinical manifestation of poliovirus infection. Virological investigations have produced evidence that a number of non-polio enteroviruses can also elicit similar clinical manifestations (Table 23.1). These were usually described as 'poliomyelitis-like diseases'. Based on these observations most recently Sabin (1981a,b) proposed to define paralytic poliomyelitis as a clinical-pathological syndrome that is caused by enteroviruses. This suggestion may be theoretically justifiable. From a practical point of view, it seems important to maintain the distinction between poliomyelitis caused by polioviruses and poliomyelitis-like diseases elicited by other enteroviruses for the following reasons: (a) paralytic disease is a usual manifestation of poliovirus infections but an exceptional one of other enterovirus infections; (b) paralytic diseases caused by non-polio enteroviruses are usually milder and more often transient than those caused by polioviruses; (c) poliomyelitis is of primary importance from an epidemiological point of view; (d) poliomyelitis is the disease, and polioviruses are the agents which can be eliminated by effective vaccinations.

Infections with enteroviruses including polioviruses may lead to a wide spectrum of clinical manifestations (Table 23.1). This is connected with pathogenetic processes characteristic to them. They enter the body by the oral or nasopharyngeal routes and the sites of their primary multiplication are the tonsillopharyngeal tissues and the small intestine with the involvement of the regional lymphonodular system. Generally no clinical signs occur when virus multiplication remains limited to these primary sites (inapparent infections), and this happens in the vast majority of cases. In certain cases the virus enters the bloodstream (viraemia) an event which may be signalled by a non-characteristic febrile illness (in poliovirus infection four to eight per cent). Through the bloodstream the virus can gain access to different organs (polioviruses invade the central nervous system in 0.01 to 2 per cent) in which secondary multiplication may occur. There is also evidence that polioviruses may gain direct access to the CNS through peripheral nerve pathways (e.g. cranial nerve filaments exposed to infection after tonsillectomy). Clinical symptoms will reflect the pathological changes caused in the secondary target organ(s). Consequently a specific enterovirus type can be responsible for different combinations of symptoms and apparently similar disease will be caused by infections with different serotypes. Nevertheless the range of diseases which may be elicited varies according to the virus type, and the ratio of actual cases to all infections depends on the serotype of the virus and on the virulence of actual strains within the types. Polioviruses for example may cause minor illness, aseptic meningitis (non-paralytic poliomyelitis) and paralytic poliomyelitis (spinal, bulbar, bulbo-spinal, encephalitic forms). Among them the type 1 viruses are the

Table 23.1 Clinical associations of enteroviruses

Syndrome or Clinical feature	Virus types associated				
	Poliovirus	Coxsackievirus A	B	Echovirus	Ungrouped
Paralytic disease	1–3	4, 7, 9,	1–5	1, 2, 4, 6–11 13, 14, 16, 18, 30, 31	70, 71
Aseptic meningitis	1–3	1–11, 14, 16, 18, 22, 24	1–6	1–11, 13–23, 25, 27, 30, 31	71
Encephalitis	(1–3)	2, 5, 6, 7, 9	1–3, 5	2–4, 6–11, 14, 18, 19, 22	71
Exanthematous disease	—	2, 4, 5, 6, 9, 10, 16	1–3, 5	1–12, 14, 16, 18–20	71
Herpangina	—	2–6, 8, 10, 22	—	—	—
Epidemic myalgia	—	4, 6, 10	1–5	1, 6, 9	—
Myocardiopathy	—	1, 2, 4, 5, 8, 9, 16	1–5	1, 4, 6, 9, 14, 19, 22, 25, 30	—
Myocarditis neonatorum	—	—	1–5	—	—
Acute respiratory disease	—	9, 16, 21, 24	2–5	1–4, 6–11, 16, 19, 20, 22, 25	68
Hepatic disturbances	—	4, 9	5	4, 9	—
Acute haemorrhagic conjunctivitis	—	24	—	—	70
Orchitis	—	—	1–5	—	—
Undifferentiated febrile conditions	1–3	1–24	1–6	1–34	68–71

most potent in causing paralytic illness, being the aetiological agents in most of the poliomyelitis epidemics. Nevertheless neurovirulence even of type 1 strains varies considerably.

Predisposing host factors also exist which influence the outcome of infections. They include

(a) Age of susceptible infected persons

The ratio of paralytic cases to infections increases with age. In temperate climates during epidemics caused by type 1 poliovirus the ratios were estimated as 1:1000 among young children and 1:75 among adults (Horstmann, 1955). Based on a recent study in Burma it is estimated that the ratio of cases to infections in recent years has been about 1:620 in the first year of life and about 1:140 in children between one and four years of age (Schonberger et al, 1981).

(b) Tonsillectomy (the reasons see above).

(c) Pregnancy

The excess manifestation is apparently associated with hormonal changes, and especially with elevated cortisone level.

(d) Intramuscular inoculations

There is strong evidence in temperate climates suggesting an increased incidence of paralytic poliomyelitis among children who have received injections of DPT vaccine within 4 weeks prior to the onset of disease. This may be true also for other injections, especially for quinine and antibiotics according to reports from African countries (Towsend-Coles and Findlay, 1953; Guyer et al, 1980).

(e) Physical exertion-trauma particularly in adults

(f) Immunological deficiencies and immuno-suppressive therapy

(g) Sex

Males usually have higher poliomyelitis attack rate than females.

It is not the aim of this chapter to describe the clinical and pathological aspects of enterovirus infections. The reader is referred in these respects to earlier publications (e.g. Bodian and Horstmann, 1965; Dalldorf and Melnick, 1965; Melnick, 1965; Steigman, 1969).

THE AGENTS

Human enteroviruses represent a large group of antigenically dissimilar but otherwise closely related agents. They belong to Enterovirus genus of family Picornaviridae. Currently over 70 human enterovirus types have been recognised. Virions of enteroviruses are small (20–30 nm in diameter) and have a single stranded ribonucleic acid core surrounded by a protein capsid built up by cubic symmetry. They are resistant to many standard disinfectants. They are sensitive to formalin (0.3 per cent formaldehyde) and chlorine (free residual level of 0.3–0.5 ppm). They are inactivated rapidly by ultraviolet light and by drying. Exposure of virions to a temperature of 50°C destroys their infectivity rapidly. Enteroviruses are stable in a deep-frozen state. They remain active for weeks at 4 to 8°C and for some days at around 20°C.

Diagnostic virology

Virus isolation is a basic technique for the detection of enterovirus infections. Faecal samples and in fatal cases autopsy specimens from the CNS or from other organs (depending on the clinical forms) are the most suitable for this purpose. Polioviruses and most of the other enteroviruses grow readily in monolayer cultures of primate epithelial cells. Relatively simple techniques can be applied for virus isolation and identification as described by Dömök and Magrath (1979) when the aim is to detect poliovirus infections. When the aim is, however, to reveal any enteroviruses which might be present, more sophisticated techniques should be used as described by Melnick et al (1979).

Serological diagnosis is based on the detection of antibody response in the course of the illness. This may mean either detection of a significant (at least four-fold) antibody titre increase by investigation of serum samples taken in the early and late phases of the illness, or detection of specific IgM antibodies — which are only transiently present following primary infection — in a serum sample originating from any phase of the illness. Unfortunately type-specific results can be obtained only by neutralization tests. These can be carried out with micro-techniques (Dömök and Magrath, 1979). IgM fractions of sera can be separated for tests by different techniques. A simple method applicable even when modest laboratory facilities are available has been described by Nagy et al (1982). Owing to the large number of serotypes of enteroviruses the serological tests can be used only for the diagnosis of infections with selected virus types (e.g. polioviruses).

IMMUNITY

Infection with poliovirus and other enterovirus types results in a long lasting homotypic immunity. The immune response does not depend on the outcome of infection. It is characterized (a) by the appearance of antibodies in the blood, and (b) by induction of local resistance of the intestinal tract to reinfection with the homologous enterovirus type.

Neutralizing antibodies are those mostly formed against the complete virions. They are type specific and have an important role in immunity by neutralization of virions entering the blood stream. Antibodies of the IgM class appear first, usually within three days after infection; their titre increases rapidly reaching a peak at two weeks, but they do not persist for more than a few months. Thus their presence indicates an actual or more recent infection. Antibodies of IgG class appear in serum somewhat later than those of IgM class; their peak titre will be attained after three to four weeks, and they persist presumably for life though with slowly decreasing levels. The appearance of IgA class antibodies in serum is irregular and they persist for a short period after infection. As neutralising IgG antibodies persist for long after infection the neutralization tests are useful for sero-epidemiological investigations.

Local resistance of the intestinal tract is mediated partly by local production of secretory IgA antibodies by immunocompetent cells located at the primary multiplication sites of the virus and partly by cellular immunity factors.

Live poliovirus vaccine elicits immunity as though to natural infection. Killed vaccine, however, induces only antibody production.

Maternal antibodies of IgG class can pass through the placenta. Thus newborns will have an antibody level in their blood similar to the maternal one. The half life time of maternal antibodies in the infants' blood has proved to be 28 days. Accordingly neutralizing antibodies of maternal origin are present in the blood usually up to six months of age. Breast milk and especially the colostrum contains secretory IgA antibodies. The probability of enterovirus infections is lessened by these antibodies in breast fed infants since a considerable part of the mucous membrane of the alimentary tract will remain covered with them for several hours after feeding.

EPIDEMIOLOGY

Source and transmission of infections

There is no independent infecting cycle in animals of polioviruses and of other human enteroviruses. Thus the source of infection is always another person without regard to whether or to how that primary infection is manifested. Since over 90 per cent of infections remain inapparent the chain of transmission cannot be followed up by epidemiological methods. The virus multiplies in the oro-pharynx for a short period, but in the intestinal tract for about four weeks. Thus virus will be present in pharyngeal excreta in the early stages of infection and can be transmitted by droplet spread from person to person for a short period. It will be excreted in the stool for several weeks and can be spread by the faecal-oral route during that time.

As enteroviruses are relatively resistant to physical and chemical influences they are readily transmitted by contaminated hands, foodstuffs, underwear, kitchen utensils and can remain active for a relatively long time.

Enteroviruses can readily be isolated from sewage samples and from latrine specimens. These viruses are also recoverable from flies and cockroaches attracted by faecal deposits. The role of these insects in transmission is, however, not essential.

Factors influencing the spread of infection

Circulation of virus types in the population or in certain age groups of the population depends upon the proportion of persons without immunity. The majority of infections occur among children of pre-school age since in any population these age groups represent the bulk of susceptibles. The antigenic experience increases with age thus infections occur with decreasing frequency as age advances. The pattern of acquisition of immunity in relation to age depends upon the intensity of spreading of infections. This is influenced by the following factors.

(a) Since the faecal-oral route predominates in transmission of infections, it follows that there is a relationship between sanitary conditions and the dissemination of polioviruses and other enteroviruses. Infections occur more often and specific immunity is acquired at an earlier age among populations or population groups living under poor sanitary conditions than in those having high standards of hygiene.

(b) Transmissibility of polioviruses and other enteroviruses is influenced by certain climatological factors. In temperate climate countries there is a marked seasonal incidence of these viruses. The vast majority of infections occur in summer and early autumn, and only a limited circulation is observable in the rest of the year. Seasonality becomes less marked in parallel with the increasing mean annual temperature and ceases in the tropics. There is no generally accepted explanation for this phenomenon. The humidity may be important, since environmental survival of polioviruses is markedly favoured by relative humidities over 40 per cent.

(c) Transmission of infections from young children to young children is the usual pattern. The transmission of infections is facilitated if children are living in a community (nurseries, kindergartens, orphanages, et cetera) or in large size families. If a virus is carried into a community of young children all the susceptible inmates will be infected within days.

(d) It is well established that poliovirus strains vary in their neurovirulence. Virulent strains besides being more able to cause disease have a greater potential for spread among susceptibles than non-virulent strains. The probable basis of this phenomenon is that many fewer virions are needed to constitute an infective dose from the virulent than from the non-virulent strains.

(e) Spreading of an enterovirus type in the population may limit the dissemination of another one by interference. Most impressive examples of the phenomenon were observed in connection with the use of live poliovirus vaccine. It has been demonstrated that a poliomyelitis epidemic can be influenced by large scale administration even of a vaccine type different from the virus type responsible for the epidemic. On the other hand, wild enteroviruses may decrease the rate of implantation of live vaccine in vaccinated persons. It should, however, be stressed that many factors influence the interfering activity of one virus with another. Thus multiple infections may equally occur.

Spreading of infections in warm climates

In warm-climate countries all factors promoting the dissemination of enteroviruses are present. The majority of the populations live in rural areas where sanitary conditions are primitive. In addition large segments of the populations of urban areas live in slums or in other populous outskirts without any benefit from modern sanitary achievements. Eating and other personal habits, as well as inter- and intra-familial associations also exist in many countries which considerably facilitate the faecal-oral transmission of infections. Large family size is a rule, thus contacts between young spreaders and susceptibles is unlimited. Climatological conditions are favourable for transmission of infections throughout the year. These factors jointly contribute to continuous high prevalence of enterovirus infections among young children in warm climate countries.

Virus excretion studies carried out in warm climate countries among young children have unanimously indicated excretion rates as high as 70 to 80 per cent of those under three years of age (Sabin et al, 1960; Parks et al, 1966). When special techniques of isolation were applied a great number of simultaneous multiple infections could also be detected. It was also demonstrated that practically all the enterovirus types can be isolated in the tropics within a relatively short period of time if sufficient numbers of stool samples are collected and investigated from young children. (Dömök et al, 1974).

Cross-sectional polio antibody surveys also brought evidence that natural infection and immunization by polioviruses occurs during the first five years of life. This is illustrated in Fig. 23.1 in respect of type 1 poliovirus for ten warm climate countries in comparison to a temperate climate country (The Netherlands) prior to vaccinations against poliomyelitis.

It is seen that the slope of curves representing the situation in warm climate countries is steep. This indicates that practically all the children became immune by five years of age. In the case of the temperate climate country the rate of subjects having antibodies reached only 55 per cent by this age.

Similar conclusions can be drawn from lameness surveys carried out in warm climate countries in most recent years. In each of these countries 76 to 99 per cent of paralytic poliomyelitis cases proved to occur before the age of five years. Table 23.2 presents data for countries where cumulative percentages for age groups under five years of age have been determined. It is remarkable that in some countries very high proportions of cases have occurred even before 12 months of age.

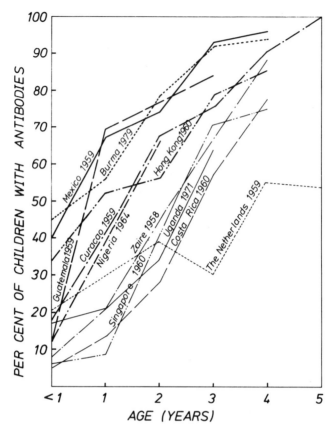

Fig. 23.1 Prevalence of polio type 1 antibodies by age in certain warm climate countries compared to that observed in the Netherlands before the introduction of vaccinations against poliomyelitis.

References. Burma: Schonberger et al, 1981; Costa Rica: Roca-Garcia et al, 1964; Curacao and Netherlands: Hofman and Wilterdink, 1960; Guatemala: Horstmann et al, 1960; Hong Kong: Franklin and Robertson, 1965; Mexico: Sabin et al, 1960; Nigeria: Poliomyelitis Commission, 1966; Singapore: Lee et al, 1964; Uganda: Dömök et al, 1974; Zaire: Plotkin et al, 1960.

Epidemiological trends of poliomyelitis

In temperate climates poliomyelitis has undergone changing epidemiological behaviour. It was endemic world-wide until the last decades of the 19th century. Then the transition from an endemic to an epidemic disease began in Scandinavia, later in North America, Australia, New Zealand and Europe. Initially small collections of cases or even large 'primary outbreaks' occurred, then gradually increasing attack rates were observed for a few years followed by severe epidemics. In epidemic years the annual paralytic poliomyelitis incidence rate surpassed even 30 per 100 000 population in certain countries. Though from the early 50s there have also been epidemics

Table 23.2 Occurrence of poliomyelitis by age based on data obtained in lameness surveys in warm climate countries*

COUNTRY Area	Cumulative percentage of cases occurring before the age (months) indicated					
	6	12	24	36	48	60
GHANA Danfa rural	1.3	22.4	64.5	79.0	90.8	96.1
National urban-rural		28.0	45.8	62.7	71.3	75.6
EGYPT Alexandria	9.8**	38.8	78.6	91.5	95.0	97.5
PHILIPPINES Urban-rural			51.0	80.0	91.0	
MALAWI Urban-rural		14.8	64.5	82.8	89.8	94.1
INDIA Vellore		49.0	64.1	74.5	87.7	89.6
NIGER Rural				70.0		99.0

* For references see Table 23.3
** Under 5 months of age

described in certain warm climate countries, the disease essentially remained endemic in this part of the world.

It was generally assumed, until only a few years ago, that while the sanitation and hygiene remained poor, the disease kept its endemic nature with extremely low incidence. This was because all infections occurred in infancy when paralysis was rare owing to partial protection by maternal immunity, to generally milder disease at this age and to the greater likelihood of infection with a poliovirus of low neurovirulence. In parallel with improvements of sanitary and hygienic conditions exposure and infection appear at increasingly older ages, when the ratio of paralytic cases to infections is considerably increased. As more and more children grow up without having immunity, the susceptible population is increased to the level needed for an epidemic to occur.

The assumption was largely based on the increase in the rates of illness with older age. Closer analysis of past epidemiological events indicated that this was insufficient to explain past epidemics of poliomyelitis in temperate climates (Nathanson and Martin, 1979). The theory does not stand up even in respect of warm climate countries. The disease remained mostly endemic and occurred in the youngest age groups (Table 23.2); but it turned out to be a fallacy that poliomyelitis was rare in these countries. Serious underreporting served for the basis of this misbelief.

Since 1974 studies of the prevalence of lameness resulting from poliomyelitis have been carried out in a number of warm climate countries in Africa, Asia and South America. Results from 12 countries are tabulated in Table 3. For comparison, the mean annual incidence rates based on

Table 23.3 Mean annual reported incidence of poliomyelitis per 100 000 population 1976–1980 and incidence estimated from lameness surveys in warm climate countries.

COUNTRY Region	Year	Surveyed age groups (years)	Subjects No	Prevalence rate per 1000	Mean annual incidence per 100 000 population Estimated from survey A	B	Reported
GHANA							
Danfa rural	1974	0–5	5885[a]	3.4	..	..	2.3
	1974	6–15	7347[a]	7.5	28	50	
National urban	1974	6–19	24011[a]	5.1	23	34	
rural	1974	6–19	50598[a]	8.2	..	55	
CAMEROON							
Youndé	1975–1978	5–11	13700[b]	8.7	46	46	1.2
Rural and semi rural		5–11	21500[b]	6.2	33	33	
EGYPT							
Alexandria	1976	0–10	524654[b]	1.7	7	9	1.8
		5–10	260141[b]	2.3	..	12	
PHILIPPINES							
Davao	1976	5–10	3000[b]	4.3	..	23	1.8
Urban-rural	1980	0–14	12055[a]	2.9	12	19	
THAILAND							
Bangkok and Southern	1978	5–10	28559[b]	0.6	2	3	1.7
Northern and Central		5–10	15982[b]	3.4	12	18	
N-Eastern and Eastern		5–10	16981[b]	1.8	6	10	

	Year	Age	No. surveyed				
INDONESIA							
Bali	1978	0–14	10332[a]	3.0	..	..	0.1
		5–9	3935[a]	3.1	..	21	
		10–14	2084[a]	1.4	..	9	
MALAWI							
Urban-rural	1979	0–15	17580[b]	0.5	28	35	1.2
INDIA							
Vellore	1979	5–17	34112[b]	3.2	10	17	2.1
Rural		5–17	18548[b]	3.2	10	17	
IVORY COAST							
Urban	1979	6–11	10847[a]	8.0	53	53	1.2
Rural	-1980	5–14	6180[a]	8.0	53	53	
Semi-urban		8–18	5717[a]	12.0	80	80	
BRAZIL							
Federal District	1980	6–7	10794[b]	2.3	..	12	1.8
		10–11	10043[b]	5.4	..	29	
YEMEN							
Urban	1980-	5–13	6039[a]	3.5	..	20	3.3
Rural	-1981	5–13	6404[a]	3.0	..	17	
NIGER							
Rural	1981	5–14	23600[a]	6.4	46	43	5.3

A = Published in original report
B = Calculated as described by LaForce et al (1980).
[a] Residual paralyses on lower limbs were surveyed. References: Nicholas et al ((1977); Ofosu-Amaah et al (1977); Sabin (1981): World Health Organization Reports of the Expanded Program on Immunization..
[b] Any kinds of disabilities probably caused by poliomyelitis were surveyed.

formal reports in the period between 1976 and 1980 are also presented. It is clear from Table 23.3 that with some exceptions the formal figures represent less than ten per cent of the number of cases estimated from the prevalence surveys. Moreover the true mean annual incidence rates are close to, or even exceed significantly those which were reported from temperate climate countries in the epidemic pre-vaccination era. This is not a new development. The distribution of the year of onset of cases detected in the surveys indicated that in warm climate countries the incidence rates have long been on such a high level and in most of the countries no major changes could be observed in annual rates showing that the disease remained endemic.

It is of note, however, that since 1950 occasional epidemics have also been described in a number of countries which might have been real epidemic flare-ups, for example in Kenya, Madagascar, Honduras, Iraq, Malaysia; (World Health Organization, 1980c), or might only reflect better recognition and reporting of cases in certain years than in the others. Examples of the latter were the epidemics reported in the Philippines from Bantayan Island in 1976 and from Cebu City in 1979. Lameness surveys later performed demonstrated that in these areas the real annual incidence rates had been high and stable in previous years (World Health Organization, 1981c).

In epidemics observed in warm climate countries the age distribution of cases remained generally the same as in endemic periods; that is the disease remained 'infantile'. Epidemics were reported in which a number of cases occurred among adolescents and adults, for example in Pakistan, (World Health Organization, 1980c).

From these data it seems plausible to assume — in agreement with a suggestion of Ofosu-Amaah et al (1977) — that the principal trend of poliomyelitis might have been uniform all over the world in this century. The ratio of cases to infections has increased gradually presumably because poliovirus strains with higher and higher neurovirulence have become successively predominant owing to mutation and selection. In warm-climate countries the disease could have remained endemic with gradually increasing incidence, since all factors except virulence of circulating virus have remained practically unchanged. In temperate climates the transmissibility of infections has been uneven due to seasonality. It has become effectively restricted by improved sanitary and hygienic conditions which resulted in periodic accumulation of susceptibles in high numbers even among older children and young adults. Whenever virulent strains became selected, being able to spread effectively even under strong restricting conditions, epidemics occurred. These affected the susceptibles in different age groups.

The occasional epidemic flare-ups in warm climate countries might have been connected with the introduction of highly virulent strains owing to population movements (wars, developmental projects, extended tourism) as suggested by Gear (1955) and Sabin (1963). It is, however, difficult to understand how epidemics can occur in three to five year cycles in certain countries (e.g. Kenya) and how a shift in the age incidence of paralytic poliomyelitis to older age groups could have occurred in certain epidemics (see above) without significant improvement of sanitary and hygienic conditions. These phenomena raise the possibility that some special factors influencing the transmissibility of infections may exist in certain populations in the warm climates (virus inhibitors?).

SURVEILLANCE

Surveillance means continuous scrutiny of all potential sources and modes of spread of infections which are pertinent to effective control. The real occurrence and spread of poliovirus and other enterovirus infections can only be studied by virological methods, since the overwhelming majority of infections remain clinically silent. Nevertheless, clinical syndromes sufficiently characteristic to be recognised are the markers of infections and poliomyelitis belongs to this category. The most important is to obtain reliable data on the impact of the disease on the health of population in order to make decisions in respect of control and prevention. Different elements of surveillance listed by the World Health Organization (1968) are applicable for this purpose. Practically all countries have some system for notification of specified communicable diseases including poliomyelitis. These systems and their reporting efficiency vary from country to country depending on the stage of development of the health services. Underreporting is a usual phenomenon even in countries with a sophisticated public health network. No wonder that data from official reporting may be seriously misleading in developing countries (Table 23.3). Here the problem is connected not only with the incomplete reporting of cases diagnosed, but with the fact that a number of cases are not even seen by physicians. In Malawi, for example, it was revealed that six per cent of patients with poliomyelitis had consulted only a traditional healer, nine per cent had not sought any medical help and a considerable proportion of patients had attended a health institution only in the pyrexial preparalytic phase (World Health Organization, 1980a).

The best available surveillance method applicable in developing countries to assess the magnitude of the problem with poliomyelitis is the clinical survey for prevalence of residual paralysis attributable to poliomyelitis among children over five years of age. An excellent description of theoretical and practical principles of lameness surveys together with a detailed technical guide on how to carry them out and how to evaluate the results has been published recently by LaForce et al (1980). Thus only a short outline of surveys will be given here.

Basic principles are as follows. (a) Residual paralyses due to poliomyelitis are distinctive and relatively easy to recognize with a high degree of probability even long after occurrence of illness (flaccid paralysis with atrophy of affected muscles and diminished, or absent tendon reflexes, without sensory loss, usually with asymmetrical manifestation, and with a history of acute onset without subsequent long time progression); (b) practically all cases of poliomyelitis have an onset before the fifth year of life in warm climate countries (Table 23.2); (c) paralysis due to poliomyelitis affects the lower limbs in about 75 per cent of cases in these age groups; (d) it can be estimated that cases with a fatal outcome, cases with residual paralysis dying before five years of age from intercurrent diseases and cases with complete recovery represent one third of total cases in developing countries.

The actual surveys can be conducted in both urban and rural areas. A search would be made for children aged five to fifteen years with lameness of the lower limbs characteristic of poliomyelitis. On the basis of the total area population in this age group the poliomyelitis prevalence rate for the five to fifteen year-olds can then be calculated. In practice, as clause (b) above suggests, this prevalence rate will reflect those infections which had already occurred in that particular cohort before the age of five. To calculate the overall true prevalence rate requires two upward corrections. The first is to multiply the lameness rate by 1.25 to account for those cases without lower extremity involvement as noted in clause (c) above.

The second correction multiplies the rate by 1.33 to account for those who either died or totally recovered as noted in clause (d). Simple recording of age of onset facilitates comparisons of annual incidence for different years. From this can also be calculated mean annual incidence and the usual age distribution of cases of poliomyelitis. A disadvantage of the surveys of the five to fifteen year-olds is that most recent poliomyelitis events in the community will not be demonstrated.

This type of survey can be carried out by teams of epidemiologists and physicians familiar with the sequelae of poliomyelitis. For initial studies a sample size of at least 6000 can be considered to be acceptable. Prevalence surveys can be performed in schools together with simultaneous intensive search for cases among non-school-attenders in the areas of the chosen schools. Surveys restricted to schools may lead to false results because only a segment of children in school age are covered owing to relatively low school attendance rates in most of the warm climate countries and because lame children may find it difficult to get there. House-to-house surveys give the most accurate data though they are time-consuming. They can be extended to children less than five years of age, and are essential if prevalence data are required for the most recent years.

Lameness surveys not only provide a measure of poliomyelitis as a public health problem but also indicate the age groups that must be covered with vaccinations.

Lameness surveys can also be adapted to measure the impact of vaccination on incidence. As poliomyelitis immunization programs become more effective within a given country, increasing attention should be given to individual cases and small outbreaks. In this phase it should be possible, for health authorities to be alerted to occurrence of multiple cases within a given locality by fostering the cooperation of all levels of existing medical services and involving even the traditional healers in surveillance. Whenever possible careful epidemiological field investigations should be carried out around the cases supported by virological investigations. The aim is to confirm that the disease in question is really poliomyelitis, to detect the poliovirus responsible for the cases, to identify factors leading to the cases including vaccination coverage in the child population, and to recommend actions to prevent further spread.

Poliovirus isolations and polio antibody surveys can play an important role in surveillance in any poliomyelitis circumstances in order to (1) verify the aetiology of individual cases; (2) determine the poliovirus type playing the main role; (3) measure the rate of poliovirus circulation among given sections of a population or in a circumscribed area; (4) determine the proportion of individuals with and without poliovirus antibodies in different age-groups; (5) determine the seroconversion rates resulting from the use of vaccine; (6) assess the possible origin of poliovirus strains isolated based on their intratypic characteristics. Laboratory examinations become especially important after institution of a large scale vaccination program to control poliomyelitis since the reasons for unexpected events can best be cleared up by virological examinations. Unfortunately most of the warm climate countries do not have laboratory facilities for virological examinations. WHO can give assistance to clear up certain situations by laboratory examinations through its collaborating virus centres. Nevertheless for an ongoing surveillance it is of primary importance to create laboratories which are able to carry out at least basic virological tests connected with polioviruses as described by Dömök and Magrath (1979).

CONTROL AND PREVENTION

Non-specific measures are ineffective to control polio- and other enterovirus infections. Improved personal hygiene, suitable housing, proper water supplies and sewage disposal can effectively limit the spread of poliovirus infections. Nevertheless — as it was outlined formerly — it leads only to postponement of exposure to a later age when the ratio of cases to infections is increased. It is a justified requirement to isolate the patients with poliomyelitis with concurrent disinfection of throat discharges and faeces as well as articles soiled with them. This measure is, however, of no community value because (a) the patients have already excreted virus in the incubation period, and (b) there are great numbers of inapparent infections in the population around the sick individuals.

The sole effective method for control and prevention of poliomyelitis is vaccination. Since the second half of the nineteen fifties both inactivated (IPV) and live oral poliovirus vaccines (OPV) have been available and used with success in the developed countries. Initially a number of countries introduced the use of IPV, but later most of them turned to the application of OPV owing to the limited epidemiological effectiveness of vaccinations with IPV products available at that time. In fact it was the use of Sabin vaccine which has resulted in almost complete elimination of poliomyelitis in the majority of developed countries. In three countries (Sweden, Finland, The Netherlands), however, good results have been achieved by the exclusive use of killed vaccine, and more recently new techniques have been developed which made possible the production of a highly potent IPV. These facts and certain problems connected with live vaccine, some of which pertain especially to warm climate countries, renewed polemics on the relative advantages and disadvantages of IPV and OPV (Salk, 1980a,b,c; Henessen and van Wezel, 1981). Seemingly it induced uncertainties in decision making in a number of warm climate countries as to the strategies to follow.

A prerequisite of effective control of poliomyelitis is to achieve and maintain a high *immunization* rate in the target population. This could have been ensured with ease using OPV in the developed countries in temperate climates since there have been facilities available for keeping the vaccine potent until its administration. Sophisticated health services have also been able to attain a satisfactory coverage of the eligible child population. Vaccinations have resulted in immunization of over 70 per cent of recipients without respect to whether the vaccine was administered in monovalent or in trivalent form, and whether the vaccinations were carried out continuously all the year round or in yearly repeated mass campaigns.

The situation is, unfortunately, different in every respect in warm climate countries. Live vaccines contain stabilizers which delay but do not prevent heat inactivation of OPV. Thus it is eminently important to keep the vaccine refrigerated until use especially in subtropical and tropical countries, otherwise only inactivated virions will be administered orally without any immunological effect. It is clear, that especially in warm climate countries there is a need for a cold-chain built up according to the guidelines of the World Health Organization (1981) before initiating any efforts in respect of vaccinations. Health services in warm climate countries are generally inadequately developed to administer the vaccine on a sufficient scale to reach an appreciable coverage rate of the target population. It is, however, only a managerial matter to incorporate lay volunteers under the supervision of health professionals into the vaccination procedures, since administration of live vaccine needs very limited skill and knowledge.

A number of studies have shown that in warm climate countries OPV was less effective in inducing antibodies than in temperate climates. This has been ascribed to various possible factors impeding the implantation and multiplication of vaccine viruses in the intestinal tract including (a) interference between widely disseminated enteric viruses and the vaccine strains (Sabin, 1980); (b) intestinal resistance without humoral immunity due to previous exposure to naturally circulating polioviruses or perhaps related viruses; (c) presence of inhibitors in the alimentary tract (Dömök et al,

1974). The role of breast feeding at six weeks of age or later during the first year of life has been excluded by studies made by Dömök et al (1974) and by John et al (1976).

Virologically controlled revaccination studies moreover demonstrated that the effects of these impeding factors may be overcome by repeated administration of the vaccine. This was substantiated by the experience with OPV used with regularity and on a sufficiently large scale to bring poliomyelitis under control even in warm climate areas (e.g. Cuba, Puerto Rico, Panama, Singapore, Hong Kong).

Experiences show that effective coverage of the entire child population cannot be achieved in most developing countries by continuous vaccinations carried out in health centres, dispensaries or by mobile teams. Most recently Sabin (1980) proposed a special strategy of using OPV to obtain optimum results in warm climates. This consists of mass vaccination campaigns which are well organised at the community level with the contribution of lay volunteers. Two campaigns are proposed to be carried out annually with an interval of two months and each lasting only for two days. During this time all children from birth to four or five years of age would be vaccinated regardless of previous vaccination history. Under these circumstances the massive dissemination of vaccine strains excreted by the vaccinated children can curtail the dissemination of wild polio- and enteroviruses. It also ensures spread to susceptible children who did not attend the vaccination posts, or who were refractory to the vaccine at the time of their own vaccination. Trivalent vaccines can be used in both campaigns, but it may be an alternative to use monovalent type 1 vaccine in the first and trivalent vaccine in the second campaign. The latter schedule provides the maximum opportunity to gain immunity against poliovirus type 1 which is responsible for the majority of paralytic cases.

The essentials for success are proper organisation with centralised national and decentralised regional planning, local implementation by the aid of a large number of easily accessible temporary vaccination posts run by lay volunteers and extensive public information. This type of national program has been applied with success in Cuba since 1962 and has been introduced in Brazil since 1980 (Sabin 198a,b).

Ample evidence exists that imminent epidemics could be prevented and existing epidemics could be terminated or at least mitigated by mass administration of live vaccine even in tropical and semitropical areas. For references see Dömök et al (1974). Thus this antiepidemic weapon should be used whenever there is a sign of unusual increase of cases. The best antiepidemic results have been obtained when homotypic vaccine was administered. If laboratory facilities are available either in the country or by WHO help the actual virus type responsible for the epidemic can be determined and the homotypic monovalent vaccine can be chosen for the campaign. Otherwise trivalent vaccine should be administered.

It has been shown that highly potent new products of killed vaccine induce high levels of circulating antibodies after a single dose even in infants in warm climates (Salk et al, 1981). This fact in itself does not mean, however, that IPV would be superior to OPV for elimination of poliomyelitis in warm climate countries. Claims have been made repeatedly in recent years (Salk 1980a,b,c; Henessen and van Wezel, 1981) which were based on experiences obtained in countries whose neighbours were themselves free from wild poliovirus circulation, where hygienic and sanitary conditions were good, the populations were highly educated, public health services were well-developed, and vaccination coverage had continuously been high. Conclusions drawn from experiences in such countries are not necessarily applicable to countries with less favourable conditions. Well-controlled large scale trials are needed to assess the value of IPV in warm climate countries. Further questions awaiting answer even if these trials would indicate the superiority of IPV to OPV are connected with the cost and availability of second generation IPV, and how to reach an appropriate coverage rate in populations in which injections are not readily accepted, and where medical manpower is scarce.

A combined program using both killed and live vaccines was instituted, in Gaza in 1978 with promising preliminary results. Conclusions on its real value and on its general applicability in warm climate countries can, however, be drawn only after final evaluation.

CONSEQUENCES

The outcome of paralytic poliomyelitis depends on localisation and extent of nerve cell damage. The case fatality rate varies between four and 10 per cent. It is influenced among others by the existence and accessibility of hospital wards well-equipped for the treatment of patients with the respiratory failure which is responsible for most of the deaths in both bulbar and spinal forms of the disease. Cases with mild muscle pareses may recover completely within several months even without special treatment. The majority of patients are, however, severely affected needing combined efforts of physicians, physiotherapists and orthopaedists at least to alleviate the consequences of the illness. Unfortunately most of the patients in warm climate countries remain untreated due to poverty, ignorance, scarcity of specialists and hospital beds, as well as complete lack of rehabilitation services. Consequently large numbers of victims are left seriously disabled needing life-long care and help of the family and of the community. The magnitude of the problem is illustrated by the experience of the small country of Uganda with a population of 10 million. About 30 000 persons are severely disabled and a further 90 000 have some residual paralysis due to poliomyelitis (LaForce et al, 1980). The price paid in human misery and in economic and social losses for natural acquisition of immunity against poliomyelitis is very high. Without any sophisticated cost-benefit analyses it is evident that control of the disease by effective vaccinations is both economically and socially desirable.

REFERENCES

Bodian D, Horstmann D M 1965 Polioviruses. In: Horsfall F L Jr, Tamm·I (eds) Viral and rickettsial infections of man, 4th edn. Lippincott, Philadelphia-Montreal, ch 18, pp 430–473

Cockburn W Chas, Drozdov S G 1970 Poliomyelitis in the World. Bulletin of the World Health Organization, 42: 405–417

Dalldorf G, Melnick J L 1965 Coxsackie viruses. In: Horsfall F L Jr, Tamm I (eds) Viral and rickettsial infections of man, 4th edn. Lippincott, Philadelphia-Montreal, ch 19, pp 474–512

Dömök I 1972 Recent progress in immunizations: Poliomyelitis. In: Proceedings of Seminar on Immunizations in Africa, Kampala, 1971, International Children's Centre, Paris, pp 80–92

Dömök I, Balayan M S, Fayinka O A, Soneji A D, Skrtic N, Harland P S E G 1974 Factors affecting the efficacy of live poliovirus vaccine in warm climates. Efficacy of Type I Sabin vaccine adminstered together with anti-human gamma globulin horse serum to breast-fed and artificially fed infants in Uganda. Bulletin of the World Health Organization 51: 333–347

Dömök I, Magrath D I 1979 Guide to poliovirus isolation and serological techniques. WHO Offset Publication No. 46, WHO, Geneva

Franklin G C, Robertson M J 1965 A mass vaccination campaign against poliomyelitis using the Sabin oral vaccine. Public Health (London), 79: 81–99

Gear J H S 1955 Poliomyelitis in the underdeveloped areas of the world. In: Debré R (ed) Poliomyelitis. WHO Monograph Series No. 26, Geneva, pp 31–58

Guyer B, Bisong A A E, Gould J, Brigaud M, Aymard M 1980 Injections and paralytic poliomyelitis in tropical Africa. Bulletin of the World Health Organization 58: 285–291

Hennessen W, van Wezel A L (eds) 1981 Reassessment of inactivated poliomyelitis vaccine. Developments in Biological Standardisation Vol 47. Karger, Basel

Hofman B, Wilterdink J B 1960 Poliomyelitis antibodies in sera from the Netherlands, Curacao, Suriname, St. Eustatius and Netherlands' New Guinea. Antonie van Leeuwenhoek 26: 397–406

Horstmann D M 1955 Poliomyelitis: Severity and type of disease in different age groups. Annals of New York Academy of Sciences 61: 956–967

Horstmann D M, Saenz A C, Opton E M 1960 Immunity to poliomyelitis in Guatemala. A serological and virological survey. Bulletin of the World Health Organization 22: 255–262

John T J et al 1976 Effect of breast-feeding on seroresponse of infants to oral poliovirus vaccination. Paediatrics 57: 47–53

LaForce F M, Lichnevski M S, Keja J, Henderson R H 1980 Clinical survey techniques to estimate prevalence and annual incidence of poliomyelitis in developing countries. Bulletin of the World Health Organization 58: 609–620

Lee L H, Lim K A, Tye C Y 1964 Prevention of poliomyelitis by live vaccine. British Medical Journal I: 1077–1080

Melnick J L 1965 Echoviruses. In: Horsfall F L Jr, Tamm I (eds) Viral and rickettsial infections of man. 4th edn. Lippincott, Philadelphia-Montreal, ch 20, pp 513–545

Melnick J L, Wenner H A, Phillips C A 1979 Enteroviruses. In: Lennette E H, Schmidt N J (eds) Diagnostic procedures for viral, rickettsial and chlamydial infections. 5th edn. American Public Health Association, Washington, ch 15, pp 471–534

Nagy G, Takátsy S, Kukán- E, Mihály I, Dömök I 1982 Virological diagnosis of enterovirus type 71 infections: Experiences gained during an epidemic of acute CNS diseases in Hungary in 1978. Archives of Virology 71: 217–227

Nathanson N, Martin J R 1979 The epidemiology of poliomyelitis: Enigmas surrounding its appearance, epidemicity, and disappearance. American Journal of Epidemiology 110: 672–692

Nicholas D D, Kratzer J H, Ofosu-Amaah S, Belcher D W 1977 Is poliomyelitis a serious

problem in developing countries? — the Danfa experience. British Medical Journal
I: 1009–1012

Nottay B K, Metselaar D 1973 Poliomyelitis: epidemiology and prophylaxis. I. A
longitudinal epidemiological survey in Kenya. Bulletin of the World Health Organization
48: 421–427

Ofosu-Amaah S, Kratzer J H, Nicholas D D 1977 Is poliomyelitis a serious problem in
developing countries? — lameness in Ghanaian schools. British Medical Journal
I: 1012–1014

Parks W P, Melnick J L, Quieroga L T, Ali Khan H 1966 Studies on infantile diarrhoea in
Karachi, Pakistan I. Collection, virus isolation and typing of viruses. American Journal of
Epidemiology 84: 382–395

Plotkin S A, Lebrun A, Koprowski H 1960 Vaccination with CHAT strain of type I
attennated poliomyelitis virus in Leopoldville, Belgian Congo 2. Studies of the safety and
efficacy of vaccination. Bulletin of the World Health Organization 22: 215–234

Poliomyelitis Commission of the Western Region Ministry of Health, Nigeria 1966
Poliomyelitis vaccination in Ibadan, Nigeria, during 1964 with oral vaccine (Sabin
strains). Bulletin of the World Health Organization 34: 865–876

Roca-Garcia M, Markham F S, Cox H R, Vargas-Mendez O, Guevara E C, Montoya J A
1964 Poliovirus shedding and seroconversion. Studies of 816 Costa Rican children fed
trivalent vaccine. Journal of American Medical Association 188: 639–646

Sabin A B 1963 Poliomyelitis in the tropics — increasing incidence and prospects for
control. Tropical and Geographical Medicine 15: 38–44

Sabin A B 1980 Vaccination against poliomyelitis in economically underdeveloped countries.
Bulletin of the World Health Organization 58: 141–157

Sabin A B 1981a Paralytic poliomyelitis: old dogmas and new perspectives. Reviews of
Infectious Diseases 3: 543–564

Sabin A B 1981b Immunization. Evaluation of some currently available and prospective
vaccines. Journal of American Medical Association 246: 236–241

Sabin A B, Ramos-Alvarez M, Alvarez-Amezquita J, Pelon W, Michaels R H, Spigland I,
Koch M A, Barnes J M, Rhim J S 1960 Live orally given poliovirus vaccine-effects of
rapid mass immunisation in population under conditions of massive enteric infection with
other viruses. Journal of American Medical Association 173: 1521–1526

Salk D 1980a,b,c Eradication of poliomyelitis in the United States I, II, III. Reviews of
Infectious Diseases 2: 228–273

Salk J, van Wezel A L, Stoeckel P, van Steenis G, Schlumberger M, Meyran M, Rey J L,
Lapinlemu K, Böttiger M, Cohen H 1981 Theoretical and practical considerations in the
application of killed poliovirus vaccine for the control of paralytic poliomyelitis. In:
Hennessen W, van Wezel A L (eds) Reassessment of inactivated poliomyelitis vaccine.
Developments in Biological Standardisation Vol. 47 Karger, Basel pp 181–196

Schonberger L B, Thaung U, Daw Khin May Khi, Than Swe, Ma Ohn Khi, Bergman D
1981 The epidemiology of poliomyelitis in Burma, 1963–1979. In: Proc. of International
Symposium on Reassessment of Inactivated Poliomyelitis Vaccine, Bilthoven, 1980
Development in Biological Standardisation Vol. 47 Karger, Basel pp 283–292

Steigman A J 1969 Infections by enteroviruses. In: Nelson W E, Vaughan V C, McKay R J
(eds) Textbook of Paediatrics, 9th edn. Saunders Co., Philadelphia-London-Toronto,
pp 669–689

Towsend-Coles W F. Findlay G M 1953 Poliomyelitis in relation to intramuscular injections
of quinine and other drugs. Transactions of the Royal Society of Tropical Medicine and
Hygiene 47: 77–81

World Health Organization 1968 Proceedings of Twenty-first World Health Assembly,
Geneva

World Health Organization 1980a Expanded program on immunization (Malawi). Weekly
Epidemiological Record 55: 60–61

World Health Organization 1980c Poliomyelitis in 1979. Weekly Epidemiological Record
55: 361–366

World Health Organization 1981c Expanded program on immunisation (Philippines).
Weekly Epidemiological Record 56: 377–384

Intestinal helminths

INTRODUCTION

Surprisingly neglected as a major area of scientific or medical research and action, infections caused by intestinal helminths stubbornly occupy a position of public health importance.

Many of these infections have high prevalences and virtually global distributions. Indeed, ascariasis, hookworm and trichuriasis are amongst the ten commonest infections existing in the world. Although morbidity and direct mortality are relatively low in proportion to prevalence, these helminthic infections can produce severe adverse effects on both the nutritional and the immune status of populations, and in particular on children. Morbidity in young rural workers, the most productive sector of the population, can be economically important, while in some areas fatal complications of intestinal helminthic infections, such as taeniasis and strongyloidiasis, can result from neurocysticercosis or dissemination within the body of *Strongyloides stercoralis*.

In the tropical and sub-tropical zones, against the general background of over-population, deficient or absent sanitation, limited access to potable water supplies, environmental conditions favouring helminth transmission and widespread socio-economic deprivation, the importance of intestinal helminthic infections deserves increased emphasis, for the life-cycles of the parasites and the principles of surveillance and control are well-understood.

Many species of helminths parasitic in man live in the human gastrointestinal tract and their life cycles are thus predictably varied. Those helminths with the simplest life cycles and the most direct routes of transmission are the most widely distributed and have the highest prevalence rates in man. In others, an extracorporeal phase of development is necessary for the production of forms infective to man and prevalences, whilst high, tend to be less ubiquitous than the directly transmitted infections since environmental conditions markedly influence their transmission.

This chapter is biased towards the intestinal nematode infections of major public health importance, that is those in which transmission occurs by the ingestion of infective eggs, *Ascaris lumbricoides*, *Trichuris trichiura* and *Enter-*

obius vermicularis, and those in which transmission follows the cutaneous penetration of infective larvae after a period of development in the earth, that is the hookworms, *Ancylostoma duodenale* and *Necator americanus*, and *Strongyloides stercoralis*. With the exception of enterobiasis, these infections are encompassed by the term, soil-transmitted helminthiases.

Only brief note will be taken of other intestinal nematodes parasitizing man which are either of lesser pathological significance, e.g. *Trichostrongylus* species, or are rare, e.g. *Oesophagostomum* species, *Capillaria philippinesis*, *Angiostrongylus* (*Morerastrongylus*) *costaricensis* and *Anisakis* and *Phocanema* species.

Trichinosis due to *Trichinella spiralis* or other genera, being primarily a zoonosis in swine, with occasional offshoots to man, will not be covered.

Only points of special epidemiological interest will be referred to in relation to diseases caused by *Cestoda*. The *Trematoda*, of which by far the most important members are the Schistosomes, are dealt with in another chapter.

PARASITOLOGY

General

Transmission to man of infection by intestinal-dwelling nematode helminths is by one of three mechanisms: (1) ingestion of infective eggs as in ascariasis, trichuriasis, enterobiasis, and visceral larva migrans (VLM); (2) cutaneous larval penetration as in the hookworm infections and strongyloidiasis; (3) ingestion of adults or infective larvae in food or plants, for example *Capillaria philippinensis* in raw fish, *Trichostrongylus orientalis* in plants, or non-human nematodes such as *Anisakis* or *Phocanema* in raw fish, gnathostomiasis from raw fish, frog, chicken or snake meat, or even from drinking water containing the primary intermediate host, a copepod, and *Angiostrongylus costaricensis* in salads contaminated by mucous secretions from the intermediate host, a slug.

Some parasites may be transmitted to man by more than one means. The cat or dog ascarids *Toxocara cati* and *T. canis*, which may cause visceral larva migrans, can enter man by swallowed dirt from ground contaminated with eggs, or by swallowed eggs adherent to fingers which have been in close contact with infected kittens or puppies.

While human trichostrongyliasis is usually acquired by eating plants contaminated with infective larvae, the infection may occasionally result from larval skin penetration.

The life history of the hookworm *Necator americanus* differs in one important respect from that of *A. duodenale*. Whereas the former is contracted percutaneously only, the latter infection may be acquired percutaneously or orally, this mode of transmission giving special emphasis to those reports of contamination of vegetables with *A. duodenale* larvae.

The recent concept of larval dormancy in muscles in *A. duodenale* infections in man (Koshy et al, 1978) has not only altered our concepts of hook-worm epidemiology, but led to the demonstration that this phenomenon occurs experimentally in pups (Schad, 1979). Thus it is possible that meat-borne ancylostomiasis occurs in nature.

Finally the phenomenon of autoinfection occurs in strongyloidiasis and enterobiasis in addition to the customary modes of transmission.

Diverse transmission mechanisms are found in infections due to cestodes. *Hymenolepis nana* is easily transmitted from person to person by ingestion of the taeniid eggs, after faecal contamination of hands or food. *H. diminuta* infection may occur in man after accidental ingestion of an infected flea or small beetle.

Infection with *Diphyllobothrium latum* in man results from consumption of raw or insufficiently cooked fish, meat, liver or hard roe. Pike, burbot, perch and ruff containing plerocercoids of the worm are the most important sources of infection in Europe and Asia.

Ingestion of the cysticerci of *Taenia saginata* or *Taenia solium* from undercooked or raw beef or pork, respectively, produces infection with the beef or pork tapeworm, *T. saginata* and/or *T. solium* taeniasis. In the latter infection accidental ingestion of eggs or segments of *T. solium* or auto-infec-tion with *T. solium* eggs gives rise to *T. solium* cysticercosis which may be a serious chronic disease carrying a definite mortality when neurocysticer-cosis is present.

Specific life cycles

Some examples are given below of the life cycles of the commonly occurring representative nematodes.

Ascaris lumbricoides

The common large roundworm is the most cosmopolitan of all helminths. Females living in the human small intestine lay fertilized but unsegmented eggs which are excreted in faeces. When deposited in moist, loose, shady, soil, a rhabditoid second stage larva develops within the egg shell after some two to three weeks incubation. If swallowed by man, larvae emerge from the eggs in the small intestine, penetrate the intestinal mucosa and are carried in the portal circulation through the liver to the lungs. After a period in which moulting occurs, the larvae migrate through the pulmonary capillaries to the alveoli and thence via the bronchioles, bronchii and trachea to the oesophagus. In this phase, considerable growth occurs and, after being swallowed, a final moult and growth to maturity takes place in the small intestine.

The time from egg-ingestion to egg-laying by adult females is 60– 80 days. The life-span of the adult worms is 9–12 months and man is the only important natural host of this species. A very closely related organism is *A. suum*, the pig roundworm. This develops better in the pig and, although able to develop in the larval tissue migratory stages in man, rarely reaches the intestinal adult stage (Phills et al, 1972). The frequency or distribution of *A. suum* infection in man is unknown.

The hookworms (Ancylostoma duodenale: Necator americanus)

The adult worms, ranging from five to thirteen millimetres in length, live in the duodenal and jejunal mucosa where they attach themselves to villi which are sucked into their buccal cavities. Fertilized eggs containing a segmented ovum are passed in the faeces. When deposited on the earth and the faeces are diluted with soil in conditions of warmth and moisture, rapid development occurs within the eggs which, in one or two days, hatch to produce rhabditiform larvae. These free-living larvae feed on faecal debris in the earth, moult twice and, under suitable conditions, are transformed in some five to eight days into sheathed non-feeding filariform larvae infective to man. In suitably warm, damp, top soils, these larvae are viable and may survive for several months. While their lateral movement is limited, vertical movement in sandy soils is some two to three feet.

Humans walking or working barefoot, or continually handling contaminated soils, are infected by penetration of the larvae through the skin. Migrating via the venous system to the right ventricle and alveoli, the larvae are then passively carried to the bronchii, trachea and oesophagus. Traversing the stomach, they arrive in the small intestine some three to five days after skin penetration. In a further four or five weeks, the worms are sexually mature and commence egg-laying. The range of their life-span has been estimated as from one to thirteen years (WHO, 1981). Whereas migrating larvae of *Necator* grow and develop in the lungs, the larvae of *Ancylostoma* do not; they undergo the same early development in the intestinal mucosa. As noted, larval dormancy may occur in ancylostomiasis. Larvae may either rest in the musculature or migrate to the intestine before becoming quiescent for about eight months after which a patent infection develops. It is thought that in *A. duodenale* infections, transmammary infections can occur.

Strongyloides stercoralis

This nematode inhabiting the small intestine has the singular property of developing in one of two different ways outside the body. Additionally, the human host is subject to autoinfection.

Parthenogenetic females, embedded in the jejunal mucosa, lay eggs from which, during the passage through the intestine, rhabditiform larvae hatch and are passed in the faeces. Eggs are seen in the stools only in diarrhoeal states or after heavy purgation.

When outside the body, rhabditiform larvae may develop either into infective filariform larvae or into a free-living generation which is the basic life-cycle of the parasite. Strongyloidiasis is, in fact, a faecally-transmitted rather than a soil-transmitted helminthiasis (WHO, 1981). Shortly after the passage of faeces, the larvae become infective and remain the focus of contamination in a humid environment for the natural life of the filariform larvae.

In unsuitable micro-environmental surroundings, each rhabditiform larva feeds, moults and develops in the soil into a filariform larva infective to man. Human infection is acquired by cutaneous larval penetration as with the hookworms and the internal migrations follow a similar pattern. Filariform larvae can survive for several weeks in soil and transcutaneous invasion of man produces adult females which reproduce parthenogenetically, eggs being laid some three weeks later.

In warm, well-watered top soils, the free-living generation develops. Rhabditiform larvae moult and form mature, free-living adult rhabditoid males and females. The females, on fertilization, lay eggs which hatch producing rhabditiform larvae which, in turn, feed on organic debris and moult repeatedly to become free-living adults. Indefinite repetition of this free-living phase can occur under suitable conditions and thus results in considerable replication of infective potential as opposed to the direct phase where each individual rhabditiform larva becomes a filariform, since under unfavourable conditions free-living rhabditiform larvae transform to the infective filariform type.

In certain clinical states, autoinfection occurs. In this syndrome, rhabditiform larvae, after development into infective dwarf filariform larvae within the bowel, penetrate the intestinal mucosa at the perianal skin and are carried by the circulation to the lungs and thence to the oesophagus to mature finally in the upper small intestine. This course is associated with heavily parasitized patients ('the hyperinfective syndrome'), who are frequently immunosuppressed — from therapeutic radiation, cytotoxic agents or immunosuppressant chemotherapy following transplant surgery — and also is seen in those patients with an underlying debilitating illness (cancer, malnutrition, the recently described acquired immune deficiency syndrome, AIDS), or a long-standing infection with repeated autoinfections. Shock and gram negative septicaemia are not infrequently the immediate cause of death.

Of the human nematode intestinal infections, strongyloidiasis and capillariasis are unique in being capable of perpetuation in man by the production of new generations of potentially infective larvae from parthenogenetic females.

Trichuris trichiura

The whipworm also has a simple life cycle. Eggs are laid by females inhabiting the caecum and large intestine and excreted in the faeces. Infective larvae form within the eggs after some four weeks development, optimum conditions being found in shaded, warm, moist soil. Man is infected by swallowing the fully embryonated eggs. In the small intestine the larvae emerge from the eggs and penetrate the villi, develop for about a week, and then re-enter the lumen to reach the caecum.

Eggs are produced some three months after the ingestion of infective eggs. The adult life span of the worm occupies many years and man is the only natural definitive host.

Enterobius vermicularis

The pinworm, seatworm or threadworm is noted here since, although not a soil-transmitted infection, transmission is by the swallowing of embryonated eggs producing enterobiasis, previously termed oxyuriasis.

A peculiarity of the life cycle is that, although adult worms inhabit the caecum and adjacent parts of the small and large intestine, gravid females migrate freely in the lumen of the gut and crawl onto the perianal and perineal skin to lay eggs. This commonly occurs at night and the vagina or bladder may be entered. Males may also be observed emerging from the anus. Eggs are only occasionally seen in the stool and the diagnosis is made by direct observation of adults, or by the demonstration of embryonated eggs using some variant of the scotch cellulose adhesive tape technique (NIH or Graham swab).

The eggs need only a few hours to mature and when swallowed by man, infective larvae are liberated in the duodenum. They then pass down the small intestine, moulting twice and sometimes temporarily occupying jejunal or ileal crypts, before reaching the caecum and developing into adults.

EPIDEMIOLOGY

Geographical distribution. Prevalence. Age. Sex. Socioeconomic factors

Ascariasis is of world-wide distribution and commonly prevalences of 50–75 per cent or greater are recorded in many African and Latin American countries. Trichuriasis is similarly common in warm, wet climates and, in populations of some tropical countries, prevalences of over 90 per cent are known. Trichuriasis is by no means rare in temperate countries. The geographical distribution of the two main hookworms, formerly regarded as reasonably distinct with A. duodenale more prevalent in Europe and South-West Asia and N. americanus predominant in the Americas and Africa, has become blurred. Both parasites are now widely distributed throughout the tropics and subtropics.

Neither sex nor race confers any protection from infection and disproportionately high prevalences in any individual sexual or racial group can be related to particular social customs or habits of work.

Age prevalence curves may be related to modes of transmission. Toddlers who crawl on faecally-contaminated earth close to the home and young children playing on contaminated ground show the highest prevalences for *Ascaris* and *Trichuris* although no age is exempt.

Given equal exposure to hookworm infection, both sexes and all ages are susceptible. An increased occupational risk is exemplified by young agricultural workers who frequently contract infection by working on contaminated farming areas or plantations.

In general, soil-transmitted intestinal infections are less frequent and of a lesser intensity in urban than in rural areas.

Intermittent excretion of *Strongyloides stercoralis* larvae in faeces and the technical difficulties in their detection, which necessitate either the use of special concentration procedures or coproculture, make the establishment of accurate prevalence figures impossible. The infection occurs in all tropical regions and is widely distributed in Eastern Europe. Vagaries of underreporting or the use of inadequate technical procedures may well be the explanation for its apparent patchy distribution.

Although exhibiting differences from the soil-transmitted helminthiases, enterobiasis has a cosmopolitan distribution. Where sanitary standards are low, prevalences are high. Enterobiasis is most frequent in pre-school and school-children and in family groupings and institutions, since crowding plays a major part in transmission. High prevalences are seen in certain groupings in the developed countries of the northern hemisphere.

Although the lower socio-economic groupings are predominantly affected by intestinal nematode infections, immunity is not necessarily conferred by rising living standards alone. The details of the important socio-economic determinants are regrettably seldom investigated and Dunn (1975) has summarized the difficulties in the study of human behavioural factors. Frequently in areas of high prevalence the living conditions are characteristically poor with over-population, a high proportion of children, absent or inadequate sanitary facilities, poor potable water supplies, illiteracy and poverty, all combining to perpetuate the vicious cycle of transmission.

Intensity of infection

Quantitative epidemiological assessment of the importance of helminthiasis in a population is related largely to the concept of intensity of infection in different age-groupings. In individuals, the load may be assessed directly by counting either the number of worms at autopsy or those expelled after specific anthelmintic chemotherapy. In samples or populations, extrapolations of intensities of infection are made from faecal egg counts performed by standard techniques.

As a generalisation, intensities of infection, in population terms, rise in parallel with prevalences. Although the wide variations in worm or egg loads found in different countries are of epidemiological interest, the reasons for the high intensities of infection are unknown. In helminthic infections, the severity of the induced pathology frequently depends on the number of parasites carried in the host. Where there is no direct multiplication of parasite within the host, as is the case in the vast majority of nematode infections, the parasite populations are greatly overdispersed and, in epidemiological terms, this is described by a truncated form of the negative binomial distribution. This means that in any population of infected humans, there are some people (who may or may not exist in clusterings or in a clumped form) carrying much higher numbers of parasites than the general mean load, and these numbers of parasites are out of proportion to those calculated on the basis of probability of contacts (Crofton, 1971).

EPIDEMIOLOGICAL VARIABLES INFLUENCING THE TRANSMISSION AND THE OUTCOME OF INTESTINAL NEMATODE INFECTIONS

A complex web of interacting variables influence the transmission and course of any intestinal parasitic infection. Stable endemicity levels of many intestinal nematode infections are the result of the interaction of loss of infections and frequency of reinfections. The latter depends on both host susceptibility acting via immunological mechanisms and parasite factors, such as the number of exposures per host in an area in a given time, the 'infection pressure' of Gemmell & Johnstone (1977).

Host factors

The important host factors involve innate susceptibility, those resulting from malnutrition or undernutrition with their resultant effects on cellular immune responses or on iron stores in hookworm, coexistent disease or the ability of the immune system to respond to antigenic stimuli, for example induced immuno-deficiency and the hyperinfective syndrome in strongyloidiasis.

Other factors are more physical than physiopathological. Embryonated eggs of *Ascaris* and *Trichuris* are swallowed usually via fingers contaminated by polluted soil, or via food or drink, especially unwashed vegetables or fruit. Young children not infrequently eat dirt. The most important human determinant of transmission is indiscriminate defaecation with seeding of the soil. Ascariasis is essentially a peridomestic infection and may be encountered in family clusters.

While soil pollution from defaecation is necessary for the transmission of hookworm, other host factors are essential. Probably the most important is the mode and extent of contact between skin and soil. Adults have higher prevalences than children, and agriculturalists or miners than urbanized workers. Usually prevalence is higher in men than in women except in those societies where the latter are responsible for the agricultural work.

The transmission of strongyloidiasis is affected by factors similar to those in hookworm although, for unknown reasons, the distribution is usually patchy.

In enterobiasis host factors are of primary importance in maintaining transmission. The most frequent method of infection is by finger contamination and the transfer of eggs from the perineum to the mouth. Soiled night clothes, bed linen, various fomites and even airborne infection have also been incriminated in the transmission cycle. Clusters of people sharing the same environment are particularly exposed to infection with this helminth.

Parasitic factors

The parasitic factors to consider are the degree of endemicity of the infection, the intensity of each infection as measured by worm load, the egg-laying capacity of the female worms and the properties of the eggs or larvae.

Since intensity of infection rises with increasing prevalence, the transmission potential is increased. All these nematodes are prolific egg-layers. A single female *Ascaris* for example, deposits about 200 000 eggs per day (Faust & Russell, 1964), and worm burdens in excess of 100 are not an uncommon clinical experience in many parts of the world. Estimates of *Trichuris* egg outputs are very variable, from 1000 to 46 000 per female per day but again, experienced practitioners have no doubts of the high intensities of infection harboured. A single female *Enterobius* deposits from 4672 to 16 888 eggs (Reardon, 1938) and loads of some hundreds of pinworms are known. In two areas of high hookworm endemicity, two rigorously conducted trials of anthelmintics in which counts of expelled worms were made, predominantly *N. americanus* in each case, demonstrated the high hookworm loads carried by individuals. In Uganda, mean worm burdens of 355 and 239 were found in small groups with severe hookworm anaemia (Hutton & Somers, 1961), and in Tanzania the mean worm load was 464 (Rowland, 1966).

In strongyloidiasis it has been impossible to reach accurate estimates of worm loads because of technical difficulties in the quantitative enumeration of larvae in the stool.

Population density is also important in helminthic infections; for each intestinal helminth there is a threshold of population size below which the host will tolerate infection with little or no pathology and above which the pathogenicity will be in proportion to the difference between the threshold and the number of infecting worms. In *Ascaris* and hookworm, in initial infections, the pathogenicity of migrating larvae is also proportional to the size of the inoculum. The mode of entry of the parasite may further influence subsequent events. Examples include the so-called Wakana disease, a pulmonary symptom complex caused by larvae of *A. duodenale* entering via the mouth and Loeffler's syndrome caused by migrating *Ascaris* larvae in areas of intermittent transmission.

Parasite virulence and adaptation to the human host may also be of importance since host specificity is relative rather than absolute and man may be a final definitive host or only an intermediate or paratenic (transfer) host. Related to this are the abnormal parasite responses to intercurrent or associated infections in man and varying parasite responses in immuno-suppressed hosts.

Environmental factors

The third great group of factors related to the outcome of an intestinal nematode infection are those of the environment which has often the most crucial role to play in transmission. The degree of contamination of the environment is enormous and is solely due to inadequate faecal disposal. For instance, the global population of adult *Ascaris* worms parasitizing man has been estimated as 7800 million (Expected No. of human hosts infected $\times$ Expected Mean No. of worms in single host) (WHO, 1981) and, since each female adult has a reproductive potential of 240 000 eggs per day, the daily global contamination of *Ascaris* eggs is some 10^{18}. A related estimate is that in 1975, in the rural areas of developing countries, excluding China, 1190 million people, that is 85 per cent of the total population, lacked adequate sanitation.

Microenvironmental factors on or within the soil determine egg or larval survival. Soil texture, structure and moisture affect the free-living stages of the intestinal-dwelling nematodes. Sandy soils are most suitable for hook-worm larvae and there is a generalized negative correlation between soil density and hookworm prevalence. Well-tilled soils contain increased amounts of air and favour larval movement by exposure to oxygen. The eggs of *Ascaris* and *Trichuris* survive longer in clay soils because of the retention of moisture and poor aeration, conditions inimical to larvae. Egg survival in cultivated soil suffers because of exposure to sunlight and drying.

Air temperature is important, its effect being related to the moisture content of the soil. Heat penetrates deeper into wet soil than into dry. Thus hookworm infections are more liable to occur in moist tropical regions. *Ascaris* eggs exposed to a temperature of $-23\,^{\circ}\mathrm{C}$ for as long as 40 days will embryonate normally when the temperature is raised (WHO, 1964). In temperate regions, *Ascaris* eggs may remain viable for many months on the ground. *Trichuris* eggs are more susceptible to low temperatures than *Ascaris* eggs.

So there is a great complex of intermingled variables affecting the outcome of these intestinal nematode infections and in any one particular area it may not be possible to unravel the threads of causation in other than a general manner although quantitative parasitological techniques used in survey and assessment will at least point to particular target populations of parasitized people as deserving priority for therapy and other intervention measures.

CLINICAL MANIFESTATIONS. MORBIDITY

Due to larval stages of human nematodes

Normal larval migrations may provoke symptoms and signs. A pulmonary inflammatory reaction occurs in ascariasis ('Ascaris pneumonia'; verminous pneumonitis) probably more often in reinfections. Hoarseness and cough reflect tracheal irritation. Pruritus or urticaria are occasionally seen.

The larvae of hookworm cause vesicular skin eruptions (Ground itch) and those of *Necator*, creeping eruption if there is repeated reinfection. Pulmonary symptoms and eosinophilia occur infrequently.

Strongyloides larvae are associated with vesicular linear lesions in the perianal area or buttocks during autoinfection. Weals or urticaria are not uncommon.

Due to larval stages of non-human nematodes

Two well recognized syndromes are caused by migrating larvae of helminths which usually parasitize domestic animals.

Cutaneous larva migrans (Creeping eruption)

Generally caused by larvae of *Ancylostoma braziliense*, a nematode of cats and dogs, *Ancylostoma caninum* of dogs, various animal strongyloids or rarely *Necator americanus* of man, sinous superficial cutaneous lesions, termed creeping eruptions, are seen. From an initial papular or vesicular lesion; irregular migration of larvae above the basal layer of the skin takes place producing serpiginous tunnels often complicated by pyoderma. Further larval development occurs only infrequently. Thiabendazole, given as a cream or orally is curative.

Visceral larva migrans

A number of clinical syndromes occur in this human infection with the dog and cat ascarids, *Toxocara canis* and *T. cati*. Rarely *Toxascaris leonina* may be responsible.

Highest prevalences occur in toddlers who have played on contaminated ground. Infective eggs are swallowed, either directly from eating dirt or via soiled fingers. Infection may result from the close contact of young children with infected puppies or kittens.

After the ingestion of infective eggs, rhabditiform larvae are liberated in the small intestine, pass through the mucosa and are transported in the portal circulation to the liver.

No further larval development occurs but the larvae may live for months. Nodules form and are composed of granulomas with a strong eosinophilic element surrounding a larva. Other organs may be involved including the lungs, heart, brain, eyeballs or striated muscles.

The severity of the condition is related to the number of infective eggs ingested and the number of larvae which reach the viscera. These may be few or miliary, and the clinical picture varies from an asymptomatic eosinophilia to the classical picture of a small toddler with persistent eosinophilia and hepatomegaly or asthma. In some tragic cases, an eye may have been enucleated under the mistaken impression of a retinoblastoma.

Diagnosis is made by histological examination of biopsy material. There is no specific treatment. Prevention lies in protecting toddlers from ground contaminated with dog or cat faeces and regular deworming of household pets.

Due to adult nematodes

Ascariasis

Since ascariasis is so widespread and prevalences are high, it is probable that many infections, perhaps even the majority, are symptomless, or the symptoms are so trivial that they are unrecognized or ignored by patient and doctor. Frequently it is only the recognition of expelled worms that calls attention to infection.

Serious morbidity in ascariasis is, however, well known. Surgical complications range from biliary obstruction to intestinal obstruction or volvulus. While heavy infections are associated with an increased frequency of symptoms, even one *Ascaris* is potentially dangerous.

Among non-surgical conditions are a variety of gastro-intestinal, respiratory or meningeal symptoms. In laboratory workers various allergic signs may be present.

Wandering adult worms may exit from mouth, nose or post operative wounds, and their internal migrations can produce a variety of disorders.

There are indirect associations between ascariasis and the precipitation and prevalence of frank kwashiorkor or less florid states of malnutrition. There seems little doubt that *Ascaris* infections can deplete the hosts' nutritional stores when a high worm load is combined with a low protein intake (Tripathy et al., 1971).

An association also exists between nematodes and microbial infections (Woodruff, 1968). In paralytic poliomyelitis, toxocaral skin sensitivity reactions were six times more frequent than in controls. Various viruses may be carried in helminth migrations and *Escherichia coli* were disseminated by filariform larvae of *S. stercoralis* (Wilson & Thompson, 1964). Toxoplasmosis was considered experimentally capable of surviving in eggs of *Toxocara cati* with subsequent transmission of *Toxoplasma gondii* (Hutchinson, 1965).

Trichuriasis

Light infections with *T. trichira* are symptom free. Heavy infections produce a fairly typical picture of a chronic diarrhoeal illness with blood-streaked stools and tenesmus. Children appear wasted since there is either loss of weight or failure to gain.

Rectal prolapse is one of the commoner complications of heavy or long-standing *Trichuris* infection.

Enterobiasis

Severe itching of the perianal and perineal skin is the hallmark, with secondary loss of sleep or a septic dermatitis caused by scratching.

Strongyloidiasis

Usually no clinical signs are evident but under certain circumstances *S. stercoralis* may produce severe morbidity or mortality. Various grades of diarrhoeal illness ranging from a mild mucous stool to an overwhelming ulcerative enteritis have been described.

A malabsorption syndrome may be encountered and opportunistic infection with serious consequences may be seen in illnesses where immuno-suppression occurs (leukaemia, reticuloses) or where drug treatment results in the same mechanism (steroids, cytotoxic agents).

Skin lesions are due to larvae in autoinfection and these may also produce visceral larva migrans.

Hookworm infection

Care must be taken to appreciate the different emphases given to hookworm infection in the individual, with whom the physician deals, and hookworm infection in the group or community, of prime interest to the epidemiologist.

Providing nutrition is adequate, mild or even moderate hookworm infections in the individual frequently cause few, if any, symptoms. If nutrition is poor a similar level of infection may be associated with symptoms. In heavy infections, symptoms and signs of anaemia are the cardinal characteristics. These differ in no way from the findings associated with any severe anaemia: pallor, dependent oedema, lassitude and easy induction of fatigue, dyspnoea on exertion, high cardiac output and tachycardia and apathy.

Epigastric discomfort or ulcer-type dyspepsia is common. The apathetic, pallid, pot-bellied child often with oedema of the feet is an everyday sight in endemic areas.

Yet in dealing with populations, cases of anaemia without heavy hookworm infection and cases of heavy infection without anaemia may be seen. Many gradations of adaptations of the host's physiological compensatory mechanisms occur in response to an infection. The interaction of the effects of other parasitic infections and the availability of dietary iron and the extent of its absorption confound the population picture. The association in a community of the prevalence and degree of iron deficiency anaemia and the prevalence and severity of hookworm infection is a statistical concept. The view that hookworm and iron deficiency anaemia of the tropics were associated has been questioned in the past on the grounds that while infection in many areas is universal, anaemia is infrequent. Detailed studies have made it plain that there is a significant negative correlation between worm load and anaemia (Roche & Layrisse, 1966), that significant losses of blood are caused by both *N. americanus* (about 0.03 ml per worm per day) and *A. duodenale* (about 0.15 ml per worm per day) (British Medical Journal, 1968) and that the hypochromic microcytic anaemia which responds to iron alone, relapses unless combined with anthelminthic treatment (Gilles, Watson Williams & Ball, 1964). Inhabitants of rural tropical areas may ingest, by customary standards, adequate amounts of dietary iron. This is frequently of vegetable origin and may be poorly absorbed, thus aggravating the constant drain on iron stores provoked and maintained by recurrent hookworm infection.

EPIDEMIOLOGICAL ASSESSMENT

Community-based epidemiological surveys are the usual means used to study the prevalence of intestinal parasites and the intensity of infection amongst different age strata. Such surveys should be performed in a programmed systematic manner. Parasitological methods of faecal examination are normally employed. Serological or cutaneous immunodiagnostic techniques find far less place. The measurement of morbidity, except in hookworm infections, is in its infancy.

Either total community surveys of small target populations or randomly selected samples of representative age-sex specific strata may be examined. It is usual to conduct surveys for the detection of multiple rather than single infections.

Parasitological techniques

Many of the simple diagnostic techniques (direct faecal smear, brine flotation, acid-ether concentration) are of ancient lineage. In the post World War II years, two major variants appeared — the cellophane thick smear and the culture of helminthic larvae from faeces. Although subsequent pragmatic modifications have improved the utility of these techniques, there have, in general, been no original inventions during the past decades that have made use of the technical revolution of the 20th century. Perhaps the improvement of immunological methods may permit the detection of specific faecal antigens and be the forerunner of a new generation of diagnostic tools? Meanwhile, epidemiological surveys rely on time-honoured parasitological methods.

The techniques of faecal examination will vary according to the precise needs of a survey. An almost universal procedure is the direct faecal thin smear in which some two mg of stool is examined as a wet preparation in water or physiological saline. It is customary to prepare two direct thin smears from each faecal sample; one in saline and the other with a temporary stain, such as iodine solution, buffered methylene blue, or merthiolate-iodine-formaldehyde (MIF) solution. Thin smears are simple to prepare, require the least equipment and are good for the identification of protozoan cysts, for example *Giardia*, haematophagous amoebic trophozoites and many helminthic eggs and larvae. Quantitation is difficult and for this the cellophane thick smear, Kato technique, Kato-Katz modification 1972, (Kato & Miura, 1954; Komiya & Kobayashi, 1966) has become increasingly popular and is now widely used. The technique is simple, is available in bulk-supply kits and has the advantage of examining a larger sample of stool (40–50 mg). It gives reasonable quantitative estimates in *Ascaris*, *Trichuris*, hookworms and *S. mansoni* and *S. japonicum* infections. As an all-purpose method of faecal examination it is used also in *Taenia* and liver fluke infections.

In surveys of endemic areas of hookworm, a quantitative estimation of egg load is essential as this must be correlated with the population haemoglobin values which are estimated simultaneously. Probably the commonest technique is still that of Stoll (1923) which has been in worldwide use for 50 years, and is a valuable epidemiological tool for comparing egg outputs in different populations. Replicated samples of five or 10 mg of stool from a specimen weighing four g are counted and a stable mean egg count can be obtained.

Species diagnosis of hookworm infections is not possible by the Stoll technique. It should no longer be customary to refer to 'hookworm endemicity' as the responses to drugs of *A. duodenale* and *N. americanus* are different. The exact species present should be diagnosed by the *in vitro* culture of nematode larvae in faeces. Different culture techniques are available but the use of a simple filter paper growth medium known as the Harada-Mori culture method is very suitable (Harada & Mori, 1951; WHO, 1963; WHO, 1981) and modifications of the original method for the processing of large numbers of stools are applicable (Sasa et al, 1965).

Other techniques such as brine flotation or formalin-ether sedimentation have been employed but quantitative examination is not so reproducible as with those noted. Stools preserved with formalin, or the merthiolate-iodine-formaldehyde fixative stain (Sapero & Lawless, 1953) may be examined.

Strongyloidiasis is not amenable to quantitative evaluation and surveys are rarely undertaken for its detection. An increased use of the Harada-Mori method of coproculture would clarify prevalence data since *Strongyloides stercoralis* larvae (and also those of *Trichostrongylus* spp.) can be differentiated from hookworm larvae. The smearing of faeces on a raised piece of filter paper in a Petri dish containing a shallow layer of water is an efficient way of isolating *Strongyloides* larvae. In the diagnosis of individual patients with strongyloidiasis, a complement-fixation test with *Dirofilaria immitis* antigen has proved a useful screening procedure (Kanani & Rees, 1970).

Epidemiological investigations of enterobiasis depend entirely on the microscopic recognition of ova on perianal swabbing with scotch cellophane adhesive tape. All members of a family should be swabbed after the detection of a case since all are likely to require treatment. Similar action is necessary for institutionalized groups of children or adults.

In the epidemiological investigation of nematode infections it may be desirable to determine the extent of ground pollution by the recovery of eggs or larvae from soil which can prove difficult, and discussion of preferred techniques is found in specialized publications.

CONTROL

Control of the soil transmitted helminthiases has been less successful than many other campaigns of preventive medicine. The combined effects of treatment and the introduction of adequate sanitation in the earlier years of this century, reinforced by health legislation, widespread education and rising living standards, diminished the prevalence of hookworm and other intestinal helminths in Europe and North America until they have become of minor importance.

One of the earliest organized campaigns against hookworm was the extensive programme conducted in Germany from 1903 to 1914 which aimed at the reduction of the prevalence of infection in mining communities. This was built around treatment of infected miners, the exclusion from underground work of those new employees discovered to have hookworm infection and the installation of sanitation. The success of the programme was instrumental in promoting control efforts in other European countries.

In the New World, the Rockefeller Sanitary Commission was established in 1909 to combat hookworm disease, and after distinguished campaigns in the Southern States of the USA, the Commission's work merged in 1915 with that of the International Health Board, one of the agencies through which the Rockefeller Foundation operated. From 1913 onwards numerous campaigns were conducted against hookworm and the areas of activity were extended to include the West Indies, Central and South America, Ceylon, India, Thailand, North Borneo, New Guinea, Papua and Australia.

Basically the problem of control is dealt with under three headings:

1. Education of the public in health and hygiene.
2. The sanitary disposal of human faeces, including the correct use of night soil, to prevent soil pollution.
3. The judicious use of population-based chemotherapy at regular intervals. The timing of chemotherapeutic intervention must be based on local epidemiological patterns of transmission.

1. Health education should be directed towards a simplified explanation of the life cycles of the parasites and the methods of acquiring infection and should be conducted by the basic units of the health care system. An explanation and demonstration of the essentials of personal hygiene and simple protective measures, such as the use of shoes and the washing of hands are necessary subsidiary activities.

Without the understanding and participation of the community, the introduction of environmental sanitation measures (latrines, safe water supplies) may not succeed in controlling helminth infections.

2. The core of the problem of control is excretal disposal. In many countries the prevalence of nematode infections has not declined with the introduction of latrines. This situation is undoubtedly related to cultural customs which are reluctantly relinquished, or, in predominantly agricultural communities, to the difficulty of providing sanitary facilities at the sites of cultivation.

Discussions of methods of disposal of faeces covering direct disposal, conservancy systems, sewerage systems and the broader aspects of the problem are found in WHO publications and other specialist sources.

One of the most difficult facets of faecal disposal is the treatment of human excreta used as fertilizers (night soil). Although composting with vegetable refuse will raise temperatures to a degree lethal to many helminth eggs, in most rural areas the use of night soil is an unsupervised family activity and the mixing of excreta and soil is no more than a random scattering. Chemical treatment of soil in rural areas, although effective, is an extremely rare activity on a world scale.

3. Chemotherapy of infected communities must be combined with these other control measures to be of maximum benefit. Large-scale population-based chemotherapy is a reinforcing agent; used alone it may make no more than a transient impression on the prevalence rates of ascariasis and hookworm infections in which there is much experience of mass drug administration. Used in conjunction with health education and the provision of sanitation, a successful control campaign is much more probable.

Failure to achieve adequate population coverage, particularly in children who contribute the major proportion of transmission potential, and failure to use chemotherapeutic drugs repeatedly, are factors contributing to the lack of success in chemotherapy campaigns. The intestinal nematodes have enormous reproductive potential and it is necessary to give drugs at frequent intervals if soil contamination with eggs is to be reduced to an unimportant level. The frequency of administration will be dictated by the pattern of transmission if this is seasonal, and by the patent period of the helminth to be attacked.

The clinical aspects of importance in mass treatment are the population tolerance to the drugs to be used, the severity of any side effects provoked by treatment, and an appreciation of the objective of mass chemotherapy which differs from that of individual treatment.

Many drugs of relatively trivial toxicity are now available for the mass treatment of helminths. It is still necessary however, carefully to weigh risk versus benefit if a drug is capable of producing severe side effects even if only in a small proportion of recipients. While individual treatment aims at eradicating a helminthic infection, the primary aim of mass chemotherapy is the reduction of the community worm load. Cure may or may not be obtained. In the mass treatment of hookworm, the object is to diminish the drain on iron stores and simultaneously to replace the lost iron by oral iron preparations. In ascariasis protein reserves can be expected to benefit after treatment. Trichuriasis and stongyloidiasis are much less amenable to chemotherapeutic attack, the former because of a lack of suitable drugs; the latter because of its patchy distribution.

Enterobiasis is usually attacked on a community basis by mass treatment but despite the high efficacy of the available drugs, the ease of reinfection necessitates repeated courses.

No attempt will be made to discuss in *depth* the many drugs available. The relative merits and demerits of chemotherapeutic agents are discussed in a monograph (Davis, 1973) and a recent review updates this information (WHO, 1981).

A variety of highly efficacious well-tolerated compounds now exist for the treatment of the common intestinal nematodes, *Ancylostoma duodenale, Necator americanus, Ascaris lumbricoides, Strongyloides stercoralis, Trichuris trichiura, Enterobius vermicularis* and the common cestodes.

Tiabendazole, one of the oldest benzimidazoles, has good activity against both adult and larval forms of tissue nematodes and is still the drug of choice for strongyloidiasis and cutaneous larva migrans. Side effects are rather common and may occur in 50 per cent or more of treated patients.

The synthetic compound mebendazole, methyl (5-benzoyl-1H-benzimidazol-2-yl) carbamate, is effective in infections caused by *Ascaris lumbricoides, Enterobius vermicularis*, the hookworms and *Trichuris trichiura*. It is usually given in doses of 100 mg twice daily for three days, irrespective of age, and clinical tolerance is extremely good. Since intestinal absorption is minimal, some 90 per cent of the drug is excreted unchanged in the faeces within 24 hours of dosage. In pregnant rodents, skeletal deformities of ribs and tail were observed but no teratogenic or embryotoxic effects were seen in dogs, sheep or horses. Mebendazole, like many other drugs, should not be used in early pregnancy if this is diagnosed and it should also be noted that children with heavy *Ascaris* infections may occasionally suffer from worm migrations with exit through mouth or nose. Mebendazole is a widely used successful drug and many examples of its large-scale use at regular intervals exist. It also is the treatment of choice for *Capillaria philippinensis* and is under trial in many centres for human hydatid disease.

The parafluor analogue of mebendazole named flubendazole has a similar range of activities and seems to produce similar therapeutic results and clinical tolerance. No teratogenic effects were seen in rats or rabbits.

Two other benzimidazoles, tetramisole and its isomer levamisole, are deservedly popular in the treatment of certain intestinal helminths and levamisole in particular has been frequently employed in large-scale campaigns in ascariasis. It should be noted that levamisole appears to possess immuno-stimulant properties. Albendazole is a recent benzimidazole and is effective against hookworms, *Ascaris*, *Enterobius*, *Trichuris* and *Strongyloides stercoralis*. There is evidence of activity in human hydatid disease and cysticercosis. The compound appears likely to be used as a single dose broad spectrum anthelmintic within the primary health care system.

A widely used drug is pyrantel pamoate, a compound of the amidine group. In a single dose, it is employed in the treatment of ascariasis and enterobiasis but in hookworm infections the drugs should be given over a period of three days. Side effects are mild and transient and there are several documented successes in maintaining massive reductions in prevalence rates of ascariasis using repeated treatments. An analogue, oxantel, is ineffective against *Ascaris* but very effective in *Trichuris* infections. The combination of pyrantel and oxantel has a wide spectrum of anthelmintic activity and may be promising for large-scale use since it is effective against *Ascaris*, *Enterobius*, *Trichuris* and hookworm infections.

In the treatment of cestode infections, praziquantel has very high therapeutic activity, in a single dose, against *T. solium*, *T. saginata*, *Hymenolepis nana* and *Diphyllobothrium latum*. For these cestode infections, niclosamide is also a widely used, well-tolerated cestocide.

Since there is in existence a wide spectrum of efficient non-toxic drugs for the treatment of human intestinal helminthic infections, the choice of drug and preferred dose régime will vary according to the species being transmitted, the community infection density, the funds available and the local delivery system.

As multiple intestinal helminthic infections are the rule rather than the exception in endemic zones, increasing use is being made of drugs active against more than one helminth species. For example, mebendazole and albendazole are active against *Ascaris*, the hookworms, *Trichuris* and *Enterobius*; pyrantel is highly effective in ascariasis, hookworm, enterobiasis and trichostrongyliasis; levamisole acts against *Ascaris* and hookworms as does bephenium. The obvious advantages of polyvalent activity are such that the increased use of such compounds can be anticipated.

REFERENCES

British Medical Journal 1968 Hookworm infection 4: 788
Crofton H D 1971 A quantitative approach to parasitism. Parasitology 62: 179–193
Davis A 1973 Drug treatment in intestinal helminthiases. World Health Organization, Geneva
Dunn F L 1979 Behavioural aspects of the control of parasitic diseases. Bulletin of the World Health Organization 57: 499–512
Faust E C, Russell P F 1964 Craig and Faust's clinical parasitology. Lea & Febiger, Philadelphia
Gemmell M A, ohnstone P D 1977 Experimental epidemiology of hydatidosis and cysticercosis. دdvances in Parasitology 15: 311–369
Gilles H M, Watson-Williams E J, Ball P A J 1964 Hookworm infection and anaemia. Quarterly Journal of Medicine xxxiii: 1–24
Harada Y, Mori O 1951 [A simple culture method for Ancylostoma duodenale] (In Japanese) Igaku to Seibutsugaku 20: 65–67
Hutchinson W M 1965 Experimental transmission of Toxoplasma gondii. Nature (London) 206: 961–962
Hutton P W 1961 A comparison of bephenium hydroxynaphthoate and tetrachlorethylene in hookworm infestation. Transactions of the Royal Society of Tropical Medicine and Hygiene 55: 431–432
Kanani S R, Rees P H 1970 The diagnosis of strongyloidiasis with special reference to the value of the filarial complement fixation test as a screening test. Transactions of the Royal Society of Tropical Medicine and Hygiene 64: 246–251
Kato K, Miura M 1954 Comparative examinations. Japanese Journal of Parasitology 3: 35 (In Japanese)
Komiya Y, Kobayashi A 1966 Evaluation of Kato's thick smear technique with a cellophane cover for helminth eggs in faeces. Japanese Journal of Medical Science and Biology 19: 59–64
Koshy A, Raina V, Sharma M P, Mithal S, Tandon B N 1978 An unusual outbreak of hookworm disease in North India. American Journal of Tropical Medicine and Hygiene 27: 42–45
Phills J A, Harrold A J, Whiteman G V, Perelmutter L 1972 Pulmonary infiltrates, asthma and eosinophilia due to Ascaris suum infection in man. New England Journal of Medicine 286: 965–970
Reardon L 1938 Studies on oxyuriasis. XVI The number of eggs produced by the pinworm, Enterobius vermicularis, and its bearing on infection. Public Health Reports 53: 978–984
Roche M, Layrisse M 1966 The nature and causes of 'Hookworm Anaemia'. American Journal of Tropical Medicine and Hygiene 15: No. 6, Part 2 of 2 parts, 1031–1102
Rowland H A K 1966 A comparison of tetrachlorethylene and bephenium hydroxynaphthoate in ancylostomiasis. Transactions of the Royal Society of Tropical Medicine and Hygiene 60: 313–321
Sapero J J, Lawless D K 1953 The MIF Stain — Preservation Technique for the identification of intestinal protozoa. American Journal of Tropical Medicine and Hygiene 2: 613–619
Sasa M, Mitsui G, Harinasuta C, Vajrasthira S 1965 A polyethylene-tube culture method for diagnosis of parasitic infections by hookworms and related nematodes. Japanese Journal of Experimental Medicine 35: 277–289
Schad G A 1979 Ancylostoma duodenale: Maintenance through six generations in helminth-naive pups. Experimental Parasitology 47: (2) 246–253
Stoll N R 1923 Investigations on the control of hookworm disease. XV An effective method of counting hookworm eggs in faeces. American Journal of Hygiene 3: 59–70
Tripathy K, Gonzales F, Lotero H, Bolanos O 1971 Effects of Ascaris infection on human nutrition. American Journal of Tropical Medicine and Hygiene 20: 212–218
Wilson S, Thompson A E 1964 A fatal case of strongyloidiasis. Journal of Pathology and Bacteriology 87: 169–176
Woodruff A W W 1968 Helminths as vehicles and synergists of microbial infections. Transactions of the Royal Society of Tropical Medicine and Hygiene 62: 446–452

World Health Organization 1963 CCTA/WHO African Conference on Ancylostomiasis. World Health Organization Technical Report Series 255

World Health Organization 1964 Soil-transmitted helminths. World Health Organization Technical Report Series 277: 13

World Health Organization 1981 Intestinal protozoan and helminthic infections. World Health Organization Technical Report Series 666: 59, 70, 77, 107, 144

Sexually Transmitted Diseases

Sexually transmitted diseases (STD) or venereal diseases are a group of infections in which the principal mode of transmission is by sexual contact involving genital organs, anus, rectum and oro-pharynx. The spectrum of these diseases has widened and includes several conditions which are usually sexually transmissible (Table 25.1).

As space constraints do not allow individual descriptions of all the sexually transmitted diseases it is proposed to adopt a more general approach.

EPIDEMIOLOGY

Geographical distribution and statistics

Accurate figures on the incidence of these diseases are hard to obtain even in the developed countries where some of these diseases are notifiable. In the developing countries where diagnosis is often based on clinical impressions or history alone, where diagnostic facilities are lacking or non-existent and where self-treatment or treatment by quacks is common, the figures are almost totally unreliable. Studies among selected populations of some rural and urban tropical areas show alarmingly high rates for example from three to 18 per cent for gonorrhoea (Arya et al 1980) and 1.7 per cent for syphilis (Lomholt 1976). These rates are about 10 to 100 times higher than those of some western countries.

Almost all the major sexually transmitted diseases are widespread in warm climate countries. Others such as lymphogranuloma venereum and granuloma inguinale have a more limited distribution — the latter being more common in South India, Papua New Guinea, South America and Central and West Africa. 'Non-specific' genital infection, which is now the commonest STD in the western countries, is less frequently recognised in many tropical areas largely because of poor diagnostic facilities. Almost half of these cases are due to *Chlamydia trachomatis*. In some studies in the western countries, 35 to 63 per cent of males and females with gonorrhoea have also been found to be harbouring *C. trachomatis* (Taylor-Robinson and Thomas, 1980., WHO, 1981).

Table 25.1 Aetiological classification of sexually transmitted diseases.

Group	Agent	Disease
Viruses	Herpes simplex	Genital herpes
	Papilloma virus	Genital warts
	Pox virus	Molluscum contagiosum
	Hepatitis virus	Hepatitis A hepatitis B non-A non B
	? Cytomegalovirus	Congenital infection: birth defects; varied manifestations in immuno-suppressed host.
Chlamydia	C. trachomatis	Non-gonococcal ('non-specific') urogenital infections Lymphogranuloma venereum
	Unknown	Acquired Immune Deficiency Syndrome (AIDS)
Mycoplasmas	? M. hominis	Non-gonococcal urogenital infections
	Ureaplasma urealyticum	
Bacteria	N. gonorrhoeae	Gonococcal infections
	Haemophilus ducreyi	Chancroid
	Calymmatobacterium granulomatis	Granuloma inguinale
	Shigella species	Shigellosis
	? Gardnerella vaginalis and anaerobes	'Non-specific' vaginitis (anaerobic vaginosis)
	? Group B streptococcus	Neonatal sepsis
	Treponema pallidum	Syphilis
Fungi	Candida albicans	Genital candidosis
Protozoa	Trichomonas vaginalis	Trichomoniasis
	Entamoeba histolytica	Amoebiasis
	Giardia lamblia	Giardiasis
Helminth	Enterobius vermicularis	Enterobiasis
Arthropods	Phthirus pubis	Pediculosis
	Sarcoptes scabiei	Scabies

Footnote
The importance and the role of sexual transmission in the epidemiology of infections associated with cytomegalovirus *M. hominis*, *G. vaginalis* and Group B streptococcus have not been finally settled.

Complicated forms of gonorrhoea such as urethral stricture, pelvic inflammatory disease (Muir and Belsey, 1980) and infertility (WHO, 1975) are a considerable drain on the resources of health services of many tropical countries.

Since the principal mode of transmission of these diseases is sexual contact, the epidemiology is largely that of sexual behaviour. The factors which determine that behaviour may be related to the environment or the host. These and some of the factors related to the agent will now be described. Many of these factors are often interrelated.

Environment

Here we are concerned with social environment comprising socio-economic socio-cultural and socio-sexual factors.

Rapid industrialisation and urbanisation in many countries has led to migration of labour, transition of tribal life to urban life, family disruption, housing problems and loneliness. This social disorganisation has been described as one of the most constant features of the transitional societies of Africa in recent times and is conducive to altered codes of sexual behaviour. Sexually active, unmarried young people form the bulk of this migrant population, a factor mainly responsible for the high incidence of gonorrhoea in big cities (Verhagen and Gemert, 1972). Other groups of young people playing similar roles are students and soldiers. Soldiers' contribution to the incidence of sexually transmitted diseases may be expected to rise with the currently increasing build-up of armies in many countries.

In some areas sexually transmitted diseases are spreading along the major routes of communication through the 'courtesy' of long distance truck drivers, joined by prostitutes.

The increased mobility is also a phenomenon of wars involving not only soldiers but also civilian populations as a result of social upheaval. The high rates of gonococcal infections among Vietnamese refugees arriving in Thailand, during wars in that part of the world in the last decade, were attributed to rapes of females during their boat journey from Vietnam to Thailand (Center for Disease Control, 1981).

The patterns of prostitution are changing in Western countries; it is no longer considered an economic necessity and hence is responsible for a comparatively small proportion of the cases of sexually transmitted diseases. It is still, however, very important in the poor countries of Africa, the Far East and South America where the large majority of STD cases are contracted from prostitutes. The latter are simply meeting the increasing demands created by the great preponderance of men over women in the rapidly expanding towns of the developing countries. Meheus et al (1974) found 51.2 per cent of the prostitutes in Butare (Rwanda) to be harbouring gonococci on the basis of only one set of tests. Khoo et al (1977) found only five per cent of the prostitutes free from an STD in Singapore where Rajan (1978) showed the prostitute to be an index case in 60 per cent of the cases.

Socio-cultural factors reflect a society's attitudes to pre-marital and extra-marital sex and promiscuity — thus accounting for tribal or racial differences in the incidence of STD. In some societies such activities are quite common and may be considered the established social norm. In one study (Arya and Bennett, 1968) 80 per cent of college students had experienced pre-marital intercourse by the age of 20.

Emancipation of women is now on the increase in the East. For example in Singapore the proportion of economically active women aged 15–44 rose from 21 per cent in 1957 to 42 per cent in 1975 (Rajan, 1978).

High bride price and polygamy have been shown to favour spread of STD and consequently sterility in some parts of Africa (Arya, Nsanzumuhire and Taber, 1973.) The former, by postponing the marriage until enough wealth has been accumulated, leads to obtaining sexual satisfaction by casual encounters, and the latter serves as a permanent reservoir of infection once the gonococcus enters the 'pool' of a polygamous family.

Some social customs such as wedding ceremonies, last funeral rites and initiation ceremonies are times of social intercourse and sexual activity — the latter being exclusively pre-marital or extra-marital (Ongom, Lwanga, Mugisha and Mafigiri, 1971), to the accompaniment of dancing, drumming and 'booze'.

Host

Demographic factors (age and sex)

The greatest number of cases of STD occur in the age group 18 to 35. Population pyramids of many warm climate countries show relatively more young people, thus keeping up the number of susceptibles. Progressively earlier physical maturity due to improving standards of nutrition may be a factor — girls maturing earlier than boys. In a recent study in Zambia 13 per cent of the female STD patients were schoolgirls (Ratnam, 1980). Age of first sexual experience seems to vary in different societies. Girls in the East start later than their counterparts in Africa or the West (Rajan, 1978). Information on age/sexual experience and STD frequency by age is essential to determine when to start the relevant health education programmes. The preponderance of male cases in the STD returns of many countries may be a consequence of resort to the pool of prostitutes by the young male population in urban centres. Men may also recognise the lesions more easily and attend for treatment in contrast to women who may be asymptomatic with no visible lesions. Out of modesty women may also be deterred from attending clinics staffed by male physicians.

Attitudes

The liberal attitude to sex already mentioned is being strengthened by the overemphasis given to the subject in the mass media and by a lack of fear of contracting STD because of the ease of effective treatment when available. The role of the *contraceptive pill* in removing the fear of pregnancy and encouraging promiscuity has not generally been demonstrated in developing countries where perhaps its use is not so widespread. Use of the *sheath* or *condom* is generally fraught with taboos and misconceptions.

Alcohol

Casual encounters are often preceded by a high intake of alcohol. Besides, in some parts of Ethiopia (Plorde, 1981) and possibly elsewhere, a female beer seller was also a prostitute. This combined occupation had been chosen by many women as a quick way to earn an income.

Knowledge and beliefs

Lack of knowledge is one of the basic factors in the upward trend of all preventable disease. However, even those individuals with formal education cannot always be assumed to have acquired the appropriate knowledge. Very high rates of STD have been reported among university students (Arya and Bennett, 1968).

In some communities STD is considered a result of bewitchment, and consequently proper treatment is not sought. There is also a belief that gonorrhoea and syphilis may be got rid of by infecting another — preferably a virgin or even a child. Such beliefs might regulate an individual's behaviour with potentially disastrous consequences.

Sexual practices

The pattern of sexual behaviour will determine the speed of the spread, the number infected, and even the site involved. A California prostitute with secondary syphilis involved 310 male contacts spread over 34 American states, Canada and Mexico (Guthe and Willcox, 1971). Changing sexual practices are reflected in the incidence of ano-rectal gonorrhoea and syphilis acquired homosexually. The possibility of oro-pharyngeal gonorrhoea as a result of oro-genital contact reported to be common in some countries is not widely appreciated in many parts of the world. Oral-anal contact commonly practised by homosexuals, may result in the acquisition of enteric infections ('gay bowel syndrome') — thus widening the spectrum of STD which now includes shigellosis, amoebiasis, giardiasis and enterobiasis. Sexual transmission of hepatitis B has been shown to be particularly common among homosexuals as is also the case with the recently recognised Acquired Immune Deficiency Syndrome (AIDS).

Occupations specially at risk are barmaids, musicians, prostitutes, sailors, salesmen, soldiers, students, taxi and truck drivers.

Other high risk groups include tourists and those with broken marriages and inadequate personalities — the repeaters. Some diseases such as chancroid are associated with poverty and poor hygiene.

Asymptomatic or 'hidden' reservoirs of infection

Over half of the women infected with *N. gonorrhoeae* or *C. trachomatis* may have no symptoms but are capable of transmitting the infection and developing complications later. A proportion of the men may also be asymptomatic carriers.

Immunity

Knowledge in this field is still incomplete. An attack of gonorrhoea does, however, not confer immunity and hence repeated infections are common. Re-infection with *Treponema pallidum* can also occur after the successful treatment of early syphilis and in cases of late untreated syphilis. As yaws came under control due to mass campaigns and better hygiene, the immunity conferred by it against venereal syphilis was being lost, resulting in rising incidence of the latter in some areas. Yaws has, however, reappeared in some parts of the tropics as a result of inadequate surveillance (WHO, 1981). Thus in such countries both venereal syphilis and yaws may be encountered, the former predominantly in urban and the latter in rural areas.

Genetic factors

Some forms of STD, e.g. tabes dorsalis, are rare in Africa. Others, such as trichomoniasis, are more common among dark skinned males than among their caucasian counterparts. These differences may have a genetic basis. Fosler and Labrum (1976) in a study of black women found significantly higher prevalence of gonorrhoea among those with blood group B.

AGENT

Agent factors include infectivity, pathogenicity, virulence, antigenic variation and sensitivity to antibacterials. *N. gonorrhoeae* has attracted considerable attention in the recent years. In many tropical areas gonorrhoea has continued to be treated by quacks, pharmacy shops and uninformed private doctors with sub therapeutic or inappropriate regimes. Such practices have continued to encourage the emergence of 'resistant' strains in several of these areas where up to 80 per cent of the gonococcal strains have now decreased sensitivity to penicillin (WHO, 1978). The emergence in 1976 of penicillinase-producing strains of gonococci has aggravated the situation. Penicillinase production is plasmid determined and these strains are totally resistant to penicillin with obvious implications in their control. They have spread to many parts of the world and have gained a footing in West Africa and the Far East (Ngeow and Thong 1979; Arya, 1981., Osoba, 1981., Rajan et al, 1981).

Genital ulcers are commonly seen in STD clinics in parts of Africa and Asia (WHO, 1981). Over 5000 such patients were being seen in a Nairobi clinic every year (Nsanze et al, 1981). *Haemophilus ducreyi*, herpes simplex virus, *Treponema pallidum*, LGV strains of *C. trachomatis*, and *Calymmatobacterium granulomatis* are the common causes. The aetiology in a considerable proportion remains undetermined. Hence, there is a lack of information on their epidemiology.

Some strains of *H. ducreyi* have been reported to have developed resistance to sulphonamides and tetracycline (Rajan and Sng, 1981).

METHODS OF CONTROL

Recognition of the problem

Knowledge of the locally operating epidemiological factors must be the basis for a rational STD control programme, which should be an integral part of the overall system of communicable disease control. The very first step towards STD control is the recognition of the problem by the health authorities. This may necessitate data collection by surveys so as to make the policy-makers aware of the problem. These surveys might include figures for uncomplicated forms of STD seen at the outpatient clinics, and complicated forms such as cases of pelvic infection, urethral stricture, ophthalmia neonatorum and congenital syphilis et cetera admitted into the hospital. The administrators and decision makers may have to be persuaded to shed their prejudices and to adopt more positive attitudes. Unless the problem is given priority, no real progress is possible.

Diagnosis and treatment facilities

In the absence of vaccine (primary prevention), early diagnosis and appropriate treatment (secondary prevention) are the essential prerequisites before any further measures such as case finding and health education can be instituted. Initially a central unit, under the care of a specialist in STD, may be established with modern facilities for diagnosis, treatment, research and training, preferably in a national or teaching hospital. This could be followed by a more wide-spread service, such as microscopy at peripheral levels and culturing and serological tests at district or provincial levels.

Improvement especially in the existing primary health care facilities in areas with high prevalence of STD must be given urgent consideration. Health centres in such areas may be staffed by medical auxiliaries trained in STD. Darkfield examination in areas with high incidence of syphilis will have to be considered. Appropriate diagnostic facilities will lead to accurate statistics and correct treatment and provide a sound basis for speedy contact tracing.

Standardised but simple methods for diagnosis and appropriate treatment are beneficial. Exclusive STD centres may be economically feasible in large cities with a high incidence of these diseases.

Contact tracing and epidemiological treatment

For every patient with STD there must be at least one contact, often more (secondary). If not traced and treated, the contacts will continue to spread the disease, may re-infect the patient and also be likely to develop complications themselves. The methods used to get the contacts to the clinics include verbal persuasion, contact slips, telephone, letter or home visiting. The communications resources available will range from the sophisticated technology of some urban centres to the messages passed from hand to hand in scattered rural communities. The pressure or cooperation of tribal leaders is helpful for case finding, essential for community surveys. Nevertheless, involvement of third parties, such as tribal leaders or members of an extended family in tracing contacts of sexually transmitted disease might result in a damaging breach of confidentiality. The methods employed will depend upon the availability of staff, the number of contacts and their literary status, and the ease of access to contacts and clinics. Health personnel already involved in the control of communicable diseases such as tuberculosis and leprosy should be quite suitable. Perhaps a start could be made with syphilis and gonorrhoea which may have greater priority in many tropical areas.

Private physicians who see the majority of patients in many countries should have access to the above facilities.

Ideally all contacts should be examined, investigated and kept under surveillance until the diagnosis is proved or excluded. But that is often not possible in many areas of warm climate countries with inadequate or non-existent diagnostic and follow-up facilities and transport problems in the case of contacts living far from health centres. Under these circumstances epidemiological treatment, that is treatment without diagnosis (or abortive treatment), of contacts, particularly of proved syphilis, gonorrhoea or 'non-specific' infection should be considered.

Case finding

Case finding entails carrying out diagnostic tests for those who are not known to have been exposed to an STD or who have attended for reasons other than STD. The value of mass screening for sexually transmitted diseases will depend upon their prevalence. The logistics will also include the reliability and acceptability of the methods used. The two main diseases to be considered are gonorrhoea and syphilis, employing smears and cultures for the former and serological tests for the latter. Serological tests are obviously more acceptable, and a simple test for gonorrhoea is a distinct possibility in the not too distant future. Screening of selected groups may be economically feasible in areas with a high incidence of the disease. These groups include pre-marital and pre-employment candidates, blood donors, pregnant women attending ante-natal clinics, women attending family planning clinics, in-patients, prisoners, prostitutes and bar girls. Screening of ante-natal women for syphilis and gonorrhoea and treating those found infected will help in the prevention of congenital syphilis and gonococcal ophthalmia neonatorum.

Personal prophylaxis

Abstinence is so rare that it need not be mentioned. Medication taken immediately before or after exposure must be discouraged; it might foster resistant strains, encourage self-treatment, predispose to unwanted side effects, and result in symptomless carriers, unless used in full doses. The only situation where prophylactic medication is desirable is the use of silver nitrate eye drops (Crede's method) for the new born child to prevent gono-coccal ophthalmia neonatorum although its efficacy has been questioned by some workers.

The use of condoms (sheaths) should be encouraged. If used properly they give good (though not 100 per cent) protection against pregnancy as well as sexually transmitted diseases. Other prophylactic methods such as vaginal preparations are being investigated.

STD vaccines

Considerable progress has been made in understanding the biology of various sexually transmissible organisms and immune mechanisms in gonorrhoea, syphilis and other STD's. Presently, however, Hepatitis B is the only sexually transmitted disease for which a safe and effective vaccine is now available (Szmuness et al, 1980., Zuckerman 1982).

Health education

Health education for STD control must be suited to the total epidemiol-ogical pattern of the sexual behaviour of the community concerned that is 'community diagnosis before treatment'. The 'treatment' or the 'educational objectives' may include abstinence or reduced sexual intercourse before marriage, use of condoms, reporting early for check-up, taking prescribed treatment and attending regularly for follow-up, co-operating for contact tracing, refraining from alcohol in sexually conducive environments and avoiding self-medication. The purpose of health education in STD is to motivate the risk takers towards the adoption of the above measures.

Space does not permit details on the various aspects of health education. The subject has been thoroughly reviewed in a World Health Organization document (INT/VDT/75,364). Education must begin early in the schools before values and attitudes relating to sex become established. It must be part of a wider education programme covering family planning clinics, maternal and child health services, school health, university health and occupational health services, general morbidity clinics and STD clinics. The evaluation, whenever possible, should be built into the programme.

Medical education

More emphasis than at present is needed in the teaching of these diseases, aimed not only at undergraduates and postgraduates including private prac-titioners but also at medical auxiliaries who provide primary care to the large majority of patients in warm climate countries. The educational content in respect of training for medical auxiliaries should include history taking, examination of the patient, diagnosis and treatment of common STD's recognition of complications to be referred to hospital, record keeping, surveillance, contact tracing, local epidemiological factors and health education.

Legislation

Legislative provisions dealing mainly with syphilis, gonorrhoea and chancroid and to a lesser extent lymphogranuloma venereum and granuloma inguinale exist in some countries (WHO, 1975). These impose obligations on both the patient and the attending physician, the former to undergo treatment and to disclose the source of infection, et cetera, and the latter to notify the specified diseases. Other aspects include pre-marital and antenatal serology for syphilis, treatment of minors without parents' consent, homosexuality, prostitution and the illegal sale of drugs.

None of the above can, however, be implemented without back-up facilities. Moreover, legislation must be suited to the local circumstances. Experiences of other countries may serve as useful guides. Prostitutes are a case in point: it is treatment and educational and alternative occupational opportunities rather than legalized status which will help in STD control. Legislation on notification of cases, to make it possible to gauge trends and evaluate control measures, may be a good starting point.

Research

Every country must have its priorities. Basic research in the field of immunology, diagnosis and other highly technical aspects requiring expensive sophisticated technology and highly skilled personnel will have to be left to those equipped for such tasks. Nevertheless, much of the operational research of more immediate concern and local relevance involving therapy, contact tracing and behavioural aspects are within the scope of many of the lesser equipped medical centres.

CONCLUSION

We have the means to control the sexually transmitted diseases. These must be vigorously applied to match human behaviour faced with the prospects of continuingly unfavourable sexual ecology (population mobility, permissiveness, prostitution, 'the pill' and promiscuity) and the emergence of resistant strains. Collaborative efforts of venereologists, dermatologists, gynaecologists, bacteriologists, public health and other interested workers will be necessary for systematic implementation of the above control measures to achieve the best results.

REFERENCES

Arya O P, Bennett F J 1968 Attitudes of college students in East Africa to sexual activity and venereal disease. British Journal of Venereal Diseases 44: 160–166

Arya O P, Nsanzumuhire H, Taber S R 1973 Clinical, cultural and demographic aspects of gonorrhoea in a rural community in Uganda. Bulletin of World Health Organisation 49: 587–595

Arya O P, Osoba A O, Bennett F J 1980 Tropical Venereology. Churchill Livingstone, Edinburgh

Arya O P 1981 Epidemiology of gonorrhoea. In: Harris J R W (ed) Recent advances in Sexually Transmitted Diseases, Number two, Churchill Livingstone, Edinburgh. ch 2, pp 35–48

Center for Disease Control 1981 Gonococcal infections among Indochinese refugees — Thailand. Morbidity and Mortality Weekly Report 30: 355–362

Fosler M T O, Labrum A H O 1976 Relation of infection with Neisseria gonorrhoeae to ABO blood groups. Journal of Infectious Diseases 133: 329–330

Guthe T, Willcox R R 1971 The international incidence of venereal disease. Royal Society of Health Journal 91: 122–133

Khoo R, Sng E H, Goh A J 1977 Incidence of sexually transmitted diseases in prostitutes in Singapore. Asian Journal of Infectious Diseases 1: 77–79

Lomholt G 1976 Venereal problems in a developing country. Tropical Doctor 6: 7–10

Meheus A, Clerq A De, Prat R 1974 Prevalence of gonorrhoea in Prostitutes in a Central African town, British Journal of Venereal Diseases 50: 50–52

Muir D G, Belsey M A 1980 Pelvic inflammatory disease and its consequences in the developing world. American Journal of Obstetrics and Gynecology 138: 913–928

Ngeow Y F, Thong M L 1979 Penicillin-resistant gonorrhoea: a report from University Hospital, Kuala Lumpur. Medical Journal of Malaysia 33: 252–258

Nsanze H, Fast M V, D'Costa L J, Tukei P, Curran J, Ronald A 1981 Genital ulcers in Kenya; clinical and laboratory study. British Journal of Venereal Diseases 57: 378–381

Ongom V L, Lwanga V N, Mugisha J K, Mafigiri J T 1971 Social background to venereal disease at Kasangati. East African Medical Journal 48: 367–371

Osoba A O 1981 Penicillinase-producing Neisseria gonorrhoeae in Nigeria. Paper presented at 1st Sexually Transmitted Diseases World Congress, Puerto Rico, Nov 15–21

Plorde D S 1981 Sexually Transmitted Diseases in Ethiopia: social factors contributing to their spread and implications for developing countries. British Journal of Venereal Diseases 57: 357–362

Rajan V S 1978 Sexually transmitted diseases on a tropical island. British Journal of Venereal Diseases 54: 141–143

Rajan V S, Sng E H 1981 Chancroid. In: Harris J R W (ed) Recent advances in Sexually Transmitted Diseases, Number two, Churchill Livingstone, Edinburgh. Ch 13, pp 201–210

Rajan V S, Thirumoorthy T, Tan N J 1981 Epidemiology of penicillinase-producing Neisseria gonorrhoeae in Singapore. British Journal of Venereal Diseases 57: 158–161

Ratnam A V 1980 Sexually transmitted diseases in Lusaka. Medical Journal of Zambia 14: 71–74

Szmuness W et al 1980 Hepatitis B vaccine: demonstration of efficiency in a controlled trial in a high risk population in the United States. New England Journal of Medicine 303: 833–841

Taylor-Robinson D, Thomas B J 1980 The role of Chlamydia trachomatis in genital tract and associated diseases. Journal of Clinical Pathology 33: 205–233

Verhagen A R, Gemert W 1972 Social and epidemiological determinants of gonorrhoea in an East African country. British Journal of Venereal Diseases 48: 277–286

World Health Organization 1975 Report of the meeting on health education in the control of sexually transmitted diseases. WHO Document INT/VDT/75, 364.

World Health Organization 1975 The epidemiology of infertility. Report of a WHO Scientific Group. Technical Report Series 582, Geneva

World Health Organization 1975 Venereal disease control — a survey of recent legislation, Geneva

World Health Organization 1978 Neisseria gonorrhoeae and gonococcal infections. Report of a WHO Scientific Group. Technical Report Series 616, Geneva

World Health Organization 1981 Endemic treponematoses. Weekly Epidemiological Record 56: 241–248
World Health Organization 1981 Nongonococcal urethritis and other selected sexually tanasmitted diseases of public health importance. Report of a WHO Scientific Group. Technical Report Series 660, Geneva
Zuckerman A J Priorities for immunisation against hepatitis B. British Medical Journal 284: 686–688

Viral hepatitis

INTRODUCTION

Viral hepatitis is a major public health problem occurring endemically in all parts of the world. The general term viral hepatitis refers to the infections caused by at least three different viruses hepatitis A (infectious or epidemic hepatitis), hepatitis B (serum hepatitis) and the more recently identified form, non-A, non-B hepatitis which is almost certainly caused by more than two viruses. There are probably several different viruses. Hepatitis A and hepatitis B can be differentiated by sensitive laboratory tests for specific antigens and antibodies and the viruses have been characterised. However, at present there are no precise virological criteria nor specific laboratory tests for non-A, non-B hepatitis.

Although other viruses such as yellow fever virus, members of the arenavirus group, several haemorrhagic fever viruses (Marburg virus, Ebola virus, Rift Valley Fever virus), and not infrequently cytomegalovirus, Epstein-Barr virus and others may cause inflammation and necrosis of the liver, these are generally excluded from the term viral hepatitis.

THE DISEASE

Infection results in acute inflammation of the liver. Inapparent or subclinical infections and infections without jaundice are common. The clinical picture ranges in its presentation from an asymptomatic infecion, a mild anicteric illness, acute disease with jaundice, severe prolonged jaundice to acute fulminant hepatitis. The incidence of individual symptoms and signs varies in different outbreaks and in sporadic cases. While hepatitis A virus does not persist in the host nor is there evidence of progression to chronic liver damage, hepatitis B and non-A, non-B hepatitis may be associated with persistent infection, prolonged carrier state and progression to chronic liver disease which may be severe. In addition, there is compelling evidence of an aetiological association between hepatitis B virus and primary hepatocellular carcinoma, which is one of the most common tumours in the world.

Hepatitis A

Epidemiology

Hepatitis A is endemic in all parts of the world but the exact incidence is not known and difficult to estimate because of the high proportion of asymptomatic and anicteric infections, differences in surveillance and differing patterns of disease. The degree of under-reporting is known to be very high. Serological surveys have shown that while the prevalence of hepatitis A in industrialised countries particularly in Northern Europe, North America and Australia is decreasing, the infection is virtually universal in most other regions, particularly in warm climate countries.

Incubation period The incubation period of hepatitis A is between 3 and 5 weeks with a mean of 28 days. Subclinical and anicteric infections are common.

Mode of spread Hepatitis A virus is spread by the faecal-oral route, usually by person to person contact, and infection is particularly common in conditions of poor sanitation and overcrowding. Common source outbreaks result most frequently from faecal contamination of drinking water and food, but waterborne transmission is not a major factor in the industrialised countries and where piped water supply has been adequately treated and chlorinated. On the other hand, many foodborne outbreaks have been reported more recently. This can be attributed to the shedding of large amounts of virus in the faeces during the incubation period of the illness in infected foodhandlers, and the source of the outbreak can often be traced to uncooked food or food that has been handled after cooking. Foodborne outbreaks have now become important epidemiologically in developed countries. The consumption of raw or inadequately cooked shellfish cultivated in sewage-contaminated tidal or coastal water, and the consumption of raw vegetables grown in soil fertilized with untreated human faeces and excreta is associated with a high risk of infection with hepatitis A virus. Hepatitis A infection is frequently contracted by travellers from areas of low prevalence to areas of high endemicity.

Hepatitis A virus is very rarely transmitted by blood transfusion or by the parenteral route, although this has been demonstrated experimentally in human volunteers and in susceptible non-human primates.

Age incidence and seasonal pattern All age groups are susceptible to infection. The highest incidence is observed in children of school age, but in North America and in many countries in northern Europe most cases occur in adults, frequently after travel abroad. In temperate zones the characteristic seasonal trend is for an increase in incidence in the autumn and early winter months falling progressively to a minimum in midsummer, but recently this seasonal trend has been lost in some countries. In many tropical countries the peak of reported infection tends to occur during the rainy season with low incidence in the dry months. A superimposed cyclic epidemic pattern with peaks every five to 10 years has been observed in several countries.

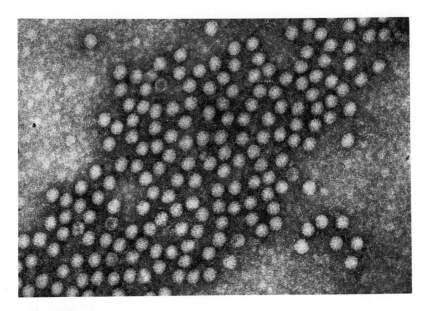

Figure 26.1 Hepatitis A virus particles found in faecal extracts by electron microscopy. Both "full" and a few "empty" particles are present. The virus measures 27–29 nm in diameter × 200,000

Reservoir host: man. More than 40 outbreaks of hepatitis A involving over 170 human cases have been reported since 1961 among handlers of newly captured apes, particularly chimpanzees. The monkeys do not suffer from a recognisable clinical illness and it seems likely that the chimpanzees contract the infection by contact with man.

Properties of hepatitis A virus and laboratory tests

In 1973, small cubic virus particles measuring about 27 nm in diameter (Fig 1) were identified by the technique of immune electron microscopy in faeces obtained during the early acute phase of illness in experimentally infected adult volunteers. The availability of the viral antigen resulted in the identification of the specific antibody and the development of specific serological tests for hepatitis A.

Hepatitis A virus is a single-stranded RNA virus possessing the features of an enterovirus and is a member of the family *Picornaviridae*. The virus is ether resistant, stable at pH 3.0 and relatively resistant to inactivation by heat. It is partially inactivated by heat at 60 °C for 10 hours and inactivated at 100 °C for 5 minutes. Semi-purified hepatitis A virus is inactivated by ultraviolet irradiation and by treatment with 1:4000 concentration of formaldehyde solution at 37 °C for 72 hours. It has been reported that hepatitis A virus is inactivated by chlorine at a concentration of 1 mg/litre for 30 minutes.

Numerous virus particles are found in faeces during the incubation period of hepatitis A, beginning as early as 9 days after exposure to infection, and shedding of virus usually continues until peak elevation of serum aminotransferases. Virus particles are also detected during the early acute phase of illness, but the number of particles decreases rapidly after the onset of jaundice. Prolonged virus excretion and a persistent carrier state have not been found.

Antibody to hepatitis A virus, initially of the IgM class followed rapidly by IgG, is detectable late in the incubation period coinciding approximately with the onset of biochemical evidence of liver damage. Hepatitis A IgG antibody persists for many years and frequently for life.

Various serological tests have been developed for the diagnosis of hepatitis A. Immune adherence haemagglutination is specific and sensitive and has been widely used. Several methods of radioimmunoassay are available and of these a solid-phase competitive type of assay is particularly convenient. Very sensitive enzyme immunoassay techniques have also been developed. Both radioimmunoassay and enzyme immunoassay for detection of hepatitis A antibodies of the IgM and IgG classes are now available. Against a very high background of past infection in warm climate countries, the diagnosis of a recent episode of hepatitis A is most conveniently and reliably established by the demonstration of hepatitis A antibody of the IgM class, which is detectable for up to about four months after infection.

One serotype of hepatitis A virus has been identified in volunteers infected experimentally with the MS-1 strain of hepatitis A, in patients from different outbreaks of hepatitis A in different geographical regions, in sporadic cases of hepatitis A and in naturally and experimentally infected non-human primates. There is considerable evidence, however, that there is an epidemic form of a hepatitis A-like illness particularly in the subcontinent of India, Burma, in the eastern USSR, parts of the Middle East and in North Africa. This epidemic and endemic strain(s) of virus is commonly transmitted by comtaminated water. There is ample serological evidence that this form of hepatitis is not caused by the recognised serotype of hepatitis A, which is not surprising since this type of hepatitis occurs in regions where most individuals are infected with hepatitis A in the first few years of life and are immune. Indeed, there is no serological evidence for reinfection of patients with hepatitis A virus. It is not known yet whether this more recently recognised type of epidemic hepatitis is caused by a virus distinct from hepatitis A, or alternatively, by a distinct but previously unrecognised serotype or serotypes of hepatitis A. Specific laboratory tests are not available.

Prevention and control

Control of hepatitis A infection is difficult. Since faecal shedding of the virus is at its highest during the incubation period and prodromal phase of the illness, strict isolation of cases is not a useful control measure. Spread of infection is reduced by simple hygienic measures and the sanitary disposal of excreta.

Normal human immunoglobulin, a 16 per cent solution in a dose of 0.02–0.12 ml/kg body weight, given intramuscularly before exposure to the virus or early during the incubation period will prevent or attenuate a clinical illness, while not always preventing infection and excretion of virus, and inapparent or subclinical hepatitis may develop. The efficacy of passive immunisation is based on the presence of hepatitis A antibody in the immunoglobulin, but the minimum titre of antibody required for protection has not yet been established. Immunoglobulin has also been used effectively for controlling outbreaks in institutions such as homes for the mentally-handicapped and in nursery schools. Prophylaxis with immunoglobulin is recommended for persons without hepatitis A antibody visiting highly endemic areas.

The successful propagation of hepatitis A virus in 1979 in primary monolayer and explant cell cultures and in continuous cell strains of primate origin has permitted the development of hepatitis A vaccines. These vaccines are at present undergoing phase I clinical trials.

Hepatitis B

Introduction and epidemiology

The discovery in 1965 of Australia antigen, now referred to as hepatitis B surface antigen, and the demonstration by B S Blumberg and his colleagues of its association with hepatitis B led to rapid progress in the understanding of this very common, important and complex infection.

In the past, hepatitis B was diagnosed on the basis of infection occurring about 60–180 days after the injection of human blood or plasma fractions or the use of inadequately sterilised syringes and needles. The development of specific laboratory tests for hepatitis B confirmed the importance of the parenteral routes of transmission and infectivity appears to be especially related to blood. However, many reports have demonstrated that hepatitis B is not spread exclusively by blood and blood products. These include the observations that under certain circumstances the virus is infective by mouth, that it is endemic in closed institutions and in institutions for the mentally-handicapped, that it is more prevalent in adults in urban communities and among those living in poor socio-economic conditions, that there is a huge reservoir of carriers of markers of hepatitis B virus in the human population and that the carrier rate and age distribution of the surface antigen vary in different regions.

There is much evidence for the transmission of hepatitis B by intimate contact and by the sexual route. The sexually promiscuous, particularly male homosexuals, are at very high risk of infection with hepatitis B virus. Hepatitis B surface antigen has been found in blood and in various body fluids such as saliva, menstrual and vaginal discharges, seminal fluid, colostrum and breast milk and serous exudates and these have been implicated as vehicles of transmission of infection. The presence of the antigen in urine, bile, faeces, sweat and tears has been reported but not confirmed. Contact associated hepatitis B is thus of major importance. Transmission of the infection may result from accidental inoculation of minute amounts of blood or body fluids contaminated with blood such as may occur during medical, surgical and dental procedures, immunization with inadequately sterilised syringes and needles, intravenous and percutaneous drug abuse, tattooing, ear-piercing and nose-piercing, acupuncture, laboratory accidents and accidental inoculation with razors and similar objects which have been contaminated with blood. Additional factors may be important for the transmission of hepatitis B infection in the tropics and in warm-climate countries. These include traditional tattooing and scarification, blood letting, ritual circumcision and repeated biting by blood-sucking arthropod vectors. Results of investigations into the role which biting insects may play in the spread of hepatitis B are conflicting. Hepatitis B surface antigen has been detected in several species of mosquitoes and in bed-bugs which have either been trapped in the wild or fed experimentally on infected blood, but no convincing evidence of replication of the virus in insects has been obtained. Mechanical transmission of the infection, however, is a possibility.

Clustering of hepatitis B also occurs within family groups but on the whole it is not related to genetic factors and does not reflect maternal and venereal transmission. The mechanisms of intrafamilial spread of hepatitis B infection are not known.

Transmission of hepatitis B virus from carrier mothers to their babies can occur during the perinatal period and appears to be an important factor in determining the prevalence of the infection in some regions, particularly in China and South East Asia. The risk of infection in the infant may reach 50–60 per cent, although it varies from country to country and appears to be related to ethnic groups. The risk is greatest if the mother has a history of transmission to previous children, has a high titre of hepatitis B surface antigen and/or e antigen. There is also a substantial risk of perinatal infection if the mother has acute hepatitis B in the second or third trimester of pregnancy or within two months after delivery. Although hepatitis B virus can infect the fetus in utero this appears to be rare. The precise mechanism of perinatal infection is uncertain, but it probably occurs during or shortly after birth as a result of a leak of maternal blood into the baby's circulation, its ingestion or inadvertent inoculation. Most children infected during the perinatal period become persistent carriers.

The carrier state

The carrier state is defined as persistence of the hepatitis B surface antigen in the circulation for more than six months. The carrier state, which may be life-long and may be associated with liver damage varying from minor changes in the nuclei of hepatocytes to chronic active hepatitis, cirrhosis and primary hepatocellular carcinoma. Several risk factors have been identified in relation to development of the carrier state. It is commoner in males, more likely to follow infections acquired in childhood than those acquired in adult life, and more likely to occur in patients with natural or acquired immune deficiencies. A carrier state becomes established in approximately five to 10 per cent of infected adults. In countries where hepatitis B infection is common, the highest prevalence of the surface antigen is found in children aged four to eight years with steadily declining rates amongst older age groups.

Survival of hepatitis B virus is ensured by the huge reservoir of carriers, estimated to number over 200 million world-wide. The prevalence of carriers, particularly among blood donors, in northern Europe, North America and Australia is 0.1 per cent or less; in central and eastern Europe up to five per cent, a higher frequency in southern Europe, the countries bordering the Mediterranean and parts of Central and South America, and in some parts of Africa, Asia and the Pacific region as many as 20 per cent or more of the apparently healthy population may be carriers. There is an urgent need to define the mechanisms which lead to the carrier state in endemic areas and to introduce methods of interruption of transmission.

Properties of hepatitis B virus and laboratory tests

Examination by electron microscopy of serum containing hepatitis B surface antigen reveals the presence of small spherical particles measuring about 22 nm in diameter, tubular forms of varying length but with a diameter close to 22 nm and large double-shelled or solid particles approximately 42 nm in diameter (Fig 2). The large particles contain a core or nucleocapsid about 28 nm in diameter. The 42 nm particle (referred to in the past as the Dane particle) is the hepatitis B virus, whereas the small particles and the tubules are non-infectious surplus virus coat protein.

The core of the virus contains double-stranded circular DNA. The molecular weight of the DNA is about 2.3×10^6 and the DNA is approximately 3200 nucleotides in length, with a single-stranded gap varying from 600–2100 nucleotides. The core also contains a DNA-dependent DNA polymerase, which is closely associated with the DNA template.

The DNA of hepatitis B virus has recently been cloned in prokaryotic and eukaryotic cells with expression of viral antigenic proteins.

Sensitive and specific laboratory tests such as enzyme immunoassay and radioimmunoassay are now available for the detection of specific serological markers of infection with hepatitis B virus. Infection with hepatitis B virus leads to the appearance in the plasma during the incubation period of hepatitis B surface antigen about 2–8 weeks before biochemical evidence of liver dysfunction or the onset of jaundice. This antigen persists during the

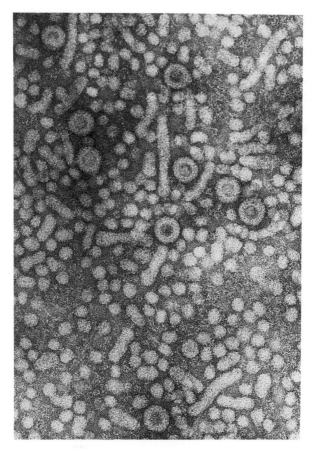

Figure 26.2 Electron micrograph of serum containing hepatitis B virus after negative staining. The three morphological forms of the antigen are shown.
(1) small pleomorphic spherical particles 20–22 nm in diameter.
(2) tubular forms.
(3) 42 nm double-shelled particles. This is the complete virus particle × 151,200.

acute illness and is usually cleared from the circulation during convalescence. Next to appear in the circulation is the viral DNA polymerase associated with the core of the virus and at about the same time another antigen, the *e* antigen, becomes detectable, again preceding serum aminotransferase elevations. The *e* antigen is a distinct soluble antigen which is located within the core and correlates closely to the number of virus particles and relative infectivity. Antibody to the hepatitis B core antigen is found in the serum 2–4 weeks after the appearance of the surface antigen, and it is always detectable during the early acute phase of the illness. Core antibody of the IgM class becomes undetectable within some months of the onset of uncomplicated acute infection, but IgG core antibody persists after recovery for many years and possibly for life. The next antibody to appear in the circulation is directed against the *e* antigen, and there is evidence that, in general terms, anti- *e* indicates relatively low infectivity of serum. Antibody to the surface antigen component, hepatitis B surface antibody, is the last marker to appear late during convalescence. Precipitating antibodies reacting with antigenic determinants on the complete virus particle have been described. These antibodies may be relevant to the clearance of circulating hepatitis B virions and the termination of the infection and their absence in patients with chronic active hepatitis may explain why the infection persists in such patients. Cell-mediated immunity also appears to be important in terminating hepatitis B infection and, under certain circumstances, in promoting liver damage and in the genesis of autoimmunity.

Antigenic heterogeneity of the surface antigen has been demonstrated by serological analysis. Hepatitis B surface antigen particles share a common group-specific antigen *a* and generally carry at least two mutually exclusive subdeterminants, *d* or *y* and *w* or *r*. The subtypes are the phenotypic expressions of distinct genotype variants of hepatitis B virus. Four principal phenotypes are recognised, *adw*, *adr*, *ayw* and *ayr*, but other complex permutations of these subdeterminants and new variants have been described, all apparently on the surface of the same physical particles. The major subtypes have differing geographical distribution. For example, in northern Europe, the Americas and Australia subtype *adw* predominates. Subtype *ayw* occurs in a broad zone which includes northern and western Africa, the eastern Mediterranean, eastern Europe, northern and central Asia and the Indian subcontinent. Both *adw* and *adr* are found in Malaysia, Thailand, Indonesia and Papua New Guinea, while subtype *adr* predominates in other parts of south-east Asia including China, Japan and the Pacific islands. The subtypes provide useful epidemiological markers of hepatitis B virus.

Hepatitis B, chronic liver disease and primary hepatocellular carcinoma

The outcome of acute hepatitis B may be either complete resolution, massive necrosis, chronic hepatitis or resolution with scarring and cirrhosis. Therefore chronic liver disease following hepatitis may be the result of necrosis, collapse of the reticulum framework, the formation of scars of nodular hyperplasia and various immunological and host factors. Patients with active chronic hepatitis with persistent hepatitis B antigens are usually male, older than patients without the surface antigen. Autoantibodies are usually absent from the serum and multisystem involvement is not present. A proportion of patients with cryptogenic cirrhosis have evidence of persistent hepatitis B infection.

In many parts of the world, primary hepatocellular carcinoma is one of the commonest human cancers, particularly in young men. There is considerable evidence for implication of hepatitis B virus in the aetiology of this important cancer. The evidence is based on the following epidemiological and geographical observations. First there is a strong correlation between hepatitis B infection and primary liver cancer. Second is the relatively constant risk of developing primary hepatocellular carcinoma in both endemic and non-endemic areas among persistent male carriers of hepatitis B surface antigen. Third the infection precedes and may accompany the development of cancer, usually in a liver with chronic damage or macronodular cirrhosis associated with hepatitis B virus. Fourth hepatitis B antigens are present in the malignant tissue and there is evidence of covalent integration of the genome of hepatitis B virus into the DNA of the tumour cells. Fifth several cell lines derived from primary hepatocellular carcinoma secrete hepatitis B surface antigen in culture and DNA has been shown to be integrated into the genome of these cells as well as RNA molecules containing specific sequences of hepatitis B virus and at least one of these cell lines has been shown to be heterotransplantable. Finally there is the finding of chronic liver damage and primary liver cancer in several animal species infected with viruses which are phylogenetically related to human hepatitis B virus.

Prophylaxis against hepatitis B

Passive immunisation   The availability of laboratory tests for hepatitis B surface antibody has allowed the selection of plasma for the preparation of hepatitis B immunoglobulin, which may confer temporary passive immunity.

The major indication for the administration of hepatitis B immunoglobulin is a single acute exposure, such as when blood or other material containing hepatitis B surface antigen is accidentally inoculated, ingested orally or splashed on the conjuctiva. The optimal dose of hepatitis B immunoglobulin is not known but doses in the range of 0.04–0.07 ml/kg have been used with success. Based on available data, two doses administered 30 days apart are required for efficacy. The timing of the first dose is important and the immunoglobulin should be administered as early as possible and preferably within 48 hours. It should not be administered after seven days following exposure.

Hepatitis B immunoglobulin administered within a few hours of birth to babies born to surface antigen-positive mothers yielded encouraging results if the baby was treated within 48 hours of birth. More recently, interruption of maternal-infant transmission of hepatitis B virus was achieved and the carrier state prevented by the administration of hepatitis B immunoglobulin within 48 hours of birth, with further doses of immunoglobulin monthly for six months, indicating that the timing of immunoglobulin was critical in determining its efficacy.

Pre-exposure prophylaxis with immunoglobulin has also been recommended in endemic settings such as haemodialysis units, where transmis sion of hepatitis B virus is known to occur and where preventive hygienic measures cannot be implemented.

Active immunisation The high rate of infection with hepatitis B virus in certain defined populations in the developed countries and among the general population in many developing countries stresses the urgent need for a hepatitis B vaccine. Among the groups which might benefit from such a vaccine are patients who require multiple transfusions, patients with natural or acquired immune deficiency and patients with malignant disease, patients and staff of haemodialysis, transplant and oncology units and residents and staff of institutions for the mentally-handicapped. Viral hepatitis is an occupational hazard among health care and laboratory personnel. High rates of infection occur in homosexual men, drug addicts and prostitutes. Reference has already been made to the high rates of perinatal transmission of hepatitis B in some regions, and protective immunisation of susceptible women of childbearing age and infants may well be the only practical way of interrupting transmission of the infection. Immunisation must also be considered for non-immune persons living in certain tropical and non-tropical areas where the prevalence of hepatitis B infection is high and where the carrier state may reach 10–20 per cent of the population, and primary hepatocellular carcinoma is common.

The inability to grow hepatitis B virus serially in tissue culture has prevented the development of conventional vaccines. Attention has therefore been directed to the use of other preparations for active immunisation. The foundation for such hepatitis B vaccines was laid by the demonstration of the relative efficacy of dilute serum containing hepatitis B virus and its antigens heated to 98 °C for one minute in preventing or modifying the infection in susceptible persons. Since hepatitis B surface antigen leads to the production of protective surface antibody, purified 22 mm spherical surface antigen particles have been developed as vaccines. These vaccines have been prepared from the plasma of symptomless human carriers. Although it is generally accepted that the preparations of 22 nm particles, when pure are free of nucleic acid and therefore non-infectious, the fact that the starting material is human plasma obtained from persons infected with hepatitis B virus means that special care must be exercised to ensure their freedom of all harmful contaminating material.

Human hepatitis B infection has been transmitted to chimpanzees, the only available susceptible non-human primate to this infection. The infection in chimpanzees is mild, but the biochemical, histological and serological responses in the chimpanzees are very similar to those in man and chimpanzees have been shown to be protected by the 22 nm particle vaccines which had been treated with formalin.

Small-scale safety tests were carried out in volunteers and trials in the United States on protective efficacy in high-risk groups such as male homosexuals, and patients and staff of maintenance haemodialysis units have shown the vaccine to be safe, potent and highly effective. There is no evidence for transmission of acquired immune deficiency syndrome (AIDS) by the currently licensed plasma-derived hepatitis B vaccines, nor by immunoglobulins which meet WHO requirements. The vaccine has been licensed in several countries and it is available in limited quantities. A course of this type of vaccine is extremely expensive (in the range of 100–150 US dollars at the time of writing). In another study the vaccine prevented the development of early carrier state of hepatitis B surface antigen in seronegative children at high risk of infection in an endemic area in West Africa. Other studies are in progress.

Considerable advances have also been made in the development of hepatitis B vaccines from the constituent polypeptides of the surface antigen in micellar preparations. The advantages of a polypeptide vaccine, derived from any source, include precise biochemical characterisation, exclusion of genetic material of viral origin, the exclusion of host or donor-derived substances, potency and ultimately the development of synthetic peptides.

Particularly attractive sources of antigenic material would be prokaryotic and eukaryotic cells expressing hepatitis B proteins as a result of cloning of hepatitis B viral DNA, and the production of significant amounts of surface antigen has recently been reported.

Non-A, Non-B hepatitis

The specific laboratory diagnosis of hepatitis A and hepatitis B has revealed a previously unrecognised form of hepatitis which is clearly unrelated to either type referred to as non-A, non-B hepatitis. It is now the most common form of hepatitis occurring after blood transfusion and the administration of blood clotting factors in some areas of the world. The infection has also been transmitted experimentally to chimpanzees. Although specific laboratory tests for identifying this new type of hepatitis are not yet available and the diagnosis can only be made by exclusion there is considerable information about the epidemiology of this infection. Non-A, non-B hepatitis has been found in every country in which is has been sought and it has a number of features in common with hepatitis B.

This form of hepatitis has been most commonly recognised as a complication of blood transfusion, and in countries where all blood donations are screened for hepatitis B surface antigen by very sensitive techniques non-A, non-B hepatitis may account for up to 90 per cent of all cases of post-transfusion hepatitis. Non-A, non-B hepatitis has occurred in haemodialysis and renal transplantation units and among drug addicts. In several countries a significant number of cases are not associated with transfusion and such sporadic cases of non-A, non-B hepatitis have been found to account for 15–20 per cent of all adult patients with viral hepatitis. In general, the illness is mild and often subclinical or anicteric. However, there is evidence that the infection may be followed by prolonged viraemia and the development of a persistent carrier state. Several recent studies of the histopathological sequelae of acute non-A, non-B infection indicate that chronic hepatitis may occur in as many as 40–50 per cent of patients after infection associated with blood transfusion or treatment by haemodialysis.

Clinical, epidemiological and experimental studies in a number of laboratories suggest that non-A, non-B hepatitis may be caused by two or more infectious agents. Clinical evidence is based on the observation of multiple attacks of hepatitis in individual patients. Epidemiologically, short-incubation and long-incubation forms of non-A, non-B hepatitis have been described, although it is possible that differences in the incubation period represent differences in the infective dose. Experimental evidence for the existence of at least two distinct non-A, non-B hepatitis viruses has been obtained from cross-challenge transmission studies in chimpanzees.

Reference has already been made to the epidemic and endemic form of hepatitis which is commonly transmitted by contaminated water and which is not caused by the recognised serotype of hepatitis A nor hepatitis B.

Serological tests for antigens and antibodies which are specifically associated with non-A, non-B hepatitis are not yet available and the causative agents have not been characterised virologically.

GENERAL REFERENCES AND SUGGESTIONS FOR FURTHER READING

McCollum R W, Zuckerman A J 1981 Viral hepatitis. Report on a WHO Informal Consultation. Journal of Medical Virology 8: 1–29
Sherlock S (ed) 1980 Virus Hepatitis. Clinics in Gastroenterology. Saunders, London
World Health Organisation 1977 Advances in viral hepatitis. Report of the WHO Expert Committee on Viral Hepatitis. Technical Report Series No 602, Geneva
Zuckerman A J 1979 The chronicle of viral hepatitis. Abstracts on Hygiene, 54: 1113–1135
Zuckerman A J 1979 Specific serological diagnosis of vi al hepatitis. British Medical Journal, 2: 84–86
Zuckerman A J 1980 Why the world needs hepatitis vaccine. New Scientist 88: 167–168
Zuckerman A J, Howard C R 1979 Hepatitis Viruses of Man. Academic Press, London and New York

ACKNOWLEDGMENT

The hepatitis research programme at the London School of Hygiene and Tropical Medicine is supported by generous grants from the Department of Health and Social Security, the Medical Research Council, the Wellcome Trust, the World Health Organisation and Organon BV. The hepatitis B vaccine development is supported by the British Technology Group (formerly the National Research Development Corporation) and the Department of Health and Social Security.

Trachoma

DEFINITION AND CLINICAL ASPECTS

Trachoma is a kerato-conjunctivitis, caused by the microorganism *Chlamydia trachomatis*. The main manifestations of the disease are the formation of conjunctival follicles, together with the ingrowth of superficial blood vessels in the superior part of the cornea — a pannus. In later stages, trachoma gives rise to conjunctival scars, which may distort the eyelids to produce a trichiasis, with the eyelashes rubbing on the cornea, subsequent corneal damage and loss of vision. Other late complications of trachoma include an advanced pannus, corneal ulcers, ptosis and dryness of the eye.

Chlamydia trachomatis is a complex microorganism, which is obligatorily intracellular for its reproduction, but has its own metabolism and contains both DNA and RNA. Thus, the *Chlamydiae* appear to be related to bacteria and *C. trachomatis* is susceptible to the action of certain antimicrobics. The organism can be demonstrated as an inclusion body in conjunctival cells, and can be grown on yolk sacs of embryonated hens' eggs or special tissue cultures. Several serotypes (A — K) of *Chlamydia trachomatis* can be isolated and types A, B and C are always associated with classic endemic trachoma.

The evolution of trachoma is usually divided into four stages, in accordance with the classification given by MacCallan. After an incubation period of five to 12 days, the first symptoms are conjunctival irritation and photophobia, when small greyish follicles can be seen on the conjunctiva of the upper eyelid. In the second stage, these follicles grow bigger, and there is a general inflammatory reaction in the conjunctiva covering the tarsus — a papillary hyperplasia — together with a pannus formation. The follicles are eventually replaced by small fibrous scars (Stage III) which look like whitish lines or stars. In the final stage of the disease, there is no further active inflammation, and only conjunctival scars remain, together with other possible complications, such as corneal opacity, trichiasis and entropion.

---

* Programme for the Prevention of Blindness, World Health Organization, *Geneva*

GEOGRAPHICAL DISTRIBUTION AND EPIDEMIOLOGY

Trachoma is an endemic disease in many developing countries, with a total of approximately 500 million cases in the world, of which probably 7–9 million are blind, and a much larger number suffering from partial loss of vision. The disease is prevalent on the African continent, particularly in North Africa and the Sahel area south of the Sahara. In the Middle East and Asia, trachoma is still a severe eye disease in certain areas of several countries. In Central and South America, the disease may be found in pockets of severe intensity, leading to blindness. In the European continent, trachoma was previously a common disorder but has gradually disappeared, and today only sporadic cases may be found.

In general, trachoma in its most severe form as a blinding disease affects rural populations, particularly those with bad living conditions and poor hygiene. Overcrowding, lack of water, bad environmental hygiene and malnutrition are factors known to be associated with prevalent and severe trachoma, but the disease is also closely related to socioeconomic conditions and the way of life in a community.

The evolution and intensity of trachoma in an individual and in a community is determined by the occurrence of repeated infections, both with chlamydial and bacterial agents, which explains the great influence of hygiene and socioeconomic factors. Children usually constitute a 'pool' of chlamydial infection in affected families, thus giving rise to repeated re-infections amongst themselves and other members of the household or in the village. Trachoma is usually transmitted by personal contact or infected personal belongings, but it is probable that flies, which are attracted to ocular discharge, play a role in this context. Epidemics of seasonal bacterial conjunctivitis, which is a regular phenomenon in many developing countries, tend to aggravate the evolution of trachoma and facilitate further re-infections. Thus, there is often a 'vicious circle' of bad living conditions and repeated chlamydial and bacterial eye infections.

In hyperendemic areas, children may already show signs of trachoma at the age of a few months, with conjunctival scarring appearing from the age of four to five years. Typically, children from two to five years of age are the most infected with trachoma, and the rate of active infections then gradually tends to decline. The late complications due to trachoma usually appear in adults, often after several years of light or inactive infection. Trachoma is usually more predominant in females being found more frequently and at a greater degree of severity than in males. Females also tend to suffer more complications due to the disease later in life. Repeated re-infections resulting from more intense exposure to, and contact with, the pool of the infectious agent in children are probably of importance in this context.

In contrast to the typical picture of blinding trachoma in a developing country, eye infections with genitally transmitted *Chlamydiae* in developed countries rarely involve the eyes severely enough to cause any complications. The term 'paratrachoma' describes the chlamydial eye disease in these cases, when the ocular manifestations only rarely progress to conjunctival and corneal scarring.

PUBLIC HEALTH ASPECTS

Trachoma is one of the most common diseases found in developing countries, where it constitutes a major cause of blindness. The widespread infection in affected communities constitutes a serious risk to ocular health throughout life for its citizens. Apart from its social and educational consequences, visual disability due to trachoma adds to the loss of the labour force afflicted by other diseases. Rehabilitative measures for the blind are expensive, and often non-existent in remote areas of developing countries. This further aggravates the consequences of any blinding disease.

Trachoma is a disease closely related to poverty and to bad living conditions. The disease has gradually disappeared in communities where there have been significant improvements in hygiene and in the standard of living. Awareness of the disease and of the factors facilitating its transmission is of great importance in this context, and trachoma is a good example of a disorder where the active participation of the community in general preventive measures is indispensable. Improved personal and environmental hygiene and health education are necessary components for the control of trachoma, complementary to medical intervention schemes. The provision of water for household use and the management of human and animal wastes to control fly breeding sites also have a great impact in trachoma control. However, economic and social advancement are often slow in rural areas of developing countries, and preventive chemotherapeutic measures to avoid blinding complications from trachoma are usually, therefore, the first steps to be taken.

TREATMENT*

(a) Chemotherapy

Tetracyclines, rifampicin, erythromycin and certain other antibiotics and sulfonamides have an inhibitory effect on the trachoma agent and on most of the bacteria which may be associated with it. These substances are known to be effective in treating active trachoma. At present, the topical application of tetracyclines (eye ointment or suspension) is recommended for mass treatment of trachoma (Table 27.1). Drugs may only be administered systematically in selected cases and under medical supervision, because of the potentially serious side-effects.

* Based on the 'Guide to Trachoma Control', World Health Organization, *Geneva* (1981)

Table 27.1 Mass treatment of active trachoma (MacCallan Stages I, II or III) of severe, moderate or mild intensity

Community Prevalence of active trachoma	Basic treatment	Additional treatment	Eye health promotion
More than 20 per cent in children under 10 years of age.	Mass treatment with topical antibiotics: topical application of a 1 per cent tetracycline ointment to the eyes twice daily for 5 consecutive days or once daily for 10 days, each month for 6 consecutive months, or for 60 consecutive days. An alternative antibiotic is erythromycin.	Selective treatment of severe or moderate intensity cases with systemic antibiotics or sulfonamides, only under medical supervision in well monitored programmes (for limitations, see footnote*). Distribution of ointment to all families for self-treatment.	Improvements in personal hygiene and community sanitation, including: fly control, improvement of water supplies & waste disposal; distribution of antibiotic ointment during annual outbreaks of purulent conjunctivitis.
From five to 20 per cent in children under 10 years of age.	Mass or selective topical antibiotic treatment.	Selective treatment as described above. Distribution of ointment to affected families for self-treatment.	As above.
Less than five per cent or sporadic cases in children under 10 years of age.	Selective topical treatment with antibiotics.	Distribution of ointment to affected families.	Case finding among family members and close contacts.

* Oral therapy with tetracyclines can be recommended only on a selective basis for severe and moderate intensity cases under medical supervision during drug administration and only for children over 6–8 years of age and adult males. For pregnant women and nursing mothers, tetracyclines are not recommended because of the possibility of adverse effections on the foetus. Other potential hazards include photosensitization (worse with dimethylchlortetracycline), staining of teeth in children under about 7 years of age (least marked with oxytetracycline and doxycycline), slowing of bone growth during the period of administration, and gastrointestinal disturbances. Systemic sulfonamides are also effective, but carry a substantial risk of allergic reactions, some of which are serious and life-threatening. Furthermore, the wide use of oral tetracyclines and sulfonamides may result in the emergence of resistant bacterial pathogens.

The most economical and effective method of mass treatment of trachoma is the intermittent topical application of antibiotics, particularly tetracycline. The methodology has been improved by the introduction of evening treatment sessions, which were found to be relatively more effective and easily acceptable to the population.

In regions where seasonal bacterial conjunctivitis occurs, the treatment schedule should include the epidemic period.

In warm climates, special attention should be given to the conditions of storage and distribution of the preparations used, as their physical properties and efficacy may deteriorate.

(b) Surgical correction of trichiasis and/or entropion

The distortion of the lids, particularly the upper lid — trichiasis (misdirection of the lashes) and entropion (inward deformation of the lid margin) — are the major, potentially blinding sequelae of trachoma. The abrasion of the cornea by the eyelashes, especially when aggravated by a minor foreign body injury or by a deficiency in tear secretion, frequently results in corneal ulceration followed by scarring and visual loss. Inturned eyelids, with eyelashes rubbing on the cornea, are most common in regions with severe blinding trachoma. The inturned eyelashes can be detected with a good light directed at the lid margin, and with the lids slightly rolled away from the eye while the patient looks up and down.

Patients with inturned eyelashes should undergo surgery of the eyelids. Such surgery does not necessarily have to be dealt with during acute episodes of disease, and so can be provided at any convenient time, either by mobile teams or at the nearest eye clinic. As a temporary measure to prevent damage to the cornea and to relieve symptoms, the inturned eyelashes should be pulled out with epilation forceps, and antibiotic ointment applied at least once daily until surgery can be carried out.

ORGANIZATION OF COMMUNITY-BASED TRACHOMA CONTROL

The primary objective of public health programmes for the control of trachoma is the prevention of blindness. Community-oriented treatment of trachoma should aim to reduce the reservoir of infection, mainly in children under 15 years of age, and to carry out surgical correction of distorted eyelids. Control programmes should be focused on communities with a substantial prevalence of blinding trachoma which can be identified by the presence of persons with severe visual loss due to corneal opacity and a predominance of potentially disabling trachomatous lesions, particularly trichiasis/entropion and moderate to severe trachomatous inflammation.

Communities with severe, hyperendemic, blinding trachoma are among the most neglected, and may not have access to any effective primary health care. In such cases, specific programmes for prevention of blindness may be required in addition to the development of primary health care facilities.

Trachoma control activities should include the following elements:

1. Assessment of the problem and establishment of priorities.
2. Allocation of resources.
3. Chemotherapeutic interventions.
4. Surgical interventions to correct lid deformities.
5. Trainirg and utilization of local health aides and other non-specialized health worke·s.
6. Health education and community participation.

Preliminary prevalence surveys should identify communities with blinding trachoma and should also assess blindness rates and other causes of blindness in the community.

The selection of target populations is a critical step in trachoma control programmes. The needs of each community change continuously and should be reviewed at regular intervals. Antibiotic treatment and economic development may reduce the prevalence of the inflammatory disease. On the other hand. in communities with a substantial amount of potentially disabling scarring, new cases of trichiasis/entropion will continue to appear; the maintenance of surveillance will, therefore, be necessary for many years after inflammatory trachoma has been controlled.

Trachoma control programmes have essentially been based on the mass administration of locally applied antibiotics. In all communities requiring intervention, especially those with the most severe blinding disease, it is desirable to plan the relevant strategy in three overlapping phases:

Phase I (Attack): Initial intensive control interventions, accompanied by public information and activities to promote eye health.

Phase II (Consolidation): Continuation of specific treatment in selected population groups or individuals, as required, with further development of information and activities to promote eye health.

Phase III (Maintenance and surveillance): Integration of specific trachoma control activities with primary health care, with provision for the treatment of individual cases.

The success of the trachoma control programme depends, to a great extent, on the work carried out by auxiliary personnel and on active community participation.

Surgical correction of lid deformities has an immediate impact in preventing blindness. Experience has shown that selected and appropriately trained medical auxiliaries can carry out most of the lid surgery needed, should there be a shortage of ophthalmologists or of general practitioners trained in this work.

Once the backlog of trichiasis and entropion has been dealt with, there will be a continuing need for surgery, although on a lesser scale, since cases of potentially blinding lid distortions will continue to occur long after infective stages of trachoma have been controlled in the community.

EVALUATION OF RESULTS

Recent investigations on chlamydial infections in a community clearly indicate that the eradication of trachoma in developing countries is not a realistic goal in the near future. The aim of trachoma control programmes must, therefore, be to prevent severe eye lesions and visual loss due to the disease. Even with such an objective, several operational aspects have to be taken into consideration, including the monitoring of results achieved in intervention schemes.

Epidemiological and clinical studies on the evolution of trachoma have shown that certain risk factors for blindness can be defined, and that the intensity of trachomatous infection seems to be of crucial importance in the eventual development of blinding lesions. A scoring system to assess the degree of papillary hypertrophy and the number and localization of follicles on the tarsal conjunctiva has been established, and can be used in the evaluation of control activities. Another useful indicator of the severity of trachoma in a population is the number and distribution of potentially disabling lesions (i.e. trichiasis/entropion) or extensive conjunctival scarring. This, together with the number of disabling lesions, in the form of severe corneal opacities, indicates the consequences of trachoma in terms of risk or actual loss of vision due to the disease in a community.

The effects of control measures against trachoma — notably the application of tetracycline eye ointment in mass campaigns — are a reduction in intensity of infection, particularly in children, and a delayed onset of the disease and its more severe stages. The prevalence of active trachoma will usually only decrease gradually over a period of several years, after which there may still be a considerable amount of trachoma of mild or insignificant intensity. However, at this stage the disease no longer represents a threat to the vision of the affected population, and only a decreasing number of old cases of severe and complicated trachoma would still need attention. Experience has shown that improved living conditions and hygiene may substantially contribute to the control of trachoma, and should, therefore, be considered in the planning and evaluation of control measures.

SELECTED REFERENCES

Bietti, G B, Freyche, M J & Vozza, R 1962 La diffusion actuelle du trachoma dans le monde. Revue internationale du Trachome, 39: 113–310

Dawson, C R, Jones, B R & Tarizzo, M L 1981 Guide to Trachoma Control. WHO, Geneva

Jones, B R 1975 The prevention of blindness from trachoma. Transactions of the Opthalmological Societies of the United Kingdom, 95: 16–33

Maichuk, I F 1973 Trachoma treatment in areas of high prevalence. Revue internationale du Trachome, 50: 55–79

Majuck, J 1976 Trachoma control in the Eastern Mediterranean Region. WHO Chronicle, 30: 97–100

World Health Organization 1975 Guide to the laboratory diagnosis of trachoma. Geneva

World Health Organization 1979 Guidelines for Programmes for the Prevention of Blindness. Geneva

Tetanus

INTRODUCTION

Clostridium tetanus is one of the few spore forming organisms dangerous to man. The spores can survive for years in soil no longer actively cultivated. Its effects as a highly fatal disease are not consequent upon active invasion of living tissue but upon production of one of the most potent exotoxins occurring in nature. In this respect it is similar to the related spore formers causing gas gangrene and botulism both of which cause disease in developing countries.

Tetanus is a common and serious disease in developing countries. It has been almost eliminated in developed countries by widespread prophylactic inoculation and good medical care. In developing countries immunisation rates are low (WHO, 1980) but the World Health Organization hopes to have immunisation available for every child by 1990.

THE AGENT — *Clostridium tetani*

Clostridium tetanus is a gram positive bacillus in young cultures, motile, spore forming and it will only grow in the absence of oxygen (anaerobic); *C. tetani* spores are at the ends of the bacilli and spherical giving a drumstick appearance; they are found in the faeces of man and in animals — in street, house and often hospital dust and particularly in manured soil. Spores remain viable for months in warm, moist soil, are very resistant to adverse influences and may resist dry heat at 150°C for one hour and five per cent phenol for two weeks (Cruickshank, 1978). They are destroyed by autoclaving at 115°C for 20 minutes and by irradiation. Heat sensitive instruments can be decontaminated by soaking in a mixture of 50 per cent methanol and sodium hypochlorite to provide 2 000 p p m of available chlorine. Povidone-iodine is suitable for skin cleansing (Warrell, 1981).

Tetanus exotoxin

C. tetanus is essentially a non-invasive organism and causes tetanus by production of a powerful neurotoxin, tetanospasmin (molecular weight 67 000) potentially lethal for a 70 kg man in a dose of 0.1 mg. From the primary wound site it reaches the central nervous system along motor nerves and possibly by the blood stream. The neurotoxin binds to gangliosides in the CNS and may persist for weeks. In the spinal cord it blocks inhibitory neurones to the alpha and gamma motor systems (Henderson K K, 1980) possibly by interfering with acetylcholine release. This results in markedly increased muscle tonus and tonic spasms. A metabolite of tetanospasmin has a stimulatory effect on the sympathetic nervous system (Bizzini, 1979).

Immunity to tetanus

There are 10 different serotypes of *C. tetani*, all produce similar exotoxins and it is antitoxic immunity that is significant in protection against tetanus. An antitoxin level of .01 U/ml serum is protective against tetanus. Antitoxin is only effective if it can combine with toxin before its fixation in the CNS. An attack of tetanus may not by itself cause production of a protective level of antibodies, relapses and second attacks of tetanus occur. Immunity is dependent upon active or passive immunisation. Rarely, people are found to have protective levels of antibody without having been immunised or having had tetanus.

THE DISEASE

The following conditions are needed to permit tetanus to develop:-
1. Contamination of a wound with spores of *C. tetani* from soil, dust, air, instruments and dressings.
2. Low oxygen tension in the area of the wound to allow of emergence of the bacilli from the spore wall, multiplication and toxin production by *C. tetani*. Such anaerobic conditions are promoted by the presence of necrotic tissue, foreign bodies, bacterial infection with other pathogens and probably by quinine and calcium salts.
3. Spread of toxin to the central nervous system.
4. Fixation of the toxin in the CNS and production of its toxic effects.

Clinical picture

The incubation period is usually six to 10 days (range one to 54 days, in 90 per cent under 16 days). There is often a history of probable portal of entry for *C.tetani* but in 30–40 per cent of cases there may be no obvious entry point. Known portals of entry are listed in Table 1.

There may be a short prodromal period with fever and malaise. In most cases the first specific symptom is inability to open the mouth due to spasm of the masseter muscles (trismus). This is soon followed by neck stiffness and tonic contraction of back and abdominal muscles with arching of the back, chest pain, abdominal rigidity and restriction of respiration. Muscle rigidity is usually followed by severe tonic spasms initially in response to external stimuli but later occurring spontaneously. Spasms can affect the larynx and are followed by temporary cessation of respiration. Muscle spasms may continue for five to 21 days- rigidity can persist for weeks. There are many serious complications of tetanus including aspiration pneumonia, respiratory insufficiency and arrest, deep venous thrombosis and pulmonary embolus, renal failure, compression fractures of thoracic vertebrae, hyperpyrexia, myocarditis, gross wasting, decubital ulcers, urinary retention, autonomic crises with hypertension, tachycardias and arrhythmias, and coma associated with treatment. Long term complications include depression, insomnia, irritability and muscle contractures.

The overall case fatality rate is probably about 50 per cent and higher in neonatal than adult tetanus.

Diagnosis

This is essentially clinical. Failure of isolation of *C.tetani* by anaerobic culture in meat broth from the wound does not eliminate tetanus as a diagnosis. The converse also applies.

Treatment

This cannot be detailed but includes administration of equine antitetanus serum (A.T.S.) or human tetanus immunoglobulin (HTIG), control of spasms and rigidity with diazepam, giving penicillin, intensive nursing care and resuscitation. In severe cases tracheostomy or intermittent positive pressure respiration after neuro-muscular paralysis may be necessary. There is some evidence that intrathecal administration of HTIG or ATS is beneficial (Gupta et al., 1980). Treatment of tetanus imposes a severe strain on resources in tropical hospitals. Most have no intensive care units.

In Haiti tetanus is a serious problem and medical resources are limited. Garnier and his colleagues (1975) have succeeded in considerably improving their treatment results by employing a standardised regime, training nursing aides especially for tetanus work and using special tetanus rooms.

EPIDEMIOLOGY

The sources of *C. tetani* are the faeces of animals particularly herbivores and man; the spores are widespread in soil and dust. Spores persist longer in warm, moist soil than in dry, cool climates. Consequently people in the tropics are at particular risk. Tetanus is especially prevalent where there are (1) An agricultural community using natural manure on their crops and where there is a substantial animal population. (2) Barefoot agricultural workers with easy liability to injury. A large proportion of wounds causing

Table 28.1 Recognised portals of entry for *C. tetani*

Portals	
The umbilical cord	Often cut with dirty implements, sometimes dressed with animal dung in the tropics.
Wounds, compound fractures	Particularly war, agricultural and automobile injuries.
Injections	Many illicit injections given in the tropics, quinine is particularly dangerous; drug addicts.
Chronic ulcers	e.g. in leprosy and guinea worm infection
Burns and firework injuries	
Human, animal and snake bites	Bite victims need tetanus immunisation (and sometimes rabies immunisation).
Surgical operations Gangrenous limbs	Dangers from contaminated theatres and catgut
Operations by traditional healers	Ritual circumcision, tribal marks, ear piercing, tatooing and uvulectomy.
Septic abortion Postparum uterus	In primitive midwifery with poor hygiene.
Chronic otitis media	Chronic discharging ears are very common where health services are poor.
Eye infections	
Dental extraction	

(References — Warrell 1981, Adams et al. 1969).

tetanus occur on the foot or leg (Habte-Gabr, et al, 1978). (3) Poor health services with primitive midwifery, poor neonatal care, inadequate wound care and a low immunisation rate against tetanus. (4) Other factors which may be inferred from Table 1 include operations and injections, drug addiction, and guinea worm infection. These conditions are commonly found in many third world countries. Tetanus (particularly in neonates) has been largely eliminated in the developed countries by immunisation and good health services.

Incidence

Statistics concerning tetanus are often inaccurate — many cases (particularly neonatal ones) are not reported. Bytchenko (1978) has suggested that world-wide there may be 1 000 000 deaths a year from tetanus including 900 000 in neonates. *True* mortality rates from tetanus in various parts of the world have been estimated as $14.7/10^5$ in Asia; $27.5/10^5$ in Africa and $0.1/10^5$ in North America (Cruickshank, 1976).

Some representative statistics from World Health Statistics (1980) are shown in Table 2.

It is suggested that 95 per cent of deaths from tetanus under one year of age are neonatal (WHO 1980[2]). Clearly neonatal tetanus is a great problem in developing countries whilst it has been eliminated in advanced countries. In Bangladesh it is believed that 75 000 neonates contract tetanus yearly and 72 000 die as a result. Immunisation of non-pregnant females in Bangladesh against tetanus could reduce neonatal mortality by one third by preventing neonatal tetanus (Black, R E et al., 1980). Males are more liable to tetanus than females even in the neonatal period when there is no clear increased exposure factor.

Transmission

Patient to patient transmission of tetanus does not occur but infected dressings and instruments should be carefully dealt with. Rigorous antiseptic cleansing of an operating theatre is needed if a tetanus patient has been operated upon.

SURVEILLANCE

The extent of the tetanus problem in a community is not always easily ascertainable. Hospital statistics show tetanus as a leading cause of adult death in African countries (Haddock, 1979) but may not reveal the toll of neonatal tetanus. Special surveys may be needed to find the extent of neonatal tetanus. Surveys would have to include rural people remote from large medical centres. From the observations of mothers, birth attendants and rural medical aids it should be possible to identify deaths from neonatal tetanus (Bergrren, et al., 1981).

THE PREVENTION OF TETANUS

Consideration of the portals of entry (Table 28.1) and the pathogenesis of tetanus (see above) indicates possible preventive interventions — 1) destroying tetanus spores on instruments, dressings and in operating theatres, 2) decreasing wound contamination with spores, 3) preventing formation of anaerobic conditions in wounds, 4) destroying *C. tetani* in the body with antibiotics, 5) neutralising toxin before fixation in the central nervous system. The objective should be universal immunisation against tetanus in infancy with maintenance of immunity by booster doses of adsorbed tetanus toxoid every 10 years. When injury occurs boosters are given if wounds are contaminated or if the patient has had no booster for over five years. Some injuries causing tetanus are too small to warrant medical attention and therefore tetanus cannot be completely eliminated by adequate wound treatment. Because of its high incidence and mortality neonatal tetanus is extremely important from the preventive aspect.

Specific measures

It is recommended that all children be given 3 Diphtheria, Pertussis, Tetanus toxoid vaccinations (DPT) at intervals of at least one month starting at 2 months of age (Stanfield 1978, WHO 1981). Malaria can suppress the immune response to tetanus toxoid — it may be advisable to give malaria prophylaxis during immunisation (Warrell, 1981). Booster doses to maintain

Table 28.2 Deaths from Tetanus

Country		Deaths per 100 000 p.a.	Total deaths 0–1 year of age	Total deaths over 1 year of age
Venezuela	1977	1.1	96	76
Honduras	1976	2.0	41	23
Peru	1973	3.7	461	74
Chile	1977	0.1	2	11
U.S.A.	1977	0.1	0	24
Phillipines	1976	9.4	3,140	1,074
Thailand	1978	3.4	866	673
Italy	1975	0.3	4	162

immunity need only be given every 10 years unless a person is injured. More frequent booster doses are not advisable as recipients can become sensitised to the toxoid. To prevent puerperal and neonatal tetanus, pregnant women should be immunised against tetanus (unless having previously had a booster within five years). Even one injection may be effective in previously non-immunised women (Black R E et al., 1980). Newborns at risk can be given ATS.

Immunisation and protection after injury

The method and need for immunisation depend on the immune status of the individual and the type of wound. (Table 28.3)

Table 28.3 Guide to Tetanus Prophylaxis in the Injured[1]

Tetanus immunisation history (No. of doses toxoid)	Clean minor wounds		All other wounds	
	Toxoid	HTIG[2]	Toxoid	HTIG[2]
Uncertain	Yes[3]	No	Yes[3]	Yes
0–1	Yes[3]	No	Yes[3]	Yes
2	Yes[3]	No	Yes[3]	No
3 or more	No[4]	No	No[5]	No

[1] Modified from Center for Disease Control; Diptheria and tetanus toxoids and pertussis vaccine. Morb. Mort. Weekly Report 26: 401–407, 1977.
[2] Use equine ATS if Humane Tetanus Immune Globulin (HTIG) is not available
[3] Complete vaccination schedule (3 doses)
[4] Unless more than 10 years since last booster
[5] Unless more than five years since last booster

If given simultaneously toxoid and HTIG or ATS are given in different arms. Equine ATS is usually given in prophylactic doses of 1500–3000 units, HTIG in doses of 250–500 units.

In developed countries there is reluctance to give prophylactic ATS because of the danger of anaphylaxis, reliance is placed on toxoid, antibiotics and wound toilet. There is no risk of anaphylaxis with HTIG but this is often unavailable in the tropics. Relatively few people in the tropics have had horse serum and the risk of anaphylaxis with prophylactic doses of equine ATS is low. Because of the high risk of tetanus from wounds in the tropics, the infrequency of previous active immunization against tetanus, the rarity of anaphylaxis and the often late presentation, it is *strongly advised to give prophylactic ATS and toxoid to non-immune injured patients* in the tropics if HTIG is not available.

Non-specific preventive measures

(a) Wound treatment

Cleansing wounds, incision of dirty wound edges, removal of foreign bodies and necrotic tissue, antibiotics and avoidance of primary suture of dirty wounds help to deprive *C. tetani* of the the anaerobic environment necessary for toxin formation. *C. tetani* are sensitive to penicillin, erythromycin and tetracycline (although penicillin resistance has been met). Early chemotherapy (within six hours) can prevent tetanus but needs to be continued for at least four days in doses large enough to penetrate poorly vascularised areas, for example Benzyl penicillin 10 MU/day (Warrell, 1981) and it should be combined with immunotherapy. Metronidazole systemically and topically has also been advocated (Public Health Laboratory Service 1982) Hellberg (1970) in South Africa has found chemotherapy without ATS effective in tetanus prevention.

(b) Reducing contact with C. tetani

C. tetani is so widespread that reduction of contract is often impracticable. However, adequate sterilisation of surgical instruments, catgut, dressings and hypodermic needles is essential. It is important to have some check on the efficiency of autoclaves.

(c) The prevention of injury

This is too large a subject to cover here. Most tetanus producing wounds in agricultural workers are on the foot or leg (Habte-Gabr, 1979). Wearing of shoes would give some protection against tetanus (and hookworm).

(d) Health education and socioeconomic conditions

Tetanus declined in many countries as the socioeconomic state improved even before the widespread use of specific preventive measures (Cruick-shank, 1976). Health education is most important as many people are unaware of the efficacy of vaccination or the connection between umbilical cord hygiene, injury and tetanus. Many deliveries in developing countries are performed by traditional midwives. It is important to instruct these women in hygienic delivery and cord care. In Haiti these midwives are given training sessions, attend monthly meetings and are given sterile packages containing razor blades, cord ties and umbilical dressings (Berggren, et al., 1981).

In many tropical countries there is a widespread belief in the necessity for injection treatment. This belief is widely abused by qualified and unqualified medical practitioners who give thousands of unnecessary injections. Tetanus following injections is common. Quinine, which is often administered, seems particularly dangerous as it may cause local muscle necrosis (Diop et al., 1977). This deplorable injection cult needs countering by Health education. Nerve damage and paralyticpoliomyelitis are also occasional consequences of injections. Drug addicts should be immunised. Tetanus may follow 'operations' by Traditional Healers — it seems somewhat doubtful if education about the perils and avoidance of tetanus would have much effect on them but it might be tried.

REFERENCES

Adams E B, Laurence D R, Smith J W G 1969 Tetanus. Blackwell Scientific Publications, Oxford
Berggren W L, Ewbank D C, Berggren G G 1981 Reduction of mortality in rural Haiti through a Primary-Health-Care Program. New England Journal of Medicine 304: 1324–1330
Bizzini B 1979 Tetanus toxin. Microbiological Re Reviews 43: 224–240
Black R E, Huber D H, Curlin G T 1980 Reduction of neonatal tetanus by mass immunisation of non-pregnant women: duration of protection provided by one or two doses of aluminium — absorbed tetanus toxoid. Bulletin of the World Health Organization 58(6): 927–930
Bytchenko B 1978 cited by Furste W In: Braude A I (ed) Medical Microbiology and Infectious Disease, International Textbook of Medicine. Saunders, Philadelphia, ch 175 p 1373–1378
Centre for Disease Control: Diphtheria and tetanus toxoids and pertussis vaccine 1977 Morbidity and Mortality Weekly Report 26: 401–407
Cruickshank R 1976 Tetanus and Diphtheria. In: Cruickshank R Standard K L, Russell M B L (eds) Epidemiology and Community Health in Warm Climate Countries. Churchill Livingstone, Edinburgh, ch 8, p 77–80
Diop Mar I, Badiare S, Sow A 1977 Le tétanos après injection intramusculaire. Bulletin de la Societ M dicale D'Afrique Noire de Lange Française 22: 72–83
Garnier M J, Marshall F N, Davison K J, Leprau F J 1975 Tetanus in Haiti. Lancet 1: 383–385
Gupta P S, Kapoor R, Gazal S, Batra V K, Jain B K 1980 Intrathecal human tetanus immunoglobulin in early tetanus. Lancet ii: 439–440
Habte-Gabr E, Mengistu M 1978 Tetanus in Gondar Public Health College Hospital, Ethiopia, a review of 72 cases. Ethopian Medical Journal 16: 53–61
Haddock D R W 1979 An analysis of adult admissions and deaths in a new teaching hospital in Southern Nigeria 1973–1976. Annals Tropical Medicine and Parasitology 73: 1–10
Hellberg B W 1970 Tetanus prophylaxis — antibiotics versus antitetanus serum. South African Medical Journal 44: 496–499
Henderson D K 1980 Tetanus. In: Yoshikawa T T, Chow A W, Guze L B (eds) Infectious

Diseases Diagnosis and Management. Houghton Mifflin, Boston, ch 54, p 435–440

Public Health Laboratory Service, 1982 Tetanus surveillance and prophylaxis. British Medical Journal 284: 1715–1716

Sénécal J 1978 Tetanus. In: Jelliffe D B, Stanfield J P (eds) Disease of children in the subtropics and tropics, 3rd edn. Arnold, London, ch 25, p 696–704

Warrell D A 1981 Tetanus. Medicine International (new series) 1: 118–122

World Health Organization 1980 (1) World Health Statistics 1980. WHO, Geneva.

World Health Organization 1980(2) Weekly Epidemiological Record 55(21): 153–157

Schistosomiasis

INTRODUCTION

In stark contrast to the progress made in the containment of some parasitic diseases in the last 20 years, the continuing spread of schistosomiasis indicates man's inability or unwillingness to protect his environment.

Despite the technical advances and refinements now at the disposal of local, national or international agencies, few serious attempts are made to control schistosomiasis. The reasons are based on the propositions that our knowledge of the disease is too scanty, and that the deficiencies in medical services and their delivery of health care are too great. These premises are not applicable solely to schistosomiasis control programmes, which in any event will invariably be of public health benefit in directing attention to water-borne infections in general.

AETIOLOGY

Although man may be infected by many species of schistosomes or blood flukes of the superfamily *Schistosomatoidea*, only four species account for the overwhelming majority of human infections.

Schistosoma japonicum and *S. mansoni* live in the pericolonic venules, lay eggs characterized by a laterally placed spine, which is rudimentary in the case of *S. japonicum*, and produce 'intestinal' or 'rectal' schistosomiasis. *S. haematobium* inhabits the terminal veins in the bladder wall or in the pelvic plexus, lays eggs with a terminal spine, and produces 'vesical' or 'urinary' schistosomiasis.

S. intercalatum deserves special mention for there is evidence that in recent years it has spread from Zaire, where it was described originally, to other states in West Africa (Deschiens & Delas, 1969; Wright et al, 1972). It appears to be a species distinct from *S. haematobium*. Although the eggs of the parasite possess a terminal spine, the clinical syndrome of infection is characterized by bowel symptoms and there are other distinguishing differences in the biology of the two species.

Infrequently, man is parasitized by schistosomes which usually dwell in other mammalian hosts, for example *S. bovis* of cattle or sheep, *S. mattheei* of many herbivora, and others. Such infections are rarely of pathological significance in humans but it has been postulated that they may confer a relative type of immunity (heterologous immunity) against *S. mansoni* and *S. haematobium* infections in areas where all species co-exist (Nelson et al, 1968; Amin et al, 1968).

Although interspecific hybridisation experiments have been conducted on African schistosomes in rodents using sibling species combinations with success in the laboratory, evidence in man and in nature that infection with hybrids produces clinically or epidemiologically important problems is lacking.

The cercariae of certain non-human schistosomes may penetrate the human skin and cause 'swimmer's itch' or cercarial dermatitis. Cercariae of the blood flukes of birds: *Trichobilharzia*, *Gigantobilharzia* and *Ornithobilharzia* may be responsible. The molluscan intermediate hosts include species of *Lymnaea*, *Physa*, *Planorbis*, *Polyplis* and *Chilina*. Outbreaks of cercarial dermatitis have occurred both in tropical and temperate areas but development of the invading cercariae into adult schistosomes does not occur in man.

PARASITOLOGY

Life cycle

All species commonly infecting man have similar life cycles with a sexual generation of adult schistosomes in the definitive vertebrate host, and an asexual phase in a fresh-water molluscan host.

Adult schistosomes inhabit small diameter preterminal intra-abdominal veins; *S. japonicum* and *S. mansoni* in the superior and inferior mesenteric veins, and *S. haematobium* in the venules of the vesical and pelvic plexuses. All three species may be found as adults in the portal vein, and may occasionally find their way into ectopic sites with unusual clinical consequences. The female genitalia, the skin and the spinal cord have all been involved. *S. haematobium* frequently lays eggs in the rectal mucosa, presumably from a site in the rectal venules but such eggs are usually non-viable.

Adult worms, of separate sex, are small, with a species variation in length of six to 28 mm, and in breadth of 0.25–1 mm. While the outer surface of the integument of the female is smooth in all species, that of the male *S. haematobium* and *S. mansoni* is covered with minute spines or tubercles. The outer surface of the male *S. japonicum* is non-tuberculated.

In all species the slender filiform females are longer than the males and are held during copulation in the gynaecophoric canal of the latter formed by the infolding of the sides of the male body. Both sexes possess oral and ventral suckers which maintain the location of the adults in the blood stream.

Eggs, the microscopic appearance of which is diagnostic of the parent schistosome species, are laid by female schistosomes intravascularly towards the periphery of the capillary venules. Details and comparisons of the measurements of the three main human infecting schistosome adult and larval stages are given in a recent WHO review (WHO, 1974). Each worm pair, dependent on the species, produces 300 — 3000 eggs per day. Adult worms may live for 20–30 years, although recent epidemiological evidence suggests that the mean life-span of the majority of worms is much shorter and varies from three to eight years (WHO, 1974).

At oviposition the eggs are partly mature. Some pass through the vessel wall into the lumen of the bladder (*S. haematobium*), or bowel (*S. japonicum*, *S. mansoni*), and reach the external world with the excreta; others, which are the pathogenic agents in the tissues, embolize from their intravascular origin to liver, lung, or other sites.

If viable schistosome eggs are excreted and reach fresh water in a suitable environment of warmth and light, the larva within each egg becomes active, the eggshell ruptures or 'hatches' through the osmotic effect of the diluting water and the larva, now termed a miracidium, emerges. These actively mobile organisms are positively phototropic and negatively geotropic and tend to reach the upper strata of water bodies where the majority of their molluscan hosts congregate. Miracidia, during a life of some 24 hours, must find a suitable fresh-water snail for continuance of the life cycle. Such snails (intermediate hosts) are specific for each parasitic species involved.

Penetration of the soft tissues of snails by miracidia is influenced by numerous factors including chemotaxis, the relative numbers and the length of contact time between miracidia and snails, water temperature, water velocity and turbulence, and ultra-violet light.

Usually, only one or two miracidia undergo further intramolluscan development with the production of a sacculate mother sporocyst which in turn produces daughter sporocysts. Migration to the digestive gland of the snail and development of cercariae then ensues. After a variable incubation period within the snail, which depends in some degree on the temperature of the water, cercariae escape from the daughter sporocysts and emerge from the snail under suitable conditions of temperature, light and pH.

Cercariae are free-swimming stages of the parasite, about 1 mm in length and, after penetration of the human skin, will develop into a male or female schistosome. Those infecting man are characterized by a forked tail and a long muscular sucker. Infected snails produce a reasonably constant number of cercariae throughout their life span and many thousands may be produced from a single miracidium. Although a proportion die of their parasitism, spontaneous cure of infected snails has been observed. Probably the size of the intermediate host is the most important factor regulating cercarial output; large snails shed more cercariae than small snails other things being equal (Barreto & Barbosa, 1959).

The life span of cercariae is 36–48 hours. They are non-feeding organisms existing on large glycogen reserves. Adverse environmental factors stimulating glycogen utilization may reduce cercarial viability.

Man is infected by exposure to water containing cercariae which penetrate the skin, although mucosal penetration in the mouth or pharynx after drinking contaminated water is possible. Cercariae traverse the skin in a few minutes losing their tails in the process and becoming schistosomula. Penetration of peripheral lymphatics or venules is followed by passage to the right heart and lungs. From here, schistosomula migrate to the portal system, some by crossing the alveolar capillary bed and being transported to the mesenteric vessels, some perhaps passing directly through the diaphragm to gain access to the portal vascular system.

Further growth occurs in the intrahepatic vessels. On sexual maturity, mating occurs and the pairs migrate to the superior mesenteric veins (*S. japonicum*), the inferior mesenteric veins (*S. mansoni*) or the vesical plexus (*S. haematobium*). Egg deposition commences and the cycle is complete.

The incubation period in man is not known accurately. The period elapsing between cercarial skin penetration and the appearance and detection of eggs in the stool or urine is very variable. A period of 30–40 days is commonly quoted although many months may elapse before egg excretion is detected.

Similarly the life span of the adult worm in the body is not known accurately. Formerly, great stress was laid on evidence of the longevity of schistosomes with periods quoted ranging from 18 to 28 years (Christopherson, 1924). More recently the pendulum has swung to the other extreme. From the results of epidemiological studies of the egg output of groups of infected people, particularly in Egypt, it has been noted that a high proportion of children cease to pass eggs in the excreta within a relatively short time, in the absence of reinfection or treatment. These observations have led to the current concept, as noted above, that the mean length of life of the female schistosome is of the order of three to eight years (WHO, 1974).

EPIDEMIOLOGY

Involving a definitive host in man, an intermediate host in various species of aquatic and amphibious snail, a freshwater environment where human contact with infested water produces transmission-sites, the epidemiology and epidemiological dynamics of schistosomiasis are both heterogeneous and complicated.

Prevalence

Although schistosomiasis is one of the most widespread parasitic infections of man, second only to malaria in socio-economic and public health importance in tropical areas, there is little reliable information on global prevalence, morbidity or mortality.

In 1965 an official estimate was 180 — 200 million infected persons (WHO, 1965). Following a global questionnaire survey distributed by WHO in 1976, it was concluded that schistosomiasis was endemic in 73 countries. Although actual prevalence figures were unsatisfactory due either to the unrepresentative sampling procedures reported or to ecological and/or social peculiarities in many countries, it was estimated that the total number of people at risk of infection in the world was 500 million (Iarotski & Davis, 1981).

Geographical distribution

S. japonicum, causing Asiatic or oriental schistosomiasis, has a restricted distribution in South-East and Eastern Asia, where some five per cent of the world's population is estimated to live in the endemic areas (Mott, 1982).

In man, the distribution of *S. japonicum* follows that of *Oncomelania* snails and ranges from the Tone River Basin in Japan to Lake Lindu in Central Sulawesi.

Schistosomiasis was formerly endemic in five areas of two of Japan's five islands but the striking success of control measures led to a marked decrease in prevalence. The infection is now found only in the Kofu Basin in the Prefecture of Yamanashi on the main island of Honshu and in parts of the Chikugo river on the island of Kyushu (Yokogawa, 1970). A small focus of human infection was discovered in 1971 in the Tone River Basin of Chiba Prefecture (Yokogawa, 1973). A high proportion of the local population of *Oncomelania* snails were infected and it was suspected that this may have arisen from local infected dairy cows. Nowhere in Japan can schistosomiasis be now said to be a public health problem of major significance.

Mainland China remains the largest area of endemic *S. japonicum* infection. Particularly difficult areas are the lakes of the Yangtze River Basin, the Yangtze delta and the provinces bordering the huge Yangtze river. While in the 1950's ten million people were thought to be infected (Cross, 1976), the cumulative successes of long-continued control measures have reduced these figures to an estimate of between one-quarter and one-third of the total.

In Taiwan, schistosomiasis is enzootic but man is not infected.

In the Philippines, six of the 13 main islands are endemic for *S. japonicum* and an estimated 655 000 people are involved (Santos, 1976). There are long-standing foci in Lake Lindu and the Napu valley in Central Sulawesi in Western Indonesia.

In Laos, Khong Island in the Mekong river was initially confirmed as an important endemic area (Barbier, 1966). A parasite resembling *S. japonicum*, with a reservoir in dogs, now known as *S. mekongi* (sp. n.) (Voge et al, 1978), transmitted through *Tricula aperta*, previously termed *Lithoglyphopsis aperta*, is the causal agent. In Cambodia, the same parasite was identified near Kratie, a floating village on the lower Mekong river (Audebaud et al, 1968; Schneider, 1976).

Rarely, transmission of *S. japonicum* occurs in Peninsular Malaysia among aboriginals via *Robertsiella kaporensis* (Greer et al, 1980).

In Thailand, a *S. japonicum*-like infection has been found at autopsy (Nidtayasudthi et al, 1975) but it is doubtful whether transmission occurs in nature.

S. mansoni, causing intestinal schistosomiasis, is distributed widely in both the Old and the New Worlds. In the Middle East it is found in the Arabian peninsula and is hyperendemic in many parts of lower Egypt and in the Nile delta. In the sub-Saharan zone of continental Africa down to the Cape Province of South Africa, there are few countries in which it does not exist.

Areas of transmission in the New World are found in South America and in the Caribbean. Brazil has numerous states of endemicity. Surinam and Venezuela are infected zones. The random distribution within the Caribbean islands is seen in its occurrence in the Dominican Republic, Puerto Rico, Guadeloupe, Martinique and St. Lucia.

S. haematobium, associated with urinary schistosomiasis, occurs only in the Old World. It is endemic over large areas of Africa south of the Sahara. In North Africa it exists in the United Arab Republic (Egypt), Libya, Tunisia, Algeria and Morocco. Endemicity is recognized in Saudi Arabia, Yemen, Aden, Syria, Iran and Iraq. Control measures in Lebanon have led to a marked reduction in prevalence. Although small foci formerly existed in Israel, Turkey, Cyprus and Portugal, current data suggest that the infection is not now a public health problem in any of these countries. There is an isolated endemic area in Maharashtra State in India, the only one in the sub-continent, although the exact status of this parasite is uncertain. Some, but not all, of the islands of the Indian Ocean are endemic zones; in particular, the Malagasy Republic, Mauritius, Pemba, Zanzibar and some other smaller islands off the East African coast.

Clinical illness

Since schistosomiasis is rarely a notifiable disease, prevalence figures usually are gross underestimates. The advanced clinical symptoms and signs associated with known cases do not represent the full pattern of infection in a community and only indicate the 'tip of the iceberg'.

Classically, *S. haematobium* infection is marked by haematuria. In fact, in an endemic zone, virtually any urinary symptom should induce suspicion of the disease. In some areas, particularly Egypt and Mozambique, the strength of the statistical association between the incidence of carcinoma of the bladder and the degree of endemicity of chronic urinary schistosomiasis has suggested a causal relationship.

Severe and repeated infection with *S. japonicum* or *S. mansoni* may, rarely, produce schistosomal dysentery. More commonly, recurrent bouts of loose motions with occasional passage of blood or mucus are seen. Heavy or long-standing infection with these parasites may lead to the syndrome of clay-pipe-stem fibrosis of the liver with increased pressure within the portal tracts, followed by splenomegaly, ascites and porto-systemic varices, commonly oesophageal, which may bleed.

It should, however, be stressed that the intensity of infections is extremely variable, and that many, perhaps the majority of cases, are uncovered either during a purposive survey or incidentally in the investigation of some other complaint.

Age and sex distribution

Neither sex nor age confers absolute immunity. Areas exist where male or female prevalences may seem disproportionate when casually related to daily practices or customs. A more penetrating investigation of water contact patterns will indicate a loading variable peculiar to the higher prevalence group. This may be occupational, frequent when male prevalences are surprisingly high, or domestic, when women use infected streams for washing or rinsing clothes.

Community-based studies of schistosomiasis usually demonstrate that age-specific prevalences are highly positively skewed, this being more marked for *S. haematobium* than for *S. mansoni* or *S. japonicum*. In urinary schistosomiasis prevalence rates rise rapidly from the age when youngsters begin to wander afield, and reach their maxima in the young teenagers. In highly endemic areas it is common for upwards of 75 per cent of the young age-groups to excrete ova. Successive decades see a progressive lowering of age-specific prevalences. Indeed if such a pattern is not seen during surveys and point prevalences remain high in the older age-groups this suggests the recent onset of transmission with no immunity in the older people.

The explanation of apparent or real reductions in prevalence among the older age-groups in endemic areas depends on a number of factors. Immunity certainly contributes, although as in other helminthic infections this immunity is of a low order compared with the acquired immunity of certain bacterial infections. Tissue fibrosis may prevent eggs from reaching the exterior. A proportion of infecting worms will have died. Exposure to infected water is likely to be less with increasing age except for occupationally exposed groups. The exact roles played by immune or ecological mechanisms and their interaction remains uncertain.

Social and economic factors

In the developing countries schistosomiasis is generally an infection of rural or agricultural areas with a low socio-economic status, poor housing, a lack of water supplies other than natural sources, substandard hygienic conditions and few if any sanitary facilities. Domestic, hygienic, recreational, occupational, and in some cases religious activities bring the population into contact with water and transmission begins. Children act as an important reservoir of infection because of their indiscriminate excretory propensities, particularly urination while swimming.

It would be a mistake to label schistosomiasis as invariably a rural disease, for there are many examples of transmission occurring within the boundaries of the modern towns of Africa. The expanding populations of the periurban fringes overwhelm the available sanitation and are at risk in these situations.

Animal reservoirs

Although many animals have been shown to be hosts of *S. japonicum*, their role in transmission in endemic areas has rarely been evaluated in detail. Some 31 wild mammals and 13 domestic animals have been found to be infected in China (Cheng, 1971).

In contrast, man is the only definitive host of *S. haematobium* and the few infections with this parasite found in the baboon, the vervet monkey and the chimpanzee can be considered as merely incidental and of no epidemiological importance.

No epidemiological studies of the significance of animal infections with *S. mansoni* have been conducted but many species have been found to be infected, for example, monkeys (Jones, 1932), baboons (Miller, 1959, 1960; Fenwick, 1969) and various rodents (Schwetz, 1956; Pitchford, 1959). In South America, high infection rates were found in rodents, opossums and the peccary (Amorin et al, 1954) and in Guadeloupe, *Rattus rattus* and *R. norwegicus* were found naturally infected with *S. mansoni* (Theron et al, 1978).

Intermediate hosts

Fresh-water snails of the family *Planorbidae* transmit *S. haematobium* and *S. mansoni*. Members of the sub-family *Bulininae* trasmit *S. haematobium* while members of the sub-family *Planorbinae* transmit *S. mansoni*. Unlike these aquatic bulinids and planorbids, the snails transmitting *S. japonicum* are amphibious and belong to the genus *Oncomelania*, there being four geographically distinct forms.

For most practical purposes, schistosome transmission is species-specific, i.e. *S. haematobium* is virtually always transmitted through snails of the genus *Bulinus* as is *S. intercalatum; S. mansoni* transmission is through the genus *Biomphalaria* while *S. japonicum* is transmitted through the genus *Oncomelania* of the family *Hydrobiidae*. Rare exceptions to these generalizations exist. For example the strain of *S. haematobium* in the small focus in India is suspected to pass through an intermediate host *Ferrisia tenuis* of the family *Ancylidae*, while the *S. japonicum*-like parasite of the Lower Mekong Basin is still associated with a snail of the family *Hydrobiidae* but not of the genus *Oncomelania*.

Although the recognition, identification and proof of transmission of the various species is usually the concern of the biologist, or a specialist malacologist, the aquatic snails have several distinctive features which should be appreciated by public health physicians.

In general, transmitting snails occur in shallow waters where conditions are favourable for feeding, sheltering, and egg-laying. They require organic material for food and are found in association with thin mud, water plants or floating debris. If a sufficient growth of unicellular algae occurs, they can adapt to stony sub-strata. Any degree of organic pollution favours snail increase.

A variety of water habitats may be colonized; small streams, ponds, swamps, marshes, irrigation channels, rice paddies, seasonal water holes, borrow-pits or flowing water. *Biomphalaria* accepts flowing water of moderate velocity while *Bulinus* prefers stagnant or very slowly moving water. In some endemic zones compact water-bodies, which may be temporary in nature, are the main transmission sites. While usually thought of in connection with small water bodies, both *Bulinus* and *Biomphalaria* may be associated with large lakes, either natural as in Lake Victoria, in East Africa, or man-made such as the Volta Lake in Ghana, Kainji in Nigeria, Lake Nasser in Upper Egypt, or Kariba in Zambia.

Local conditions dictate transmission patterns and the potential permutations of man-water-snail contact are great, ranging from lake shores, small irrigation canals, drains, swamps or overgrown marshes to water bodies of a temporary nature occurring only in the rainy season. It is important to appreciate that in any large area of transmission microhabitats frequently exist where the environmental conditions are most favourable to snails.

There is great variation in snail resistance to dry conditions. If stranded on dry land by a falling water level due to evaporation or drainage, many aquatic snails die. Snails which can survive dry conditions may be carried for considerable distances in mud attached to transplanted bushes, shrubs or trees, the bodies of cattle or the feet of wading birds, and populate previously mollusc-free areas. In nature, in parts of Africa and South America, snails may aestivate, that is undergo a dormant phase in the hot season. They burrow into mud and although many die, a proportion may survive and are capable of recolonizing the habitat when it fills with water again.

The amphibious snails of the genus *Oncomelania* possess an operculum or lid which can fairly effectively seal the opening of the shell in a dry environment. The aquatic snails of the species *Bulinus* or Biomphalaria are non-operculated and are less resistant to adverse conditions.

While cross-fertilization is usual amongst aquatic species, all the intermediate hosts of *S. haematobium* and *S. mansoni* are hermaphroditic and thus capable of self-fertilization. In general the life span of these species does not exceed one year but there is a marked degree of individual species variation. Each population of snails has its own particular rate of increase dependent on the environmental variables of habitat size, the degree of crowding, food supply, temperature, pH, and the intrinsic variables of natural birth and death rates.

The oncomelanid intermediate hosts of *S. japonicum* are of male or female sex and copulation occurs repeatedly. The average life span ranges from four weeks to over twelve months in different species in different countries. Full details of mollusc biology can be found in standard works on schistosomiasis (Jordan & Webbe, 1982).

EPIDEMIOLOGICAL ASSESSMENT

Such assessments are necessary preliminaries to a projected control scheme or may be part of enquiries into local or regional endemic or epidemic morbidity studies. In the schistosomiases, each of the three epidemiological components, the definitive human host, the molluscan intermediate host and the environment, is subject to considerable variability. Thus the epidemiology presents interactions not usually encountered in other communicable diseases.

Perhaps the major difficulty is that in endemic areas, schistosomiasis is not a rapidly fulminating dramatic disease causing a high direct mortality. It is a chronic insidious infection with debilitating effects resulting in the reduction of the capacity of the infected person to contribute to the local and national economy. Many health administrations remain unconvinced of either the long-term pathological effects at the population level although they may agree that the individual, subject to repeated and heavy infections, is at considerable risk of grave sequelae. Nor do they concede that expensive control measures are justifiable when many other pressing public health problems exist. Yet Farooq (1967), in commenting on schistosomiasis in Egypt, estimated a minimum prevalence of 14 million people in a total population of, at that time, 30 million, a 35 per cent reduction in individual labour output in those infected, and a yearly economic loss to the country of some 560 million US dollars.

The methods of epidemiological study include both cross-sectional and longitudinal surveys and are dealt with conveniently under three headings.

Man — the definitive host

In the epidemiological assessment of the human population, the primary information needed is whether the disease is absent or present in a population or area, and if present, whether transmission is focal or diffuse. Four essential measurements are the prevalence of infection, the incidence of new cases, the intensity of infection and the morbidity produced.

Since these measurements depend on the accurate detection of numerator and denominator elements, the initial step is a census of the local population. The preparation of adequate maps of the area and a precise enumeration of all residents, with age and sex tabulations, in theory differs in no way from censuses conducted for other purposes. In practice, the fact that schistosomiasis is often associated with rural areas and primitive agricultural populations makes the collection of the necessary information more difficult.

While the ratio of the number affected to the total population gives a point prevalence estimate of infection, further data are needed to give a clear understanding of transmission patterns. Among these are maps showing the relationships of dwelling places to water sources and a continuing study of human-water contact patterns, which may be invaluable in explaining any clustering of infection.

The techniques used to obtain the epidemiological measurements are divisible into two groups, immunological and parasitological, each of which has advantages and drawbacks.

Immunological procedures (of which there are many) have, in practice, proved both disappointing and expensive. While numerous diagnostic techniques exist, ranging from the simple circumoval precipitin reaction test (COP), to various modifications of the enzyme-linked immunoabsorbent assay (ELISA), the multiplicity of the antigens used, the 'high technology' of the equipment necessary in many cases, and the expense of the tests, render them of more use to the research laboratory than to actual operations in the field. Although, undoubtedly reasonably sensitive and specific (Mott & Dixon, 1982), the overwhelming constraint of these immunological techniques is their failure to provide an adequate correlation with 'intensity of infection', which is essential to provide planners with a strategy for control. A recent review is provided in Jordan & Webbe (1982) and an up-to-date comparison of the performance of multiple techniques and antigens is given by Mott & Dixon (1982).

At some stage, despite their disadvantages (accuracy varies with the microscopists; the specialized equipment needed; time consumed), parasitological techniques will be used to isolate schistosome eggs. Indeed they are essential because they provide the only means of demonstrating directly the prevalence, the incidence and the intensity of infection.

There are several commonly used excretal examination techniques which are deservedly popular although comparative trials of their efficacy are lacking. Whichever technique is used the one essential requirement is that it must be quantitative. It is not enough to conduct qualitative examinations. Epidemiological sensitivity is increased disproportionately to the amount of effort involved in counting the number of eggs in excretal specimens.

Urine should be collected about noon since it is between approximately 10 am to 3 pm that there is both maximal egg excretion and minimal variability of the daily egg output in *S. haematobium* infections. The eggs in subsamples from the total bladder content are counted microscopically or a filtration technique may be used. While the early filtration procedures used filter papers, staining with Ninhydrin, Nile blue or carbol fuchsin and microscopic counting of eggs on the filter paper, recent advances have rendered these methods, if not obsolete, seldom indicated. Currently urine filtration techniques use plastic filter supports and polycarbonate (Nuclepore®) or nylon (Nytrel®) filters. The numerous advantages of these quantitative filtration techniques include rapidity of performance, low cost and reproducibility of results between technicians.

Alternatively, eggs may be hatched and the miracidia enumerated, a simple and highly accurate index of viable egg excretion.

The examination of stools by the direct faecal smear is too insensitive for routine use and it is preferable to employ a filtration-staining technique in which the eggs are collected, stained and counted on filter paper, or some variant of the Kato thick cellophane smear which is easily performed under field conditions and is suitable for the examination of large numbers of specimens.

Descriptions of diagnostic techniques are given in Jordan & Webbe (1982) and full technical details with addresses of supply agents are provided on application to the Parasitic Diseases Programme, World Health Organization, Geneva, Switzerland.

In the majority of epidemiological assessments the measurement of morbidity in man has not been attempted for there are considerable technical difficulties to be overcome in this field. The studies of the Ross Institute team in Tanzania (Forsyth & Bradley, 1964) were outstanding in demonstrating, by mass urography, the complications of *S. haematobium* infections at population level, and similar findings have now been recorded from various parts of the African continent. The subject is discussed at length in a WHO publication (1967) devoted to the public health importance of schistosomiasis.

Incidence and intensity of infection are the two most important measurements made for an assessment of man's part in the epidemiological cycle. Incidence may be measured in two ways: (a) by repeated prevalence surveys for positivity on excretal examinations; (data correction is required for subjects passing eggs initially but not on subsequent surveys and it must be ascertained whether such results are due to technical reasons such as method insensitivity or to irreversible loss of infection); (b) by detecting the occurrence of infections in a cohort of inhabitants of a suspected area known to be uninfected previously. Children should be examined since they rapidly acquire the highest prevalence rates in any area of transmission and they do not possess acquired immunity which may blur results in older age-groups.

The intensity of infection, expressed as the number of eggs excreted per standardized unit of excretal material, rises parallel with prevalence. Particularly in the younger age-groups, changes in intensity of infection are a sensitive indicator of the degree of transmission. When measuring the intensity of infection by a standard technique of egg counting, it is also useful to investigate the mean proportion of eggs which hatch under laboratory or simulated field conditions. This is a simple technique which provides an estimate of one variable for a mathematical model for the evaluation of control measures. When large human samples or populations are measured for their egg output, the resulting distributions of egg counts are of log-normal form for both intestinal and urinary schistosomiasis.

There may be particular areas, particularly in *S. japonicum* endemic zones and to a lesser degree in *S. mansoni* areas, where surveys of lower animals are necessary to detect reservoir hosts and their contribution to the transmission cycle.

Molluscan hosts

Systematic searches for snails and their collection and identification are preliminary essentials. If identification is impossible locally, suspected vectors should be forwarded to a malacological reference centre. Full details of procedures are given in WHO publications.

The identification of a snail as an intermediate host is within the scope and functions of all public health physicians. By crushing the shell and mincing the snail with dissecting needles, the tissues can be examined microscopically for daughter sporocysts and cercariae. Oncomelanid snails are rarely infected with other trematodes but confusion in cercarial identification may arise in examination of planorbids or bulinids. The exact taxonomic status of cercariae may require expert advice, but for the unaided medical officer conducting such investigations, the presence of fork-tailed cercariae whose tail length equals body length is practically diagnostic of schistosome cercariae capable of infecting man.

An alternative, rather more cumbersome method of identifying snails as carriers of cercariae, is to place them in small amounts of water, subject them to artificial light and examine for cercarial shedding after a few hours. If cercariae are shed, the snails can then be placed in individual tubes, the procedure repeated and the carrier(s) identified.

Others methods of incriminating a suspected vector involve more complex procedures and the skills of the field biologist. Cercariae may be isolated, used to infect mice or hamsters and the adult worms identified at autopsy. Eggs may be isolated from human excreta and used to infect laboratory reared snails to demonstrate that transmission is possible under laboratory conditions in the suspected intermediate host(s).

In the majority of epidemiological assessments the services of a professional biologist will be essential, as are laboratory facilities for snail maintenance, for the establishment of breeding colonies or for transmission experiments. The sampling design for snail collections and the proper use of the correct snail collecting device are only two of the essential steps. Measurements of snails are made to judge their age and to assess growth rates. The study of snail population dynamics and any seasonal trends in reproduction or mortality demands specialized malacological knowledge. For the construction of life tables of differing species under varying environmental conditions, accurate quantitative assessments of many variables in the molluscan life cycle are essential.

Allied to the epidemiological study of the molluscan hosts are certain techniques used for the identification of the free living stages of the parasite in the transmitting habitats. These techniques demand biological expertise. 'Clean' laboratory-bred snails may be exposed in field habitats for 24 hours. The snails are then placed in a holding laboratory for 12–14 days after which they are examined by standard techniques for sporocysts (Upatham, 1972). Any resulting schistosome infection indicates the degree of miracidial contamination of snail habitats.

The detection of cercariae in natural waters (cercariometry) is difficult and, despite a considerable amount of effort, returns have been disappointing. The exposure to natural waters of sentinel laboratory animals in cages has been used frequently but the technique may fail to detect low cercarial densities, and is expensive for routine surveys as a holding laboratory is needed where exposed animals are kept prior to autopsy. In addition to mouse exposure tests, a recent review listed the advantages and disadvantages of four methods of filtering large volumes of water to recover cercariae on filter paper, and a method of recovery based on the cercarial phototaxic response (Rowan, 1965). Water turbidity may impair the efficiency of these methods and it may be difficult to identify the cercariae of different species.

Improvements in these techniques can be anticipated and their utility thereby enhanced. A significant series of observations arising out of cercariometry was the demonstration of a daily cercarial periodicity in natural waters. In Puerto Rico *S. mansoni* cercarial densities were minimal in the early morning and evening and consistently maximal in the middle part of the day. Similar patterns have been seen in Africa and Brazil. This is of considerable importance with regard to human exposure and, ideally, cercariometric studies should always be combined with human-water contact observations and epidemiologic prevalence investigations to provide a complete picture of transmission.

The environment

Surveys of snail habitats, whether actual or merely suspected, depend on the accurate delineation of all water courses within a given land area. Good maps are essential and details of all permanent or temporary water bodies are plotted with other additional observations, the scope of which will vary in different circumstances. Population concentrations are of obvious importance.

Physical geographical details, fluctuations in climatic factors such as rainfall, temperature and humidity, must be collected since they may be important determinants of snail population behaviour.

The chemistry of water bodies attracted much attention in former times, but enthusiasm waned when it was appreciated that multiple interactions of individual environmental components rather than an overwhelming influence of any single factor, were of more importance in predicting or explaining the characteristics of snail populations.

Ecological descriptions of the environment remain of prime importance and should include comments on the types of water habitats existing, hydrographic factors (flow rates, permanence, dimensions), the nature of the bed, the aquatic plants, sources of pollution by man or animal and human-water contact patterns.

CONTROL

Control is not a rigid concept and must not be confused with eradication which is the complete and permanent cessation of transmission. With present methods this will rarely be achieved.

Less ambitious programmes, however, may achieve reduction in the level of transmission, in the clinical consequences of infection, and may ameliorate the socio-economic sequelae of schistosomiasis.

The aims of any control programme must vary with the characteristics of the endemic zone, the interest of the administering health authority and the personnel, time and facilities which can be allotted.

To forestall misconceptions in the minds of both the lay and professional inhabitants of an endemic area, it is essential that the objectives of a schistosomiasis control programme be clearly stated. Even a modest success is worthwhile and seldom fails to provide peripheral benefit. Nevertheless an environmental Elysium rarely follows a programme of schistosomiasis control.

In the vast majority of locations, it is extremely difficult to 'control' transmission and therefore to eradicate the infection. The reasons for this are:
— the expense of repetitive mollusciciding;
— the failure of molluscicides to achieve total kills of snails and their eggs in operationally difficult terrains;
— the restricted choice of molluscicides and the lack of incentive for industry to invest in research on new compounds;
— the lack of skilled personnel to undertake control operations;
— the unchanging, or only slowly changing, socio-economic status of the human population which perpetuates the social and domestic use of potentially infected and infective water bodies;
— the unchanging or only slowly changing environment;

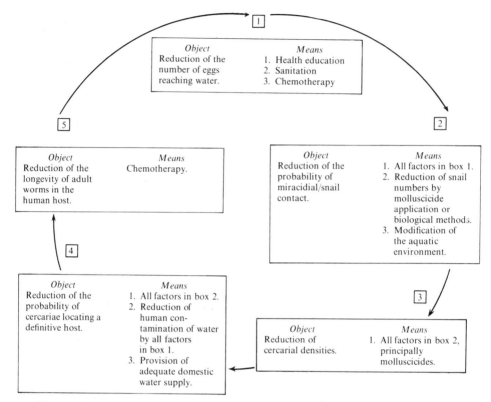

Fig. 29.1 The objects, means of attainment and their interrelationships in the control of schistosomiasis.

— the fact that maximal prevalences of infection are reached in the younger age groups whose water contact and potential for contamination of water bodies is greatest of all the different population age-groupings.

As can be seen from the schematic summary of control methods presented in Figure 1, there is much overlapping of different control techniques. These various control techniques must not be considered as individual tools although their individual values will vary under different environmental conditions.

Undoubtedly the two most valuable practical control measures are the employment of population-based chemotherapy to cure the infection in the human host or at least to reduce the intensity of infection and hence the morbidity, and the application of molluscicides to eradicate or, more commonly, to reduce the population-density of the intermediate host molluscs.

Chemotherapy

By chemotherapy is meant purposeful, large-scale, population-based drug treatment of schistosome infection in man. The treatment of individuals, or even infected groups, under normal public health policies is not regarded as an essential control tool and is unlikely to influence prevalence rates.

In few other parasitic diseases have there been advances in therapy comparable to those which have occurred in the treatment of schistosomal infections during the last 15 years. A variety of alternative drugs has become available — curative efficacy has improved markedly and side-effects of treatment have diminished in frequency and severity. That this should have occurred in a period of steadily rising research and development costs and of increasingly stringent national and international standards of drug safety, combined with uncertain prospects of market returns, is surprising. Hopefully it indicates that the chemotherapy of schistosomiasis and, indeed, of parasitic infections generally, still commands the interest of certain specialised sectors of the pharmaceutical industry.

Compared with the therapeutic scene a decade ago, treatment nowadays is a relatively simple procedure and increasing attention is being paid to the more complex clinical situations encountered.

For medically pragmatic purposes, schistosomiasis control means the prevention and control of schistosomal disease in the human population by means of operational programmes which will be implemented until it is considered that the infection and the disease it produces are no longer of major public health importance.

At that stage, previously planned surveillance and maintenance operations must be introduced with the eventual aim of incorporating these preventive and control measures into the routine public health practice of the country and within the capabilities of the local health care system.

It should be firmly stressed that schistosomiasis is a parasitic manifestation of a socio-economic syndrome with multiple symptoms resulting from ecological and social deprivation and human behavioural patterns. Naive expectations that modern technology will cause it to disappear overnight must be resisted and replaced by a balanced appreciation of the potential possibilities of the available, and future, tools for schistosomiasis control.

The time scale of the operation of schistosomiasis control is not short but the remarkable advances in antischistosomal chemotherapy of the last 20 years have reduced the active attack phase of population-based chemotherapy to two to three years if motivated and supported teams are available to undertake schistosomal morbidity control and to teach lower echelon health workers simultaneously.

One fact is certain: if ignored, endemic schistosomiasis, particularly if due to S. mansoni, worsens, transmission dynamics increase in intensity, clinical morbidity slowly becomes more serious and the increasing human reservoirs of infection act as foci to spread transmission to previously schistosome-free areas. Thus schistosomiasis control exemplifies preventive medicine in its broadest sense.

Control of schistosomiasis is neither cheap nor simple to implement.

Technical expertise and persistence in operational activities are essential. Simultaneous health education and transfer of practical technology to a broader stratum of health para-professionals must be pursued from the start to ensure continuing activities in prevention and control at the population and primary health contact levels.

The principles on which the control of schistosomiasis rests are well known but only infrequently used. They comprise:

1. Accurate demographic and epidemiological survey techniques to delineate the numerator of infections over the population denominator. Standardized quantitative parasitological, biological, epidemiological and sociological techniques should be employed to determine the relationships between intensity of infection and clinical morbidity by comparisons between different geographical areas and to provide reliable baseline data for studies on chemotherapy, malacology, sociology, and contamination patterns within defined communities. These basic data will provide the precise information necessary for control programmes to utilize in their strategies of operation and assessment.

2. The necessity of community participation, an essential element of any schistosomiasis control project. National interest should be promoted once the schistosomiasis problem is considered of high priority. Organized national efforts through acceptable mechanisms for community participation is the responsibility of those national governments and communities which undertake to implement schistosomiasis control programmes.

Important contributions to control measures can be obtained from local people if there is an adequate community organization and if the possibility exists of reaching the concerned communities through the existing political and technical structures.

Community participation must be organized as an integral part of basic health care activities and the primary health agents must be prepared to assume their responsibilities at the local level.

3. The employment of population-based chemotherapy. For the immediate future, chemotherapy will play the predominant role in schistosomiasis control and, in particular, the control of schistosome-induced morbidity in man. Although focal mollusciciding will always be a desirable input at human water-contact sites, where epidemiologically feasible, the rising costs of chemicals, the necessity for repeated application, the possibility, even though remote, of resistance in the intermediate snail hosts and the logistic difficulties of application will make chemical control of snails a subsidiary tool in transmission control and will, paradoxically, focus attention on chemotherapy.

The use of chemotherapy in control requires a clear definition of aims, selection of the appropriate chemotherapeutic agent, decisions on the dosage and time-course to be followed, and on the organization of the delivery system.

Whereas the other means of schistosome control only reduce transmission, with any effects on human worm load a secondary and delayed consequence, chemotherapy can have two immediate effects: by reducing the output of live eggs from man it diminishes transmission and by killing worms within the body it reduces the risk of disease in the treated individuals and allows recovery from such lesions as are reversible. It is important to distinguish between these two beneficial effects. The second benefits only those who are treated; the first helps the whole community. Conversely, when the reduction in transmission is incomplete, the fall in disease risk may still be considerable. Chemotherapy is thus a tool for primary (transmission, infection) and secondary (morbidity) prevention of schistosomiasis.

The strategy of primary prevention is clearly to minimise egg output, especially by those most likely to pollute transmission sites. Where egg output reduction is incomplete, we do not know the level of persisting egg excretion that can be ignored. Some epidemiological models suggest that egg production is so great relative to what is needed for continued transmission that even a small residual percentage of egg output will suffice to maintain transmission at a considerable level. It is not yet possible to say whether a few individuals with high egg excretion rates are epidemiologically more or less of a problem than many with a low egg output. It follows that the goal of primary prevention must be to reduce the egg output of as large a part of the population as possible to as near zero as can be obtained within the constraints, logistic and otherwise, of operational field practice (WHO, 1980).

Where an infected community is to be treated actively, in contrast to the passive programmes of treatment of those sick people presenting at health care facilities with symptoms, two main approaches are possible. In one, the whole population is examined parasitologically and those found infected are treated. This is termed selective population chemotherapy (SPC), that is the treatment of all the infected cases within the population. Various modifications of SPC can be used in particular epidemiological situations, for example, SPC in a specific age group; in an occupational high risk group and so on. One variant of SPC is the so-called 'targetted' chemotherapy strategy where therapy is directed to those with high excretal egg outputs who are at particularly high risk of severe morbidity. This has not yet been tested adequately in the field. Treatment is basically related to individual risk of morbidity and many important questions on the efficiency of the parasitological detection procedure and its cost arise when the efficacy of the treatment is assessed in an overall evaluation.

In an alternative approach to population-based chemotherapy, sample parasitological surveys for infection are conducted in populations. Where the prevalence and intensity of infection reach a predetermined level, which must be decided individually for each epidemiological setting, then treatment is given to the whole population or to a particular predetermined segment based on age, sex, or occupation whether a particular individual within that group is infected or not. This may be termed a group risk approach. In general the first alternative is preferable, but where prevalences and intensities of infection are very high in samples then it may be wasteful of scarce resources to continue surveying and the second group approach would be adopted (WHO, 1980).

Available chemotherapeutic compounds

A variety of highly effective drugs now exist for the treatment of schistosomiasis. Traditionally, drugs were either antimonials or non-antimonials, but since the use of the former has declined markedly in parallel with the advent of new compounds, the classification has outlived its utility.

The great majority of uncomplicated cases of schistosomiasis can, with modern drugs, be treated in the home, the out-patient clinic or the rural dispensary.

For *S. haematobium* infections, metrifonate is cheap and well-tolerated but has the disadvantage of necessitating repeated doses. Praziquantel is highly efficacious in a single oral dose. Standard niridazole and antimony therapy are second choices and experience with Oltipraz is as yet limited.

S. mansoni infections can be treated easily with oxamniquine, with good patient tolerance, and praziquantel is again an effective agent. Oltipraz is also highly effective in a single oral dose. One of the major therapeutic advances of recent years is in the provision of highly effective yet well-tolerated drugs which can be used to treat complicated cases of late *S. mansoni* infection such as advanced hepatosplenic schistosomiasis (Farid et al, 1980) or diffuse colonic polyposis (Farid et al, 1976), conditions which until only a few years ago posed difficult problems in management. As with (*S. haematobium*) infections, niridazole or antimony can be used if no alternatives are available, but care must be taken and troublesome side-effects anticipated.

Persons doubly infected with *S. mansoni* and *S. haematobium*, of frequent occurrence in the Egyptian Delta, the Sudan and many areas of sub-Saharan Africa, can be given praziquantel, effective against both parasites and well tolerated, or combined oxamniquine and metrifonate treatment. Oltipraz promises to offer another choice of drug. A third alternative in otherwise healthy adults would be hycanthone and, finally, niridazole or antimonials are available.

In *S. japonicum* infections, the treatment of which was always unsatisfactory, praziquantel is the treatment of choice. It is too early to assess the future role of amoscanate but there is little doubt of its efficacy. Finally, niridazole and antimonials can be used although with care and in the dual knowledge of rather poor cure rates and the occurrence of troublesome side-effects.

For the treatment of *S. intercalatum* or other more exotic species infections, praziquantel will be the primary drug.

Detailed reviews of the chemotherapy of schistosomiasis have been produced recently (Davis, 1982a,b).

Population-based chemotherapy will rapidly reduce the prevalence, intensity and morbidity of schistosomal infection but, unless a surveillance system is instituted and due attention paid to intermediate host dynamics, the indices of infection will rise gradually so necessitating repeated chemotherapy, the timing of which will be dependent on the local epidemiological dynamics.

Molluscicides

The use of molluscicides in control is a specialized field. The selection of one of the available compounds, the determination of dose and exposure time productive of maximum effect at minimum cost, the preferred formulation to apply, the appreciation of both short and long-term side effects on the biota of snail habitats, must all be considered. The general strategy of mollusciciding and the physical method of application is likely to vary with the water habitats encountered.

Where transmission is limited to well-defined small areas, focal control by periodic molluscicide application may be favoured. Where transmission is widespread then blanket control (area control) may be the only feasible approach.

Synthetic molluscicides are virtually restricted nowadays to one compound, niclosamide ('Bayluside®'). For detailed reference, use should be made of the latest specialist textbook (Jordan & Webbe, 1982).

In view of the rising costs of chemical molluscicides, interest has been reactivated in those of plant origin (Webbe & Lambert, 1983) but the practical outcome of research into these compounds is likely to occupy many years and the eventual outlook is blurred.

It should be understood that although mollusciciding *per se* can control transmission (WHO, 1978), such programmes are long-term commitments. This point is not always appreciated. In theory, control by molluscicides alone may take up to 20 years (Macdonald, 1965), but the addition of chemotherapy will shorten this interval immensely. Even so, continuation of molluscicidal activities must be maintained for many years in order to eradicate (or diminish) transmission.

Other control measures

While stress has been laid on the two major control tools of molluscicides and chemotherapy, the other forms of control, modification of the environment, provision of sanitation and health education must be regarded as essential but the time scale of their effects is longer. The provision of piped water supplies will reduce human contact with infected water markedly. This has been demonstrated in both St. Lucia and South Africa. Prevalence and incidence may be expected to fall slowly over some years.

The provision of latrines as a sole control measure was shown to be ineffective in a classical field study in Egypt in 1938 (Scott & Barlow, 1938) and Macdonald in 1965 again stressed that it would have little effect on the worm load in the community. Transmission can be maintained by minute amounts of contamination. Nevertheless the provision of adequate sanitation increases the chances of success of other control measures and carries peripheral benefits.

Many attempts have been made to use biological agents to control the intermediate hosts of schistosomiasis but with little success. The difficulties of ensuring supervision of the activity and spread of natural parasites or predators of snails gives little hope that biological control methods will play any major role in the containment of the disease. The most successful of such methods has used the ampullarid snail *Marisa cornuarietis* to reduce populations of *Biomphalaria glabrata* but this tends only to achieve adequate results in impounded waters with a low background of aquatic vegetation.

In summary the evidence suggests that schistosomiasis will rarely be controlled by any single measure although there are examples of success where the epidemiological circumstances are favourable, e.g. chemotherapy of *S. haematobium* in Iran; molluscicides in certain areas of Japan.

Combinations of control measures are essential for optimum success rates and the comprehension and participation of the affected communities is necessary. Barbosa (1972) has vividly emphasized the desirability of a comprehensive rural health service as part of broader programmes of community development and to serve as a base for control campaigns in schistosomiasis.

THE FUTURE

Undoubtedly, the next ten years will see the use of large scale chemotherapy in the control of morbidity in human schistosomiasis. Whether this will have a parallel effect in diminution of transmission of infection is, as yet, unknown. Perhaps the resultant diminution in human morbidity will enable populations to live in a 'reasonable symbiosis' with the schistosomes?

REFERENCES

Amin M A, Nelson G S, Saoud M F A 1968 Studies on heterologous immunity in schistosomiasis. 2.Heterologous schistosome immunity in rhesus monkeys. Bulletin of the World Health Organization 38: 19–27
Amorin J P de, da Rosa D, Lucena D T de 1954 Ratos silvestres, reservatorios do Schistosoma mansoni no nordeste do Brasil. Revista Brasileira de Malaciologia e Doencas Tropicais 6: 13–33
Audebaud G, Tournier-Lasserve C, Brumpt V, Jolly M, Mazaud R, Imbert X, Brazilo R 1968 Premier cas de bilharziose humaine observé au Cambodge (Région de Kratié). Bulletin de la Société de Pathologie Exotique 61: (5)778–784

Barbier M 1966 Détermination d'un foyer de bilharziose artérioveineuse au Sud Laos (Province de Sithadones). Bulletin de la Société de Pathologie Exotique 59: 974–983

Barreto A C, Barbosa F S 1959 Qualidades de vetor dos Lospedeiros de S. mansoni no nord-este do Brasil. 4.Eliminaçao de cercarias de Schistosoma mansoni por Australorbis glabratis de diametros diversos. Anais da Sociedade de Biologie de Pernambuco 16: 13

Cheng T H 1971 Schistosomiasis in mainland China. A review of research and control programs since 1949. American Journal of Tropical Medicine and Hygiene 20: (1) 26–53

Christopherson J B 1924 Longevity of parasitic worms. The term of living existence of Schistosoma haematobium in the human body. Lancet 1: 742–743

Cross J H 1976 Schistosomiasis japonica in China: a brief review. South East Asian Journal of Tropical Medicine and Public Health 7: 167–170

Davis A 1982a Management of the patient with schistosomiasis. In: Jordan P, Webbe G (eds) Schistosomiasis. Epidemiology, Treatment and Control, William Heinemann Medical Books Ltd, London, p 184–226

Davis A 1982b Available chemotherapeutic tools for the control of schistosomiasis. Behring Institute Mitteilungen, Behring Institute Research Communications 71: 90–103

Deschiens R, Delas A E 1969 L'extension géographique de la bilharziose à Schistosoma intercalatum en Afrique tropicale. Transactions of the Royal Society of Tropical Medicine and Hygiene 63: (4) Suppl. 557–565

Farooq M 1967 Progress in bilharziasis control. World Health Organization Chronicle 21: 175–184

Fenwick A 1969 Baboons as reservoir hosts of Schistosoma mansoni. Transactions of the Royal Society of Tropical Medicine and Hygiene 63: (5) 557–567

Forsyth D M, Bradley D J 1964 Irreversible damage by Schistosoma haematobium in schoolchildren. Lancet 2: 169–171

Greer G J, Ow-Yang C K, Singh K I, Lim H K 1980 Discovery of a site of transmission and hosts of a Schistosoma japonicum-like schistosome in Peninsular Malaysia. Transactions of the Royal Society of Tropical Medicine and Hygiene 74: (3) 425

Iarotski L S, Davis A 1981 The schistosomiasis problem in the world; results of a WHO questionnaire survey. Bulletin of the World Health Organization 59: (1) 115–127

Jones S B 1932 Intestinal bilharziasis in St Kitts (B.W.I.). Journal of Tropical Medicine and Hygiene 35: (9) 129–136

Jordan P, Webbe G (eds) 1982 Schistosomiasis. Epidemiology, Treatment and Control, William Heinemann Medical Books Ltd, London, pp 361

Macdonald G 1965 The dynamics of helminth infections, with special reference to schistosomes. Transactions of the Royal Society of Tropical Medicine and Hygiene 59: 489–506

Miller J H 1959 (Correspondence) East African Medical Journal 36: 56–57

Miller J H 1960 Papio doguera (dog-face baboon), a primate reservoir host of Schistosoma mansoni in East Africa. Transactions of the Royal Society of Tropical Medicine and Hygiene 54: 44–46

Mott K E 1982 S. japonicum and S. japonicum-like infections. In: Jordan P, Webbe G (eds) Schistosomiasis. Epidemiology, Treatment and Control, William Heinemann Medical Books Ltd, London, p 128

Mott K E, Dixon H 1982 Collaborative study on antigens for immunodiagnosis of schistosomiasis. Bulletin of the World Health Organization 60: (5) 729–753

Nelson G S, Amin M A, Saoud M F A, Teesdale C 1968 Studies on heterologous immunity in schistosomiasis. I. Heterologous schistosome immunity in mice. Bulletin of the World Health Organization 38: 9–17

Nidtayasudthi T, Jaroonvesama N, Dharamadhach A 1975 Schistosomiasis from a new locality in Thailand: a case report. Journal of the Medical Association of Thailand 58: (10) 542–546

Pitchford R J 1959 Natural schistosome infections in South Africa rodents (correspondence). Transactions of the Royal Society of Tropical Medicine and Hygiene 53: (2) 213

Rowan W B 1965 Ecology of schistosome transmission foci. Bulletin of the World Health Organization 33: 63–71

Santos A T 1976 Prevalence and distribution of schistosomiasis in the Philippines: a review. South East Asian Journal of Tropical Medicine and Public Health 7: 133–136

Schneider C R 1976 Schistosomiasis in Cambodia: a review. South East Asian Journal of Tropical Medicine and Public Health 7: 155–166

Schwetz J 1956 Role of wild rats and domestic rats (Rattus rattus) in schistosomiasis of man. Transactions of the Royal Society of Tropical Medicine and Hygiene 50: 275–282

Scott J A, Barlow C H 1938 Limitations to the control of helminth parasites in Egypt by means of treatment and sanitation. American Journal of Hygiene 27: 619–648

Theron A, Pointier J P, Combes C 1978 Approch eécologique du problème de la responsabilité de l'homme et du rat dans le fonctionnement d'un site de transmission à Schistosoma mansoni en Guadeloupe. Annales de Parasitologie Humaine et Comparée 53: (2) 223–234

Upatham E S 1972 Exposure of caged Biomphalaria glabrata (Say) to investigate dispersion of miracidia of Schistosoma mansoni Journal of Helminthology XLVI: 297–306

Voge M, Bruckner D, Bruce J I 1978 Schistosoma mekongi sp. n. from man and animals, compared with four geographic strains of Schistosoma japonicum. Journal of Parasitology 64: (4) 577–584

Webbe G, Lambert J D H 1983 Plants that kill snails and prospects for disease control. Nature 302: (5911) 754

World Health Organization 1965 Expert Committee on Bilharziasis. World Health Organization Technical Report Series 299: 7

World Health Organization 1967 Measurement of the public health importance of bilharziasis. World Health Organization Technical Report Series 349

World Health Organization 1974 Immunology of schistosomiasis. Bulletin of the World Health Organization 51: 553–595

World Health Organization 1980 Epidemiology and control of schistosomiasis. World Health Organization Technical Report Series 643: 31–35

Wright C A, Southgate V R, Knowles R J 1972 What is Schistosoma intercalatum Fisher 1934? Transactions of the Royal Society of Tropical Medicine and Hygiene 66: 28–64

Yokogawa M 1970 In: Sasa M (ed) Recent Advances in Researches on Filariasis and Schistosomiasis in Japan, University of Tokyo Press, Tokyo. University Park Press, Baltimore, Maryland and Manchester, England, pp 23–255

Yokogawa M 1973 Symposium II. Recent advances in research on schistosomiasis. Epidemiology of schistosomiasis japonica. Japanese Journal of Tropical Medicine and Hygiene 1: (2)129

Epidemiology and control of malaria

INTRODUCTION

Malaria has compelled the attention of public health workers throughout the world ever since, more than three quarters of a century ago, Ross showed how it was transmitted. After the Second World War the availability of residual insecticides and new antimalarial drugs heightened interest in control measures and in the past 14 decades malaria has claimed a greater share of the world's scientific and financial resources than has any other disease. Yet, today, malaria remains a major, in developing countries probably the major, health hazard. Its ability to strike back in devastating fashion during eradication campaigns when pressure against it is relaxed prematurely is now well recognized and has emphasized that such campaigns must only be planned in the light of full and detailed knowledge of the epidemiology of malaria in the area under consideration. This brief review is presented as a broad and very general account of some of the more important factors that shape the epidemiological pattern of the disease and of current concepts regarding its control and eradication. There already exists a voluminous literature on both these aspects of malaria, much of which is admirably summarized and assessed with appropriate references in textbooks and manuals. Recommendations for further reading are made as perhaps the best way of facilitating access to this information.

The epidemiology of malaria

The following map shows the World Health Organization's epidemiological assessment of the world malaria situation in December 1980 and also provides an indication of the known limits of malaria transmission.

The epidemiology of malaria may vary from country to country and between different areas of a single country. At one extreme it may be unstable, occurring in epidemics separated by regular or irregular intervals of low incidence. At the other extreme it may persist in a stable state where little difference in incidence occurs from year to year. Between these two extremes a range of intermediate forms occur.

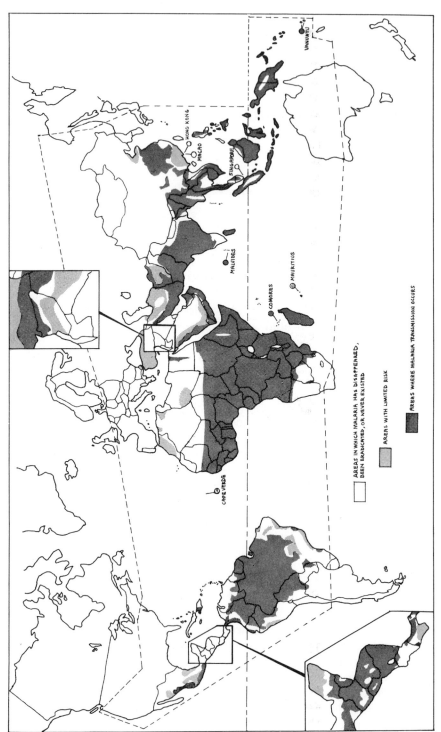

Fig. 30.1 Malaria situation, December 1980

Unstable malaria results from the sudden development of circumstances which favour the transmission of infection at levels far above those that usually prevail. It presents as an acute febrile illness which affects all age groups in the community more or less equally. Occurring in clear-cut epidemics, its effect in terms of morbidity and mortality and its adverse influence upon the economy of the affected area are usually severe and unmistakable. Levels of communal immunity, which may be relatively high in the immediate post-epidemic period, decline until they are virtually non-existent by the time the next epidemic occurs. The epidemics that have been described from some regions of Ethiopia constitute an example of this epidemiological form. In late 1958 one such epidemic ravaged an area of 100 000 square miles and caused some three million cases of which 150 000 proved fatal.

Stable malaria occurs where transmission rates remain high year after year. Transmission may be perennial or influenced markedly by season but must be intense enough to ensure repeated reinfection of the entire community within the period of a single year. Communal immunity is in consequence maintained at a high level and clinical malaria is usually restricted to young childhood where acute, febrile episodes occur separated by long or short periods of relatively asymptomatic parasitaemia. As childhood advances the frequency and duration of febrile illness diminishes and gradually an ability to restrict even asymptomatic parasitaemia is developed. In adult life, febrile malaria is infrequent and usually mild but low grade parasitaemia remains demonstrable at a prevalence of about 25 per cent. Against this background of widespread parasitaemia the effects of stable malaria on health and economy are difficult to evaluate. Mortality directly due to malaria may be as high as 10 per cent over the first three years of life. The indirect effects have never been satisfactorily assessed but, since parasitaemia has been shown to suppress the immune response of young children to certain bacterial antigens, and since immune complexes are now known to form and circulate in the course of infections they may well be considerable. At older ages the effects of malaria become even more blurred. Adults in intensely malarious regions develop an immunity which is strong enough to maintain productivity at an economic level. The cost to health of maintaining that immunity, however, is unknown and, although assertions are sometimes made to the contrary, the extent to which the productivity of immune adults can be increased by freedom from malaria is by no means clear.

FACTORS WHICH INFLUENCE THE EPIDEMIOLOGY OF MALARIA

Many factors combine to shape the pattern of malaria within a community. Some, including climatic influences, are essentially environmental, some derive from intrinsic characters of the parasite and its vectors while probably the most important of all is man's immune response to infection. Careful study and evaluation of these factors are essential to the understanding of malaria in any area. Ross recognized this and advocated the mathematical consideration of these variables. He was the first to produce mathematical formulae by which the epidemiological state of malaria in a locality could be appraised rationally. This line of approach was, in more recent years, greatly extended by the late Professor George Macdonald, and has been further developed in the Savannah area of Africa to assist in the selection of control measures that are locally appropriate.

Environmental factors

Wherever anopheline mosquitoes coexist with a reservoir of infection, transmission is primarily influenced by the interaction of atmospheric temperature, rainfall and humidity. Since the mosquito is poikilothermic, none of the four plasmodial species that infect man can develop in it successfully when the constant air temperature falls below 15 °C. Thus, the limits of the distribution of *P. vivax*, probably the hardiest of the human parasites, lie within the 15 °C summer isotherms, while those for *P. falciparum*, which has more exacting requirements, lie within the 20 °C isotherms. Temperature also influences the rate of development of the parasite's extrinsic cycle. At 16 °C, *P. vivax* requires 55 days for full development but at 28 °C the cycle is reduced to seven days. High temperatures are detrimental to parasite development in the mosquito; those in excess of 32 °C tend to be lethal. Optimal temperatures are probably in the region of 27 °C.

Temperature also influences mosquito activity. In countries possessing a well marked cold season or winter, fall in air temperature may cause mosquitoes to hibernate until the return of warmer weather. When air temperatures are high the relative humidity or, more accurately, the saturation deficit, or drying capacity of the air, becomes most important. Mosquitoes are extremely sensitive to dehydration and in a hot and arid environment their longevity is reduced and they must drastically curtail their activities or perish. Until recently it was not understood how vectors could seemingly disappear during a long, hot, dry season and yet reappear suddenly to recolonise pools formed when the rains returned. Studies in the central Sudan, where the hot rainless season lasts for nine months, have now shown that some female *A. arabiensis* survive by aestivating in selected micro-climates and, although they continue to blood-feed as the opportunity presents and therefore to transmit malaria at a low level, they manage to retard or suppress egg development until the rains provide breeding places.

Rainfall, too, is important. Where distinct wet and dry seasons occur the duration of rains may largely determine the extent of the malaria season. The effects of amount and distribution of precipitation are complex and will vary according to the bionomics of the vectors in the area. Heavy rainfall may damage or flush out larvae with a subsequent diminution in transmission. Alternatively, it may cause the formation of many new breeding sites capable of supporting the customary main vector or of favouring the rapid multiplication of an important, but not usually prevalent, vector species with the result that transmission is enhanced.

Man-made alterations to the environment can cause climatic changes which may alter epidemiological patterns. The introduction, for example, of extensive irrigation systems into areas where vector activity usually declines to low levels during a dry season may serve to maintain *Anopheles* density and longevity at a level at which substantial transmission can occur.

Factors involving the vector

Only *Anopheles* mosquitoes transmit malaria and to be efficient vectors they must possess four characteristics. First, they must be moderately susceptible to infection by gametocytes. Second, they must feed frequently upon man. Third, they must live long enough to permit development of the extrinsic cycle of the parasite. Fourth, they must be present in adequate numbers to maintain transmission.

Studies in laboratories involving infection of *Anopheles* have often indicated considerable variation between different species in their susceptibility to infection, while field investigations have shown that genetically distinct, but almost morphologically identical members of a single species complex may have very different habits. Species A (A. *gambiae* [*sensu stricto*]) and B (A. *arabiensis*) of the A. *gambiae* complex, which each appear to have different breeding habits, feed frequently upon man and are consequently good vectors while species C (A. *quadriannulatus*) is believed to feed mainly on animals and to be of little importance as a vector of human malaria.

The ability of a vector to change the epidemiological pattern of malaria in an area is well exemplified by the accidental introduction of A. *gambiae* (*sensu lato*) into Brazil in 1930. An epidemic ensued which was more severe than any the country had experienced beforehand and which was associated with such high mortality that some districts became almost totally depopulated. It is thought that A. *gambiae* (*sensu lato*) proved to be a much more efficient vector than the resident Brazilian anophelines and that the increase in transmission rates it produced was the principal factor which triggered the epidemic.

Factors involving the parasite

Given equal environmental conditions some plasmodial species complete their development in mosquitoes faster than others. At 25 °C, for example, *P. vivax* will complete its extrinsic cycle in 10 days while *P. falciparum* requires 12 days, *P. ovale* 16 days and *P. malariae* 28 days. The ability to render infective mosquitoes of moderate longevity is epidemiologically important and explains why *P. vivax* and *P. falciparum* can rapidly become epidemic while *P. malariae* rarely becomes so.

The four species vary in their capacity to multiply within man and so differ in lethality. In both the exo-erythrocytic and erythrocytic phases *P. falciparum* multiplies faster than the other species and rapidly produces extremely dense parasitaemia which often overwhelms the defences of the host with fatal results. Epidemics of *P. falciparum*, therefore, are usually marked by high mortality rates. The other three parasite species have slower rates of multiplication and infections with them are not usually fatal.

Differences also occur in gametocyte production and consequently in the ability to infect mosquitoes. In infections with *P. vivax* and *P. falciparum* gametocyte production is profuse while in infections with the other two species it is scanty. Furthermore, gametocytaemia in primary infections occurs within two or three days of the onset of asexual parasitaemia in infections with *P. vivax* but in the case of *P. falciparum* it tends to occur much later, at a time when asexual parasitaemia is declining. Profuse, early gametocytaemia favours the rapid and progressive epidemic spread of *P. vivax* while late gametocytaemia in the case of *P. falciparum* enforces slower epidemic development.

Differences may exist between infections caused by a single plasmodial species. Vivax infections in different parts of the world may show striking variations in the duration of the incubation period which may sometimes be as long as nine months, and also in the length of periods of latency that precede relapses.

Finally, the longevity of parasites within man is variable. *P. falciparum* is the least persistent and most infections with it do not appear to last more than a year although some may persist for more than three years. *P. vivax* infections are more persistent and, although most die out within three years, some may last for more than five. *P. malariae* infections are the most long-lived and records exist indicating persistence in the absence of reinfection for periods of more than 30 years. The longevity of *P. ovale* is probably similar to that of *P. vivax*. The mechanism by which the parasite can survive within the host for long periods is not known.

Factors involving man

Man himself is the principal source of the malaria parasites that infect him and although certain other primates can be infected experimentally there is as yet little evidence to indicate that these animals constitute an important reservoir of infection in natural circumstances.

Humans are not all equally susceptible to plasmodial infection and today several genetically controlled polymorphisms, notably of the erythrocyte, are recognised as important factors in the shaping of epidemiological presentations of malaria within communities. The capacity of merozoites to penetrate erythrocytes successfully is dependent on the presence of appropriate receptor sites on the red cell membrane. Glycophorin A and glycophorin B appear to constitute receptor sites for merozoites of *P. falciparum* and erythrocytes lacking these sialoglycoproteins resist invasion by this species. For the merozoites of *P. knowlesi* and probably also of *P. vivax* there is evidence that the route of invasion involves the antigens of the Duffy blood group, and the relative absence of *P. vivax* infections over much of West Africa is today attributed to the high prevalence of the Duffy negative phenotype (Fy-Fy) in residents of that area.

Factors within the red cell are also important. Heterozygosity (HbAS) for the sickle cell gene is generally accepted as conferring on the host a survival advantage in *P. falciparum* infections. In this instance the mechanism appears to involve the selective destruction of parasitized erythrocytes in conditions of low oxygen tension, thus limiting the rate of parasite replication. Erythrocytes deficient in the enzyme glucose-6-phosphate dehydrogenase (G-6-P-D) are prone, when infected, to damage by oxidants generated by the parasite so that G-6-P-D deficiency may also confer survival advantage by restricting plasmodial replication. In some areas of the world the consumption of potent dietary oxidants, e.g. fava beans, may potentiate the effects of G-6-P-D deficiency and thus materially enhance host protection against the lethality of *P. falciparum* infections. Other genetic conditions which have been considered to contribute to innate immunity to malaria include HbF, the haemoglobinopathies, HbC and HbE, thalassaemia and ovalocytosis. The bases of protection in these latter conditions and their practical significance in terms of host survival are not well understood at present.

However, the most important single factor which shapes the epidemiological patterns of malaria within human populations is the acquisition of immunity which follows intense and prolonged parasitaemia. In areas of instability malaria transmission and, consequently, parasitaemia is too inconsistent to stimulate any effective level of immunity throughout the community and so in all ages from the youngest to the oldest infection usually produces acute febrile illness. Even newborn infants may show clinical infections which have been congenitally acquired. On the other hand, where malaria is stable transmission is frequent enough to stimulate effective immunity which is evident at all ages apart from early childhood. The immune response to naturally acquired infections appears to be effective only against asexual erythrocytic stages of the parasite and even strongly immune individuals continue to be capable of infecting mosquitoes, albeit at low levels. Acquired immunity in man involves complex interactions between cellular and humoral components which probably activate both specific and non-specific effector mechanisms. The precise locations of parasitic destruction are not known with certainty, although the liver and the spleen are probably both important organs in this respect. Specific malarial antibodies occur in the immunoglobulin (Ig) G, M and A fractions of immune human sera. Those of the IgG isotype have been shown to be protective; the function of those belonging to IgM and IgA is not yet known. Antibodies of the subclasses IgG1, IgG3 and IgG4 cross the human placenta with facility and high concentrations of IgG with antimalarial specificity are to be found in the cord blood of infants born in highly malarious regions. Antibodies passively acquired in this way are currently believed to account for two important features of stable malaria, namely the rarity of clinical malaria resulting from congenitally acquired infections, and the relative freedom from infection which the newborn enjoys for the first few months of life.

It seems likely that the degree of immunity acquired in areas of stable malaria is governed by the number of viable sporozoites inoculated by the mosquito at the time of feeding. Thus in areas where sporozoites are frequently inoculated in large numbers higher levels of effective immunity may be attained than in areas where the magnitude of sporozoite infection is usually of a low order. Such a hypothesis could account for the increased malarial morbidity in indigenous populations which has been sometimes observed as the result of the introduction of a new and more efficient vector or which has followed the large scale immigration of non-immunes, causing a subsequent sharp increase in the gametocyte reservoir.

Acquired immunity is species-specific and largely strain-specific. Immunological techniques are not yet sufficiently developed to permit any estimate of the number of different strains that may exist in a single locality or to compare the antigenic identities of strains of the same species obtained from different geographical areas. Thus, while the introduction of a new and virulent strain of parasite could theoretically adversely affect host-parasite equilibrium in an area of stable malaria, the importance of the event cannot yet be estimated with accuracy.

The measurement of malarial endemicity

The measurement of splenic enlargement has for decades provided one of the classical indices in malariometry.

For the past 25 years the percentage of children aged two to nine years showing enlargement of the spleen (spleen rate) has been used as an index of the prevalence of malaria. The classification is shown in Table 30.1. It

Table 30.1

Endemicity		Spleen rate (children 2–9 years)
Low	(Hypoendemic)	10 per cent or less
Moderate	(Mesoendemic)	11–50 per cent
High	(Hyperendemic)	Constantly over 50 per cent and associated with high spleen rates in adults
Very High	(Holoendemic)	Constantly over 75 per cent and associated with low spleen rates in adults

is not entirely satisfactory. In warm climates diseases other than malaria can cause splenic enlargement and even when these can be discounted it is frequently impossible from spleen rate data alone to decide whether an area should be classified as hyperendemic or holoendemic.

More pertinent are age-specific parasite rates, i.e., the prevalence of parasitaemia by age. Where malaria is intensely endemic and where treatment facilities are few, parasite rates rise rapidly in early childhood and may be in the region of 100 per cent at three to four years. In older childhood they begin to fall and tend to level off in adult life at about 20–25 per cent. In areas of lower endemicity lower parasite rates are found in young children but higher rates may occur in adults. Parasite rates should be based on the examination of stained thick blood films. At least 100 oil immersion fields

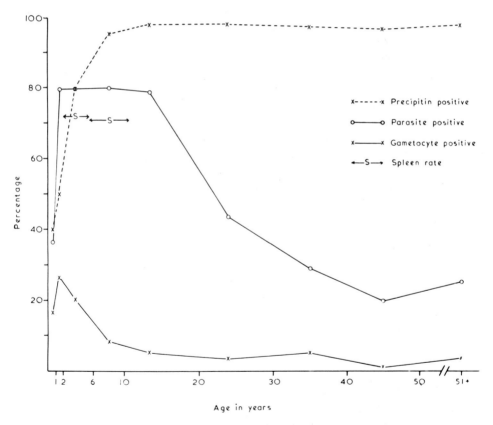

Fig. 30.2 Assessment of the endemicity of malaria in a rural Gambian community.
    The pattern, high in childhood, low in adult life, of parasitaemia and gametocytaemia, the high rates of splenic enlargement in children aged two to nine years and the widespread prevalence in serum of precipitating antibodies to malaria indicate a high level of endemicity. Children under the age of three months have been excluded since antibodies in their sera are more likely to have been acquired passively than actively.

should be examined or, alternatively, each film should be examined for at least five minutes. Parasite rates in infants at different seasons of the year are valuable indices of transmission and may be used to calculate the frequency of infective inoculations. When blood films are being examined the percentage of persons harbouring gametocytes (gametocyte rate) should be noted as an indication of the extent to which feeding *Anopheles* may become infected.

In recent years serological methods have been used to assess endemicity. Techniques of complement fixation, immunohaemagglutination, immunofluorescence, immunoprecipitation and immunoabsorption have been used to detect and quantify specific malarial antibodies in sera. As these tests become positive in the course of infection and remain so for some time after parasitaemia has been eliminated, they can provide valuable information on the recent malaria experience of an individual or a community. Where malaria is highly endemic and where the use of protective drugs by the population is not widespread antibody prevalence at birth may be 100 per cent. It then declines but begins to rise again in the second half of the first year and at ages older than two years may again approximate to 100 per cent. Changes also occur in antibody concentrations. Titres in areas of high endemicity are high in newborns, fall in the early weeks of life and then slowly rise again through childhood to reach maximum values in adult life. Immunofluorescence has been widely used to study malarial endemicity and has proved reliable, although comparisons of the results of different investigations is frequently impossible because of variations in the techniques used.

When the methods described above are used to assess endemicity care must be taken to ensure that the sample of the population studied is representative of the community as a whole so far as age and sex distribution is concerned.

Finally, entomological data may be used to assess endemicity. These include the percentage of mosquitoes found infected and capable of transmitting malaria (sporozoite rate), the longevity of vector mosquitoes as estimated by ovarian dissection, the house resting density of *Anopheles* and their degree of dependence upon man as indicated by the percentage of freshly fed adults whose stomach contents give a positive precipitin reaction for human blood.

The control of malaria

In the years following the Second World War extensive use of the residual insecticide, DDT, showed that where the interruption of transmission of malaria could be achieved and maintained for several years by carefully conducted spraying operations, the parasite reservoir tended to become so depleted that spraying could be discontinued without the resurgence of malaria even where competent anopheline vectors again became numerous.

This observation gave rise to the concept of malaria eradication as opposed to control. Eradication implies the interruption of transmission and the elimination of the parasite reservoir by intensive, meticulously conducted operations that are limited in time. Control, on the other hand, implies measures which will reduce transmission to low levels but which will require to be maintained indefinitely.

In 1955 the World Health Assembly endorsed the concept of world-wide eradication of malaria. Since then eradication campaigns have produced variable results. In developed countries and particularly where malaria was epidemiologically unstable, spectacular successes have been achieved. In many developing countries however, where the disease was stable, results have tended to be unsatisfactory. Many reasons have been advanced to explain the failures but usually the principal cause was the lack of basic health and administrative services capable of supporting the complex, extensive operations that eradication entails. Thus global strategy, which still aims ultimately at world-wide eradication, today recognizes that many countries are in no position to initiate eradication programmes and accepts that in these areas antimalarial measures will, for some time to come, be aimed no higher than control. For countries which have achieved eradication this prospect is not reassuring for it means that constant vigilance on their part will be required to prevent the reimportation of malaria by travellers returning from endemic areas.

By mid-1980 it was estimated that 759 million people lived in areas that have been freed from malaria, while another 1958 million lived in areas where malaria control or eradication programmes were in operation. However, 378 million still lived in malarious areas which were not protected by any antimalarial measures. Most of these areas are in Africa south of the Sahara.

CONTROL MEASURES

Control by antimalarial drugs

Although many effective plasmodicidal drugs are currently available their value as a means of controlling malaria is limited by the difficulties that oppose their widespread, well directed administration. Intermittent administration combined with vector control and timed to coincide with spraying cycles may sometimes be effective but regular administration at weekly or fortnightly intervals is not usually feasible on a large scale. Weekly doses of chloroquine or amodiaquine (300 mg base for an adult and proportionately less for children) or of pyrimethamine (adult dose 25–50 mg) have been used to protect special stress groups such as pregnant and nursing women, pre-school children and school children. Pyrimethamine being tasteless is more acceptable to children than bitter drugs like chloroquine but its use has become obsolete on account of widespread parasite resistance.

However, a paediatric preparation of amodiaquine has proved to be quite acceptable to children.

Combinations of drugs may be selected for special purposes. Formulations of pyrimethamine with dapson or pyrimethamine with sulfadoxine are used in areas with chloroquine-resistant *P. falciparum*, the former for prophylaxis, the latter for treatment and prophylaxis. Their widespread, uncontrolled use is not recommended because of the risk of inducing resistance in parasites and prevalent bacterial pathogens. Combinations of chloroquine or amodiaquine with primaquine attack the parasite both in its exoerythrocytic and erythrocytic stages and exert gametocytocidal action against *P. falciparum*. Quinine and tetracycline are at present the last resort for treating multiresistant falciparum malaria, but the introduction of mefloquine should alleviate the situation in the near future.

The effective use of protective drugs on a large scale must be expected to interfere with the development and maintenance of immunity to malaria. This is not important so long as drug cover is maintained but it becomes so if drugs are withdrawn while the disease is still highly endemic. In such a situation the gains to health from prolonged protection could be swiftly lost and, were levels of immunity in adults substantially reduced, the economy of the community could be adversely affected.

An alternative to fully effective prophylaxis has been sought which, while offering relative freedom from symptoms, might permit the development or maintenance of protective immunity. For instance, the monthly administration of pyrimethamine (25 mg) to children aged less than five years together with the treatment with chloroquine of any supervening acute, febrile illness has been suggested as a means of shielding children while giving them an opportunity to develop some degree of protective immunity. Pyrimethamine in monthly doses does not protect fully and the object of this regimen is to restrict parasitaemia to low and non-lethal levels which are still capable of evoking an immune response. Its value has not yet been adequately assessed.

In areas with unstable malaria and a low intensity of transmission, detection and radical treatment of malaria cases may result in a reduction of malaria incidence.

Vector control

Successful malaria control by anti-vector measures calls for much specialized knowledge and should never be undertaken without detailed understanding of the bionomics of the local vectors. This is a field in which the World Health Organization has a wealth of experience and countries planning large scale operations should not hesitate to seek its advice. The method of choice is usually the spraying of surfaces of buildings with a residual insecticide at a dosage and frequency sufficient to make these surfaces lethal to resting adult mosquitoes. DDT at a rate of 2.0 g/m^2 is widely used but in each project the insecticide chosen should be one known to be effective against the local vectors.

Other anti-vector measures may be directed against mosquito larvae and include elimination of breeding places by drainage or filling, the application of larvicides and biological methods e.g., the introduction of larvivorous fish such as Gambusia. Anti-larval measures tend to be most successful when breeding places are not extensive and in such circumstances they may represent the cheapest form of control. Neither larvicides nor biological methods should be used on a large scale without first ascertaining what adverse ecological changes may follow their use. Chemicals intended to kill larvae may also kill fish and wildfowl and the establishment of Gambusia in a country may be at the expense of other fish possessing an economic value.

At the present time it is widely thought that new methods of vector control are required which in cost and practicability are more suited to the needs of developing nations. One such method under study entails the introduction into a mosquito population of large numbers of males sterilized by ionizing radiation or chemosterilants. These males then compete with fertile males and the reproduction rate of the population is drastically reduced. This method of control has proved successful in the case of some other insects but to be effective the sterile males must outnumber the fertile ones. As in the case of larvicides, it is most likely to prove successful when breeding places are not extensive.

Also the biological control by ecologically compatible larval pathogens such as *Bacillus thuringiensis israeliensis* offers some prospects for malaria control.

Control by immunization

Experimental studies have shown that man and animals can be effectively immunized against malaria and it is, therefore, possible that in the future control or even eradication of the disease may be achieved by the use of selected vaccines. Many investigations involving animals have proved that vaccines which employ as antigen extra-cellular forms of the parasite, i.e. sporozoites, erythrocytic merozoites or gametes, can each induce an effective but strictly stage-specific immunity. Because of difficulties in securing adequate supplies of purified extra-cellular forms from currently available cultivation techniques, extensive tests of vaccine efficiency in man have not been made. At the present time hybridoma-derived monoclonal antibodies of defined specificity are being employed to identify and recover the surface antigens of extra-cellular parasites which are concerned with the induction of protective immunity. In parallel, attempts are being made to synthesize or to produce by recombinant DNA technology the specific, protective antigens that are associated with the different developmental stages of the parasite. So far as man is concerned, interest in artificial immunization resides in its promise; vaccines have no practical part to play in control operations at the present time.

MALARIA CONTROL PROGRAMMES

The eradication of malaria from areas in which it still persists remains today a valid and desirable objective. In some countries, particularly those in which malaria is epidemiologically unstable, this objective may be attainable by short- or medium-term programmes employing currently available methodologies providing that technical, financial and administrative support is adequate. However, in many economically weak countries where malaria is highly endemic, particularly those countries in Africa south of the Sahara, eradication is unlikely to be achieved in the near future. The need to protect populations resident in such countries against the onslaught of malaria has, therefore, caused the World Health Organisation to review its strategy and to define, in order of priority, the following objectives for control in areas where time-limited eradication is impracticable at present:-
1. the elimination of mortality from malaria;
2. the reduction of morbidity from malaria;
3. the reduction of malaria incidence and prevalence.
The first two goals may be achieved through the systematic, judicious use of antimalarial drugs, especially for treatment. The effectiveness of drug usage, however, is dependent on the degree of population cover it attains and on the willingness of the public to utilize the drugs provided. Best results can be expected where health facilities, for example, primary health care services, are well developed and extensive and are particularly orientated to special risk groups such as infants, young children and pregnant women. The realisation of the third objective, the reduction of incidence and prevalence, will probably necessitate the application of vector control measures and, in consequence, greater financial commitment. The choice of specific control methods will be influenced by environmental factors, the ecology and bionomics of local vectors, the degree of control to be attained, the availability of adequate resources in terms of trained personnel and finance and, by no means least, the active and sustained co-operation of the population.

Malaria control may be implemented nationwide or be restricted to specific areas. It may be advantageous to begin a programme in areas of greatest economic importance and gradually to extend it to cover an entire country. In doing so the health planner must strive to counter any sense of injustice or deprivation which peripheral communities may feel and which may, if unrelieved, lead to undesirable population migrations.

It must be emphasised that present techniques of malaria control are not sufficiently effective to achieve eradication in some areas where very high rates of transmission prevail, for example in large tracts of Tropical Africa. In such areas, the ultimate conquest of the disease must await the introduction of new methodologies and the promotion of health infrastructures to a level which permits their effective utilization.

CONTROL MEASURES IN COUNTRIES INTENDING TO EMBARK UPON ERADICATION

Experience from eradication programmes in different parts of the world has shown that governments are often tempted to 'economize' and reduce financial support once malaria ceases to be a prevalent health hazard but before it has been eliminated. It is therefore important that no government should contemplate initiating eradication operations without being firmly resolved first, to support them from beginning to end and second, to allocate the necessary financial provision. When a firm decision to proceed has been taken, plans for eradication should be prepared and scrutinized for feasibility. There should be evidence from studies made within the country to indicate that the methods proposed are likely to prove technically effective. The application of the anti-malarial measures in the manner specified and precisely at the planned times should present no insuperable obstacles. Communications, for example, should be good enough to permit movement of the eradication teams even in the worst weather. In the malarious area special study of the habits and customs of the population, particularly those related to migrational movements, should be made to assess their possible influence on eradication operations. Professional and skilled manpower resources should be examined to assess whether the country is capable of organizing and directing the operations defined in the eradication plan. In particular, the health and general administrative services of the country must be sufficiently developed and organized to fulfil their part in the campaign. Finally, the government's ability to support the programme to a successful conclusion in the face of competing claims from other aspects of the country's development plan must be fully assessed.

If these studies show the plan to be feasible it can then be implemented.

THE MALARIA ERADICATION PROGRAMME

The time taken to achieve eradication will vary according to the complexity of the operations but these are usually expected to be completed within eight to 15 years. As long drawn out, ill planned operations appear to favour the development of insecticide resistance in mosquitoes, campaigns should aim at achieving success in the shortest possible time. Eradication programmes are planned in four phases, preparation, attack, consolidation and maintenance. The objectives of these phases have already been fully described (Pampana 1969; WHO 1972) and will be only briefly summarized here.

The preparatory phase, which usually lasts six to 18 months is devoted to creating the organization that eradication operations require and in collecting the base line entomological and parasitological data against which subsequent changes will be measured. The attack phase is usually expected to last about four years and although mass drug administration and anti-larval operations may be incorporated, the main weapon is usually residual spraying conducted with such efficiency that an effective, lethal deposit of insecticide is maintained on possible mosquito resting sites within all buildings. Progress is monitored by serial parasite surveys, by entomological observations and by serological studies which record changes in the prevalence and concentration of specific malarial antibodies. As the parasite reservoir becomes depleted, parasite surveys become less sensitive in detecting malaria cases and gradually an extensive case detection system is introduced throughout the malarious area. Detection may be passive or active. The former involves the compulsory notification by medical practitioners of confirmed malaria cases and of febrile illness which might possibly be malaria. In addition blood films should be taken from suspected cases and sent to the nearest approved laboratory for examination and the patient then given an appropriate course of anti-malarial treatment as recommended by the eradication services. Active case detection comprises the house to house search throughout the malarious area for fever cases at regular intervals by members of the eradication services. Cases detected have blood films taken for examination and then are treated with a single dose of a drug combination specified by the eradication services which is intended to suppress asexual parasitaemia and also render the patient incapable of infecting mosquitoes for some weeks. When slide examination confirms the presence of malaria the patient is again visited and given a course of treatment designed to eradicate the infection. The attack phase lasts until adequate surveillance of the entire area has been in operation for at least one year and until a number of criteria — one of which is the total absence of any new indigenous malaria cases within the preceding 12 months — are fulfilled.

In the consolidation phase spraying operations are discontinued and consequently vectors may become sufficiently numerous and long-lived to reestablish transmission. It is therefore necessary to maintain surveillance at a level that permits the detection and treatment of such new blood infections or relapses of old infections that may occur before these can infect mosquitoes. Should transmission be shown to have occurred, residual spraying operations may be resumed over as large an area as is thought necessary. In this phase and also in the succeeding one antibody detection tests can be of assistance. Although there is little information available concerning the rate at which malarial antibodies decay and disappear from serum following the eradication of the infection from the host's body, there is considerable evidence that antibody titres remain high so long as the infection persists. Thus, when the trend is towards too low or even non-existent antibody levels in the general population the detection of high titres in some individuals is strongly indicative of persisting infection and justifies the administration of radical treatment. In blood transfusion services all potential donors should be screened routinely and no one whose serum contains a high titre of antibody should be accepted without first receiving adequate treatment. The consolidation phase lasts until the criteria for its fulfilment are attained. One of these is the absence of any indigenous case of malaria other than a relapse within a three-year period during which adequate surveillance has been maintained.

The maintenance phase lasts as long as malaria transmission exists in any part of the world, and entails the continuation of facilities for the detection, treatment and epidemiological investigation of malaria cases, the prevention of reintroduced infection by immigrants or visitors from malarious areas and regular reviews of the epidemiological situation.

Throughout the consolidation and maintenance phases the danger is ever present that nations may relax their efforts against malaria prematurely. In 1967 and 1968 when most of the country was in the consolidation or maintenance phases Sri Lanka experienced a sharp epidemic resurgence in which more than a million cases occurred. Currently, in areas of north and central India residual spraying has had to be reintroduced on a huge scale to combat renewed transmission. These examples are reminders that the price of eradication is constant vigilance.

REFERENCES AND FURTHER READING

Boyd M F (ed) 1949 Malariology. Saunders and Company, Philadelphia and London: Vols 1 and 2
Bruce-Chwatt L J 1980 Essential malariology. Heinemann, London
Kreier J P (ed) 1980 Malaria. Academic Press, New York and London: Vols 1–3
Macdonald G The epidemiology and control of malaria. Oxford University Press, London
Malaria. British Medical Bulletin 1982 38: 115–212
Molineaux L, Grammicia G 1980 The Garki Project. Research on the epidemiology and control of malaria in the Sudan savanna of West Africa. World Health Organisation, Geneva
Pampana E 1969 A textbook of malaria eradication. Oxford University Press, London: 2nd edition
UNDP World Bank WHO 1979 Immunodiagnostic techniques in malaria. Special programme for research and training in tropical medicine. World Health Organisation, Geneva
World Health Organisation 1967 Prevention of the re-introduction of malaria. World Health Organisation, Geneva, Technical Report Series: 374
World Health Organisation 1972 Manual of planning for malaria eradication and malaria control programmes. World Health Organisation, Geneva, Mimeographed Document: ME/72.10
World Health Organisation 1974 Malaria control in countries where time limited eradication is impossible at present. World Health Organisation, Geneva, Technical Report Series: 537
World Health Organisation 1979 Expert committee on malaria Seventeenth report. World Health Organisation, Geneva, Technical Report Series: 640
World Health Organisation 1981 Chemotherapy of malaria. World Health Organisation, Geneva, Monograph Series: 27

Lymphatic filariasis

INTRODUCTION

Human lymphatic filariasis is caused by three species of nematode parasites — *Brugia malayi*, *Brugia timori* and *Wuchereria bancrofti*. About 250 million people in the world are infected (WHO, 1974). All three parasites are mosquito borne, live in the lymphatic system in their mammalian hosts and evoke similar host-parasite responses. They can however be separated into distinct species and strains on morphologic and epidemiologic grounds.

Filariasis was probably known in the period 600 to 150 B. C. as Buddhist texts referred to the exclusion of people with elephantiasis from the priesthood (Laurence, 1967). Microfilariae were first found in hydrocoele fluid by Demarquay in 1863 and in chylous urine by Wucherer in 1868. Bancroft in 1877 found adult female worms from a lymphatic abscess in Brisbane and Cobbold in 1877 named the parasite *Filaria bancrofti*, now known as *Wuchereria bancrofti*. In 1884 Manson working in Amoy, China, demonstrated the development of *W. bancrofti* from the microfilarial to the infective larval stages in the mosquito. Brug (1927) described a new microfilaria species from the Malay Archipelago as *Filaria malayi*. The adult worms were first described by Rao and Maplestone (1940) from specimens in India and Buckley and Edeson (1956) named the parasite *Brugia malayi*.

Filariasis is still an important cause of morbidity both in urban and rural areas in the tropics and subtropics. In many countries there are now filariasis control programmes utilising mass or selective chemotherapy with diethylcarbamazine citrate (DEC-C) and vector control. While there has been a decrease in prevalence of the disease in some countries as a result of control programmes, urban *W. bancrofti* infections increased in some areas concomitant with the proliferation of *Culex quinquefasciatus* mosquitoes in overburdened severage systems resulting from uncontrolled and unplanned urbanization. In other areas the increase in the prevalence of microfilaraemic patients is more apparent than real as with accessibility of remote areas, infected patients have been more easily detected.

Nevertheless, in other places, as in Indonesia, real increases in filariasis among transmigrants to endemic areas of *B. malayi and B. timori* have occurred.

THE AGENT

Life Cycle

The life cycles for these three human lymphatic filarial parasites are essentially the same. Microfilaraemic carriers serve as the source of infection for vector mosquitoes which vary depending on the species and strain of the parasite involved and the geographic locality. A wide range of *Culex, Anopheles* and *Aedes* spp. transmit bancroftian filariasis while *Mansonia, Anopheles* and *Aedes* spp. transmit *Brugian* filariasis.

Microfilariae taken in by the mosquito exsheath and migrate from the midgut into the haemoceole usually within a few minutes of the uptake. They then go to the thoracic muscles of the mosquito where they become the first larval stage. Growth and development occurs here with the larvae undergoing two moults as they pass from the first to the third stage (infective stage or L_3). The duration of the first stage is approximately three days, that of the second stage from the fourth to the eighth day. By the tenth day the infective stage is normally attained under most tropical climatic conditions. Under unfavourable conditions such as low temperature and humidity, the infective stage may only be reached two to three weeks after the uptake of the microfilariae. The infective larvae migrate to all parts of the body but mainly to the proboscis where they await transmission to the definitive host. Infective larvae are deposited onto the host's skin surface during the process of probing and penetration of the mosquito proboscis. Active migration of the infective larvae into the puncture wound occurs after the withdrawal of the proboscis. They will then migrate to the lymphatic system (afferent lymphatics and subcapsular sinuses) where they undergo the third moult approximately nine to 10 days later to become the fourth stage (L_4). The final moult occurs approximately 35–40 days after the introduction of the infective larvae when the parasite becomes a juvenile adult (Edeson and Buckley, 1959). Sexual maturity occurs two to three months post-infection in *Brugia malayi* infections with pre-patent periods (from infection to microfilaraemia) of about 80 days in cats and jirds (Edeson and Wharton, 1967; Ash and Riley, 1970). The pre-patent period for *W. bancrofti* in monkeys is about eight to 18 months (Cross *et al.*, 1979). In man the pre-patent period for *B. malayi* infection is about $3\frac{1}{2}$ months (Edeson and Wharton, 1957) while that for *W. bancrofti* is about 11 months (Colwell *et al.*, 1970).

Morphology

Wuchereria bancrofti can easily be distinguished from *B. malayi* and *B. timori* at the microfilaria, infective larva and adult stages (Table 31.1). The microfilariae of *W. bancrofti* are longer than those of *B. malayi*. Unlike the two *Brugia* spp. there is no terminal nucleus seen in the tail end of the microfilaria. Another important character is the ratio of the length of the cephalic space to the width at the first nucleus, this being approximately 1:1 in *W. bancrofti*, 2:1 in *B. malayi* and about 3:1 in *B. timori*. The nuclei in the body of *W. bancrofti* are distinctly separated from each other while those in the two *Brugia* spp. tend to overlap. The microfilaria of *W. bancrofti* is disposed in smooth, graceful curves while secondary, irregular curves are normally seen in *Brugia* spp. *B. timori* microfilaria is longer than that of *B. malayi* and unlike the latter, its sheath is normally unstained with Giemsa stain. The periodic form of *B. malayi* may sometimes shed its sheath under normal drying conditions. More than 50 per cent of the microfilariae of the periodic form shed their sheaths compared to less than eight per cent in the subperiodic form (Sivanandam and Dondero, 1972). However, on the basis of recent findings in Malaysia and Indonesia, it appears that this is not a constant character and is therefore an unreliable measure alone of the periodicity of the parasite.

The infective larvae of *B. malayi* and *B. timori* can easily be distinguished from those of *W. bancrofti* (Table 31.1). However infective larvae of *B. timori* cannot be differentiated from those of *B. malayi* on morphological characters. *W. bancrofti* infective larvae can be mistaken for those of *Cardiofilaria* spp. The latter has similar caudal papillae but a smaller anal ratio (Wharton, 1957) this being 2.2 — 2.8 (Dissanaike and Niles, 1967) compared to 4.0 in *W. bancrofti* (Yen *et al.* 1982).

The adult worms are filiform in shape, white in colour and except for minute cuticular bosses at the posterior end of females, have smooth cuticles. The males are easily differentiated on the basis of the morphology of spicules, and the number and arrangement of the genital papillae (Table 31.1).

Periodicity

An important character of the filarial parasite is the tendency of some strains to show a rhythmic variation in the microfilarial density in the peripheral blood during the 24-hour cycle. Strains that show such variations are termed periodic whereas those that do not are called non-periodic. On the the basis of whether the peak density is at night or in the day it is termed nocturnally or diurnally periodic respectively. To determine the periodicity of a particular strain it is necessary to obtain the microfilarial count in a fixed volume of peripheral blood (40 or 60 ul) taken at regular intervals (two or four hourly) over a 24-hour period. A statistical method has been developed to classify and compare microfilarial periodicity (Sasa and Tanaka, 1974;

Table 31.1 Morphological characters and mean measurements* of *Brugia malayi*, *Brugia timori* and *Wuchereria bancrofti*

Species	*Brugia malayi*	*Brugia timori*	*Wuchereria bancrofti*
Microfilaria			
Reference	Mak and Yen (1976)	Purnomo et al. (1977)	Harinasuta et al. (1970)
Sheath	Present	Present	Present
Terminal nucleus	Present	Present	Absent
Length	222 (205–240)	310	311 (295–330)
Cephalic space			
Length:width	1.9:1	2.7:1	1.3:1
Infective larva			
Reference	Yen et al. (1982)	Purnomo et al. (1976)	Yen et al. (1982)
Length	1533 (1250–1730)	1530 (1350–1749)	1755 (1530–2000)
Maximum width	26.8	29 (25–39)	27.2
Caudal papillae	3 mere protuberenace (2 sublateral, 1 subterminal)	3 broadly based, gently rounded (1 dorsal, 2 ventrolateral)	3 prominent, bubble-like
Adult worm			
Reference	Buckley and Edeson (1956)	Partono et al. (1977)	Dissanaike and Mak (1980)
Male			
length	18.3 (13.5–23.3) mm	16.9 (13.4–22.8) mm	27.5 (23.8–30.6) mm
maximum width	75 (70–80)	72 (67–80)	108.1 (90–120)
spicular length:			
left	342 (290–365)	385 (352–419)	596.1 (560–630)
right	106 (100–120)	124 (110–142)	235.6 (220–250)
ratio left:right	3.3:1 (2.4–3.8:1)	3.1:1 (2.8–3.6:1)	2.5:1 (2.3–2.9:1)
Genital papillae	12–17	13–25	24–26
Female			
length	48.2 (43.5–52) mm	26.7 (21.1–39.2) mm	44.3 (42.3–46.3) mm
maximum width	148 (130–170)	99 (80–140)	174 (160–188)

* All measurements in micrometers unless indicated. Range in parentheses.

Tanaka, 1981). The microfilarial wave over the 24-hour period is considered to correspond to a harmonic wave described by the formula $= m + a \cos 15 (h-k)°$ where the microfilarial ratio (y) at a given hour

$$= \frac{\text{microfilarial count}}{\text{mean count of observations over 24 hours}} \times 100$$

m = mean microfilarial ratio of all patients at a given hour,
a = periodicity index, h = hour and k = peak hour. Through trigonometric conversion the formula becomes
$Y = m + b \cos 15h° + c \sin 15h°$ and allows for easier calculation
$(a^2 = b^2 + c^2, b = \dfrac{2 \Sigma y \cos 15h°}{n}, c = \dfrac{2 \Sigma y \sin 15h°}{n}$, n = number of observations in 24 hours, $\tan 15° k = \dfrac{b}{c})$.

By this method the microfilarial periodicity of a particular strain can be defined by its periodicity index and the peak hour. These two indices are summary measures of the periodicity of a particular microfilaria and allow comparison with those of another. These indices describe the periodicity of a strain more precisely than the earlier terminology of periodic, subperiodic and non-periodic, and should be used in its characterization. Thus nocturnally periodic *W. bancrofti*, *B. timori* and *B. malayi* have periodicity indices of about 100 and peak hours around midnight. The nocturnally subperiodic form of *W. bancrofti* from Thailand and subperiodic *B. malayi* have periodicity indices of about 50 and the peak hour from 20.5 — 22.00 hours. The South Pacific form of *W. bancrofti* has a periodicity index of about 25 and peak hour of 16.00 hours.

The microfilarial periodicity is closely related to the biting cycle of vector mosquitoes and therefore its definition is of importance in the understanding of the transmission dynamics.

Vectors and hosts

The ecotype of a particular endemic area determines to a large extent the complex combination of parasite species and strains, vectors and mammalian hosts present (Table 31.2). In some countries in Southeast Asia (especially Malaysia), subperiodic *B. malayi* can be zoonotically transmitted from wild animals and domestic cats. Leaf monkeys (*Presbytis* spp.) are the most important wild animal reservoirs as they live in relatively close proximity with man and in some areas 90 per cent of these monkeys may be infected (Mak *et al.* 1980, 1982). The control programmes using mass chemotherapy with DEC-C in these areas have therefore been affected by reinfections of man from monkeys. In these areas the development of an effective method of chemoprophylaxis would be useful.

Table 31.2 Relationships between filarial species and strains, ecotype, hosts and vectors

Species	Brugia malayi		Brugia timori	Wuchereria bancrofti		
Strain	periodic	subperiodic		urban	rural	
Vectors	Anopheles spp. Aedes spp. Mansonia spp.	Mansonia spp.	Anopheles barbirostris	Culex quinquefasciatus	Anopheles spp. Aedes spp.	
Hosts	Man	Man Monkeys Domestic cats Carnivores	Man	Man	Man	
Ecotype	Established agricultural areas e.g. ricefields	Swamp forest habitat	Irrigated ricefields	Urban areas	Hilly forest regions	

PATHOLOGY AND IMMUNOLOGY

Pathology

Although elephantiasis is a vivid manifestation of the pathological process in filariasis, it represents only one of the many possible final outcomes of the host-parasite interaction. Although in the hyperendemic areas probably 90–100 per cent of people are infected (Connor, 1932) not all infections result in such drastic sequelae, and the wide spectrum of clinical response reflects the interaction of a multiplicity of factors of which those of host (genetic, immunologic) and parasite (species, strain, infective dose) will determine to a great extent the disease pattern. While clinical manifestations may differ, the pathological processes are essentially similar in filariasis due to *W. bancrofti* and *Brugia* spp. All stages of the parasite in man may cause damage under certain conditions.

Experimental studies on the histopathology of early *Brugia* spp. infections (Schacher and Sahyon, 1967) have advanced our understanding of the immunopathological process. The invasion of the lymphatic system by infective larvae evokes hyperplasia of the secondary lymph follicles and reticular cells of the stroma of the lymph node. There is a reduction of lymph flow due to medullar oedema and obliteration of the peripheral sinus. At the moulting of the infective larvae to the fourth and fifth stages one and three weeks respectively after infection, there are widespread thrombotic and inflammatory reactions to the shed cuticle and moulting fluid in afferent lymphatics and in the node. Granulomatous reactions with foreign body giant cells, histocytes and epitheloid cells surrounding the sheaths and dead parasites occur, followed by healing with fibrosis and recanalization. At two months after infection, in addition to the organization of lesions with fibrosis, acute lesions consisting of parietal and polypoidal thrombo-lymphangitis may be seen around infertile ova, microfilariae and fibrinous, amorphous materials.

As many as 50 adult worms may be present in some patients (Connor, 1932). Worms are mostly found in the periglandular tissues, the lymphatic vessels or the cortical sinuses. The mechanical presence of the worms in the lumen and the subsequent changes which they evoke in the walls and surrounding tissues produce varying degrees of lymph stasis. In genital lesions worms are perdominantly found in the eipdidymimary and paraepididymary locations rather than in the cord or testis.

When worms are viable and intact few inflammatory cells are present and lymph vessel dilatation is minimal. With death and disintegration of worms, inflammatory reaction with granuloma formation occur followed by scarring (Galindo *et al.* 1962). Healing with fibrosis of granulomatous lesions may cause complete loss of architecture and obliteration of the lymph node and lymphatic vessel (Connor, 1932). Elephantiasis has been postulated to result from the above reactions to the death of the adult worms in the lymphatic system (Jordon, 1955).

In tropical pulmonary eosinophilia (TPE) there is a patchy inflammatory reaction to dead and degenerating microfilariae in both exudative and granulomatous lesions in the lungs. The exudative lesions are characterized by amorphous eosinophilic material, eosinophils and other chronic inflammatory cells, and the granulomatous lesions are distinguished by foreign body giant cells and fibroblasts (Danaraj *et al.* 1966).

Immunology

People who live in an endemic situation are constantly being exposed to infective larvae of animal and human origin. While the parasites may not establish themselves, they may survive long enough to modify the immune system. Whether this modification is sufficient to induce protection without causing disease will depend on a number of factors of which cross reactivity of parasitic antigens and the intensity of the immune response are important. It has been shown that sera from exposed but apparently normal subjects living in endemic areas are able to promote antibody dependent cell-mediated cytotoxicity (ADCC) of *B. malayi* infective larvae (Sim *et al.* 1982). A similar but more intense reaction is present with sera of patients with tropical pulmonary eosinophilia, elephantiasis and those amicrofilaraemic patients with clinical evidence of filariasis.

Immunoglobulin levels in *B. malayi* microfilaraemic patients are not significantly higher than those of clinically and parasitologically negative subjects living in endemic areas (Mak *et al.* 1979). Microfilaraemic patients have depressed lymphocyte responses in the lymphocyte transformation tests to *B. malayi* adult worm (Otteson *et al.* 1977) and microfilarial antigens (Piessens *et al.* 1980). Unlike other clinical states of filariasis, microfilaraemic patients' sera do not promote the *in vitro* ADCC reaction using normal buffy coat cells to infective larvae. It is hypothesized that repeated exposure to infective larvae could induce desensitization and a loss in the capacity to respond effectively to filarial antigens. This specific loss of antigen recognition might then allow the establishment of chronic filarial infections, resulting ultimately in clinical and pathological changes. In chronic filarial disease states (elephantiasis, hydrocoeles) especially those associated with persistent microfilaraemia, there is a specific cellular unresponsiveness to filarial antigens.

Tropical pulmonary eosinophilia is believed to be due to a hyperresponsiveness to filariasis infection. IgE levels in these patients are found to be very much higher than in those with classical filariasis (Ezeoke *et al.* 1973). The pathogenesis of the disease though not completely known is believed to be due in part to immediate hypersensitivity (Type I responses) and antibody-antigen complexes (Type II responses) (Otteson, 1975).

CLINICAL MANIFESTATIONS

The signs and symptoms of lymphatic filariasis follow predictably upon the pathologic processes described earlier and may be grouped as acute-inflammatory, chronic-obstructive, or hypersensitive in character. There are, however, considerable variations in disease manifestations among affected persons in the same community, between populations in different geographic areas, and between persons infected with bancroftian or *Brugia* spp. parasites.

Filarial adenolymphangitis and fever

The acute attack of lymphadenitis and lymphangitis, with fever, is the hallmark of lymphatic filariasis. In the usual episode there is a rapidly developing onset of pain and tenderness in a single node or small group of adjacent nodes at a superficial inguinal, axillary, or epitrochlear site. This is accompanied by systemic symptoms of fever, sweats, chills, headache, weakness, and generalized mild muscle and joint pains. Retrograde lymphangitis affects major afferent vessels, and lymphoedema may accumulate in the distal part. Less frequently, the focus of inflammation is found to be in cervical, pectoral, mammary, popliteal or other superficial nodes.

The uncomplicated filarial attack is generally mild and lasts for a few days only. In some instances, however, an abscess develops at the site of inflammation. These abscesses may persist for a period of one to several weeks prior to their rupture or involution. The resulting ulcer heals by granulation quickly and without complication, leaving a characteristic scar overlying a sclerotic vessel.

A common feature of filarial adenolymphangitis is its irregularly recurring nature. Some persons experience only one or a few attacks in a lifetime, others experience one or two attacks a month during the periods of greatest activity of their disease. In endemic communities, episodes are most frequent and severe among persons in late adolescence and early adulthood. The frequency of attacks may increase during periods of hard physical labour.

Filarial orchitis, epididymitis, and funiculitis

Bancroftian parasites have a propensity to establish themselves within lymphatic channels of the testis, epididymis and spermatic cord. Acute attacks of inflammation come on suddenly with pain, swelling and tenderness in the affected structure and surrounding tissues. The pain frequently radiates up the spermatic cord and, less commonly, to the inguinal nodes. High fever, chills and other constitutional signs are common. The acute symptoms usually persist for three to five days only, but may continue for one to two weeks.

Hydrocoele

Hydrocoele, or chylocoele, depending upon whether the exudate is serous or chylous, is a major sign of chronic bancroftian filariasis, and may be found to affect 35 per cent or more of the adult males in an endemic community. Scarring and hypertrophy of the epididymis and spermatic cord are commonly found in association with hydrocoele. Filariasis due to *Brugia* spp. is not a documented cause of urogenital disease.

Lymphoedema and elephantiasis

Lymphoedema of the distal part typically first appears during an acute attack of adenolymphangitis. In early episodes, the swelling is usually slight and resolves completely over several weeks. With repeated attacks, the swelling may increase and resolve more slowly. When it persists for more than six months it is considered to be elephantiasis, with or without the chronic thickening of the skin frequently associated with the term. In endemic situations, there is a slow and steady rise in the prevalence of elephantiasis beyond the age of 20 years, with the peak incidence between the ages of 25 to 45 years. The legs are most commonly affected, followed in frequency of occurrence by elephantiasis of the arms and scrotum. The breasts, penis and labia are less commonly involved. Although at first confined to the distal portion of the extremity, the swelling may progress proximally to involve the entire limb. The oedema does not usually advance beyond the knee or elbow in filariasis due to *Brugia* spp., and the deformity is 'water-bag' in appearance.

Other less common signs of chronic obstructive bancroftian filariasis include chyluria, chylous ascites, lymph scrotum and varicocoeles, varicose nodes and vessels.

Atypical, hypersensitivity disease

Tropical (pulmonary) eosinophilia (TPE) describes a complex of symptoms arising from hypersensitivity to microfilariae of the lungs and the reticulo-endothelial system, especially the lymph nodes and spleen. Useful criteria in arriving at a diagnosis of TPE are: recent residence in a filariasis endemic area, especially South and Southeast Asia; hyper-eosinophilia, usually exceeding 3000 per cu mm peripheral blood; paroxysmal nocturnal cough, with scanty sputum production but with dyspnea and with course rhonchi and rales of wheezing; increased bronchovesicular markings and diffuse miliary mottling in roentgenograms of the chest; and, elevated IgE and high titers of anti-filarial antibodies. Circulating microfilariae are almost never found, and the symptom complex has been appropriately described under the term 'occult filariasis' (Lie, 1962). There is usually a prompt and favourable response to treatment with DEC-C.

TREATMENT

Diethylcarbamazine citrate (DEC-C), a piperazine derivative, is the treatment of choice of lymphatic filariasis. DEC-C (Hetrazan, Banocide, Notezine, Filarizan) is an efficient microfilaricide, with a slower and less complete action against adult worms. The usual dose of DEC-C in treating individual cases is four to six mg per kg body weight daily in single or spaced doses given after meals for 14 to 21 days. Most infections will be cured with this regimen, although in some persons low levels of microfilaraemia may persists. Re-examination of the blood is recommended to establish the parasitological response. The drug is rapidly excreted and relatively non-toxic, and retreatment may be safely given a month following completion of a previous course.

Untoward effects of treatment with DEC-C are of two types: those arising directly from toxicity of the drug itself, and those resulting from destruction of the parasite. Symptoms of toxicity to the drug include dizziness, weakness, and nausea. These symptoms are generally mild and last for a few hours only. Reactions to the death of parasites, however, may be more severe. The rapid destruction of microfilariae often produces a systemic reaction with fever to 41°C, headache, pains in muscles and joints, nausea and vomiting, weakness, dizziness and, less commonly, asthma. These symptoms develop within the first two days of treatment, often within 12 hours of the first drug dose, and persist over the following two to four days of drug administration. They are less common and less severe in children than in adults. Attacks of adenolymphangitis and lymphatic abscess arising during treatment are presumed to be caused by reactions to damaged or dead adult worms.

The incidence and severity of reactions is directly related to microfilarial density and adult worm burden. Systemic reactions are usually most severe in persons infected with *Brugia* spp. Treatment seldom needs to be interrupted, but drug recipients should be clearly told in advance of the possibility of reactions. The drug is contraindicated in pregnancy, and in persons with cardiac and renal disease. Special care should be exercised in treating persons from areas in which there is loaisis and onchocerciasis, since reactions among persons infected with these parasites may be life-threatening. Reactions in persons with lymphatic filariae are self-limiting and may be reduced somewhat by starting treatment with low or spaced doses; symptoms are almost always relieved with simple analgesic-antipyretic compounds. Antihistamines and steroid preparations appear to have little value.

Adenolymphangitis and filarial abscesses can usually be managed conservatively with analgesics, antipyretics, and antibiotics. Hydrocoeles are temporarily relieved by aspiration. Lymphoedema and elephantiasis are managed by reducing periods of dependancy of the part and by firm bandaging. Excision of the redundant tissue of scrotal elephantiasis may afford considerable relief, but operations upon elephantoid limbs should be performed with caution. Surgical biopsy and excision of lymphatic nodes and vessels is generally contraindicated.

EPIDEMIOLOGY

Geographical distribution

Lymphatic filariasis is found throughout much of the warm and humid tropics and subtropics between latitudes 40 °N and 30 °S. The range of the most prevalent form, bancroftian filariasis, circles the globe within the *zona torridae* (Fig. 31.1). The endemic range of those species of the genus *Brugia* which normally infect man is, on the other hand, limited to the Oriental biogeographic zone, from India in the extreme west to Korea in the northeast (Fig. 31.2).

Lymphatic filariae are particularly favoured by conditions that have longexisted in the tropical lowlands of the Indo-Malayan region; nowhere else is there found a wider variety of parasites, mosquito vectors, mammalian hosts, and ecotypic associations. It is possible that important radiation from this site has followed trade and migration routes, with adaptation of the parasites to local mosquitoes in the course of the movement of the human reservoir east and west.

In Asia, *W. bancrofti* is found in both urban and rural foci on the Indian subcontinent, the island of Sri Lanka, and in Burma; in scattered rural foci in Thailand and Indo-China; extensively in the south and eastern alluvial plains of China; among indigeneous peoples of the hill forests of the Malayan peninsula, northern Borneo, and in varied forest and agricultural ecotypes of the Philippine islands. In Indonesia, the parasite is found in a

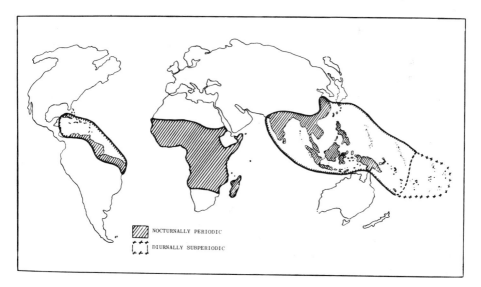

NOCTURNALLY PERIODIC

DIURNALLY SUBPERIODIC

Fig. 31.1 World-wide distribution of *W. bancrofti* within the *Zona torridae*. The interrupted line demarcates the limits of the diurnally subperiodic strain in the South Pacific region east of longitude 170°.

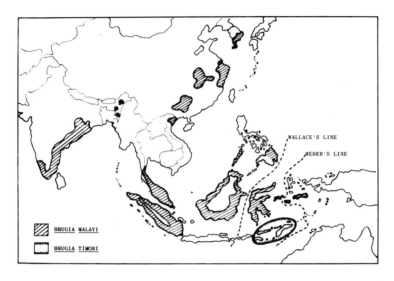

Fig. 31.2 Distribution of filariasis due to *B. malayi and B. timori*.The subperiodic and the periodic strains of *B. malayi* occur in Malaysia, Indonesia and the Philippines. *B. timori* is found only in Southeastern Indonesia.

generally low prevalence in low-lying hill forests of Sumatra, Kalimantan, and Sulawesi, and along the coasts of small islands east of Lombok. The urban form only is present in Java. In the South Pacific, the parasite is highly prevalent in low-lying areas of the island of New Guinea, and in many islands of Melanesia, Micronesia and Polynesia. The parasite is vectored by *Aedes* spp. and is of the diurnally subperiodic form throughout Polynesia, New Caledonia and the Loyalty Islands.

The second major endemic zone of bancroftian filariasis is in sub-Saharan Africa, where it is transmitted by *An. gambiae* and *An. funestus* in a patchy distribution throughout the equatorial belt between 25 ° N and 20 ° S. The parasite is adapted to *Culex* spp., as well as to anophelines, along the East African coastal plains and offshore islands, and is found there in urban as well as rural foci. Bancroftian filariasis is endemic in the southern Sudan, adjacent lowland Ethiopia and in the Nile Delta.

The parasite was brought by African migrants to the New World. It is now of importance only in Dominica, the Guyanas, and coastal Brazil, where *Culex quinquefasciatus* is the vector.

The population affected by *Brugia* spp. is much less than that affected by *W. bancrofti*, and is limited to rural areas. In India, the periodic form only is found, especially in Kerala and a few scattered rural foci elsewhere. In peninsular Malaysia, the periodic strain is most commonly found in open swamps and rice-growing areas of the west coast, where it is transmitted by *Anopheles campestris* and various *Mansonia* spp. The nocturnally subperiodic form is endemic along the lower reaches of the major rivers of both coasts.

It is associated with fresh-water swamp forest ecotypes favourable for the breeding of *Mansonia bonneae* and *M. dives*, and for the maintenance of an important zoonotic reservoir in several endemic leaf monkeys of the genus *Presbytis*.

Brugia spp. are widespread in Indonesia. Subperiodic and periodic forms occur throughout lowland Sumatra, the island of Borneo, Sulawesi and smaller islands as for east as the Mollucas.

Periodic *B. malayi* is endemic in the Red River Valley of Viet Nam and in the eastern alluvial rice-growing areas of China, where *Anopheles sinensis* is the vector. The parasite occurs in the southern tip of the Korean Peninsula and in a few offshore islands. *Aedes togoi* is a vector in coastal foci of Korea and China.

Brugia timori, a nocturnally periodic parasite closely related to *B. malayi*, is endemic in low-lying riverine and coastal strip areas of Timor, Flores, Sumba and other small islands surrounding the Savu Sea. It is transmitted by *Anopheles barbirostris*, and it is responsible for considerable morbidity in affected populations.

Vector factors

The geographic distribution of lymphatic filariasis is due largely to the adaptability of the parasites to endemic mosquito species, themselves limited to specific ecotypes and characterized by differing vectorial capacities; the whole producing a widespread but focal pattern of occurrence with major differences in intensity of transmission.

Factors which determine the vectorial capacity of a mosquito species include the man-biting density and proportion of feeds obtained from humans (the man-biting index); the timing of feeding as related to the rhythmic circadial fluctuations in density of microfilariae in the peripheral blood of man; the degree of concentration of parasites in the blood meal and the amount of blood ingested and retained; the frequencey of feeding and the longevity of the vector, taking into account the efficiency with which it supports parasite development to the state of infective larvae and then delivers these larvae to man. This is best summarized in the Annual Transmission Potential (ATP), which is the estimated number of infected larvae to which a person is exposed by a mosquito species during one year.

Host factors

The signs and symptoms of filariasis are unevenly distributed amongst exposed persons in endemic communities. In heavily exposed populations, the rates of microfilaraemia generally increase rapidly beyond the age of five years to a plateau of prevalence in the age grouping 10 to 20 years, gently rising or falling thereafter. The curves inscribed by plotting the frequency distributions of signs and symptoms of acute filarial illness usually trail somewhat behind, demonstrating peak prevalence and incidence rates in the second and third decades of life.

In those unusual circumstances in which a population is newly exposed to infection, such as agricultural migrants settling in an endemic focus, or military personnel being exposed during operations, the pattern of infection and disease may be quite different. This is particularly well described for American servicemen exposed to *W. bancrofti* in the South Pacific during WWII. In this circumstance, acute, focal adenolymphangitis was most frequently manifest within six to 12 months of first exposure, and, although adult worms were recovered by biopsy, microfilaraemias were rarely detected and chronic sequelae were unusual (Beaver, 1970). Hypersensitivity reactions to infection as manifest by high eosinophilia and bronchopulmonary symptoms (tropical eosinophilia), were sometimes seen.

As noted earlier, host immune factors play an important role in determining the parasitological and clinical-pathologic outcomes of exposure to infection. The immune response is, however, imperfectly protective, and the pattern and intensity of exposure seems to be a major factor in determining the profile of established infection and disease in communities.

Infection may be dependent upon occupational and other activities. For example, rubber and oil palm plantation workers in Malaysia may be heavily exposed to bites of forest-breeding *Mansonioides*; similarly, workers in abaca plantations in the Philippines and in coconut plantations in Polynesia may be unusually exposed to bites of vector *Aedes* spp. which breed in axils of the abaca plant in the former, and in discarded coconnut husks and tree holes in the latter. Filariasis is mostly a condition of persons of the lower socioeconomic levels, due to inadequate personal protective measures and to associations with environmental conditions favourable to the breeding of vectors. Further, lack of knowledge on filariasis by the population at risk can unwittingly lead to infection and disease-promoting behaviours, including unnecessary exposure to vector mosquitoes, poor environmental sanitation practices, non-use of personal protective measures, non-seeking of treatment of symptoms and poor compliance with community control and treatment programmes.

Parasite factors

A large number of parasite factors act to facilitate transmission. Adaptability of the parasite to vector mosquitoes is a function of such variables as microfilarial periodicity and the efficiency with which microfilariae develop into infective larvae, taking into account the rates of maturation and effects of the parasite upon survivability of the vector. Little is known of the dynamics of infection within man, but the infection is generally chronic and has incubation and pre-patent periods of several months or years. Observations on *W. bancrofti* infections in Samoa suggest that the mean duration of microfilarial patency from a single worm pair is about two to four years, producing a theoretical maximum density of 70 microfilariae per 60 μl of peripheral blood. The mortality rate of mated female worms was calculated to be 0.02 to 0.05 per month, with an average load of fecund pairs in microfilaraemic individuals of about seven for men, six for women and three for children (Hairston and Jachowski, 1968). There are enormous differences in efficiency of transmission between various vector-parasite combinations. On the one hand, it is estimated that 15,500 bites by infective *Culex quinquefasciatus* in Rangoon resulted, on average, in one new patent *W. bancrofti* infection in man (Hairston and DeMeillon, 1968) while studies in East Africa suggest that less than 200 infective bites a year per person by *Anopheles* spp. maintain transmission at endemic levels (White, 1971). About 30 infective bites annually per person has been described in highly endemic foci of sub-periodic *B. malayi* (Wharton, 1962).

COMMUNITY DIAGNOSIS

Community diagnosis is best established with an epidemiologic survey by a trained team. Essential features include: (1) examination of local health records; (2) geographic reconnaissance, especially as related to breeding of vector mosquitoes; (3) census and registration of the target population; (4) selection of a representative study sample, preferably by probabilistic methods; (5) administering of a health questionnaire; (6) the performing of a physical examination designed to detect adenolymphangitis, scars of previously ruptured abscesses, sclerotic vessels and varices, genital lesions, and lymphoedema; (7) collection of blood for identifying microfilariae, using measured quantities of 60 μl for thick films, and one to five ml for concentrating methods; (8) determination of microfilarial periodicity; (9) identification of man-biting mosquitoes and their breeding and feeding habits, and determination of man-biting densities under various conditions of time and place; (10) dissection of potential vectors in order to identify developing larvae and to calculate the infection and infectivity rates; and (11) examination of animals as a source of blood meals for vectors and as reservoirs of infection.

Useful tabulations and measures in assessing the endemicity of the local situation include: (1) age and sex-specific rates of acute and chronic symptoms and signs of filariasis; (2) similarly stratified rates of microfilaraemia; (3) median microfilarial densities as determined by the log-probit method (the MFD_{50}) (WHO, 1974); (4) the infectivity index of the human population as determined by the density distribution of microfilariae among carriers (WHO, 1974); (5) man-biting density of vector species as estimated in the Annual Biting Rate (ABR), and the infectivity rates of these vectors; (6) the Annual Transmission Potential (ATP) of the important vector species; and, in sub-periodic *Brugia malayi* endemic sites, (7) the rates of infection in domestic cats and local monkey species.

Assessment of the public health impact of filariasis can be made by determining the restriction of activities due to elephantiasis, the number of man days of labour lost in a community per annum from acute attacks of filarial illness, and the demands made upon health services for treatment, control and prevention.

LABORATORY DIAGNOSIS

Although it may be easy to recognise classical obstructive filariasis, many who are infected have no symptoms or signs of infection. Laboratory confirmation of the infection will therefore be important. Parasitological, histopathological and immunological techniques are available for this purpose. Parasitological techniques are used to demonstrate circulating microfilariae or their presence in various body fluids as in hydrocoele fluid and chylous urine. Normally a thick blood film is made from a quantitated volume (60 μl) of peripheral blood taken at night (except for non-periodic *W. bancrofti* where it may be taken in the day time). This is then allowed to dry, preferably overnight, or for at least an hour and then stained with diluted Giemsa stain (one to two ml in 100 ml buffered distilled water pH 7.2). Field's stain can also be used (Sivanandam and Mak, 1975). The dried blood smear is dehaemoglobinized for two minutes in water, dried, and then fixed with methanol for 30 seconds. After rinsing in water it is stained in Field's stain A for one to two seconds, washed, stained in Field's stain B for one to two seconds, washed and restained in Stain A for one to two seconds. The film is then dried and ready for examination.

The thick blood film technique may not be sensitive enough to demonstrate low density microfilaraemia. Concentration techniques are needed in such situations. Filtration techniques using membrane filters efficiently concentrate microfilariae from large volumes of blood collected with anticoagulant. A modification of the technique by Dennis and Kean (1971) has been developed and is being used routinely in some laboratories (Mak, 1981).

One ml of blood collected with anticoagulant is diluted with nine ml of normal saline. This is then passed through a 25 mm diameter Swin-Lok Holder assembly containing a polycarbamate membrane with five μm pore size. A further 10 ml of normal saline is then passed through followed by 10 ml of air. The membrane is removed and dried on a microscope glass slide. This is then fixed with methanol and stained with Giemsa or Field's stain as described above. The stained membrane can be examined directly or mounted in a drop of immersion oil with a cover slip before examination. Although the technique is extremely valuable in the demonstration of low density microfilaraemia, the relatively high cost of the membrane and the need for venepuncture to obtain the one ml of blood has restricted the use of this technique to special situations.

Histopathological techniques are employed to demonstrate worms in lymph nodes and other organs, for example lesions in lungs or subcutaneous nodules, and in confirming the filarial aetiology in such states as in occult filariasis where granulomatous lesions surround degenerating microfilariae.

Immunodiagnostic techniques range from the now abandoned Sawada skin test to the currently used indirect fluorescent antibody (IFA) and the indirect enzyme-linked immunosorbent assay (ELISA) techniques. These tests have their limitations. In most endemic areas, populations are exposed to mosquito borne animal as well as human filarial infective larvae. The resultant sensitization will make difficult the interpretation of serological tests for individual diagnosis and for epidemiological purposes. Furthermore the detection of circulating antibodies does not distinguish between current or past infections. Tests which detect circulating antigens and therefore current infection are still being developed. The IFA techniques using both frozen sections of adult worms and microfilariae (papainized or sonicated) should be used simultaneously (Mak 1981). The IFA test using frozen sections of *B. malayi* worms is found to be a useful indicator of active infection while that using microfilarial antigens are correlated with disease (Grove and Davis, 1978).

PREVENTION AND CONTROL

The systematic control of filariasis is almost everywhere a function of national disease control programmes which generally follow established principles put forth in WHO guidelines (WHO, 1962; WHO, 1967). The three primary strategies: (1) vector suppression and control; (2) chemo-therapeutic reduction of the parasite reservoir in man; and, (3) promotion of personal protection from the bites of mosquito vectors are variously effective alone, and they are best applied in combination. Larviciding of polluted breeding sites and sanitary engineering at the municipal and house-hold level are important methods for control of the *Culex*-borne bancroftian filariasis. Source reduction, and larviciding of the peridomestic breeding sites of *Aedes* spp. (e.g., coconut husks, discarded tins, drums, tyres), is used in the South Pacific in conjunction with mass treatment. Residual indoor spraying of insecticides in malaria control is effective in reducing the density of most anopheline vectors of *W. bancrofti* and of periodic *B. malayi*, and in some instances has alone resulted in significant reductions of filariasis in the community (Webber, 1979). Similar anopheline control efforts might be expected to reduce transmission of *B. timori*. Drainage of open swamps and control of water plants which sustain the developing stages of *Mansonia* spp. is used in the control of periodic *B. malayi*, but, to date, there are no known practical and effective methods of suppressing the swamp-forest breeding *Mansonia* vectors of sub-periodic *Brugia malayi*. Due to the chron-icity of filarial infection, vector control measures alone can be expected to take three or more years to bring about a detectable reduction in the parasite reservoir.

Diethylcarbamazine citrate (DEC-C) is used widely in community control on a mass and case-selective basis. Its main disadvantages are that multiple doses over time are required, and that death of parasites during treatment frequently causes unpleasant but self-limited systemic and local reactions of the host in response to injury or death of parasites. These factors may deter public cooperation with filariasis control teams, and a new emphasis is being laid on community education and participation in control methods.

Mass treatment with DEC-C is recommended for all otherwise healthy, non-pregnant individuals two years of age and above in a community in which 5 per cent or more of its members are found to be microfilaraemic by standard survey techniques. When the microfilaraemia rate is less than 5 per cent, it may be more practical to treat selectively only those individuals who are parasite positive or who experience signs and symptoms of infection. There are many differing schedules of treatment employed throughout the world, variation being applied to balance parasitologic effectiveness, drug tolerance and programme cost. The usual daily doseage in field programmes is five to six mg per kg body weight (at doses of eight mg per kg or greater the incidence of drug intolerance markedly increases), and the total drug dose varies between 36 mg per kg to 72 mg per kg body weight. In general, bancroftian parasites are less sensitive to treatment than *Brugia* spp., and communities with higher rates and densities of microfilaraemia require greater dosage for effective control than communities in which these parameters are of lower value. The drug is effective when given at close or widely spaced intervals; in some situations, once and twice-yearly single doses are being used with promising result. The drug has been applied effectively in selected circumstances as a medicated household salt.

Monitoring and long-term evaluation of control programme effectiveness is based upon repeated measurements of the vector population, particularly as related to the man-biting density, infectivity rate and the transmission potential; determining the incidence, prevalence, and median microfilarial density of patent infections in the community; and, defining trends in filarial illness, to include study of the health impact.

The value of DEC-C in prophylaxis is not yet known; recent studies in monkeys, however, show that the drug is highly effective against developing larvae under experimental conditions (Mak, unpublished data).

Protective clothing, repellants, bed-netting, avoidance of mosquito biting environments and improved housing are common sense elements in prevention and control. The keys to the implementation of these personal measures are health education and socioeconomic advancement.

REFERENCES

Ash L R, Riley J M 1970 Development of subperiodic Brugia malayi in the jird, Meriones unguiculatus, with notes on infections in other rodents. J Parasit 56: 969
Bancroft J 1877 Discovery of the adult representative of microscopic filariae. Lancet 2: 70
Beaver P C 1970 Filariasis without microfilaremia. Amer. J Trop. Med. Hyg. 19: 181
Brug, S L 1927 Filaria malayi n. sp., parasitic in the Malay Archipelago. Trans VII Congr. Far East Ass. Trop. Med. 3: 279

Buckley J J C, Edeson J F B 1956 On the morphology of Wuchereria sp. malayi? from a monkey Macaca irus and from cats in Malaya and on Wuchereria pahangi n.sp. from a dog and a cat. J Helminthol 30: 1

Cobbold T S, 1877 On Filaria bancrofti. Lancet 2: 495

Colwell E J, Armstrong D R, Brown J D, Duxbury R E, Sadun E H, Legters L J 1970 Epidemiologic and serologic investigations of filariasis in indigenous populations and American soldiers in South Vietnam. Amer. J. trop. Med. Hyg., 19: 227

Connor F W 1932 The aetiology of the disease syndrome in Wuchereria bancrofti infections Trans. roy. Soc. trop. Med. Hyg., 26: 13

Cross J H, Partono F, Hsu M Y K, Ash L R, Oemijati S 1979 Experimental transmission of Wuchereria bancrofti to monkeys. Amer. J. trop. Med. Hyg., 28: 56

Danaraj T J, Pacheco G, Shamugaratnam K, Beaver P C 1966 The etiology and pathology of eosinophilic lung tropical eosinophilia. Amer. J. trop. Med. Hyg., 15: 183

Demarquay J N 1863 Note on a tumour of the scrotal sac containing a milky fluid (galactocoele of vidal) and enclosing small wormlike beings that can be considered as hematoid helminthes in the embryo stage. Helminthologie Gaz. Med. Paris, 18: 665

Dennis D T, Kean B E 1971 Isolation of microfilaraemia: report for a new method. J. Parasit Parasit, 57: 1146

Dissanaike A S, Mak J W 1980 A description of adult Wuchereria bancrofti rural strain from an experimental infection in the long-talied macaque, Macaca fascicularis (Syn. M. irus). J Helminthol, 54: 117

Dissanaike A S, Niles 1967 On two infective filarial larvae in Mansonia crassipes with a note on other infective larvae in wild-caught mosquitoes in Ceylon. J Helminthol, 41: 291

Edeson J F B, Buckley J J C 1959 Studies on filariasis in Malaya: on the migration and rate of growth of Wuchereria malayi in experimental infected cats. Ann. trop. Med. Parasit., 53: 113

Edeson J F B, Wharton R H, 1957 The transmission of Wuchereria malayi from man to the domestic cat. Trans. roy. Soc. trop. Med. Hyg., 51: 366

Ezeoke, A, Perera, A B, Hobbs, J R 1973 Serum IgE elevation with tropical eosinophilia. Clin. Allergy, 3: 33

Galindo L, von Lichtenberg F, Baldizon C 1962 Bancroftian filariasis in Puerto Rico: infection pattern and tissue lesions. Amer. J. trop. Med. Hyg., 11: 739

Grove D I, Davis R S 1978 Serological diagnosis of Bancroftian and Malayan filariasis. Amer. J. trop. Med. Hyg., 27: 508

Hairston N G, DoeMeillon B 1968 On the inefficiency of transmission of Wuchereria bancrofti from mosquito to human host. Bull. Wld. Hlth. Org., 38: 935

Hairston N G, Jachowski L A 1968 Analysis of the Wuchereria bancrofti population in the people of American Samoa. Bull. Wld. Hlth. Org., 38: 29

Harinasuta C, Guptavanij P, Bell D R, Wilson T, Ramachandran C P, Sivanandam S 1970 Studies on the nocturnally subperiodic strain of Wuchereria bancrofti from West Thailand. Southeast Asian J. trop. Med. Publ. Hlth., 1: 152

Jordon P 1955 Notes on elephantiasis and hydrocoele due to Wuchereria bancrofti. J. trop. Med. Hyg., 58: 113

Laurence B R 1967 Elephantiasis in Greece and Rome and the Queen of Punt. Trans. Roy Soc. trop. Med. Hyg., 61: 612

Lie K J 1962 Occult filariasis: its relationship with tropical pulmonary eosinophilia. Amer. J. trop. Med. Hyg., 11: 646

Mak J W 1981 Filariasis in Southeast Asia. Ann. Acad. Med. Singapore, 10: 112

Mak J W, Cheong W H, Yen P K F, Lim P K C, Chan W C 1982 Studies on the epidemiology of subperiodic Brugia malayi in Malaysia: problems in its control. Acta trop., 39: 237

Mak J W, Singh M, Yap E H, Ho B C, Kang K L 1979 Studies on human filariasis in Malaysia: immunoglobulin and complement levels in persons infected with Brugia malayi and Wuchereria bancrofti. Trans. roy. soc. trop. Med. Hyg., 73: 395

Mak J W, Yen P K F 1976 The possible zoonotic significance of the filarial parasite, Brugia pahangi. Proc. Inst. Med. Res. Sci. Meetings, 1975–1976, Inst. Med. Res., Kuala Lumpur. pp 153

Mak J W, Yen P K F, Lim K C, Ramiah N 1980 Zoonotic implications of cats and dogs in filarial transmission in Peninsular Malaysia. Trop. Geog. Med., 32: 259

Manson P 1884 The metamorphosis of Filaria sanguinis hominis in the mosquito. Trans. Linn. Soc. Lond., 2: 367

Otteson E A 1975 Eosinphilia and the lung. In: Kirk batrick, C H and Reynolds, H Y Immunologic and Infectious Reactions in the Lung. pp. 289–332. Marcel Dekker, New York 1975

Ottenson E A, Weller P F, Heck L 1977 Specific cellular immune unresponsiveness in human filariasis. Immunology, 33: 413

Partono F, Purnomo, Dennis D T, Atmosoedjono S, Oemijati S, Cross J H 1977 Brugia timori sp. n. Nematoda: Filarioidea from Flores Island, Indonesia. J. Parasit., 63: 540

Piessens W F, McGreevy P B, Piessens P W, McGreevy M, Koiman I, Saroso J S, Dennis D T 1980 Immune responses in human infections with Brugia malayi. Specific cellular unresponsiveness to filarial antigens. J. Clin. Invest., 65: 172

Purnomo, Dennis D T, Partono F 1977 The microfilaria of Brugia timori Partono et al. 1977 = Timor microfilaria, David and Edeson, 1964: morphologic description with comparison to Brugia malayi of Indonesia. J. Parasit., 63: 1001

Purnomo, Partono F, Dennis D T, Atmosoedjono S 1976 Development of the Timor filaria in Aedes togoi: preliminary observations. J. Parasit., 62: 881

Rao S S, Maplestone P A 1940 The adult of Microfilaria malayi Brug, 1927. Indian med. Gaz., 75: 159

Sasa M, Tanaka H, 1974 A statistical method for comparison and classification of the microfilarial periodicity. Japan J. exp. Med., 44: 321

Schacher J F, Sahyoun P F 1967 A chronological study of the histopathology of the filarial disease in cats and dogs caused by Brugia pahangi Buckley and Edeson, 1956. Trans. roy. soc. trop. Med. Hyg., 61: 234

Sim B K L, Kwa B H, Mak J W 1982 Immune responses in human Brugia malayi infections: serum dependent cell-mediated destruction of infective larvae in vitro. Trans. roy. soc. trop. Med. Hyg., 76: 362

Sivanandam S, Dondero T J 1972 Differentiation between periodic and subperiodic Brugia malayi and Brugia pahangi on the basis of microfilarial sheath casting in vitro. Ann. trop. Med. Parasit., 66: 487

Sivanandam S, Mak J W 1975 Some problems associated with the processing and staining of blood films for filaria diagnosis. J. Med. Hlth. Lab. Tech. Malaysia, 2: 25

Tanaka H 1981 Periodicity of microfilariae of human filariasis analysed by a trigonometric method Aikat and Das. Japan J. exp. Med., 51: 97

Webber R H 1979 Eradication of Wuchereria bancrofti infection through vector control. Trans. roy. soc. trop. Med. Hyg., 73: 722

Wharton R H 1957 Studies on filariasis in Malaya: observations on the development of Wuchereria malayi in Mansonia Mansonoides longipalpis. Ann. trop. Med. Parasit., 51: 278

Wharton R H 1962 The biology of Mansonia mosquitoes in relation to the transmission of filariasis in Malaya. Bull. Inst. Med. Res. Fed. Malaya, 11: 114 pp

White G B 1971 Studies on transmission of bancroftian filariasis in North Eastern Tanzania. Trans. roy. soc. trop. Med. Hyg., 65: 819

World Health Organization Expert Committee on Filariasis (1962) Wld Hlth Org. techn. Rep. Ser. 233.

World Health Organization Expert Committee on Filariasis (1967) Wld. Hlth. Org. techn. Rep. Ser. 359.

World Health Organization Expert Committee on Filariasis (1974)Wld. Hlth. Org. techn. Rep. Ser. 542.

Wucherer D E H 1868 Preliminary report on a species of worm as yet undescribed, found in the urine or patients with tropical haematuria in Brazil.

Noticia preliminar solre vermes de uma especre ainda nao descripta, encontrados na urina de doentes de hematuria inter-tropical no Brazil. Gazeta Medica de Bahia, 3: 97.

Yen P K F, Zaman V, Mak J W 1982 Identification of some common infective filarial larvae in Malaysia. J Helminthol., 56: 69.

Onchocerciasis

INTRODUCTION

Definition

Onchocerciasis is caused by a threadlike nematode worm, *Onchocerca volvulus* (Leuckart 1893), occurring in Central- and South America, tropical Africa and at the southern tip of the Arabian peninsula. It is transmitted by blackflies of the genus *Simulium* acting as intermediate host. No animal reservoirs of the parasite are known. The infection may exist for many years without any symptoms. Clinical signs are pruritus, inflammatory and degenerative skin lesions, subcutaneous nodules the size of 3–50 mm known as onchocercomata, containing the adult parasite and eye lesions that may lead to blindness. Diagnosis is usually made by demonstrating microfilariae (larvae of the parasite) after they have left snips of skin immersed in a suitable liquid for sufficient time. Onchocerciasis can be treated chemotherapeutically with suramin and diethylcarbamazine (DEC) and surgically through the excision of palpable onchocercomata. Because of its economic importance, programmes to control the infection have been organized by international and bilateral agencies in many endemic areas. They aim to eliminate the parasite by controlling the vector and thus breaking transmission.

Economic importance

In a very typical way onchocerciasis demonstrates the problems of health care in rural areas of the third world. Although it is estimated that between 20 000 000 and 50 000 000 persons are infected globally, the importance of the disease was not realized until fairly recently. Even now it is not uncommon to find medical personnel in areas with a near 100 per cent prevalence in the adult population quite unfamiliar with its clinical appearance and diagnosis.

Geomedical studies have demonstrated that onchocerciasis is the single most important factor forcing West-African populations to leave fertile areas in river valleys near vector breeding places thus abandoning almost a tenth of the arable land. Overcrowding in adjacent areas leads to a vicious cycle of agricultural overexploitation, diminishing production, malnutrition and disease.

DISEASE

The prepatent period between the inoculation of a third stage larva and the first detection of microfilariae in skin biopsies is at least seven months and may be as long as three years in mild infections (Prost 1980). Adult worms are not only found in onchocercomata but also free in the connective tissue (Van den Berghe 1936). Pathology is mainly caused by microfilariae, either directly as mechanical damage when they migrate through the body or in the form of inflammatory reactions around dead microfilariae. They are known to occur in all parts of the body. In heavy infections it is not rare to find them in the urine (Buck et al 1971) and they may even pass from the maternal body to the embryo *in utero* (Brinkmann et al 1976).

Clinical signs

The systemic character of onchocerciasis has been described by Buck (1975). The infection correlates with a reduced general and nutritional state, it has been linked to a form of dwarfism in Uganda and may cause lymphadenitis and scrotal elephantiasis (Connor et al 1970, Connor 1974).

Onchocercomata are nodules ranging in size from three to 50 mm. About 50 per cent of them may be detected by palpation of the scalp, the thorax, the pelvic area and the knees.

Onchocerciasis causes intense pruritus and dermatitis with a tendency to become chronic. In this later stage, often called onchodermatitis the inflammatory reactions lead to degenerative processes affecting the pigment layers of the skin and the elastic fibres. The clinical picture is characterized by lichenification, scaling, superinfected eroded papules and disturbed pigmentation. The lower legs of dark skinned persons often show a typical spotted or maplike depigmentation. Generalized atrophy is the last stage.

Special forms of onchocerciasis skin lesions are hanging skin folds as in elastosis, called 'hanging groins' after their site of predilection by Nelson (1958), and the hyperreactive localized condition originally only known from the Arabian focus as 'sowda'. Microfilariae can be observed in great numbers in the cornea and in the anterior chamber of the eye. Inflammatory reactions around dead parasites lead to sclerozing keratitis. Other ocular lesions common in onchocerciasis patients are iritis leading to secondary glaucoma, chorioretinitis and optic atrophy. Anterior as well as posterior lesions may result in blindness. Onchocerciasis eye changes have been described by Thylefors (1978) and Rodger (1981). A more detailed description of clinical onchocerciasis is contained in the book edited by Buck 1974.

Diagnosis

An easy, sensitive and specific way to diagnose onchocerciasis is to excise a small superficial snip of skin at the iliac crest and submerge it in normal saline for 24 h. Microfilariae that have left the specimen can be detected unstained at a magnification of × 25 to × 50. For a quantitative determination of microfilarial density, the skin snip should be weighed previous to submersion. This technique has been described and discussed by Braun-Munzinger et al (1977).

Other more complicated diagnostic methods are the demonstration of microfilariae in the urine or the anterior segment of the eyes, serological tests and tests based on skin reactions either following the oral application of the microfilaricide DEC (Mazzotti-test) or the local use of antigen-preparations.

Therapy

A definite treatment of the infection consists of a primary reduction of microfilariae using DEC at gradually increasing doses from 25 mg the first day to 200 mg on the fifth day for a total of 14 days, followed by suramin. If a test dose of 0.1 g suramin is tolerated 1.0 g is injected once weekly to a total of five to seven grammes. The excision of onchocercomata is beneficial as an adjuvant. Because of the high toxicity of suramin and severe side-reactions to DEC, treatment should only be administered by trained physicians on an individual basis. The reader is recommended to consult the paper by Duke et al (1981) expressing current views on the chemotherapy of onchocerciasis. It is available on request from WHO.

PARASITE, VECTOR AND LIFE CYCLE

Adult *O. volvulus* worms have a life span of up to 15 years. One or several of them usually live coiled up in onchocercomata. The smaller males (length 3–6 cm) move possibly from nodule to nodule to fertilize the considerably longer females (length 30–60 cm). One female parasite produces about one million microfilariae per year.

Microfilariae are unsheathed, they are 0.3 mm long. If they are not ingested by the vector they may live about 18 months. Those that have been taken up by a blackfly, traverse its stomach wall and develop through two larval stages to infective larvae (third stage larva) that, upon reinoculation mature to male or female adult worms in the human host. The development inside the vector is dependent on the outside temperature. It is stopped below 18°C. At 25–30°C it takes six to eight days. A morphological description of *O. volvulus* based on scanning-electron microscopy has been given by Franz (1980).

Investigations of Bain (1981) have shown that *O. volvulus* is phylogenetically most closely related to onchocerca species parasitizing cattle in Africa. It is therefore very probable that the human parasite differentiated in the savanna areas of this continent. Since then however enough time has passed for the sub-species of *O. volvulus* to have developed.

Onchocerciasis is transmitted by various simulium species. Most important among them are *S. ochraceum* in Central America, *S. exiguum* and *S. metallicum* in South America, the *S. damnosum* complex in West-, Central-, East-Africa and Yemen. The biology of *Simulium* has been described by Le Berre (1966) and Philippon (1978). Female insects lay their eggs in batches of 250 at waterlevel on vegetation in fast flowing water. The larvae live in a depth of not more than 50 cm firmly attached to the ground or plants. Nutrition is obtained with the help of fans near the head. Larval development is dependent on the outside temperature. In tropical rivers it takes about one week. After a pupal stage the adult insect hatches and leaves the water. Blackflies are exophile and active during the day. As they are dependent on the humidity in the air they are found closer to rivers during the dry season. Garms et al (1979) have proved that infected flies may be carried by monsoon winds over distances up to 500 km. In savanna areas blackflies breed in rivers whereas in the forest small streams may also be used as breeding sites.

EPIDEMIOLOGY

The distribution and spread of onchocerciasis in a population is determined by the intensity of transmission, which in turn is dependent on ecological conditions, the vector species and its vectorial capacity, the level of endemicity, the density and distribution of the human population and socio-economic factors like migration, nutrition, agriculture et cetera with a bearing on exposure and the general state of health. Although there is no protective immunity to onchocerciasis, in each individual living in an area of transmission a balance is struck between the worm-load and the bodily defense mechanisms with age which is usually equivalent to the duration of residence.

Geographical aspects of onchocerciasis

Distribution

Although onchocerciasis is counted among the most important diseases in the third world and has received much attention in the last 20 years the knowledge of its distribution is extended almost every year. It is not yet a decade since it was first identified in the Amazon basin and Saudi Arabia. There are indications that hitherto unknown foci exist in Peru. Figure 32.1 is based on a map incorporating all informations available to WHO by the end of 1975 (WHO 1976) with recent additions.

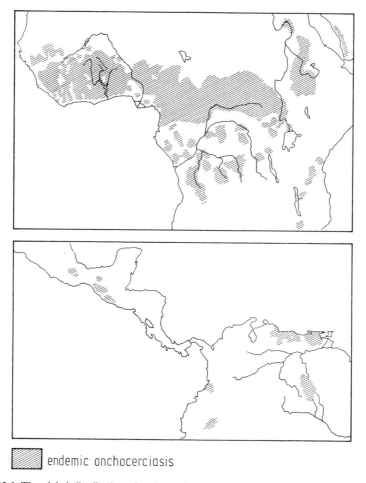

endemic onchocerciasis

Fig. 32.1 The global distribution of onchocerciasis

Except for the focus in South-Arabia onchocerciasis is not known in either Asia or the Pacific. Its main occurrence is in Africa. The foci in Latin-America are usually small. Since larval development in the vector is halted below 18°C onchocerciasis is restricted to tropical areas between roughly 15° north and south of the equator and below an altitude of 1500 m. Since the vector depends on fast flowing rivers for breeding places and on sufficient air-humidity for survival and as man is the only reservoir of the parasite, the distribution of onchocerciasis is highly focal.

Onchocerciasis and cyclic migrations

The inexperienced may form a totally wrong impression of the fertility of tropical soils when judged from the luxuriant growth encountered. In fact the land in the African savanna has to lie fallow for many years between the short periods it may be tilled. Using traditional methods of agriculture a high amount of physical labour is required to achieve adequate harvests. In this delicately atuned balance between population density, working capacity and soil fertility, onchocerciasis can be the proverbial grain that causes the cart to break. A generally decreased state of health and an increasing proportion of adults disabled by visual impairment and blindness are more than a community can bear for a long time. Hunter (1966) in Northern Ghana and Bradley (1976) in Nigeria have described cyclical migrations with a duration of three to four generations. They result when populations with a low prevalence of onchocerciasis settle in river valleys, profiting initially from the better soil and the availability of water. These settlements diminish to total abandonment after the infection has spread and its impact is felt.

Geographical variants of onchocerciasis

When prevalence rates for various signs of onchocerciasis, especially blindness, are compared there are striking differences. In Africa blindness can be 2.5 times as frequent in savanna areas as in the forest zone. Savanna onchocerciasis is further characterized by higher skin concentrations of microfilariae, more skin lesions, more microfilarial invasion of the eye and much higher prevalence of sclerozing keratitis (Anderson et al 1974, Prost et al 1980). Higher rates for onchocercomata, lymphadenopathy and hanging groins are typical for the savanna type in West-Africa and for the forest type in Cameroon. Microfilariae from patients of the forest area in Cameroon developed poorly in *S. damnosum*. s.l. from the savanna, and vice versa microfilariae from patients of the savanna did not develop well in forest flies. Experimental inoculation of microfilariae in the eyes of rabbits showed that microfilariae of the 'savanna strain' were more pathogenic for the cornea than those of the 'forest strain' (Duke 1981). In Guatemala and Mexico head nodules are much more frequent than in Africa. Although microfilarial density is equivalent to Africa skin lesions and lymphadenopathy are less frequent and milder. Whether the low rates of blindness are a success of control programmes or a characteristic of Central American onchocerciasis can presently not be determined.

Reviewing the subject, Duke (1981) concluded that neither nutritional nor environmental factors could explain the phenomenon and that intrinsic strain differences are the most favoured hypothesis. Morphological and biochemical evidence for different strains of *O. volvulus* however is still scarce and not very satisfactory.

Quantitative aspects of transmission

Arbitrarily one may start the cycle of transmission with a blackfly feeding on an infected person. About four minutes are necessary for the insect to obtain about one milligramme of blood. It takes longer in patients with skin lesions. The number of microfilariae ingested is proportional to skin density (Campell et al 1980). The age-groups between 11 and 30 years contribute most to the infection of the vector (Duke & Moore 1968). Due to a peritrophic membrane forming around the ingested blood in the gut of the insect only few of the microfilariae reach the haemocoele. This phenomenon, known as 'limitation' was first described by Philippon (1977), it means that the number of infective larvae that develop eventually is not proportional to the density of microfilariae in the skin.

Of the microfilariae that have reached the haemocoele 25–33 per cent die within the first 24 hours. Of those remaining, another 15 per cent will die during larval development. Low temperatures at night may increase their mortality to 33 per cent. The gonotrophic cycle of the insect is shorter than the development of the parasite. As a consequence of this superinfections are possible on one hand and the vector may not take a bloodmeal for several days after the parasite has completed larval development. While feeding on plant juices during this time up to 50 per cent of the infective larvae may leave the insect. When biting man 68 per cent of infective larvae leave the *Simulium* vector.

As an index to measure the intensity of transmission Duke (1968) has proposed to use the number of infective larvae potentially transmitted per person per year. It correlates with the prevalence of infection and morbidity and is widely used as it can be determined on the spot. It is usually referred to as ATP (annual transmission potential). It should not be overlooked however that ATP's usually appear unrealistically high since they are determined using one fly catcher close to a simulium breeding place. Simulium density may in the absence of severe pollution be regarded as constant. Increasing the human population therefore means that the number of bites per person per unit of time decreases. With regard to the aforementioned cyclic migrations this also explains that transmission becomes more intense the more population diminishes. ATP's are also increased as larvae of *O. ochengi* cannot be distinguished from those of *O. volvulus*.

No data exist concerning the proportion of larvae that mature to adult parasites and mate after they have been inoculated. Duke et al (1974) observed that villages are abandoned if ATP's exceed 4400. Thylefors et al (1978) were not able to determine a minimum level of transmission at which no more severe eye-lesions occur in the population.

A mathematical model to describe transmission has been designed but it is still based on a number of parameters that cannot be determined with accuracy and whose interdependence and thus mathematical connexion is unclear.

Prevalence of infection and morbidity

Because of the longevity of the parasite and the resulting long duration of the infection, incidence is hardly if ever used in onchocerciasis. It can only be determined indirectly.

The overall prevalence of infection in a given area is usually roughly grouped into hyperendemic (66 to 100 per cent), mesoendemic (33 to 65 per cent) and hypoendemic (less than 33 per cent). This corresponds to perennial exposure of all members of the community to transmission (hyper-), transmission limited seasonally and/or to certain areas outside the villages (meso-) and sporadic transmission (hypoendemic). Figure 32.2 demonstrates the increase of all signs and symptoms of onchocerciasis with age except for microfilaruria. In hyperendemic areas of the African savanna blindness becomes noticeable beyond the age of 30. From four per cent (30–39 years) the prevalence increases to 13 per cent (50 + years). In hypoendemic areas

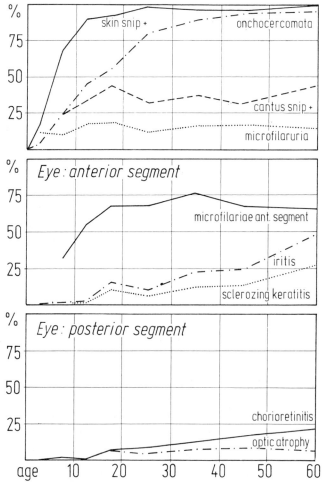

Fig. 32.2 Prevalence of signs and symptoms and age in onchocerciasis.

blindness) caused by *O. volvulus* is rare. Prevalence is not a good index as it depends on the age-structure of the population. A better way to express endemicity is Knüttgen & Büttner (1969) AI_{50}, the age at which 50 per cent of the population have overt infection. Personal characteristics like sex, occupation, ethnic group et cetera influence prevalence only in meso- or hypoendemic areas and only if they increase or reduce exposure. This changes from place to place and no general rule exists.

Risk factors

Although large numbers of persons in onchocerciasis areas develop signs of sickness and an economically important proportion becomes disabled by blindness astonishingly many remain free of all adverse objective signs despite high parasite loads. With limited means of chemotherapy prohibiting mass application on one hand and a large proportion of the population in definite need of treatment on the other, it is necessary to identify those individuals most likely to develop eye-lesions (Scharlau 1981). In the absence of long term observations, only the results of cross-sectional studies can be used for this purpose. A definite sign of ocular risk is the presence of microfilariae in the anterior segment of the eye (Thylefors & Brinkmann 1977) but it is not easy to diagnose. Microfilaruria has been proposed by Ba et al (1981). The value of various parasitological signs for the identification of risk patients is discussed in more detail by Brinkmann (1982). If the presence of more than 100 microfilariae per skin snip at the iliac crest and/or a positive skin snip at the outer cantus of the eye and/or the presence of microfilariae in 10 ml urine and/or five or more onchocercomata can be palpated are taken as criteria the proportion of persons with eye-lesions in the groups thus defined is shown in figure 32.3. It is based on the examination jointly with Thylefors of 1577 persons in Ghana and Togo.

SURVEILLANCE

For an epidemiological assessment of the prevalence and importance of onchocerciasis in a given area baseline data are required on the distribution of infection and morbidity in the population together with entomological investigations of vector breeding places, vector species and the annual transmission potential (ATP). At least in part the first can be done through basic health services; the second requires the specially trained personnel attached to large control programmes or specialized institutions.

In most areas where onchocerciasis is endemic, prevalence studies have been performed. Only a few have been published in scientific journals. Unpublished reports may be located at Ministries of Health, at WHO programme coordination offices, regional offices or headquarters, through World Bank, FAO or bilateral agencies. In Franco-phone countries organisms like O.C.C.G.E., O.R.S.T.O.M. and the Service des Grandes Ende-

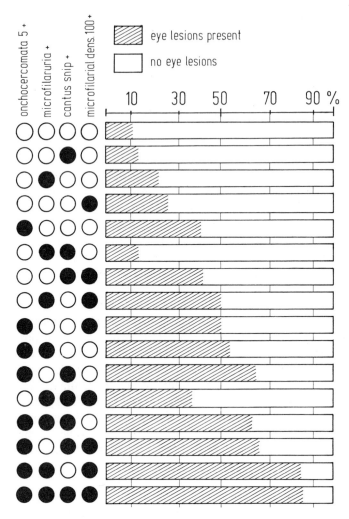

Fig. 32.3 Parasitological signs and the risk of eye lesions. Dark circles indicate the presence of one of the parasitological risk signs and possible combinations.
The graph is based on the examination of 1577 persons in Ghana and Togo.

mies possess valuable information. It is sometimes worth consulting local offices of tax-collection. In Mali and Upper Volta blind persons are exempted from taxes.

Onchocerciasis surveys are conducted as cross-sectional studies. The sampling unit is ideally a village of about 300 inhabitants. Everybody in this cluster should be examined. Since blind people may find it difficult to reach the place of examination, special enquiries should be made to ensure that their drop-out rate is not too high. In larger villages or towns the cluster can be a section of the desired size. Stratification is important in onchocerciasis surveys because of the focality of the disease. It is done with regard to endemicity or proximity to rivers (vector breeding places if they are known).

Infection is diagnosed by examining two skin snips from the right and left illiac crest. The most simple way to take them is to raise the skin with a pin and snip off a piece three to five millimetres in diametre. It is faster and less painful to employ Walser (or Holth) type corneal scleral punch instruments. Detailed descriptions of the method can be found in the articles of Braun-Munzinger et al (1977) and Awadzi et al (1980).

It is useful to record morbidity if time and resources permit. It has been shown above (fig. 3) that the number of onchocercomata is a very good indicator of the severity of the disease. Bodily inspections for onchocercomata and skin lesions require well lit rooms providing privacy, so that patients can undress completely. A simple way to classify skin lesions is to identify acute unspecific dermatitis, sowda, chronic dermatitis (onchodermatitis), atrophy, depigmentation, elastosis (instead of 'hanging groin' as elastosis has also been seen on other parts of the body). A survey-technique for the detection of microfilariae in the urine has been described by Ba et al (1981). In addition to the recording of personal data like age and sex, it is important to ask about migrations and the location of farms in relation to possible vector breeding places.

When the results of onchocerciasis surveys are presented, it is better to have narrow age-groups below 15 years, in adults a width of 10 years is usually sufficient. Rates should be standardized for age and sex by the direct method. This is only meaningful if there are at least 10 persons in each group. Microfilarial densities of populations are characterized by their geometric mean, since their distribution is approximately log-normal.

CONTROL

The only effective macrofilaricide that can be used therapeutically is suramin. Because of its high intrinsic toxicity it cannot be recommended for mass-campaigns even if it is used at low doses. The use of regular application of DEC again at low doses to diminish microfilarial density to the point that transmission is broken is not feasible because of resulting skin reactions (Duke et al 1981). Nodulectomy as a means to control onchocerciasis has been used in Mexico and Guatemala for more than 40 years without affecting prevalence. In short there are at present no means to control onchocerciasis by the elimination of the parasite through medical treatment.

Because of the longevity of the parasite, schemes to diminish onchocerciasis by breaking transmission through vector control have to be maintained for about 20 years and they have to cover a large enough area (blackflies have been carried over distances up to 500 km by monsoon winds). It goes without saying that they are very expensive, require an efficient management, international cooperation and are constantly endangered by the development of insecticide resistance. Attack has to be directed against the larvae of the vector since breeding places at least in savanna areas can be mapped whereas fighting the adult fly would require aerial spraying of immense proportions. Since 1973 WHO has organized an onchocerciasis control programme (OCP) in seven West-African countries covering about 1 000 000 km². Its annual costs are presently in the order of U.S.-dollar 15 000 000. Additional programmes are planned west of OCP to cover Sierra Leone, Guinea, Senegambia and western Mali, east of OCP in Nigeria and in Guatemala (Ogata 1981). The disease has been largely controlled in foci of Mexico and Venezuela. It was successfully eradicated from Kenya. Le Berre (1981) has recently published an account of problems and prospects of antivectorial campaigns to control onchocerciasis.

PREVENTION

No chemoprophylaxis is known to prevent the infection with onchocerciasis. DEC at weekly doses of 200 mg may be used as a suppressive therapy. Preventive measures are either the diminuation of exposure through protective clothing and insect repellents or the destruction of vector breeding places. For example spillways of dams should be constructed in such a way as to enable a complete interruption of the flow of water for at least 24 hours per week. Sometimes it may be possible to destroy rapids by canalizing a river. If possible villages should not be constructed close to vector breeding places.

CONSEQUENCES

The consequences of onchocerciasis for the structuring and organization of health services are to put more emphasis on opthalmological diagnosis and care in rural areas. Facilities for the detection and care of risk cases have to be provided. The rehabilitation of blind persons must become a regular part of basic health programmes in endemic areas.

REFERENCES

Anderson J, Fuglsang H, Hamilton P J S, Marshall T F de C 1974 Studies on onchocerciasis in the United Cameroon Republic II. Comparison of onchocerciasis in rainforest and sudan savanna. Transactions of the Royal Society of tropical Medicine and Hygiene 68: 209–222

Awadzi K, Roulet H, Bell D R 1980 The chemotherapy of onchocerciasis. V: A standard method for the determination of microfilarial density in skin snips. Annals of tropical Medicine and Hygiene 74: 363–366

Ba O, Rolland A, Marshall T F de C 1981 Microfilarurie et lésions oculaires onchocerquiennes. Tropenmedizin und Parasitologie 32: 181–183

Bain O 1981 Les éspeces du genre Onchocerca et principalement O. volvulus, envisagees du point de vue épidemiologique et phylogenique. Annales belges de la Médecine tropicale 61: 225–231

Bradley A K 1976 Effects of onchocerciasis on settlement in the Middle Hawal Valley, Nigeria. Transactions of the Royal Society of tropical Medicine and Hygiene 70: 225–229

Braun-Munzinger R A, Scheiber P, Southgate B A 1977 Simplifying modifications to the microtitration plate technique for onchocerciasis surveys. Transactions of the Royal Society of tropical Medicine and Hygiene 71: 548–549

Brinkmann U K 1982 Onchozerkose in West-Africa, Verlag Peter Lang, Frankfurt M., Bern

Brinkmann U K, Krämer P, Presthus G T, Sawadogo B 1976 Transmission in utero of microfilariae of O. volvulus. Bulletin World Health Organization 54: 708–709

Buck A A (ed) 1974 Onchocerciasis, symptomatology, pathology, diagnosis, World Health Organization, Geneva

Buck A A 1975 Host factors. World Health Organization, unpublished document ONCHO/WP/75.28

Buck A A et al 1971 Microfilauria in onchocerciasis. Clinical and epidemiological follow-up study in the Republic of Chad. Bulletin World Health Organization 45: 353–369

Campbell C C, Collins R C, Houng A Y, Figueroa Marroquin H 1980 Quantitative aspects of the infection of Simulium ochraceum by Onchocerca volvulus: The relation of skin microfilarial density to vector infection. Tropenmedizin und Parasitologie 31: 475–478

Connor D H 1974 Pathology of onchocerciasis and main geographical and local characteristics of the disease. Pan American Health Organization Scientific Publication 298, 11–24

Connor D H et al 1970 Onchocercal dermatitis, lymphadenitis, and elephantiasis in the Ubangi Territory. Human Pathology 1: 553–579

Duke B O L 1968 Studies on factors influencing the transmission of onchocerciasis. IV. The biting-cycles, infective biting density and transmission potential of 'forest' Simulium damnosum. Annals of tropical Medicine and Parasitology 62: 95–106

Duke B O L 1981 Geographical aspects of onchocerciasis. Annales belges de la Médecine tropicale 61: 179–186

Duke B O L, Moore P J 1968 The contributions of different age groups to the transmission of onchocerciasis in a Cameroon forest village. Transactions of the Royal Society of tropical Medicine and Hygiene 62: 22–28

Duke B O L, Anderson J, Fuglsang H 1975 The O. volvulus transmission potentials and associated patterns of onchocerciasis in four Cameroon Sudan-savanna villages. Tropenmedizin und Parasitologie 26: 143–154

Duke B O L, Thylefors B, Rougemont A 1981 Current views on the treatment of onchocerciasis with diethylcarbamazine citrate and suramin. World Health Organization unpublished document WHO/ONCHO/81.156

Franz M 1980 Electron microscope study of the cuticle of male and female Onchocerca volvulus from various geographic areas. Tropenmedizin and Parasitologie 31: 149–164

Garms R, Walsh J F, Davies J B 1979 Studies on the reinvasion of the Onchocerciasis Control Programme in the Volta River Basin by S. damnosum s.l. with emphasis on the South-Western areas. Tropenmedizin und Parasitologie 30: 345–362

Hunter J M 1966 River blindness in Nangodi, Northern Ghana: A hypothesis of cyclical advance and retreat. The geographical Review 56: 398–416

Knüttgen H J, Büttner D W 1967 Die altersspezifische 50%-Mf-Rate (AI_{50}) ein Index für das Onchozerkosevorkommen in einer Bevölkerung. Zeitschrift für Tropenmedizin und Parasitologie 20: 303–310

Le Berre R 1966 Contribution a l'étude biologique et écologique de S. damnosum Theobald, 1903 (Diptera, Simuliidae). Memoires O.R.S.T.O.M. 17

Le Berre R 1981 La lutte contre les simulies vectrices d'onchocercose en Afrique. Annales de la Societe belge de Médécine tropicale 61: 187–192

Nelson G S 1958 'Hanging groin' and hernia, complications of onchocerciasis. Transactions of the Royal Society for Tropical Medicine and Hygiene 52: 272–275

Ogata K 1981 Preliminary report of Japan-Guatemala Onchocerciasis Control Pilot Project. In: Marshall Laird (ed) Blackflies, The future for biological methods in integrated control. Academic Press, London New York Toronto Sydney San Francisco

Philippon B 1977 Étude de la transmission d'O. volvulus (Leuckart 1893) (Nematoda Onchocercidae) par Simulium damnosum Theobald, 1903 (Diptera, Simuliidae) en Afrique tropicale. Traveaux et Documents O.R.S.T.O.M. No. 63

Philippon B 1978 L'onchocercose humaine en Africque de l'ouest, ORSTOM Initiations Documentations techniques No. 37, Paris

Prost A 1980 Latence parasitaire dans l' onchocercose. Bulletin World Health Organization 58: 923–925

Prost A, Rougemont A & Omar M S 1980 Charactères épidémiologiques, cliniques et biologiques des onchocercoses de savanne et de forêts en Afrique occidentale. Revue critique et éléments nouveaux. Annales de Parasitologie 55: 347–355

Rodger F C 1981 Eye disease in the tropics. Churchill Livingstone, Edinburgh London Melbourne New York. h 3, p 22

Scharlau G 1981 Onchocerciasis-chemotherapy: a risk approach. Tropical doctor 11: 8–14

Thylefors B 1977 Vision screening of illiterate populations. Bulletin World Health Organization 55: 115–119

Thylefors B 1978 Ocular onchocerciasis. Bulletin World Health Organization 56: 63–73

Thylefors B, Brinkmann UK 1977 The microfilarial load in the anterior segment of the eye. A parameter of intensity of onchocerciasis. Bulletin World Health Organization 55: 731–737

Thylefors B, Philippon B. Prost A 1978 Transmission potentials of O. volvulus and associated intensity of onchocerciasis in a Sudan-savanna area. Tropenmedizin und Parasitologie 29: 346–354

Van den Berghe L 1936 Note préliminaire sur la localisation extranodulaire de 'O. volvulus' chez l'homme. Annales Societe belge Médécine Tropicale 16: 539–551

Trypanosomiasis

Primarily because of geographical and linguistic barriers, studies on the two great human trypanosome diseases of the world — Chagas' disease in America and sleeping sickness in Africa — have largely developed separately. Nevertheless, these two diseases have much in common and development of comparisons and contrasts between them has resulted recently from modern improvement in communication and from initiative on the part of the World Health Organization. The present review has been written by authors with special experience of Chagas' disease (PDM) (Marsden, 1971) and of sleeping sickness (WHRL) who, however, are also familiar with each other's fields.

American trypanosomiasis — Chagas' disease

INTRODUCTION

This disease is caused by infection with *Trypanosoma (Schizotrypanum) cruzi*, which is transmitted from one mammal host to another mainly by blood-sucking bugs of the subfamily Triatominae of the family Reduviidae. Transmission is 'posterior station', 'contaminative', i.e., the infective forms occur in the faeces of the bugs and gain entrance to new mammal hosts *via* skin abrasions or *via* mucous membranes, often the conjunctiva. Besides man, a wide variety of other animals, both domestic and wild, may be infected, and in some situations these other 'reservoirs' of infection may be important epidemiologically.

The World Health Organization has estimated that seven million people are infected and 30 million exposed to the risk of infection. The available evidence suggests that an individual, once infected, remains so for life. Only a small proportion (five to 15 per cent) of these infected persons, however, develop clinical signs of Chagas' disease. These are usually chronic myocarditis, causing weakness of heart muscle function, and gut dilatations ('mega' syndromes).

Human infections are usually acquired in childhood and most of the acute recognized infections are in children under the age of 10 years. Unilateral bipalpebral odema (Romaña's sign) is a common sign where the conjunctiva is the portal of entry but the infecting organisms in bug faeces may invade the host through any skin abrasion, causing often a local indurated swelling, the chagoma. Although acute infections with fever, tachycardia, lymphadenopathy and hepatosplenomegaly are sometimes clinically recognizable, the rarity of diagnosed acute cases in highly endemic areas indicates that many infections are initially asymptomatic. Usually acute cases are easily diagnosed because trypanosomes are abundant in the peripheral blood and may be demonstrated by microscopy. After the first couple of months the parasitaemia falls and decades may then elapse before the emergence of the clinical signs of the chronic disease, such as cardiac insufficiency and gut dysfunction, in a small proportion of infected persons. During this period and after the cardiac and gut signs appear, trypanosomes are very scanty in the blood and as a rule can only be demonstrated by xenodiagnosis (feeding clean bugs on the patient and examining their gut contents for organisms some 30 days later). Heart failure and arrhythmias tend to occur mostly in males, and in the third to fifth decades of life. About half the patients presenting with heart failure die within a year. Sudden death from heart failure, is a proverbial event in Chagas' disease affected areas.

The other group of clinical manifestations of Chagas' disease are the 'mega' syndromes of the gut dysfunction and these have an uneven geographical prevalence; e.g., they are quite common in Brazil but virtually unknown in Venezuela. This uneven geographical distribution may be related to strain differences of *Tryp. cruzi*. Although the predisposing factor which determines whether an individual will develop these serious late complications is not definitely known, Köberle (1968) has suggested that it may be the destruction of parasympathetic ganglia in the acute phase of the disease. The degree of ganglion destruction, and of the consequent aperistalsis, determine whether 'mega' syndromes develop. The oesophagus and colon are most commonly affected but other hollow viscera, bronchi, bladder, etc., may also be involved.

The incapacitation or mortality which the disease causes, because it affects mainly males in the most economically productive decades of their lives, are, for poverty-stricken large families existing in subsistence agricultural economies, tragic. This crippling effect is the direct social result of the disease, but it exerts a wider indirect effect in that the disease is feared, being known as a frequently fatal infection for which no really effective chemotherapy is as yet available.

EPIDEMIOLOGY

The infection is restricted to the Americas, especially South America, where the vector bugs mainly occur. In South America every country is affected but Romaña (1963) has pointed out that the infection is particularly prevalent in Brazil, Venezuela, Argentina and Chile. Estimates of human infection rate are based on serological reactions detected usually by a complement fixation test, by the indirect fluorescent antibody test or by the ELISA test (Anthony et al 1979). Chagas' disease has been quoted as the commonest cause of myocarditis in the world.

In the countries in which the disease is commonest, there exist highly domiciliated bug species such as *Panstrongylus megistus*, *Rhodnius prolixus* and *Triatoma infestans*. Less information is available from other countries but Chagas' disease is an important public health problem in Peru, Ecuador and Bolivia. Cases of Chagas' disease have also been found in many Central American countries and in Mexico. Two human cases have been reported in Texas, but although infected bugs are widely distributed in the southern United States, human infections are rare because the bugs live in association with sylvan animal hosts and the standard of housing is high. Also, North American *Tryp. cruzi* strains have a low pathogenicity for laboratory mice suggesting they may also be poorly pathogenic to man.

Why certain bug species have developed an affinity for living in houses is not altogether clear but it may be that man has killed off so many of the natural animal hosts that the bugs enter houses in search of a blood meal. The bugs are entirely dependent on blood (either mammalian or avian) for survival and reproduction. They can, however, survive for many months without feeding.

Basically Chagas' disease affects poverty-stricken families living in houses of poor construction. In Brazil the walls are made of wooden poles covered with mud frequently with a palm leaf roof. The mud walls tend to crack along both the horizontal and vertical wooden supports, leaving myriad connecting channels that are colonized by the bugs. Although adult bugs are winged, how often an infection is initially established in a house by an infected bug flying into it is not known, and must vary with species. Bugs are probably frequently transferred from house to house in clothing and bedding.

The intensity of transmission in any epidemiological situation depends on a variety of factors. These include the predilection of the local bug species for entering or becoming established in houses and in what numbers, the extent of their contact with extra-human reservoirs of *Tryp. cruzi*, their propensity to develop *Tryp. cruzi* infection, their preference for feeding on man, and so on. Some examples are illustrative of the complexities of the epidemiology. *P. megistus* is very sluggish and may remain immobile in the same crack in a wall for many days; total populations of this species in houses, as established by demolition, seldom exceed 600. *Triatoma infestans*, on the other hand, is more active and is found in larger number; over 8000 bugs were taken from a single hut in one instance. *T. infestans*, in contrast to *P. megistus*, is frequently found in the roof as well as in the walls of houses. Little is known of the dynamics of domestic bug populations under natural conditions in relation to the availability of blood meal sources, methods of migration, seasonal effects, etc. Some bug species are predominantly sylvan, some vary in this characteristic from place to place; *P. megistus* is often found in the field in the south of Brazil but is fully domiciliated further north. Extra-human cycles of *Tryp. cruzi* transmission occur among dogs, cats, opossums, rodents and many other mammals. The distribution of bugs in houses relates to the source of blood meals; for example, with *P. megistus* faecal smears of whitish or greenish colour, indicating the presence of bugs, can be seen on the pillow of a sleeping child. The face is probably most frequently attacked because it is the only part exposed; the bite of the bug seldom wakes the sleeper. Bugs engorge rapidly and ingest many times their own weight of blood. They appear to be non-selective feeders and will feed on any warm-blooded host. In areas of uniformly poor housing bugs may occur particularly in some houses but not in others, and it is not clear why this is so. Minor variations in bug behaviour may be important. In some bug species defaecation accompanies feeding and engorgement and so the infective trypanosomes discharged at this time are likely to contaminate the wound made by the mouth parts of the bugs; in other species defaecation is delayed until the bug has left the host. The fact that some children may live in a house with a large infected bug population and remain uninfected suggests that, on many occasions, even if skin contamination occurs, infection does not supervene. *Trypanosoma cruzi* does not withstand desiccation and a minimum number of organisms may be necessary to initiate infection.

Tryp. cruzi will infect most mammalian species in the laboratory and a multitude of wild animal reservoirs have been recorded. Dogs and cats are highly susceptible and important domestic reservoirs; young animals are particularly susceptible. Pigs, cattle and horses are comparatively resistant. Guinea pigs, reared for food, may provide a reservoir host. Bugs often feed on chickens but birds do not maintain *Tryp. cruzi* infection. Chick embryos will support the growth of *Tryp. cruzi* but infections die out rapidly after hatching. This insusceptibility may be related to their high body temperature. It appears that *Tryp. cruzi* is originally an infection of wild animals and that man has intruded into the natural cycle at a relatively late stage (zoonosis). The profusion of domestic and wild animal species which have been found to harbour *Tryp. cruzi* would appear greatly to complicate control measures but evidence from the iso-enzyme characterization of strains indicates that *Tryp. cruzi* is heterogeneous and that many of these 'reservoir' strains may be ecologically isolated from man (Miles, 1979).

CONTROL

The construction of houses with modern building materials such as concrete and corrugated iron reduces the chances of bug infestation but requires considerable expenditure and, apart from Venezuela, where many rural communities have been rehoused, most governments cannot afford such an expense and so rely on residual insecticides. Individual house owners often attempt to deal with the problem with a varying degree of success by walling the bugs in with fresh mud, and killing any bugs they find. If it is decided to abandon an infested house, the new house should be built some distance away from the old house and all articles should be inspected and treated with insecticides on transfer. The old house must be destroyed by fire.

The main method of controlling transmission is by the use of residual insecticides. DDT is not very effective against bugs so that a malaria control programme with this insecticide cannot be relied on to control Chagas' disease as well. However, other organochlorines, namely benzene hexa-chloride (BHC, Gammexane) and dieldrin are effective. BHC is widely used by the health authorities in Brazil and elsewhere.

In Brazil a control programme is carried out in three phases. First the area is mapped, and houses are searched for bugs using a pyrethrum spray to drive them out of their hiding places. This establishes where house infes-tation exists. In the second or attack phase, insecticide (BHC) is applied to all houses and out-houses in localities where bugs have been found. Both infested and non-infested houses are sprayed since live bug capture is but a crude index of bug presence. In many houses infestations are light and no bug can be captured. BHC exhibits bug killing activity up to three months depending on the type of surface sprayed. One spraying with BHC is not sufficient since eggs can survive this period and hatch; also, recently fed bugs deep in the wall may not come into contact with the insecticide before its activity is lost. A second, selective, spraying is, therefore, done more than 90 days after the first; only houses known to have had bugs are resprayed. Respraying of houses with persistent bug populations continues until the number of localities affected falls below five per cent, when the third, vigilance, phase is instituted. Vigilance consists of periodic searches for bugs in houses in the area by Ministry of Health personnel and the setting up of a series of information posts where a responsible member of communities of more than 25 houses has been trained to catch bugs and send them to a central collecting point, where they are idendified; appro-priate house spraying is arranged. SUCAM (Superintendencia de Campanhas de Saude Publica), the field arm of the Ministry of Health, set up initially to control malaria, is responsible for these programmes in Brazil. Spray teams usually consist of 2 spray men, a driver for the jeep and an inspector. They usually average four houses per man per day. Compression back-pack sprayers deliver $0.5g\ m^{-2}$ ie gram per square metre of BHC emul-sion. The inside of the roof and the inner and outer walls are sprayed. In Mambai — Goias — Brazil where such a programme was initiated in 1980, the cost per house spraying was approximately 250 cruzeiros (5 U.S. dollars); many visits may be necessary.

BHC has been the principle insecticide used against *T. infestans*, the most important vector of Chagas disease in Brazil, Argentina, Chile, Paraguay, Uruguay, Bolivia and Peru. It is cheap, of low toxicity and relatively effec-tive. Dieldrin was found to be better against *Rhodnius prolixus* in Venezuela

(1.0 g m^{-2}) but is more toxic. Many new insecticides are now available. An organophosphorous compound (malathion) has controlled *T. infestans* in Argentina. The carbamates (propoxur) and pyrethroids (decamethein) are effective but expensive.

Because such control programmes are so expensive research continues on finding ways of reducing costs so that more afflicted communities can be covered. The initial spraying kills the great majority of bugs and the possibility exists that by stimulating community participation the number of visits of Ministry personnel (an expensive business) could be reduced. One approach already mentioned is the information posts to notify the presence of bugs.

House improvement is even more costly and should be reserved for families with infestations persisting after insecticide application. The largest programme of new house contruction was carried out in Venezuela where *R. prolixus* is introduced repeatedly into the houses in palm fronds traditionally used for roofing. Roof replacement with corrugated iron had a beneficial effect. In Brazilian houses replastering of walls reduces man-bug contact, though bugs tend to escape into the roof through cracks around the wooden uprights. The composition of the mud plaster is critical to avoid early cracking; a binding agent such as cow faeces can be beneficial.

Specific drug treatment of *T. cruzi* infections remains unsatisfactory. Nifurtimox, a nitroturazone compound, is the most active drug available. The only solid indication for such treatment is in the acute phase of the disease. As such, treatment of patients has no place in a control programme and a vaccine is a very distant prospect. Transmission by blood transfusion can be prevented by accepting blood only from sero-negative donors. If the prevalence of infection is so high that this cannot be done, the addition of 1/4000 gentian violet to the blood at least 24 hours before transfusion is trypanocidal.

African trypanosomiasis — sleeping sickness

INTRODUCTION

Sleeping sickness is caused by *Trypanosoma (Trypanozoon) brucei*. It has been known in tropical Africa for centuries; some of its salient clinical signs, such as the enlargement of the posterior cervical triangle lymph nodes (Winterbottom's sign) were well known to slavers in the eighteenth century. However, it was only in the early twentieth century that the disease was related to its causative organisms. *Tryp. brucei* is transmitted 'inoculatively' by the 'anterior station', i.e., it is an organism in which the infective forms are developed in the proboscis of a blood-sucking insect or in its salivary glands and so are inoculated into the vertebrate host by its bite. The vectors are *Glossina* spp. (tsetse flies); the infective forms are injected into the host along with the salivary secretion.

There are three 'subspecies' of *Tryp. brucei,* all morphologically identical, and the epidemiology and control of the infections which they cause are determined by their differing biological characteristics. These are:

Tryp. b. brucei This subspecies is by definition non-infective to man and will be excluded from consideration in this review except in so far as it complicates the study of the epidemiology of the human disease; as it is morphologically identical to the man-infecting subspecies, it cannot be distinguished from them when it occurs in extra-human situations, such as in wild animals and in wild vectors. It does not cause human disease, but it is indirectly important to man as a cause (with other non-man-infecting trypanosome species) of *nagana,* a cattle disease which prevents the raising of cattle in huge areas of subsaharan Africa, so leading to protein deprivation in human populations. The area so deprived exceeds the total area of the United States of America.

Tryp. b. gambiense and *Tryp. b. rhodesiense* are causative organisms of human sleeping sickness, both by definition being able to infect man. They differ biologically from one another in causing, generally, diseases of different clinical picture. *Tryp. b. gambiense* sleeping sickness is a 'slow' disease, with an incubation period which may extend to several years; it is lethal only after a similarly protracted illness. *T. b. rhodesiense* sleeping sickness is, on the other hand, an acute infection, manifesting itself clinically in a few weeks and lethal, if untreated, in a very few months. These are typical rates of progression of the two diseases and although there are intergradations, these two different syndromes are fundamental and are associated with differences in many aspects of the diseases which they, respectively cause — e.g., clinical signs, pathology, epidemiology and control. The two diseases will, therefore, be mostly considered separately, with initial and final considerations of aspects common to them both.

Nagana, the trypanosome disease of cattle mentioned above, is practically coextensive in its distribution with the distribution of the tsetse flies. The human diseases are focal within the distribution of the tsetse flies, depending on local ecological conditions. *Tryp. b. gambiense* sleeping sickness occurs mainly in West and Central Africa from about 18°N to 18°S latitude, eastwards to about the western Rift Valley. It involves practically all the countries in that region, from The Gambia in the west to Zaire and Uganda in the east. *Tryp. b. rhodesiense* sleeping sickness occurs mainly in eastern Africa extending from some 8°N of the Equator to about 20°S, from Ethiopia to Zimbabwe.

The foregoing is the traditional view of the relationships of the *Tryp. brucei*-caused diseases and is still valid as a general concept for descriptive purposes. However, recent studies on the enzyme polymorphism of these morphologically-identical organisms have afforded objective intrinsic characters for their subspecific identification (Gibson et al., 1980). A new classification of the organisms on the basis of 'zymodemes' is in the process of development. A practical application of these studies already in use is the pinpointing of the wild animal species important as reservoirs of the human disease by finding man-infective zymodemes circulating in their blood.

The problems of the diagnosis of sleeping sickness are essentially the same for both types of the disease. Serological tests are indicative but not pathognomic and demonstration of the organism necessarily precedes treatment, as the specific drugs available are all highly toxic. Organisms may be abundant in early cases and easily found by the microscopy of Giemsa-stained thick blood films (TBF) or of wet or Giemsa-stained films of the aspirate from enlarged lymph nodes. But often, particularly in *T. b. gambiense* cases and in the later stages of both diseases, organisms are scanty and difficult to demonstrate by direct microscopy. Epidemiologically the main diagnostic requirement is the rapid recognition of *T. b. gambiense*-infected individuals in large rural populations, many of whom may be clinically unaffected, so that they may be treated and so stopped from acting as sources of infection for tsetse flies. Over most of the affected areas of Africa only the micro scopical methods mentioned above are available; these are laborious and miss many cases. Where more sophisticated methods are available, populations are first screened serologically, by immunofluorescent antibody tests (IFAT) or by immunosorbent enzyme-linked assays (ELISA) carried out on fingerprick blood samples collected on absorbent paper and dried. Serologically suspect individuals are examined intensively protozoologically on a second visit. If centrifugation is not available, the Giemsa-stained thick blood film is used. Two more sensitive methods depend on centrifugation: the microhaematocrit buffy-coat microscopy (MBCM) method, in which 50 µl samples of finger-prick blood are centrifuged at about 12 000 g; trypanosomes are concentrated in the buffy coat and in the immediately superjacent plasma and may be seen by microscopy either *in situ* in the tube or after expressing the buffy coat on to a microscope slide (Murray *et al.*, 1977): the miniature anion-exchange/centrifugation (MAEC) method in which 200 µl samples of blood from finger pricks are passed with appropriate buffer solutions through 2 ml columns of DEAE cellulose; blood cells are retained in the column while trypanosomes pass through and can be detected by microscopy of the deposit from the centrifuged (600 g) eluate (Lumsden *et al.*, 1981). Both these methods, and particularly the MAEC method, are much more sensitive than the TBF and have the additional advantage that they give immediate results without laborious microscopy.

TRYP. B. GAMBIENSE SLEEPING SICKNESS

Although a primary lesion at the site of bite — the 'trypanosome chancre' — may occur in *Tryp. b. gambiense* sleeping sickness, this lesion is seldom noticed, probably because the patient does not associate it with the subsequent disease because of the very long incubation period. The disease thus usually presents in its 'early' or 'blood-lymphatic' stage during which multiplication of organisms is taking place widely in the body, not only in these tissues, but also in tissue spaces generally. Lymphadenopathy and hepatosplenomegaly may be present. Typically there are bouts of fever associated with lassitude, with remissions for periods of days or months during which the patient feels quite well; or the infection may be quite cryptic. Only after a minimum period of some months do 'late stage' signs indicative of CNS involvement begin to appear — blunting of higher cerebral function, hand tremors, choreiform or athetotic movements of the limbs and trunk. It is likely, however, that the brain is invaded early (Apted, 1970).

Epidemiology

The slow clinical progress of *Tryp.* (*T.*) *gambiense* sleeping sickness is reflected in its epidemiology. Because of this slow progress, a situation may arise in which a large proportion of the population is infected before clinical cases are recognized. These unnoticed cases are, nevertheless, infective to tsetse flies and so epidemics may reach considerable proportions, even near medical centres, before the presence of the disease is suspected (Scott, 1970). Maintenance of transmission is possible by purely intrahuman cycles and this belief is supported by the distribution of the disease where the prevalence is high — cases are grouped together and correspond with ecological situations in which the people are repeatedly bitten by tsetse — and by the results of mass survey and treatment. Nevertheless, there is a long standing suggestion that domestic pigs are important as reservoirs and this has recently received support by the finding of *T. b. gambiense* zymodemes among the trypanosomes isolated from pigs in Liberia (Gibson *et al.*, 1980).

Tryp. b. gambiense transmission is particularly likely to arise when human populations are living close to river courses in regions otherwise arid. In this situation the vector tsetse flies, usually *Glossina palpalis palpalis* or *Glossina tachinoides* are restricted in their distribution to the riverain forest bordering the river courses; they cannot seek blood meals far outside this forest, which affords them a humid refuge in the otherwise arid country. The same flies will then tend to bite repeatedly any host entering the forest. If this is man, for the purposes of obtaining water for cooking or washing, then the stage is set for frequent man-to-man transmission. In this epidemiological situation all categories of the human population may be involved but usually mostly women and children, as it is these groups which spend most time in the river bed.

Control

The near restriction of the vertebrate component of the cycle to man and of the insect component to *Glossina* spp. of restricted environments offers the best possibilities for the control of the disease. The use of drugs has been already mentioned. According to Waddy (1970) an exclusively human infection should be eradicable by the protection of a high proportion, not necessarily 100 per cent, of the population by chemoprophylaxis and this procedure, using pentamidine, has been adopted in most endemic areas of West and Equatorial Africa. The recommended dosage (WHO, 1962; Waddy, 1970) — 4 mg of pentamidine base per kg body weight, up to a maximum of 300 mg — affords virtually complete protection in previously uninfected individuals for at least six months. However, experience indicates that *Tryp. b. gambiense* sleeping sickness is never eradicted by chemoprophylaxis alone; the procedure is unpopular and the mobility of male African population is extensive (Waddy, 1970).

Besides the use of drugs, the *Tryp. b. gambiense* sleeping sickness transmission cycles can sometimes be readily attacked by vector control methods. Restricted areas of forest can be economically cleared; it may be sufficient to clear only the stretches of the water course visited by the people for drawing water or doing their washing, or road crossings. The *Glossina* spp. inhabiting riverain forest are also susceptible to economical attack by the use of insecticides; Burnett (1970) gives the doses required for such linear habitats; in general, DDT and dieldrin are applied by spraying on trunks, stems and exposed roots, sometimes also leaves.

TRYP. B. RHODESIENSE SLEEPING SICKNESS

In this type of sleeping sickness the primary lesion, the trypanosome chancre, is more frequently noticed, because the onset of the developed clinical disease, with pyrexia, temporal and frontal headaches, rigors and vomiting, takes place within a few weeks. The chancre is an area of induration some three to 10 cm in diameter, inflamed or bluish, sometimes painful, which gradually subsides over some 14 days by a process of scaly desquamation. The part of the body in which chancres occur sometimes can be used to denote the *Glossina* spp. concerned as a vector. For example Robertson and Baker (1958) deduced from the common occurrence of chancres on the legs of fishermen on the north-east coast of Lake Victoria that the main vector was *G. pallidipes* which preferentially attacks the legs.

In *Tryp. b. rhodesiense* sleeping sickness, with a natural duration of the untreated infection of only some eight months to death, the later stage nervous manifestations which are so characteristic of *Tryp. b. gambiense* sleeping sickness are less often seen. Similarly, the classical brain histopathology described for *Tryp. b. gambiense* sleeping sickness — perivascular cuffing, occurrence of morular cells both in the brain substance and in the cerebrospinal fluid, round cell infiltration — although essentially similar in *Tryp. b. rhodesiense* sleeping sickness, is characteristically less advanced at death than in the *Tryp. b. gambiense* disease.

Epidemiology

With this acute clinical picture, human cases cannot for long continue to play a part in the epidemiology of the disease. As sources of infection, infected humans are soon removed either by hospitalization and treatment, or by death. The trypanosome chancre is, for example, well known to the fishermen of Lake Victoria who seek early treatment as soon as they recognize, by its occurrence, that they have been infected. In such a situation, maintenance of transmission of the organism solely by intrahuman cycles is an impossibility and alternative cycles of transmission must be sought for. On a basis of the circumstantial evidence that infection is usually acquired in uninhabited country, it is believed that the maintenance transmission cycles occur among wild artiodactyls (mainly antelopes) by *Glossina* spp. which are of savannah, wide-ranging, habit, adapted to live at low population densities in huge areas of sparse woodland and relying for their blood meals on these mammal hosts similarly distributed at low population densities over these large areas. Examples of the *Glossina* spp. of this habit are *G. morsitans*, *G. swynnertoni* and *G. pallidipes* which mainly feed on wild antelopes and wild pigs. On this hypothesis, a certain number of strains capable of infecting man (i.e. not *Tryp. b. brucei*) circulate silently among wild animals and the *Glossina* spp. which feed upon them; they declare their presence only on the infrequent occasions on which a *Glossina* carrying metacyclic infective forms in its salivary glands happens to bite a non-immune human. In this epidemiological pattern, the persons who are infected are those who, for one reason or another, invade environments, normally uninhabited by man, in which these transmission cycles are in progress, e.g., indigenous people who enter the normally uninhabited woodland for the purposes of hunting, fishing, gathering of wild honey and so on. Recently a new category of 'invader' has been added to the list — the tourist who, attracted by the prospect of seeing or photographing wild animals in their natural haunts, joins a 'wild-life safari' and enters the woodland in a motor vehicle. 'Savannah' species of *Glossina* are particularly attracted to moving objects and so are likely to follow and enter a vehicle when it stops or to bite the occupants when they emerge from it. Except for this instance, in which both male and female tourists are likely to be equally exposed, the incidence of *Tryp. b. rhodesiense* sleeping sickness is predominantly among adult males as it is this category of the indigenous population which invades the wild woodland habitat. Among the fishing communities of the north-east coast of Lake Victoria for instance, infection is practically confined to adult males and incidence is related to fishing activity, not directly to seasonal factors, such as *Glossina* population size as determined by rainfall or temperature. Fishing activity is seasonal but it is determined not directly by climatic factors but secondarily by changes in the stratification of the water in the lake. At certain seasons, when the lake waters are stratified, the main food-fish species cannot survive in the deoxygenated deeper waters and so move to marginal, shallow waters. At this season they are, therefore, more easily netted and so this season is one of maximum fishing activity — and consequently, also, of maximum incidence of *Tryp. b rhodesiense* infection among the fishermen.

Control

As compared with the *Tryp. b. gambiense* epidemiological situation, the *Tryp. b. rhodesiense* one is much less susceptible of control. Because of the huge extent of the savannah woodland infested by the *G. morsitans* group tsetse flies concerned in this epidemiological pattern, clearing of vegetation and insecticide application are rarely possible economically, and if they were, they might well destroy the environment's main productive aspects — its display of wild 'game' for hunting or for spectacle, and wild honey. Secondly, chemoprophylaxis is rarely justified in people entering these environments. With a disease which, if acquired, soon declares its presence, it is better, as with syphilis, to allow infection to declare itself and then cure infected persons with the efficient specific drugs available, rather than suppress infection with the attendant danger of the suppression being incomplete, simply concealing the disease till it manifests later on in the more intractable late stage.

CONCLUSION AND GENERAL CONSIDERATIONS

Possible measures for the control of African sleeping sickness fall into four main categories:
(a) control of the vertebate host;
(b) chemotherapy and chemoprophylaxis;
(c) control of the insect vector;
(d) immunization.

Applications of some of these methods have been discussed in relation to particular epidemiological situations but some comments may usefully be made on the general principles involved in these measures.

Control of the vertebrate host was the only real prophylactic measure available up until about 1920. Neither specific chemotherapy nor efficient insecticides were available and so virtually the only measure possible was to move populations out of the infected areas. This method was effective in halting the epidemics in East Africa at the beginning of the century — mass evacuation of the human population from infected areas was imposed. Such measures are, however, in default of better ones and may lead to more-or-less permanent depopulation — several of the famous game parks of East Africa are areas from which the human population was removed because of sleeping sickness.

Efficient chemotherapeutic agents specific for trypanosomes date only from about 1920 when suramin, an analogue of trypan red, was found to be effective in the early stages of sleeping sickness and, tryparsamide, a pentavalent aromatic arsenical, in cases with neurological involvement. These drugs greatly altered the epidemiological picture and eliminated the need to evacuate populations from infected areas. They were ineffective in West Africa only in some late stage infections with tryparsamide-resistant *Tryp. b. gambiense* and in East Africa in late stage *Tryp. b. rhodesiense* cases. Drugs effective in these situations date only from the 1940s, when melaminyl drugs, particularly melarsoprol, were found effective.

Suramin has a prophylactic effect — a dose of 2 gm will protect for at least three months — but later infections tend to be of a cryptic insidious type (Waddy, 1970). However, pentamidine, an aromatic diamidine, is preferred as a prophylactic drug; one dose of 4 mg base per kg body weight (WHO, 1962) is effective for at least six months in persons not infected before drug administration.

Control of trypanosomiasis by control of the insect vector has been the main aim of extensive researches into the ecology of *Glossina* spp. Very important improvements in techniques of bush clearance and of insecticide application have stemmed from this work but still, and particularly in *Tryp. b. rhodesiense* situations, the most economical measures possible are often disproportionate to the economic productivity of the lands concerned. And vector control measures require continuous vigilance against regrowth of bush and reinvasion by fly.

Although there is evidence that some immunity to infection may be acquired by populations living in contact with trypanosomiasis the mechanism of this immunity is not yet understood. The immunology of trypanosome infections is being actively studied at the present time but the prospect of preparing vaccines by classical methods seems poor, mainly because of the ability of trypanosome populations in mammal hosts to alter their antigenic constitution every few days, apparently over very extended periods.

REFERENCES

Anthony R L, Johnson C M Sousa O E 1979 Use of micro-ELISA for quantitating antibody to Trypanosona cruzi and Trypanosoma rangeli. American Journal of Tropical Medicine and Hygiene 28: 969–973
Apted F I C 1970 Clinical manifestations and diagnosis of sleeping sickness. In: Mulligan H W (ed) The African Trypanosomiases. George Allen and Unwin, London
Brener Z. Andrade Z A 1979 Trypanosoma cruzi e doenca de Chagas. Editora Guanabara Koogan, S A, 463pp. Rio de Janeiro, Brasil. Abstracted in Tropical Diseases Bulletin 76: 1009. 1979
Burnett G F 1970 Control by insecticides. In: Mulligan H W (ed) The African Trypanosomiases. George Allen and Unwin, London
Cancado J R (ed) 1970 Doença de Chagas. Impresa Oficinal de Estado de Minas Gerais, Belo Horizonte, Brazil
Gibson W C, Marshall T F de C, Godfrey D G 1980 Numerical analysis of enzyme polymorphism: a new approach to the epidemiology and taxonomy of trypanosomes of the subgenus Trypanozoon. Advances in Parasitology 18: 175–246

Koberle F 1968 Chagas' disease and Chagas' syndromes. Advances in Parasitology 6: 63–116

Lumsden W H R, Kimber C D, Dukes P, Haller L, Stanghellini A, Duvallet G 1981 Field diagnosis of sleeping sickness in the Ivory Coast. 1. Comparison of the miniature anion-exchange/centrifugation technique with other protozoological methods. Transactions of the Royal Society of Tropical Medicine and Hygiene 75: 242–250

Marsden P D 1971 South American trypanosomiasis (Chagas' disease). In: Woodruff A W Lincicome D R (eds) International Review of Tropical Medicine: 497–121. Academic Press, New York and London

Miles M A 1979 Transmission cycles and the heterogeneity of Trypanosoma cruzi. In: Lumsden W H R , Evans D (eds) Biology of the Kinetoplastida, Vol 2. Academic Press, London and New York

Murray M, Murray P K, McIntyre W I M 1977 An improved parasitological technique for the diagnosis of African trypanosomiasis. Transactions of the Royal Society of Tropical Medicine and Hygiene 71: 325–326

Robertson D H H, Baker J R 1958 Human trypanosomiasis in south-east Uganda. 1. A study of the epidemiology and present virulence of the disease. Transactions of the Royal Society of Tropical Medicine and Hygiene 52: 337–348

Romaña C 1963 Enfermedad de Chagas. Lopez, Buenos Aires, Argentina

Scott D 1970 The epidemiology of Gambian sleeping sickness. In: Mulligan HW (ed) The African trypanosomiases. George Allen and Unwin, London

Waddy B B 1970 Chemotherapy of the human trypanosomiases. In: Mulligan H W (ed) The African trypanosomiases. George Allen and Unwin, London.

Leishmaniasis

THE PARASITE

Leishmaniasis is the term used for a number of different diseases caused by protozoan flagellate parasites of the genus *Leishmania*. The diseases may be classified into two main types: visceral leishmaniasis in which the parasites are restricted to the deep organs of the body, and cutaneous leishmaniasis in which parasites are found in skin macrophages (histiocytes) at the site of a granuloma of the dermis. Reliable figures of the incidence of leishmaniasis are notably difficult to obtain but recently it has been suggested that there are approximately 400 000 new cases of all types each year (Chance, 1981). In the mammalian host leishmanial parasites are present as amastigotes, round or ovoid bodies which do not possess an external flagellum but are characterised by the possession of two DNA containing organelles — the nucleus and kinetoplast. The latter is a bizarre form of mitochondrial DNA which is readily stained and observed in Giemsa stained preparations. In general the cytoplasm is relatively poorly stained in such preparations.

Amastigotes are restricted to macrophages, only very rarely being found in other cell types and thus are found in those tissues which contain large numbers of macrophages, that is the mononuclear phagocyte (reticulo-endothelial) system. This includes the liver, spleen, bone marrow and lymph nodes.

Leishmaniasis is transmitted by arthropod vectors, sandflies of the genus *Phlebotomus* in the Old World and *Lutzomyia* in the New World. When a female sandfly takes a bloodmeal from an infected person amastigotes are taken up either from the peripheral circulation in the case of visceral leishmaniasis or from the cutaneous tissue in the case of the cutaneous disease. Once in the sandfly midgut the ingested amastigotes transform to elongated flagellated forms known as promastigotes which are about 20μm in length. The promastigotes divide in the lumen of the midgut and, as this fills, move forward into the anterior station of the gut. By a mechanism as yet unknown, when the now infective sandfly takes the next bloodmeal; parasites are introduced into the individual on which the sandfly is feeding. The injected promastigotes are taken up by phagocytic cells and become established in macrophages transforming immediately to amastigotes in which form division takes place and thus a new infection becomes established.

Non sandfly mediated transmission is extremely rare, a few cases of infection due to blood transfusion are known and it has also been suggested that the nasal discharge containing amastigotes sometimes seen in Sudanese visceral leishmaniasis may be a means by which infection by contagion may occur. In the past there has been much confusion regarding the identity of *Leishmania* due in the main to the lack of distinguishing features between the various assumed species of *Leishmania*, with the result that the taxonomy of this genus was not based upon features of the organism but somewhat unsatisfactorily upon the clinical features produced in man, together with the geographical distribution of the diseases. In the last ten years the application of the techniques of biochemical taxonomy has lead to a much clearer understanding of the subdivision within the genus (Chance, 1979). The species of *Leishmania* infecting man are as follows:

Old World *Leishmania*

The causative organism of visceral leishmaniasis is *L. donovani*; the distribution of which is shown in Figure 34.1 and which includes the north east and east of the Indian subcontinent, western Kenya and southern Sudan. In this latter focus rodents have been implicated as reservoirs of the infection but in India and Kenya man appears to be the only reservoir. Visceral leishmaniasis is also seen in the countries surrounding the Mediterranean Sea where the parasite is sometimes referred to as *L. infantum* because of the age distribution of the disease in which children under ten years old are the predominant age group. Dogs form the reservoir of the Mediterranean disease as they do in South America where again the disease is infantile in its age preference. The parasite of South American visceral leishmaniasis has been referred to as *L. chagasi* but modern practice includes both *L. chagasi* and *L. infantum* within *L. donovani*. Visceral leishmaniasis also extends from the Mediterranean through Iraq and Iran into Central Asia. A further Asian focus is north east China which was previously very active.

L. major (= *L. tropica major*) causes cutaneous leishmaniasis, usually a rural disease characterised by large wet sores which cure relatively rapidly, and which is widely distributed from West Africa to Central Asia, including the Sahelian belt and parts of North and East Africa. The parasite is also found in the Middle East, Iran, southern USSR, Afghanistan and North West India. Throughout most of this range it is known that cutaneous leishmaniasis is a zoonosis with rodents identified as the reservoir.

L. tropica (= *L. tropica tropica* = *L. tropica minor*) is also responsible for cutaneous leishmaniasis in the Old World and is often considered to be an urban parasite causing a longer lasting dryer lesion than that due to *L. major*. In reality in many areas the distributions overlap and often the distinction between the two clinical forms is not clear cut.

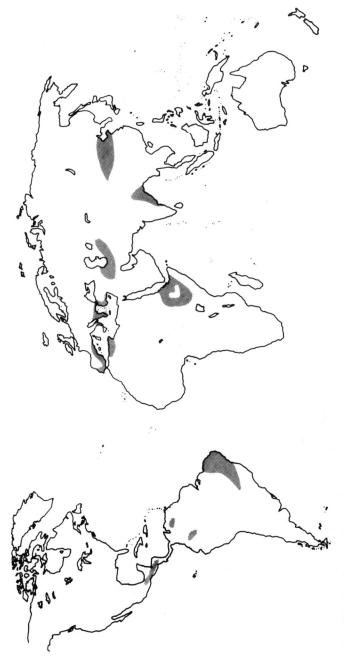

Fig. 34.1 Distribution of visceral leishmaniasis

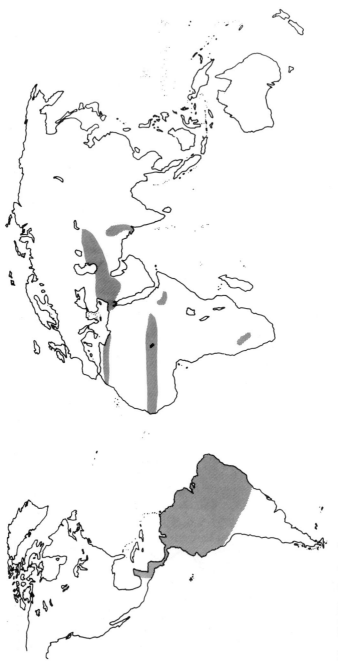

Fig. 34.2 Distribution of cutaneous leishmaniasis

Transmission of this parasite is apparently mainly from man to man and the distribution is from the southern USSR, Afghanistan, North West India through the Middle East in to the countries of the eastern Mediterranean and parts of North Africa.

In the highlands of Ethiopia and on the geographically separate Mt. Elgon of Kenya cutaneous leishmaniasis is caused by *L. aethiopica* which has an animal reservoir, the hyrax. The geographical distribution of cutaneous leishmaniasis can be seen in Figure 34.2

New World leishmaniasis

In addition to visceral leishmaniasis (see above) the cutaneous leishmaniases present in Central and South America are caused by two parasites *L. mexicana* and *L. braziliensis* both species being subdivided into a number of subspecies. *L. mexicana* is distributed from the Southern USA, a few autochthonous cases having been recently seen in Texas, through Central America into Venezuela and the eastern Amazon region of Brazil. Though the parasite is seen in a variety of forest rodents and marsupials the infection in man in some regions is comparatively rare though when it does occur it produces, in perhaps as many as 30 per cent of cases, diffuse cutaneous leishmaniasis.

L. braziliensis is widespread throughout the rain forest of Central and South America. Recent studies have shown that tree dwelling endentates, the sloth and the lesser tamadua (anteater) are reservoir hosts of this parasite.

In the highlands of Peru *L. b. peruviana* which is tentatively described as a subspecies of *L. braziliensis* causes a form of cutaneous leishmaniasis known as uta which is self curing with no chronic complications. The domestic dog forms the reservoir of this disease.

THE DISEASE

Visceral leishmaniasis

The incubation period is not easy to determine in natural conditions but would appear to be between three and six months. There is, however, a wide variation with times of a few weeks or a few years being occasionally reported.

At the site of introduction of the parasites there may be either no obvious response, or the formation of a transitory leishmanioma which may vary from a minute papule to a cutaneous ulcer identical in appearance to cutaneous leishmaniasis. A significant proportion of infected persons may cure at this point, the evidence of this being somewhat circumstantial, but in others the parasites become centred in the macrophages in the liver spleen, bone marrow and lymph glands (Manson-Bahr, 1982). Again self cure may take place before the onset of full blown visceral disease but in those who do progress to full disease self cure is probably a very rare event. The disease is characterised by a persistent fever and marked hepatosplenomegaly in which the spleen enlarges rapidly and may extend as far as the iliac crest and become massive. Emaciation and respiratory or gastrointestinal intercurrent infections are noticeable features as the disease progresses.

There are also profound changes in the blood with the red cell count falling to perhaps 3.0×10^{12} litre^{-1} and a marked leucopenia in which, in 95 per cent of the cases, the white cells are reduced below 3×10^9 litre^{-1}. There is thrombocytopenia which results in a tendency to spontaneous bleeding.

It is also seen that there is an enormous rise in immunoglobulins with IgG being raised sufficiently to reverse the normal globulin-albumin ratio.

Once severe symptoms have become established it appears that mortality may be as high as 90 per cent.

There are a number of intriguing differences between the distinct geographical forms of visceral leishmaniasis in terms of clinical features. There is a marked dissimilarity in age distribution in different regions. In India and Africa the disease is mostly seen in young adults 10–20 years of age, whereas in the Mediterranean region and in north east Brazil the disease is mostly seen in infants and children less than five years of age. Amastigotes can be detected circulating in the blood stream either free or inside mononuclear cells in a relatively high proportion of cases in the Indian form of the disease, in a smaller proportion of African cases and virtually never in the Mediterranean form. In the African form there is a generalised lymphadenopathy with enlargement of the inguinal and femoral glands which is only occasionally seen in Indian and Mediterranean forms.

As a sequel to visceral leishmaniasis a cutaneous form known as post kala-azar dermal leishmanioid sometimes occurs in which the parasites are present in skin nodules which may in some cases contain numerous parasites. The proportion of kala azar patients in India who develop this condition is variously reported as between five and 20 per cent. Untreated the condition may last for 20 years. The presence of persistent parasites in the skin readily accessible to feeding sandflies is considered to form an effective reservoir of the disease and to explain the maintenance of the parasite in an area during inter epidemic periods. The condition is much more common in India than other areas where visceral leishmaniasis occurs, being rare in Africa and unknown in the Mediterranean and South American areas.

Cutaneous leishmaniasis

In contrast to visceral leishmaniasis the parasites usually remain at the site of introduction into the dermis by the infecting sandfly where they multiply initially within the resident macrophages, the histiocytes. Following recruitment of monocytes the area becomes congested with macrophages and the infiltration of plasma cells and lymphocytes leads to parasite destruction and to ulceration of the dermis (Mauel and Behin, 1982). Ulcers may be found at any site but are most commonly found on parts of the body exposed to sandfly bites such as arms, legs and face. Ulcers may be single or multiple with two or three lesions being present — in extreme cases over 100 lesions may be present. It is usually thought that multiple lesions arise from multiple infecting sandfly bites though in some cases they may be due to metastasis. The usual outcome of cutaneous leishmaniasis is spontaneous cure though this may take several months leaving rather a characteristic scar. In some cases however chronic infections become established. In leishmaniasis recidivans apparently healed lesions break down at the margin giving rise to satellite lesions which continue to spread. Some persons infected with *L. mexicana* or *L. aethiopica* have a specific defect in which they appear incapable of mounting a cellular response to *Leishmania* antigen. The parasites become widely disseminated over the surface of the body (diffuse cutaneous leishmaniasis) forming disfiguring nodules which are not usually ulcerated. Undoubtedly the most destructive chronic form of cutaneous leishmaniasis is espundia or mucocutaneous leishmaniasis due to some subspecies of *L. braziliensis* in which the cartilaginous parts of the nose, mouth and pharynx are eroded leading to gross deformities. The condition is due to the metastatic spread of the parasite from a cutaneous lesion at some other site on the body, the condition being activated perhaps as many as 30 years following the resolution of the primary infection.

DIAGNOSIS

The only definite diagnosis of visceral leishmaniasis is the detection of amastigotes in Giemsa stained preparations. The most reliable tissue to examine is obtained by spleen puncture which does, however, have attendant dangers, particularly since the thrombocytopaenia associated with visceral leishmaniasis may be marked. A safer but more painful procedure is to examine bone marrow obtained from either the sternum or the iliac crest (particularly in children). In the African form of the disease the puncture of the lymphatic glands of the groin commonly yields amastigote-containing material. If the number of amastigotes present are too few to be revealed by microscopy their presence may be revealed by culturing spleen or marrow aspirates in NNN medium at 27°C. Any amastigotes present will in most cases transform and grow and multiply as promastigotes in culture and be visible within four to seven days. NNN medium comes in many varieties but is essentially nutrient agar containing for preference rabbit blood at a concentration of about 10 per cent v/v (Lainson, 1982). A number of immunodiagnostic techniques such as IFAT, ELISA, and CIEF are very sensitive methods for the detection of antibodies to *Leishmania*. They do suffer, however, from lack of specificity being prone to false (and unpredictable) positive reactions with a number of cross reacting organisms such as *Trypanosoma* and *Mycobacterium*.

The marked hyperglobulinaemia associated with visceral leishmaniasis is taken advantage of in the useful, simple, but non-specific formol gel test in which 1 ml of clear serum is thoroughly mixed with a few drops of 40 per cent formaldehyde. After about 20 mins the immunoglobulin, if present, forms a firm opaque gel similar to a boiled egg white.

In cutaneous leishmaniasis, material for microscope examination is obtained from the raised edge of a lesion and is prepared as a smear. In some cases, particularly in mucocutaneous leishmaniasis, amastigotes are present in low numbers and are difficult to detect microscopically or by culture because of their poor *in vitro* growth. The recognition of amastigotes in tissue sections can prove very difficult and because of this there is little justification in removing the large piece of tissue necessary to prepare sections. Antibody titres are usually fairly low in cutaneous leishmaniasis but a cell mediated response can be demonstrated early in the infection by the intradermal introduction of killed *Leishmania* promastigotes suspended in 0.5 per cent phenol saline. The site of introduction is examined after 48 hours for a delayed hypersensitivity reaction. A positive *Leishmania* reaction only becomes apparent in visceral leishmaniasis several weeks following recovery.

The differential diagnosis for visceral leishmaniasis includes all febrile conditions in which hepatosplenomegaly is apparent, and for cutaneous leishmaniasis all causes of chronic non painful ulcers.

The treatment of visceral leishmaniasis is usually with pentovalent antimonials, either Pentostam or Glucantime, though cases which do not respond to antimony may be treated with either diamidines or amphotericin B. Antimonials also appear to be the most reliable means of treating cutaneous leishmaniasis though a number of other drugs have been used. Mucocutaneous leishmaniasis is sometimes completely refractory to treatment though good results may be obtained with amphotericin B.

EPIDEMIOLOGY AND CONTROL

Visceral leishmaniasis

Case detection and treatment

In those areas where the transmission of *L. donovani* is from man to man with no involvement of an animal reservoir, control has centred on a two pronged attack on the parasite, case detection and treatment, and the control of the sandfly vector. Individual protection is not possible since no immuno- or chemoprophylactic measures are available.

Case detection presents some problems due to the invasive nature of the diagnostic procedures for the demonstration of the parasite and the considerable degree of skill needed to demonstrate amastigotes microscopically.

There is a great need for a simple, cheap and above all specific immuno-diagnostic procedure which can either be used with sufficient confidence to allow the commencement of treatment or at least allow the identification of probable kala-azar patients from which spleen or bone marrow aspirates may be obtained. The formol gel test which has been used in this role is, of course, completely non specific but when performed when visceral leishmaniasis is present in a community may produce strong circumstantial evidence of infection.

Treatment of individuals may prove problematic because of the scale, the availability of drug and the length of treatment necessary. In China the anti kala-azar campaign which was instituted following liberation involved some 1400 personnel who up to 1952 treated at least 150 000 cases free of charge, the scale of the problem being indicated by a 1951 survey which estimated perhaps 530 000 cases at an endemicity of 1–5 per thousand (Zahar, 1979). During the outbreak in Bihar in the 1970s it is thought that there were about 100 000 cases with perhaps 4500 deaths. The scale of this epidemic initially caused problems over the availability of drugs with many poor patients not completing a full course of treatment due to the cost of the medication and subsequently relapsing. Eventually sodium antimony gluconate was made available free of charge at primary and other health centres. The parasite causing visceral leishmaniasis in India is relatively sensitive to antimonial drugs, only six days treatment being required, hence there are only moderate problems of adequate treatment but in other areas especially East Africa, 30 days of treatment may be necessary and there is the danger of incompletely treated patients absconding as soon as the worst symptoms are alleviated.

Vector control

Many control programmes aimed against visceral leishmaniasis have included attempts to control the vector in which insecticide resistance has not yet been reported. Spraying need only be carried out at restricted foci due to the short flight range of sandflies. In India it is generally believed that the virtual disappearance of visceral leishmaniasis during the 20 years following 1950 can be accounted for by the coincidental destruction of peridomestic *P. argentipes* by antimalarial DDT spraying. It has been suggested that spraying banished the vector to unsprayed outhouses, particularly cattlesheds, and that a reversal in behaviour of *P. argentipes* to reinfect human dwellings may have been one of the features which precipitated the latest epidemic. Since spraying is usually combined with case detection and treatment it is usually difficult to unravel the relative contributions of these two methods of control. In Bihar these two measures lowered the overall prevalence rate from 0.23 per cent in September 1977 to less than 0.02 per cent in February 1979. There is some evidence to suggest that spraying on its own is not sufficient to control the spread of the infection. In part of the campaign against the vector the spraying of inner surfaces was restricted to a height of 6 feet (180 cm) at a dose of 1 g m^{-2} which was found as equally effective as total spraying and which reduced DDT consumption to about half. A successful spraying campaign against *P. chinensis* was conducted in the early 1950s which saw the use of DDT at 1.5 g m^{-2} and gamma HCH at 0.12 g m^{-2}. Single sprayings were sufficient to reduce sandfly populations to very low levels for several years. In contrast to the spraying pattern in India the upper two thirds of walls were sprayed emphasising the importance of knowledge of vector behaviour and resting sites.

The avoidance of non domiciliory transmission "hot spots" will obviously break the vector-man contact cycle. Examples of lessening the chance of infection are avoiding the building of dwellings near termite hills in Kenya or entering the *Acacia-Balonites* forest in Sudan. The use of insecticides in these two particular areas has provided interesting results. In the Kenyan situation 2670 termite hills were sprayed with DDT which resulted in an overall reduction of about 90 per cent in the number of sandflies caught at the termite hills. Unfortunately kala azar transmission in the area in question was almost non existent making it impossible to determine the effect upon human infections. The Sudanese experiment of spraying *Acacia Balonites* forest produced only a minimal reduction in sandfly numbers due to the rapid reinvasion of the forest emphasising again the necessity of understanding fully sandfly behaviour in a particular situation.

Reservoir control

In those parts of the world where the dog is the reservoir of human visceral leishmaniasis considerable attention has been paid to controlling this reservoir of infection. Extensive surveys of dog populations have been carried out either serologically or parasitologically. In China for example, in the early 1950s about 120 000 dogs were examined. If found to be infected dogs should be destroyed but obviously obtaining the owners' permission may be difficult especially if the dog has some economic value, such as a hunting dog. The control programme in Brazil initiated by Professor Deane involved the killing of about 750 000 dogs and the use of DDT spraying of houses. Despite these vigorous measures kala-azar was seen to return to some foci within two years.

Old World cutaneous

Urban anthroponotic cutaneous leishmaniasis due to *L. tropica* has been virtually eliminated from the cities of the southern USSR either as an incidental by-product of antimalarial spraying or the control of sandfly fever or in a programme aimed directly against leishmaniasis which included case detection and treatment. This indicates that the control of *L. tropica* is an attainable goal. The control of zoonotic cutaneous leishmaniasis is a much more challenging problem which nevertheless has been achieved in parts of the USSR. Non-immune individuals such as agriculturalists and civil engineers become infected at rates as high as 40 per cent in their first season of exposure when intruding into the rodent-sandfly cycle (Sergiev, 1977). Because of this, development projects may be hindered by the incapacitation caused by lesions due to *L. major*. In Israel and the USSR vaccination is carried out using virulent strains of *L. major*. After natural healing of the induced lesions a solid immunity is developed. There is a danger that large and long lasting lesions may be produced in a small number perhaps 5 per cent of those treated in this manner (Greenblatt, 1980). This coupled with a time delay of about three months after inoculation before immunity develops limits the usefulness of this strategy for control.

The most impressive control programmes directed against zoonotic cutaneous leishmaniasis are those seen in Soviet Central Asia. It was found that DDT spraying of the burrows of the great gerbil *Rhombomys opimus* was ineffective at reducing sandfly densities as was the placing of DDT impregnated cloth at the burrow entrances even though this material was taken into the burrows by the gerbils. Measures directed against the gerbil, however, were extremely successful at eliminating this reservoir. This was achieved by either poisoning with zinc phosphide animals which had previously having been dosed with an anticoagulant or by ploughing the burrow complexes to a depth of 0.5 m. The gerbils were eliminated from large tracts of land. It has been reported that five workers eradicated all the gerbils in an area of 700 km^2 in a period of one year. Reinvasion which otherwise might have been rapid has been prevented in one large project by integrating the control programme with an irrigation project in which the control area was surrounded by irrigation canals to prevent the movement of gerbils back into the area in question. Though projects of this nature are very effective, perhaps reducing the morbidity in non-immunes in some area from about 40 per cent to virtually nil in one or two years, they do require a tremendous effort in the mapping and treatment or destruction of burrows. In addition, perhaps the Russian workers have been aided by a less tenacious hold on their territory by *Rhombomys opimus* than is normally seen with rodents. In those areas where physical barriers have not been constructed continued surveillance for and elimination of reinvading rodents is necessary.

In some areas avoidance of close contact with infected rodents by siting human habitation away from rodent burrows may give some measure of protection since sandflies are not likely to be widely dispersed from rodent burrows.

New World cutaneous leishmaniasis

The control of cutaneous leishmaniasis in the New World presents almost insuperable problems (Marinkelle, 1980). Only in Peru has control been achieved with the fortuitous control of uta as a consequence of DDT spraying campaigns directed against the vector of human bartonellosis (Carrion's disease).

In general those individuals involved in the economic exploitation of the jungle are those exposed to infection with L. mexicana and L. braziliensis. It is probably true that the vectors of L. mexicana are poorly attracted to man, thus although the parasite may be widely distributed among forest rodents and marsupials, infection in man may be extremely rare as for example, in Panama where human infection with this parasite is unknown. Where infection with L. mexicana is common, as in the case of chiclero's ulcer this is presumably due to the long exposure in the forest of these gum collectors.

The vectors of L. braziliensis are in contrast much more anthropohilic, aggressively biting man by day or night. Lutzomyia umbratilis the vector of L. b. guyanensis in North Brazil and the Guyanas, rests in large numbers on the trunks of large trees. Consequently any person involved with tree felling is particularly at risk even more so since the infection rate in the vector may be as high as 7 per cent. Insecticide spraying of the bases of large trees has not been found effective in reducing sandfly densities. In general the practical problems of insecticide spraying in dense jungle have discouraged any attempt at control on a large scale. Personal protection by means of insect repellants is not feasible in a hot humid climate, also control of rodents and marsupials in the case of L. mexicana or edentates in the case of L. braziliensis is not possible nor necessarily desirable in ecological terms.

Wholesale landscape modification would of course eliminate both vector and reservoir. This approach apart from the ecological disaster it might precipitate is not without its dangers with respect to leishmaniasis. Any open terrain generated might be colonised by Lu. longipalpis the vector of visceral leishmaniasis in the New World (Lainson and Shaw, 1978).

Safe effective vaccination is not available against South American leishmaniasis which coupled to the fact that cross immunity does not seem to exist even between subspecies of L. mexicana or L. braziliensis means that no personal protection is available.

CONCLUSION

Successful control measures designed to combat leishmaniasis depend upon a clear understanding of all the aspects of the biology of the vector and reservoir. Unfortunately this self evident principle is sometimes impossible to apply owing to our incomplete knowledge of essential details such as the resting sites or flight range of the vector or, in extreme cases, a complete lack of knowledge about the identity of the vector or reservoir. The essential principles of control may be summarised as follows:
1) Detection and treatment of human disease
2) Vector control

3) Reservoir control
4) Vaccination may be possible against Old World cutaneous leishmaniasis
5) Limiting man-vector contact by careful siting of settlements away from heavy concentrations of sandflies.

REFERENCES

Chance M L 1979 The identification of Leishmania. In: Taylor A E R, Muller R (eds) Problems in the Identification of Parasites and Their Vectors. Blackwell, Oxford. p 55–74
Chance M L 1981 Leishmaniasis. British Medical Journal 283: 1245–1247
Greenblatt C L 1980 The present and future of vaccination for cutaneous leishmaniasis. In: Mizrachi A, Herman I, Klingberg M A, Kohn A (eds) New developments with human and veterinary vaccines. Progress in Clinical and Biological Research Vol 47. Alan Liss, New York p 259–285
Lainson R 1982 Leishmanial parasites of mammals in relation to human disease. Symposium of Zoological Society of London 50: 137–179
Lainson R, Shaw J J 1978 Epidemiology and ecology of leishmaniasis in Latin America. Nature 273: 595–600
Manson-Bahr P E C 1982 Leishmaniasis. In: Manson-Bahr P E C, Apted F I C (eds) Manson's Tropical Disease, 18th ed. Bailliere Tindall, London. p 93–115
Marinkelle C T 1980 The control of leishmaniasis. Bulletin of World Health Organisation 58: 807–818
Mauel J, Behin R 1982 Leishmaniasis: immunity, immunopathology and immunodiagnosis. In: Cohen S, Warren K S (eds) Immunology of Parasite Infections. Blackwell, Oxford, p 299–355
Sergiev V P 1977 Control measures against leishmaniasis. Colloques Internationaux du CNRS No. 239: 321–323.
Zahar A R 1979 Studies on leishmaniasis. Vectors/reservoirs and their control in the Old World. WHO/VBC/79.479; WHO/VBC/80.776; WHO/VBC/80.786; WHO/VBC/81.825.

Arthropod infestations of man

INTRODUCTION

In this short chapter it is not possible to include all the arthropods which live in close association with man. The four groups selected are lice, fleas, mites and ticks, all of which are widely distributed in warm climates and live for a time attached to man or in his clothing or his home. Bed-bugs have been excluded since although they are of public health concern they are not vectors of parasitic infections. Triatomine vectors of Chagas' disease in the Americas are also excluded since they are of more restricted interest geographically.

It is not the intention to provide descriptions of the selected arthropods; if details are required they may be found in other textbooks. The main objectives are to provide guidance on the main features of their ecology, on alternative methods of control and on their role in the transmission of disease agents to man.

The pattern of infections transmitted by arthropods is not fixed, and disease incidence fluctuates both with time and with geographical region. The situation concerning such major arthropod-borne infections as plague and louse-borne typhus is regularly reviewed by the World Health Organization in its Weekly Epidemiological Record, the WHO Chronicle and in the Technical Report Series. These publications form an invaluable source of new information.

LICE

Lice are present in all human communities, and although both the head louse, *Pediculus humanus capitis*, and the pubic louse, *Pthirus pubis*, are of importance, it is the body louse, *P.h. corporis*, which, as a vector of epidemic typhus, trench fever and relapsing fever, presents the greatest potential danger to man. Body lice are now uncommon in highly-developed countries (though the head louse is still well established), but they are still prevalent in some countries with low standards of hygiene. Where people are crowded and unable to wash and change their clothing regularly, body lice, and their infections, will spread. Lice are most host-specific, and for practical purposes those on man cannot live on an alternative host. Body lice spend most of their time on clothing, especially underwear, on the fibres of which the eggs are laid, and they move to the skin to feed. If they are deprived of a blood meal, they die within a few days.

They can multiply rapidly. Under suitable conditions a single egg can give rise within three weeks to a female which will itself be egg-laying. This female will continue laying several eggs each day until her death about a month later, by which time the offspring will have become adult and will themselves be egg-laying daily. In theory, the louse population within about 3 months might number some thousands, but in nature the numbers are regulated and reduced, most often by human activities such as changing and washing clothes. Under very unhygienic conditions, where facilities for changing and washing clothes are restricted, louse populations might reach abnormal numbers.

Louse-borne typhus

The causative organism of typhus is *Rickettsia prowazeki*, and after the rickettsiae are ingested by the louse while it feeds on an infected individual they invade the cells of the insect gut where they multiply. Subsequently, the cells become greatly distended and, after a few days, rupture, releasing the rickettsiae into the lumen of the gut. The cellular damage caused by the rickettsiae usually results in the death of the louse some seven or 10 days later.

The rickettsiae in the gut are excreted in the louse faeces; the salivary glands do not become infected, and there is therefore no transmission by bite. The infected faeces contaminate clothing and bedding, and since the rickettsiae can remain viable and infective for at least two months in dry faeces, all clothing and bedding associated with individuals with typhus should be regarded as hazardous and treated with great care. The dry rickettsiae can infect people through cuts and abrasions, or they may be scratched into the skin, and it is thought that they might also infect through the conjunctiva and mucous membranes.

Vaccines are available against louse-borne typhus, and infected individuals can be effectively treated with some antibiotics.

The epidemics of the past have been associated with such conditions as occur in war, famines, prison camps, and the like, where people have been crowded together in unhygienic conditions with limited facilities for washing and changing clothing. They have also been associated with temperate countries, as in Europe, or in high altitude regions of tropical areas, where people wear many items of clothing. In more recent times, and associated with a low general level of hygiene, outbreaks are reported mainly from the highlands in tropical zones, for example in Ethiopia, Burundi and Rwanda in Africa and in Bolivia, Ecuador and Peru in South America.

In 1979, 18 359 cases of louse-borne typhus were notified to the World Health Organization (World Health Organization, 1981).Of this number, 95 per cent were derived from Ethiopia. A few years earlier large numbers of cases were reported from Burundi and Rwanda (10 204 cases with 156 deaths in 1974; 10 266 cases with 146 deaths in 1975), but there has been a decline in those areas. In 1980 a total of only 7506 cases were notified (including 18 deaths) and of these Burundi reported 101 and Rwanda only 46 (World Health Organization, 1982). The highlands of Bolivia, Ecuador and Peru have long been associated with persistent endemic foci and small numbers of cases are reported annually.

Louse-borne relapsing fever

Relapsing fever is caused by *Borrelia recurrentis* and is transmitted by lice. When the spirochaetes are ingested with a blood meal, most of them die in the gut of the louse, but a few survive and penetrate the stomach wall to reappear in the haemocoele. There they multiply, but they do not infect the salivary glands and they are not therefore transmitted by bite. The spirochaetes can only infect man when the louse is crushed, for example between the fingers or between the teeth, and the infected haemocoelic fluid contaminates scratches and abrasions. This infection has been responsible for seven major epidemics during this century, with more than 16 million cases and five million deaths (World Health Organization, 1976); those epidemics were associated with wars or famines. The infection is now confined to some remote regions of the world, including parts of Ethiopia.

Control of lice

Where a community is exposed to a possible outbreak of louse-borne disease, the louse population must be reduced as quickly as possible. The most effective means is by applying an insecticide in dust form to the inner clothing of all members of the community. 10 per cent DDT powder has proved most effective in the past, but, owing to the wide usage of DDT, resistance of lice to this compound is now common. DDT is no longer effective, for example, in Korea, Iran, Egypt and in many of the refugee camps of the Middle East. Alternative insecticidal dusts include one per cent gamma HCH, one per cent malathion, two per cent temephos, one per cent propoxur and five per cent carbaryl. Reports of resistance to HCH and to malathion are increasing and the pattern is changing with time and insecticide usage. Periodic detailed reviews are published by the World Health Organization, for example that of Brown & Pal (1971). The reports of the W.H.O Expert Committee on Vector Biology and control, for example that of 1980 (World Health Organization, 1980a) usually include up-to-date statements on the spread of resistance and on recommended vector control measures.

For the treatment of individuals, about 30 g of the dust or powder should be applied from sifter-top cans to the under-clothing, with particular attention being paid to treating the inner seams. The seams of outer garments should also be dusted, as should socks.

Large groups of people can be treated without removal of their clothing by the use of hand-operated dusters or by means of motor-driven compressors with a series of duster heads. About 50 g of powder is applied to clothing through neck and waist openings and through sleeves. In treating women, the application around the waist is usually omitted and an extra quantity of powder is introduced down the neck of their garments. Treatment of socks, head-wear, spare clothing and bedding should not be neglected.

A thorough treatment of individuals and their clothing and bedding is often sufficient to eliminate the louse population. If some lice persist, retreatment may be required after three or four weeks. If HCH or pyrethrins, whose residual life is short, are used, weekly applications are recommended until the infestation is eliminated.

The possibility of resistance of the lice to the insecticides available should always be kept in mind. There has been no very recent global survey of the resistance spectrum, but it is likely that DDT-resistance is now widespread, and perhaps also HCH-resistance. Malathion may still be effective in most areas, but there have been reports of resistant strains in Egypt, Ethiopia and Burundi (see, for example, Sholdt et al, 1977). Head lice are best controlled by treatment of the hair with insecticidal lotions. After treatment the hair should be allowed to dry naturally and to remain unwashed for at least 12 hours. Shampoos are less effective than lotions. Lotions containing 0.5 per cent malathion or carbaryl are effective both against the eggs and the immature and mature lice and one treatment is usually sufficient to eliminate an infestation. Although there is some residual action of these insecticides, which are bound to the hair, re-infestation may occur within a few weeks. The key to successful control lies therefore in community treatment rather than treatment of individuals as infestations become recognized in a random fashion.

FLEAS

As adults, fleas spend part of their time on their host and part free-living in the home or burrow of the host. The proportion of time spent on the host varies according to the species of flea. The immature stages are in the burrow. The species of most concern to man is *Xenopsylla cheopis*, the tropical rat flea, which associates with commensal and with wild rodents. It is a major vector of plague and murine typhus, and if given the opportunity it feeds readily on man. Besides *X. cheopis*, however, there are many other fleas which are found living with wild rodents but which, following an intrusion of new hosts into their environment, will readily adapt to these hosts for blood meals.

Plague

The bacilli of plague, *Yersinia pestis*, multiply in the portion of the flea gut known as the proventriculus, which acts as a valve regulating the passage of blood into the stomach. When the bacilli have multiplied in the proventriculus, they may form a blockage so that blood is unable to pass. Fleas with such a blockage are especially dangerous, since during their frequent attempts to feed, the plague bacilli are dislodged and some pass forwards to contaminate the mouth-parts and subsequently are transferred to the vertebrate host. Such blocked fleas often die of starvation, though in some the blockage is cleared, but before their death they may infect several hosts during their efforts to feed.

The permanent reservoirs of plague are different species of wild rodent, such as rabbits, ground squirrels, gerbils and voles. During ecological disturbances the contact between these animals and commensal rodents and man may be greatly increased. In many of the plague epidemics of the past the infection has passed in the first instance from wild rodents to commensal rodents via the flea vectors. Thereafter, since domestic rats usually die of the infection, the fleas (often *X. cheopis*) leave their dead or moribund hosts and readily pass to man, in whom the infection is severe and often fatal. The contact between wild rodents and man may at times be more direct. In 1944–45 in Botswana, for example, there was an epidemic of plague among villagers which had its origins in an unusual animal migration following flooding (Pollitzer, 1954). The flooding caused an unusually large population of multimammate mice to leave their burrows in the swamps, and it is thought that these mice acquired plague from gerbils, which were suffering an epizootic at the time, and then brought the infection into the villages which they invaded during their migration. More recently, in October 1974, there was an outbreak of plague in Ovamboland in Namibia also associated with a mass migration of rodents. In this case the rodent migration followed a bush fire and the outbreak, with 102 cases and five deaths, was ascribed to the subsequent close contact between man and the rodents and their fleas (World Health Organization, 1975).★

Although plague has declined as a major public health problem during this century, except in South Vietnam from which the great majority of human cases and deaths are reported, the number of foci of wild or sylvatic plague has probably changed very little. There are still many human cases reported annually from the Americas, Africa and Asia which have their origins in sylvatic foci, and such foci should be recorded and mapped in all areas susceptible to ecological change.

★ Owing to the sporadic nature of cases plague vaccine is useful only in highly exposed individuals and then tetracycline prophylaxis may be preferred — D. Robinson.

Murine typhus

Murine typhus (*Rickettsia mooseri* or *R. typhi*) is another infection of rodents which is transmissible by fleas to man. However, it is more sporadic than the related louse-borne form, and it is of less danger than plague. The rickettsiae multiply in the cells of the stomach of the flea, and are subsequently released back into the lumen of the gut when the cells rupture. Transmission occurs when the flea is crushed by the host and the released rickettsiae contaminate scratches or abrasions or when infected flea faeces are scratched into the host.

Murine typhus occurs in many parts of the world — from Manchuria, China and South-east Asia to South and West Africa and the Americas. The vector to man is most commonly *X. cheopis*; however, *R. mooseri* has been recovered from many kinds of wild rodent and no doubt several species of flea play a part in its transmission. It has been associated primarily with the commensal rat, *Rattus norvegicus*, and where populations of this rat are high there is always a risk of transmission to man. Owing to difficulties in diagnosis, data on the incidence in most countries are not available. In the United States, where data have been gathered and analysed (Pratt, 1958), there has been a marked fall in the number of human cases since 1944, when 5401 cases and 193 deaths were reported, owing largely to a programme of rat flea control using DDT coupled with the introduction in 1949 of chloramphenicol for treatment. However, the infection has remained in the rat population, and in a survey of Atlanta, Ga., in 1957, although the level of infection in rats was very low, the average flea index was 2.4 *X. cheopis* per rat, and in some areas the index was as high as 30–40 fleas per rat. Where such high flea indices occur, there is a great risk of transmission to man, particularly if there is any ecological disruption in the area.

The difficulties of diagnosing murine typhus, which has some clinical similarities to the louse-borne form, have undoubtedly led in the past to under-notification. There was an outbreak in 1978 in Kuwait which was initially thought to be louse-borne typhus until detailed epidemiological and serological studies demonstrated that the infection was murine typhus.

Control of fleas

Surveillance of plague and murine typhus foci is a primary requirement in areas subject to natural or man-made ecological changes. And an important part of surveillance concerns the vector fleas. The organization and requirements for plague surveillance have been described in detail by the World Health Organization (1973, 1980b), which laid great stress on factors which bring human beings into contact with the vertebrate reservoirs and the vectors of the plague bacillus. Bahmanyar and Cavanaugh (1976) have given good descriptions of field survey methods and laboratory methods relating not only to fleas but to mammals and the plague bacillus.

The destruction of rodents will in time cause a reduction in the flea population, but since fleas quickly leave dead hosts and transfer to living animals a campaign against rodents may result in an increase in the numbers of fleas attacking man. Consequently, in a plague outbreak, or where one may threaten, it is essential to attack the flea population first.

The generous application of insecticidal dusts to rodent runs, to the entrances to burrows, and to all possible resting and foraging areas is the best method of flea control. The dust is picked up on the feet and fur of the rodent and carried to its nest where it is transferred, during grooming, over its body.

Dusts of 10 per cent DDT or three per cent HCH have been used most successfully in the past. However, resistance of *X. cheopis* to DDT and to HCH has been reported from many parts of Asia, Africa and the Americas, and in emergency situations two to five per cent carbaryl (Sevin) dust is the most certain to be effective. In an Indian village trial (Krishnamurthy et al, 1965) carbaryl caused a reduction of the flea index on rodents to zero and a zero or very low index was maintained for three months. Carbaryl has also given equivalent results in the United States. If two per cent diazinon, three per cent fenthion or five per cent malathion dusts are available, these should prove satisfactory.

Hand-carried dusters specially designed for dusting are available, but in an emergency any form of tin-can with a perforated lid can be used. The aim is simply to apply a liberal layer of dust on all rodent pathways. If the burrows can be detected, about 30 g of dust should be blown into the entrance; some of this may penetrate sufficiently to reach the flea larvae in the nest.

The period of efficacy of a single treatment is influenced by the amount of exposure to sunlight, wind and rain, but one treatment will commonly be effective in holding the flea population at a low level for two or more months.

Control measures against fleas of domestic or commensal rodents present fewer difficulties than those against fleas of wild rodent populations. In the latter circumstances, besides dusting the burrow entrances and any recognisable pathways, it is useful to treat bait-boxes with about 100 g of powder. The boxes should have an ample supply of easily accessible bait, and when the rodents visit the bait their feet and fur are contaminated with the insecticidal powder.

THE SCABIES MITE

Although in some respects it is of secondary importance, the scabies mite, *Sarcoptes scabiei*, deserves mention and consideration. The mite is world-wide in distribution, and in addition to the severe irritation which might be caused during the infestation of the horny epidermis of the skin there may also be associated secondary skin infections which result from scratching the affected area. The mites are concentrated mostly on the hands and wrists, but they may be found elsewhere on the body. Scabies has been described as a familial infection, readily spreading from parent to child and child to child. Transmission and spread are likely to be greatest in autumn and winter, perhaps because people then sleep in closer contact. At those times also they generally wash less often, and although washing does not affect the mite in its burrow, infrequent washing may increase the prevalence of secondary infections. The areas of severe secondary infection do not correspond with the distribution of the mites on the body; nor does the distribution of the scabies rash correspond with the mite distribution.

New cases of scabies are not usually recognised until about four weeks after infection; at that time the signs of infestation are easily recognised. In general, therefore, an increase in scabies may be inapparent for some weeks, but the probability of increased transmission in crowded conditions should be anticipated.

Control of scabies

The successful control of scabies is greatly helped by early and accurate diagnosis of the infection. If scabies is present in a community, and the conditions are such as to favour transmission, early treatment can obviate much distress. Infected individuals require the application of a mite-killing compound over the whole surface of the body, excluding the head. The most widely-used compound has been benzyl benzoate, and 'painting' the body with a 25 per cent emulsion, allowing the patient to dry in warm surroundings and discouraging him or her from bathing for 24 hours, will prove most effective. Sometimes a second treatment is required a few days after the first, but in most cases a single treatment is adequate for the elimination of an infestation.

TICKS

There are two main groups of ticks. The soft ticks, chiefly *Ornithodoros*, live in close association with their hosts in the home or burrow of the host. Hard ticks, on the other hand, live outdoors widely distributed in a range of habitats. Both groups have a long life-cycle, which may be completed in several months or extend to several years. Adults can survive long periods unfed, and adult soft ticks have been known to survive for 10 years or more. Since viruses, rickettsiae and spirochaetes may be transmitted through the successive life stages of the ticks and from the adult female through the eggs to the next generation, the ticks themselves are a main reservoir of infection.

Tick-borne relapsing fever

Tick-borne relapsing fever caused by *Borrelia* is maintained and transmitted by soft ticks of the genus *Ornithodoros*. There are many strains of *Borrelia* distributed over much of Central and Southern Africa, Central Asia, the eastern Mediterranean and the Americas, and the main vertebrate hosts are rodents. Localized foci of infection may persist for very many years, and caves, which commonly support rodents and other wild animals and their ticks, form such foci. Travellers and refugees inhabiting caves are at high risk of infection.

Transmission may be by injection of infected salivary secretions during feeding or via infected coxal fluid, which is a watery fluid secreted by the tick following concentration of the haemoglobin and serum proteins of the blood-meal.

Ornithodoros ticks attach to their hosts and feed for short periods commonly of 15–20 minutes.

O. moubata in East, West and Central Africa is closely associated with man, living in cracks in the mud walls and floors of village houses.

Tick-borne viruses

Viruses transmitted by hard ticks are most prevalent in northern latitudes. The primary hosts are rodents and birds; man is usually an incidental host. One group of virus infections is characterized by haemorrhagic disease, for example Crimean-Congo haemorrhagic fever and Kyasanur Forest Disease. The second group includes the tick-borne encephalitides such as Russian spring-summer encephalitis of the Siberian forests and tick-borne encephalitis of Western Eurasia. Several genera of ticks are responsible for virus maintenance, and transmission is from the salivary glands whilst the ticks are feeding. Hard ticks are slow feeders and it may be two to three weeks before they are engorged.

Tick-borne rickettsiae

Hard ticks of many genera and species are the chief vectors and reservoirs of such rickettsial infections as *Rickettsia rickettsi* (Rocky Mountain Spotted Fever, Sao Paulo Fever), *R. siberica* (Asian or Siberian Tick Typhus), *R. conori* (Boutonneuse Fever, Kenya Tick Typhus, Indian Tick Typhus, etc.), *R. australis* (Queensland Tick Typhus) and *Coxiella burnetti* (Q fever). The rickettsiae are transmitted by bite, but tick faeces can be infectious so that crushing ticks in the fingers may be hazardous, especially if there are scratches or abrasions on the hands. The main vertebrate hosts of the ticks are wild rodents and birds of many species. However, wild animals seem in general to sustain a transitory rickettsial infection. Dog ticks have often been found infected with rickettsiae. The larval, nymphal and adult stages of the tick may transmit the infection, which is passed through the eggs to larvae of the next generation, but rickettsiae are seldom transmitted during the first hour or two after the ticks attach to the host.

Control of ticks

Tick control is far from easy. Where natural shelters are occupied by man, for example in emergency situations, a liberal application of insecticidal dusts, such as HCH or malathion, on the floor of the shelter would be recommended. Similar treatments should be applied to housing where *Ornithodoros moubata* may be present. Control of hard ticks in vegetation by outdoor applications of insecticides is generally expensive and relatively ineffective. Protection of individuals may be achieved by repellents, especially if they are used to impregnate clothing. Compounds that have proved effective include deet (N, N-diethyl-m-toluamide), Indalone, dimethyl carbate and dimethyl phthalate. M-1960 was formulated for military personnel in the United States. It contains 30 per cent of 2-butyl-2-ethyl-1, 3-propanediol for repelling mosquitoes and biting flies, 30 per cent benzyl benzoate for mites and fleas, 30 per cent N-butyl acetanilide for ticks and 10 per cent of a nonionic emulsifier. Synthetic pyrethroids may also be effective and in a trial in the United States permethrin performed well in comparisons with M-1960 and deet and gave no complaints from test subjects with regard to odour or irritancy (Schreck et al, 1980).

REFERENCES

Bahmanyar M, Cavanaugh D C 1976 Plague manual. World Health Organization, Geneva
Brown A W A, Pal R 1971 Insecticide resistance in arthropods. World Health Organization Monograph Series No. 38
Krishnamurthy B S, Putatunda J N, Joshi G P, Chandrahas R K, Krishnaswami A K 1965 Studies on the susceptibility of the oriental rat fleas, *Xenopsylla spp.* to some organophosphorus and carbamate insecticides. Bulletin of the Indian Society for Malaria and other Communicable Diseases 2: 131–138
Pollitzer R 1954 Plague. World Health Organization Monograph Series No. 22
Pratt H D 1958 The changing picture of murine typhus in the United States. Annals of the New York Academy of Science 70: 516–527
Schreck C E, Snoddy E L, Mount G A 1980 Permethrin and repellents as clothing impregnants for protection from the Lone Star tick. Journal of economic Entomology 73: 436–439
Sholdt L L, Seibert D J, Holloway M L, Cole M M, Weidhaas D E 1977 Resistance of human body lice to malathion in Ethiopia. Transactions of the Royal Society of Tropical Medicine and Hygiene 70: 532–533
World Health Organization 1973 Technical guide for plague surveillance. WHO Weekly epidemiological Record 48: 149–160
World Health Organization 1975 Plague in 1974. WHO Weekly epidemiological Record 50: 317–319
World Health Organization 1976 Imported louse-borne replapsing fever. WHO Weekly epidemiological Record 51: 269–270
World Health Organization 1980a Resistance of vectors of disease to pesticides. WHO Technical Report Series No. 655
World Health Organization 1980b Plague surveillance and control. WHO Chronicle 34: 139–143
World Health Organization 1981 Louse-borne typhus in 1979. WHO Chronicle 35: 188–189
World Health Organization 1982 Louse-borne typhus in 1980. WHO Weekly epidemiological Record 57: 45–46

Rickettsiae

INTRODUCTION

Epidemic louse-borne typhus has been one of the captains of the men of death since antiquity. It has always been associated with poverty, war and famine. Zinsser (1935) estimated that there were 25 million cases of typhus in the Soviet republics between 1917 and 1921 with nearly 3 million deaths. Major epidemics of typhus also occurred in Eastern Europe during and after the second world war. The threat of typhus was even used in Poland to prevent the deportation of Poles as slave labour to Germany. Lazowski and Matulewicz (1977) describe how a formalin-killed proteus OX19 strain was used as a 'vaccine' to give falsely positive Weil-Felix tests in people who might otherwise have been deported. At present louse-borne typhus is chiefly reported from the highlands of Ethiopia, Rwanda and Burundi with small numbers of cases reported from other African states and from the Andean highlands of South America (WHO, 1982)

If louse-borne typhus is less prevalent than previously the importance of some other rickettsial diseases is only now being recognised. Murine typhus is probably much commoner and more widespread than has been thought whilst scrub typhus is a common cause of undifferentiated febrile illness among people admitted to hospital in South East Asia (WHO Working Group on Rickettsial Diseases 1982). Q fever due to the rickettsia-like organism *Coxiella burnetii* differs from the typhus group in that its transmission does not depend upon an arthropod vector but is usually by the inhalation of an aerosol from infected domestic animals such as sheep during parturition. Q fever may present as a pyrexia of undetermined origin, as a respiratory illness or as atypical pneumonia. It sometimes leads on to a chronic endo-carditis. It will not be discussed further in this short chapter.

THE RICKETTSIAE

These organisms were formerly thought to be intermediate between bacteria and viruses. We now appreciate that they are closely related to gram negative bacteria although they can only grow within living cells. Rickettsiae can survive for long periods in the faeces of the louse or flea and can then infect man by inhalation. Except in the case of louse-borne typhus man is not essential for the survival or transmission of rickettsiae but is merely an accidental host. The major rickettsial infections and their reservoirs and vectors are summarised in Tables 36.1 and 36.2.

Sporadic cases of rickettsial infection can be very difficult to recognise without appropriate tests. Unfortunately infection can easily be acquired in the laboratory so that attempts to isolate rickettsiae should only be made by skilled staff in secure laboratories. Serological tests are usually the only ones available. The serendipitous discovery by Weil and Felix that serum from patients with typhus agglutinated certain strains of Proteus bacteria isolated from urinary tract infections led to the Weil-Felix test which is still widely used. More specific serological tests including micro-agglutination and complement fixation tests are preferable but the most practicable test is usually the indirect fluorescent antibody (IFA) test although it does not reliably differentiate louse-borne from murine typhus or between the members of the spotted fever group. Paired sera are required for confirmation of the diagnosis.

Louse-borne typhus

Louse-borne typhus (LBT) occurs among poor people who wear unwashed clothes infested with the body louse *Pediculus humanus corporis*. At present LBT is almost confined to mountainous areas in the tropics but if conditions deteriorate epidemics can occur in any area where heavy clothing is worn. Illness begins after an incubation period of from one to two weeks, usually 12 days. After a prodromal mild illness of one or two days there is a rapid onset of fever with chills, severe headache and muscle pains. Mental dullness may be striking and there is conjunctival injection. About the fifth day a rash of rose coloured macules which often become papular and haemorrhagic appears on the trunk and spreads to the limbs usually sparing the palms and soles. In the untreated patient fever continues for about two weeks and delirium or frank encephalitis may occur. Death is due to bronchopneumonia, peripheral vascular collapse, renal failure or peripheral gangrene from vascular occlusion. Mortality rates vary but can reach 40 per cent in older or malnourished people. Co-incident infection with louse-borne relapsing fever is not uncommon.

Infection takes place by scratching body fluids of a crushed infected louse or louse faeces through wounds in the skin or mucous membranes. *Rickettsia prowazekii* can remain alive in louse faeces for many months and infection is sometimes acquired by inhalation of infected dust. Lice tend to leave a febrile or dead patient and seek another host. The lice are killed by the rickettsial infection and do not transmit infection transovarially so they cannot act as a reservoir.

Recurrences of LBT may occur many months or years after the initial

Table 36.1 Typhus Group of Rickettsial Diseases

Disease	Organism	Vector	Reservoir or Mammalian Host	Transmission	Distribution
Louse-borne typhus	Rickettsia prowazekii	Louse	Man Flying squirrel?	Infected crushed louse or louse faeces through broken skin or mucosae	Worldwide Tropical highlands
Brill-Zinsser disease	R. prowazekii	None	Man	Late recrudescence of LBT	Worldwide
Murine typhus	R. typhi	Rat flea	Rodents	Infected flea faeces or crushed flea through broken skin or mucosae	Worldwide
Scrub typhus	R. tsutsugamuchi	Mite chigger	Mites Rodents	Chigger bite	Asia Australasia

Table 36.2 Spotted Fever Group of Rickettsial Diseases

Disease	Organism	Vector	Reservoir or Mammalian Host	Transmission	Distribution
Rocky Mountain Spotted fever	R.rickettsii	Ixodid tick	Small mammals, ticks	Tick bite or via mucous membranes	Americas from Canada to Brazil
Boutonneuse fever) African tick typhus)	R.conorii	Ixodid tick	Ticks, rodents, dogs	Tick bite	Mediterranean littoral Africa Indian sub-continent
Siberian tick typhus	R.siberica	Ixodid tick	Wild rodents	Tick bite	Siberia, Mongolia
Queensland tick typhus	R.australis	Ixodid tick	? rodents marsupials	Tick bite	Queensland
Rickettsial pox	R.akari	Mite	House mice, mites	Mite bite	USA, USSR Korea,? Africa

illness and it is in this way that man acts as a reservoir of disease. Recurrent typhus or Brill-Zinsser disease is a milder version of the initial infection with a very low mortality and can occur in the absence of lice. If body lice are present however they may become infected and begin an epidemic. Patients are infective to lice whilst they are febrile and perhaps for two days afterwards. Lice can pass an infection if they are crushed within a few hours of feeding on an infected person whilst rickettsiae appear in their faeces within two to five days.

Previous infection with LBT confers useful immunity to reinfection so that typhus may affect mainly the younger members of populations in hyperendemic areas. The disease is usually mild in children. In the United States *R. prowazekii* has been isolated from the flying squirrel *Glaucomys volans* and mild typhus-like illness in humans has been attributed to this source (Bozeman et al 1975; Duma et al 1981). So far this is the only reliably reported animal reservoir of LBT and its relevance to the usual epidemiology of the disease is doubtful.

Control

Cases of suspected LBT should be reported at once to the national health authority and to the World Health Organization under International Health Regulations. Establish active surveillance of the surrounding population by regular visits to search for cases. The most important control measure is to delouse cases and contacts with an effective residual insecticide powder such as one per cent malathion or five per cent carbaryl depending on the local pattern of susceptibility. If necessary whole populations can be rapidly deloused without removing their clothes. Details are given by Macdonald in Chapter 35. LBT responds rapidly to treatment with tetracyclines. Under epidemic conditions a single dose of doxycycline 200 mg for adults and 50 mg for children swallowed under supervision is usually effective. Close contacts should be kept under surveillance during the incubation period where possible.

Immunisation with vaccines prepared from rickettsiae grown on egg yolksacs and formalin killed are often protective by modifying disease and reducing mortality. Yearly booster doses are needed and these vaccines are currently difficult to obtain. A live attenuated vaccine (E strain) proved protective in a field trial in Burundi and is undergoing further development. Immunisation is useful to protect medical and nursing staff from the danger of inhaled rickettsiae. The long term control of LBT depends on improved conditions for the population at risk with education and provision of facilities for bathing and washing clothes. Insecticides by themselves will not keep human populations free from lice and resistance develops readily.

Murine typhus

Murine typhus (M.T.) is a worldwide infection due to infections with

R.typhi (= *R.mooseri*). The clinical picture is like that of mild LBT or may present as an undifferentiated febrile illness. Recent experience using specific tests suggests that it is a much commoner disease than formerly appreciated (Traub, Wisseman, Farhang-Azad 1978). In Kuwait from April to August 1978 there was an outbreak with 254 cases most of whom were men between 15 and 44 years of age and belonging to the lower socio-economic groups (Al-Awadi et al 1982).

MT is essentially a disease of rodents transmitted by fleas or other ecto-parasites. Cats, opossums and other small animals are sometimes briefly infected. Rats including *Rattus rattus* and *Rattus norvegicus* do not suffer from the infection but are important reservoir hosts. Man is usually infected by the rat flea *Xenopsylla cheopis* which defecates whilst it feeds. *R.typhi* present in the flea faeces gains access through scratches, wounds or mucosal surfaces. Occasionally infection is transmitted by inhalation of infected flea faeces. The rat flea is not harmed by the rickettsia and remains infective for life. Occasionally other rat ectoparasites may transmit infections to man.

Human infections occur inside buildings where people are in close contact with rats. People are often infected sporadically within sharply defined localities such as a single house or building (shop typhus). MT is often seasonal in late summer or autumn following the grain harvest or whenever rodent populations and their ectoparasites increase. Infection confers lasting immunity. There is no man to man transmission nor is there transmission from one generation of fleas to the next.

Control

Control measures are directed against rodents and their fleas. Rat fleas must be killed first or at the same time as the rats or the fleas will tend to transfer to man for their blood meals. Fleas can be eliminated by dusting rat runs and holes with an effective residual insecticide such as carbaryl five per cent or fenitrothion two per cent. After this rat control is by the use of baited tubes or rat poisons. Bait tubes combined with an insecticide dust are some-times used to control fleas and rats together. Rat proofing of buildings is a longer term measure. Murine typhus responds well to tetracycline treat-ment over several days but as yet there is no vaccine available for prophy-laxis. The LBT 'E' vaccine is not reliable in the prevention of M.T.

Scrub typhus

Scrub typhus (ST), chigger-borne rickettsiosis or tsutsugamuchi disease is a widespread and important disease in Asia and the Pacific islands. The enzootic cycle of *Rickettsia tsutsugamuchi* (= *R.orientalis*) is known from the Primorski Krai region in the far east of the Soviet Union in the north to Northern Australia in the south and as far as Afghanistan and Pakistan in the west. First infections especially in non-indigenous people often cause a severe illness with an appreciable mortality. There is an eschar at the site of attachment of the mite, high fever with headache and lymphadenopathy and an often evanescent typhus-like rash spreading from the trunk to the extremities. The incubation period is from one to three weeks and usually about 12 days. Second infections with a different strain of R.tsutsugamuchi often give rise to a fever without specific signs. In one hospital in rural Malaysia specific tests showed that ST was the cause of 23 per cent of febrile illnesses although only a minority showed the classical rise in the OXK titre of the Weil-Felix test (Brown et al 1976).

R. tsutsugamuchi is present in mites of the Leptotrombidium deliense complex passing from one generation of mites to the next transovarially so that infection can be maintained for very long periods. The chiggers or larval mites are the only parasitic phase and generally feed on rodents only once; so that although rodents are important as hosts of the chiggers and frequently become infected they probably do not often pass on this infection. Infection occurs as a 'zoonotic tetrad' where rats, chiggers, suitable secondary vegetation and R. tsutsugamuchi co-exist (Traub and Wisseman 1974). This is often in quite localised areas or 'mite islands' in areas of transitional vegetation such as old farmland returning to scrub, oil palm estates, the banks of rivers or river islands, mountain slopes with Kogan grass, coralline coastal areas or even grassy gardens as in the Pescadore islands (Audy 1968).

Man is infected through the bite of a chigger when he wanders into one of these mite islands. The chigger attaches firmly to the skin, it does not suck blood but injects a digestive fluid that lyses cells locally. Clinical infections are commonest in adult males with occupations that take them into the bush. ST is a particular problem for the military and caused many casualties during the second world war and in Vietnam. Taiwanese troops in the Pescadore islands have often been infected in recent years. When troops move into an area with mite islands sharp outbreaks of ST affecting as many as fifty per cent of the soldiers can occur, although there is no person to person transmission. Serological testing of indigenous populations suggests that many infections in childhood are asymptomatic or associate with only mild illness. Infection with a single strain of R. tsutsugamuchi provides good immunity against illness from the same strain but heterologous strains frequently cause recurrent illness after a few months, however the illness may be less severe.

Control

The control of chiggers is difficult except in localised areas around new settlements, development projects or military camps. In these situations vegetation should be cleared to discourage rodents and mites and fogs or emulsions of an ascaricide applied around the site. Dieldrin or fenthion can be sprayed from knapsack sprayers or even as ultra low volume mists from aircraft. Anti-rodent measures should also be taken. Personal protection is afforded by wearing clothes impregnated with benzyl benzoate which kills chiggers and by using repellants such as diethyltoluamide on exposed skin surfaces.

Chemoprophylaxis with 200 mg doxycycline taken once weekly was successful in a trial in Taiwanese troops in the Pescadores (Olson J G et al 1980). This method should only be used in special circumstances. Cases of S.T. respond satisfactorily to treatment with tetracyclines or chloramphenicol. A single dose of 200 mg doxycycline has often proved sufficient but relapses can occur and it is usually better to treat with a daily dose of 200 mg until two or three days after the fever has settled. Because of the many different serogroups of *R. tsutsugamuchi* there is as yet no commercially available vaccine.

Tick-borne rickettsioses (spotted fever group)

This group of rickettsioses is focally present in every continent where there are pathogenic organisms and suitable hard tick vectors which bite man. Infection is generally passed transovarially from one generation of tick to the next but rodents may also act as disease reservoirs. Clinically the infections vary considerably so that Rocky Mountain Spotted Fever is often fatal if untreated while some cases of African tick typhus are quite mild. New varieties of spotted fever rickettsiae are being differentiated, for example *R. israeli*. In most spotted fever infections in man there is a small ulcer (eschar or tache noir) at the site of attachment of the ticks with local lymph node enlargement, a febrile illness with headache and conjunctivitis with a rash which begins on the limbs and may become haemorrhagic.

Rocky Mounted Spotted Fever is due to infection with *R. rickettsii*. Despite its name it now occurs most commonly in the south east of the United States (Centre for Disease Control 1982) and in other American states from Canada to Brazil. The major vectors are ixodid ticks such as the wood tick *Dermacentor andersoni* and the dog tick *Dermacentor variabilis*. Infections are usually sporadic during the summer months.

Rickettsia Conori Infections occur in a wide area from southern Europe and the Mediterranean littoral, through Africa to the Indian sub-continent. There are many local names including fièvre boutonneuse, Kenya tick typhus, South African tick typhus and Indian tick typhus. Fièvre boutonneuse is an infection of dogs transmitted to man by the bite of the dog tick *Rhipicephalus sanguineus*. It is a sporadic infection often occurring in urban areas. In Italy the infection appears to have increased recently and this has been attributed to agricultural chemicals interfering with the natural predators of ixodid ticks (Bellissima P, Farrugia G, Zuccaro I, 1981). In southern Africa tick typhus is often acquired from the ticks of cattle or wild game picked up during safaris through the veldt.

Control

It is generally not possible to control the ixodid ticks of rodents or wild game in an economic fashion. Prevention depends upon the use of repellents such as dimethyl phthalate whilst exposed to tick bites. Skin surfaces should be inspected regularly about every four hours and any attached ticks removed at once with forceps or a handkerchief. Transmission of infection generally takes some hours from the time of attachment of the tick. Take care to avoid contamination with the body fluids of crushed ticks. Domestic dogs should be kept free of ticks by regular inspection and removal and the use of insecticide powders or collars.

At present there are no vaccines against infections with spotted fever rickettsiae although work on *R. rickettsii* vaccines is in progress. Early recognition and treatment with tetracycline is particularly important in Rocky Mounted Spotted Fever.

CONCLUSION

Although epidemic louse-borne typhus has only been a problem in a few highland tropical areas in recent years the potential for serious epidemics remains wherever clothing is worn and standards of personal hygiene fall. Scrub typhus is a disease of major importance in the Pacific and Asian regions. It is the cause of a high proportion of febrile illnesses in patients admitted to hospital in some countries and carries a significant mortality rate. The disease is much under recorded unless specific diagnostic methods are used; vaccines are not yet routinely available but tetracyclines are highly effective in treatment. Flea-borne murine typhus is another much under-diagnosed zoonosis and is widespread throughout the world especially in urban areas. It is readily controlled by measures against rodents and their ectoparasites. Tick-borne rickettsioses vary enormously in severity but are widely prevalent in most tropical areas.

REFERENCES

Al-Awadi A R, Al-Kazemi N, Ezzat G, Saah A J, Shepard C, Zaghlou T, Gherdian B 1982. Murine typhus in Kuwait in 1978. Bulletin of the World Health Organization 60: 283–289
Audy J R 1968. Red mites and typhus. University of London, Athlone Press
Bellissima P, Farrugia G, Zuccaro I 1981. La febbre bottonosa nel caltagironese nel 1979–80. Revista di Parassitologia 42: 333–335
Bozeman F M, Masiello S A, Williams M S, Elisburg B L 1975. Epidemic typhus rickettsiae isolated from flying squirrels. Nature 255: 545–547
Brown G W, Robinson D M, Huxsoll D L, Ng T S, Lim K J Sannasey G 1976. Scrub typhus a common cause of illness in indigenous populations. Transactions of the Royal Society of Tropical Medicine and Hygiene 70: 444–448
Centers for Disease Control 1982 Rocky mountain spotted fever — United States, 1981. Morbidity and Mortality Weekly Report 19: 261–263
Duma R J, et al 1981. Epidemic typhus in the United States associated with flying squirrels. Journal of the American Medical Association 245: 2318–2323

Lazowski E S, Matulewicz S 1977. Serendipitous discovery of artificial positive Weil-Felix reaction used in 'private immunological war'. ASM News 43: 300

Olson J G, Bourgeois A L, Fong R C Y, Coolbough J C, Dennis D T 1980. Prevention of scrub typhus: prophylactic administration of doxycycline in a randomised double blind trial. American Journal of Tropical Medicine and Hygiene 29: 989–997

Traub R, Wisseman C L 1974. The ecology of chigger-borne rickettsiases. Journal of Medical Entomology 11: 237–303

Traub R, Wisseman C L, Farhang-Azad A 1978. The ecology of murine typhus — a critical review. Tropical Diseases Bulletin 75: 237–317

World Health Organization 1982. Louse-borne typhus in 1980 WHO Weekly Epidemiological Record 57: 45–46

World Health Organization Working Group on Rickettsial Diseases 1982. Rickettsioses: a continuing disease problem. Bulletin of the WHO 60: 157–164

Zinsser R H 1935. Rats, lice and history. Routledge, London

Introduction to the zoonoses

Infections and parasites transmissible in nature between man and vertebrate animals have been called *zoonoses*. Over 150 have already been recognized but the list is growing with the discovery of new pathogens (Marburg/Ebola disease, Lassa fever, Philipine capillariasis) and with the clarification of transmission cycles and zoonotic relationships (toxoplasmosis, babesiosis, African trypanosomiasis, simian malaria). In other cases recent knowledge has underlined the greater importance of zoonoses which were previously considered to be minor or only locally important (*Campylobacter* and *Yersinia* infections).

Zoonoses now constitute the majority of the known infections and parasites of man and their causal agents include all groups of pathogens such as viruses, rickettsiae, mycoplasms, bacteria (including spirochaetes), fungi, helminths and arthropods. Evenomation caused by poisonous reptiles, fishes and other vertebrates is not considered a zoonosis, the term being restricted to infections. Additional infections common to man and animals and which are derived from the environment or other common source (tetanus, melioidosis, rhinosporidiosis and certain fungal infections) are not zoonoses in the strict sense. They are, however, animal related and their control is usually the task of the health agency responsible for the control of zoonoses; sometimes they are called *sapro-zoonoses* and listed with the zoonoses.

The animal hosts of zoonoses are spread throughout the different classes of vertebrate animals but the most important sources of infection for man are farm animals, companion animals (pets) and those living in or around human habitations or places of work and recreation (rats, mice, pigeons, etc.). Most of the zoonoses derived from these animal groups are widespread in the world and constitute important hazards to human health as well as serious economic problems.

Although all members of the community are exposed to one or other of the zoonoses at some time, certain sections of society are at special risk. In general, persons in direct contact with animals or animal products, and those living or working in areas where reservoir animals and vector arthropods are not controlled, run the highest risk of infection. In warm climates and in non-industrialized societies where the majority of the population live in rural areas or are nomads, and where others live in over-crowded cities with unsatisfactory sanitation and preventive services, the proportion of the exposed population may be as high as 80 or even 90 per cent.

In any society children run a special risk of infection because of their tendency to touch animals, their naivety, their ignorance of risk, and in most cases their higher susceptibility to infection. Many zoonoses (rabies, hydatidosis, toxocariasis) are therefore more common in younger age groups.

The occupational groups which are at risk include livestock farmers, animal attendants, abattoir and dairy workers, hide, wool and fur handlers, wildlife workers, foresters, hunters, campers, fishermen, pet owners and dealers, veterinarians and their assistants, dog catchers, zoo staff, physicians, nurses and laboratory workers. In most countries, only a few zoonoses are legally recognized as occupational but this situation is changing. In recent years, protective measures for exposed persons (particularly immunization) have also been improved although their use is still restricted largely to industrialized countries.

The exact public health significance of the zoonoses and the economic losses which they occasion have been grossly underestimated or have remained unknown for most countries. This stems from the lack of national surveillance programmes, and particularly of diagnostic facilities. Laboratory aids to diagnosis are particularly important as many zoonoses may produce mild, sub-acute or chronic illness or may occur as sub-clinical infections, especially in animal reservoir hosts. Obscure diseases (fevers, encephalitides, diarrhoeas, nephritides) classed as those of 'unknown etiology' may often be zoonoses. Even where the disease is diagnosed, it may not be officially or even voluntarily notifiable.

The ebb and flow of human illness attributable to zoonoses is generally a reflection of the level of activity of the infective agent in the animal reservoir. This relationship is particularly notable in the case of vector-borne infections. In a recent epidemic of Rift Valley fever in a north-African country (18 000 cases with 598 deaths), retrospective studies showed that abortions and deaths due to this infection had occurred in livestock six months before the disease appeared in man. Outbreaks of Japanese encephalitis have also been observed in pigs before people were affected. In these and other similar instances, surveillance of the infection in animals and implicated arthropod vectors would be essential in order to take preventive measures before human infection began to occur. It would also be necessary for information about zoonoses observed in animals by the veterinary services or diagnosed in the slaughter houses or veterinary laboratories to be passed on promptly to the health agency responsible for the control of these diseases in man.

Apart from the widespread human illness and death, several zoonoses, especially those involving cattle and other large domesticated animals cause very large economic losses. It has been estimated that animal diseases may reduce the productivity of farm animals by from 20 per cent of potential yields in developed countries to 67 per cent in developing countries. Zoonoses rank high among the diseases which reduce production. This reduction is occasioned not only by death of the animals but also by depression of yields of milk*, meat, eggs, wool and other products. The loss of these high quality protein foods often has a serious effect on the nutritional status of the people especially of children. In areas where animal power is used for cultivation and draft, there may be serious losses in crop production. Meat, milk and other products from affected herds may carry dangerous pathogens (such as *Brucella*, *Mycobacteria*, *Salmonella* and *Trichinella*) the detection and elimination of which would increase the cost of production. This would also interfere with national and international trade and might therefore hamper national development and tourism.

Reliable quantification of losses caused by zoonoses and of the cost of control programmes has not been done in most countries. Some recent estimates from Latin America and the United States may, however illustrate the enormity of these losses. In Latin America bovine rabies is responsible for an estimated yearly loss of US$ 50 million. In the United States brucellosis and bovine tuberculosis cost US$ 25 million and 100 million respectively. Brucellosis in Latin America and the Caribbean costs annually US$ 600 million. Cost-benefit ratios of brucellosis control programmes have been calculated to be between 1:5 and 1:8 in the USA and between 1:6 and 1:140 in Latin American countries. It is disconcerting to observe that in spite of the foregoing facts very few zoonoses control programmes of significance are being undertaken in warm climate countries.

The prevention and control of zoonoses, as of other communicable diseases, require constant surveillance and prompt notification of the disease in man as well as in animals. Only then can the transmission from animals to man and among animals and human beings be interrupted by appropriate measures. Most of the control measures need to be taken against the infection present in the animal reservoir, against the animals which constitute that reservoir and against the invertebrate vector where one exists. Such action presents some organizational problems as in most countries the veterinary and public health services work in isolation and in different governmental departments. A close collaboration of these services is necessary for the surveillance and control of zoonoses and to assure that the food supplies are safe and free from pathogens derived from animals and from food handlers.

In developed countries the major zoonoses (brucellosis, tuberculosis, anthrax, rabies, ornithosis-psittacosis, hydatidosis and taeniasis) have been successfully controlled so that the incidence of these infections in man is low and losses in animals are relatively minimal. It is heartening to see that some

---

* FAO has estimated that zoonoses contribute significantly to the loss of about 30 million tons of milk attributed annually to diseases of milk animals. This quantity would provide two glasses of milk daily for some 200 million children.

important zoonoses have also recently been brought under control in some developing countries, for example, rabies in Malaysia, Taiwan and some islands in the Philippines, Japanese encephalitis in China, equine encephalitis in central and south America and hydatidosis in Cyprus. Rabies is also being brought under control in large areas of south America and many large cities in Africa. The experience gained in these control programmes can be invaluable for other countries embarking on similar programmes.

Many of the major zoonoses (arbovirus infections, trypanosomiasis, leishmaniasis, some diarrhoeal diseases, Marburg/Ebola infections, et cetera) are dealt with in other chapters in this book. Others specifically associated with companion animals (pets) and farm animals are described in the succeeding chapter. A number of other infections are left out for lack of space but are dealt with in the publications listed in the bibliography at the end of this chapter.

SUGGESTED READING

A number of useful publications on zoonoses in general and on individual zoonoses have appeared in recent years. The reader may find the following publications in the English language of interest, in addition to those cited as references in the text of the later chapters.

Acha P N, Szyfres B 1980 Zoonoses and communicable diseases common to man and animals, Pan American Health Organization, Washington DC

Edney A T B 1981 WHO/WSAVA guidelines to reduce human health risks associated with animals in urban areas, VPH/81.29 World Health Organization, Geneva

Hubbert W T, Schnurrenberger P R (eds) 1980 Update to zoonoses, 1980, Iowa State University, Ames

Steele J H (ed) 1979 and 1980 CRC Handbook series in zoonoses, Vols I + II, CRC Press Incorporation, Boca Raton, Florida

WHO Expert Committee with the participation of FAO 1982 (in press) Bacterial and viral zoonoses, Technical Report Series No. 682 World Health Organization, Geneva

Infections from companion animals (pets)

INTRODUCTION

Companion or pet animals have been defined by the European Economic Community as 'animals belonging to species normally nourished and kept, but not [generally] consumed* by man, except animals bred for fur'. Dogs and cats are the traditional pets but a large number of other species such as monkeys, lambs, rodents, cage and aviary birds, fishes, tortoises and many others are also kept as pet animals. These animals live in close association with their owners, particularly children and women, and are very beneficial as they fulfil real mental health needs. They can, however, also represent a health hazard to the owners and the community, being sources of zoonotic infections and pollution and they may cause physical injuries as well as allergies. In the following pages only the more important zoonoses of companion animals are dealt with; a fuller account will be found in the publications listed in the preceding bibliography. Most of these zoonoses occur also in wild animals and farm animals and these aspects are also covered in this section.

Rabies (Syns. hydrophobia, lyssa)

This acute viral encephalitis, which is almost always fatal, is well known for its fearful symptoms common among which is the spasm of deglutition muscles. Many patients experience this spasm simply when seeing a liquid and avoid drinking it or swallowing their saliva (hydrophobia). Transmission is through bites of rabid animals particularly dogs and other carnivores and sometimes bats. The relatively long incubation period, two to eight weeks, sometimes much longer, allows time for the exposed person to be immunized and protected before the virus reaches the central nervous system. Control depends upon elimination of the reservoir animals, particularly dogs and upon immunization of those which have to be kept.

---

* In some parts of the world, the distinction between pets and food or free roaming animals is not always clear.

Disease in man and animals

In Man, the initial symptoms consist of irritation and pain at the site of the animal bite, anxiety, headache and sensory changes. These arise two to eight weeks following the bite; though longer, and rarely, shorter, incubation periods have been reported. Further development of the disease is characterized by hyperaesthesia, dilatation of the pupils, excess salivation, difficulty in swallowing resulting from spasms of deglutition and respiration muscles followed by general convulsions. In most cases, there is a generalized paralysis and death resulting from respiratory failure, two to six days after onset of the disease.

In *dogs*, the incubation period is 10 to 60 days but, rarely, it may extend to several months. Early signs of the disease are a change in behaviour, a tendency to hide in corners or under furniture and an enhanced excitability. In the next stage, the animal becomes greatly agitated and aggressive and tends to bite anything it can take in the mouth including inanimate objects and it attacks other animals and man. Salivation is profuse but the animal is unable to swallow and its voice becomes hoarse. It has a tendency to run away from its usual habitat and may develop convulsions, incoordinated movements and paralysis before death, which takes place in five or six days, often earlier. In the so-called dumb form of the disease, the excitement and agitation is absent or very brief and paralysis predominates starting with the head and neck and descending to the trunk and extremities. The disease in *cats* is usually similar to the furious type in dogs. In *cattle* and other farm animals, there is generally a short or variable stage of excitement followed by paralysis which manifests itself as incoordination of movements, difficulty in swallowing and general paralysis. In pigs, there is marked agitation and the signs are similar to those in dogs.

The diagnosis in man is generally based on the history of an animal bite and by the characteristic symptoms. It can be confirmed by immunofluorescence test of corneal impressions, frozen skin sections or biopsied pieces of brain. These tissues expecially brain can also be used in the mouse inoculation test, the results of which are, however, available only after a few days.

In dogs and other animals direct immunofluorescence test on brain tissue gives rapid and specific results in experienced hands. The mouse inoculation test can be used for confirmation. In many warm climate countries, microscopic examination for Negri bodies is still widely used but is less sensitive than the foregoing methods. (For techniques see Kaplan and Koprowski, 1973). Suspected dogs which are involved in human exposure, can be isolated and kept under observation for up to 10 days during which period they may develop characteristic signs of the disease and die. Animals remaining healthy during this period are regarded as non infective. (This method is not applicable to wild animals.)

The agent

Rabies virus belongs to the group of rhabdoviruses and has generally been regarded as antigenically singular. However, recent studies using a mono-clonal antibody method have identified what appear to be antigenic variants isolated from persons whom vaccination failed to protect. Even so, most of the strains obtained from human beings and animals in a given area react uniformly to monoclonal antibody. The exact significance of these rare variants needs further clarification. Some other strains show variations in their biological properties and pathogenecity.

In Africa, several viruses of the rabies sub-group have been identified, two of which (Mokola and Duvenhage viruses) were isolated from human beings dying of rabies-like illness. It is doubtful if current antirabies vaccine would protect against these particular viruses.

Epidemiology

Rabies is primarily a disease of animals and occurs in all continents except Australasia and the Antarctic. Several countries in the other continents have eliminated the disease and have remained rabies-free for many years. The more important reservoir animals are canines (dogs, foxes, jackals, coyotes, wolves, et cetera) other carnivores (cats, mongooses, skunks, raccoons) and bats (vampires and insectivorous bats). Herbivorous animals, both domes-ticated and wild are usually unimportant in the transmission cycle, as also are rodents and lagomorphs. In central Europe, strains of rabies virus with low infectivity have been isolated from apparently healthy field mice but their epidemiological significance is still unknown.

Dogs are the most important sources of human infection and areas of high incidence of the disease in man generally have large populations of stray or pariah dogs. In these animals, the disease shows seasonal variations, the highest incidence being in late spring and early summer, following the mating season. A second, shorter, peak is observable in some countries in autumn. In addition, epizootics occur in cycles of three to five years (or longer) unless checked by control programmes.

Transmission from infected vampire bats to cattle and other animals on which they feed occurs in central and southern America (North Mexico to North Argentina and Trinidad) but the bats rarely attack man. Sporadic human infections result from bites of insectivorous bats in the USA and Canada. Bat rabies is extremely rare and insignificant in other continents.

Human exposure occurs through deposition of the virus-laden saliva in a bite wound or through contact of infected material with the conjunctiva or other mucous membrances. Bites on the head and neck are more dangerous than those on extremities and children (5–14 years) are bitten more often than adults; they may kick or handle a street dog or bring home a pariah puppy of unknown origin. Owners sometimes open and look for a bone in the mouth of a dog that has difficulty in swallowing and get bitten in the process. Rabid wolves have a tendency to attack people sleeping in the open and tend to bite them on the head and neck as they would in catching their prey.

It should be remembered that not all rabid dogs excrete the virus in their saliva. Also in some cases superficial abrasions especially if caused by bites through clothes may not have enough virus to cause infection. On the other hand dogs often start to excrete the virus in their saliva two, three or even five days before onset of recognizable signs of rabies and continue to do so during the course of the disease. Abortive or inapparent infection in dogs should be regarded as a medical curiosity.

In rare cases infection with airborne virus through inhalation has occured in a closed space, for example bat cave, and confirmed by animal experiments but this may be regarded as an exceptional mode of transmission for humans.

Surveillance

Currently, most warm climate countries report rabies on the basis of data from hospitals though only a small proportion of such cases are admitted. Compulsory notification of such deaths (even where physicians are not available to certify) increases the rabies reported as people in endemic areas are familiar with the disease.

Surveillance in animals should cover not only domesticated carnivores but also strays and wild animals as the latter constitute an important reservoir. Laboratory examination of tissues is the only sure way of diagnosing the disease in animals dying under suspected circumstances. Canines found dead in the wild and those killed on the road should also be examined.

An efficient surveillance system is necessary not only for control programmes but also for evaluating the animal bites for prophylactic treatment of exposed persons.

Control

Control of rabies in the community depends on its elimination from the animal reservoirs especially dogs which are responsible for the vast majority of human infections. This is achieved by elimination of stray and pariah dogs (and cats) and by immunization of the remaining animals in as short a time as possible. Transmission stops if the level of the immunized population reaches 70 per cent or more. Thereafter, vaccination of new comers and re-vaccination of older animals has to be carried out to ensure the immune status of the dog (and cat) population. Elimination of unwanted dogs is sometimes rendered difficult by the socio-cultural resistance of the community but it can be overcome by judicious education of the public.

A number of vaccines are now available for the immunization of dogs. In the early stages of control programmes in endemic areas, one of the modified live virus vaccines may be used as their cost is reasonable and the period of immunity is long. Later, when the disease has been brought under control, one of the inactivated virus vaccines may be used. In all cases, the vaccine should have been tested for potency and safety.

Rabies-free countries may prohibit the importation of dogs and cats from infected areas or may keep them in quarantine for four to six months following immunization with an inactivated vaccine at the time of entry.

Rabies in wild carnivores (foxes, jackals) is controlled by reducing their numbers by gassing litters in the lairs. Vaccination of foxes by oral administration of modified virus is still in the experimental stages. Vampire bats are eliminated by using anticoagulants smeared on the bodies of captured individuals which are then released and are licked clean by other bats during mutual grooming. Insectivorous bats are useful to agriculture and the decision to reduce their numbers should only be taken after due consideration of the risk posed by them.

Prevention of rabies in man

It is important that people in endemic areas should be informed about the risks of handling both pets with changed behaviour and free living animals which appear to be excited, paralyzed or otherwise unwell. Children should be warned particularly not to pick up pets in the streets and elsewhere outside their homes.

In case of a bite, the animal should if possible be secured alive for observation and diagnosis and when it dies or is killed, the brain should be sent for laboratory examination.

The bitten person should be treated as soon as possible by washing the wound thoroughly with soap and water. Later the physician can decide if specific treatment is required. (The guide included in the Sixth Report of the WHO Expert Committee on Rabies, 1973, as revised by a group of WHO consultants in 1980, mimeographed document WHO/Rabies/80 188, Annex I is extremely useful for this purpose.)

The bite wound should be cleaned and infused with antirabies serum or its globulin fraction which should also be injected in the surrounding area. The wound should not be sutured unless absolutely necessary. Thereafter a course of antirabies vaccine should be started with or without a single inoculation of serum or immune globulin (vide the WHO Guide) at the start only.

There are a number of inactivated vaccines available for use in man. In warm climate (developing) countries, vaccines derived from nervous tissues of adult (sheep, goats, rabbits) or newborn animals (rabbits, mice, rats) are commonly used. Other vaccines are prepared from virus grown in avian embryos (chicken or duck) or in cell cultures. Of the latter a vaccine prepared with virus grown in human diploid cells is highly potent and relatively safe but its high cost hinders its large scale use. The high potency of this vaccine permits the course of inoculation to be shortened as compared to nervous tissue vaccine.

Persons occupationally exposed to rabies (laboratory workers, dogs-catchers, veterinarians, et cetera) can be immunized with one of the fore-going vaccines but the risk of infection has to be carefully weighed against the risk of side effects of the vaccine. On subsequent exposure, a shortened course of vaccination is still necessary besides the local treatment of the bite wound as described above.

Psittacosis (Syns. ornithosis, avian chlamydiosis)

At one time this infection was much feared because of an outbreak in 1929–1930 affecting nearly 1000 persons with 200–300 deaths in 12 countries where psittacine birds had been imported from South America. Currently the disease has become milder and occurs sporadically, as small familial outbreaks and rarely as an extended outbreak in poultry plants.

Human infections generally result from inhalation of the airborne caus-ative agent (*Chlamydia psittaci*) in contaminated premises. Apart from pet owners who may be infected by cage or aviary birds, pigeon lofts and house-hold poultry, most cases occur among employees in pet shops, workers in poultry (including turkey) processing plants and those who pluck ducks and geese. The incubation period extends over one to two weeks and the disease may be inapparent or mild in most cases. In fact, the fever, chills, headache and cough may be attributed to other respiratory diseases. In some cases there may be atypical pneumonia, chest radiographs showing small patches of consolidation in lower parts of lungs, later developing into broncho-pneumonia. There is dry cough with scanty expectoration. In the elderly, the disease is more serious with endocarditis and hepastosplenomegaly.

In the birds also the disease is usually inapparent or mild but under conditions of stress such as prolonged transport, crowding, malnutrition or intercurrent disease, the birds may develop conjuctivitis, fever, diarrhoea, emaciation and respiratory distress.

The causative agent is excreted via the gastrointestinal tract and dried faeces infect both birds and man. Ingestion may be an additional route of infection in birds (coprophagia, cannibalism). Man-to-man transmission is rare but physicians and nurses may be infected while attending psittacosis patients.

Diagnosis is confirmed by serological tests especially the complement fixation test on paired serum samples to show significant increase of anti-body in convalescent serum. Care should be excercised in interpreting the results if only a single serum is available as *Chlamydia psittaci* cross-reacts with *Ch. trachomatis* which is prevalent in many warm climate countries. The agent can be isolated from human sputum or from the organs of birds in laboratories equipped with the necessary safety measures. Microscopic examination of Giemsa or Macchiavello stained smears of serous exudate or organ smears of suspected birds may show the agent.

Surveillance of poultry, and pigeon flocks and aviaries helps to identify foci of infection. Examination of free ranging birds is less useful as the results cannot be put to any practical use.

Control of the infection is based on suppressing the infection in birds by the administration of tetracyclines. Psittacines and other birds are treated with 0.5 per cent chlortetracycline in their feed for 45 days. Unaffected birds on infected turkey and poultry farms should similary be fed tetracyclines for three to four weeks before being sent for slaughter.

There are no vaccines to protect humans or birds.

Echinococcosis (hydatidosis) (Syn. hydatid disease)

Echinococcosis (hydatidosis) is the infection of man with the larval stage (hydatid) of the dog tapeworm *Echinococcus granulosus* and related species. It is widely distributed in the world. Human infection takes place through infection of the eggs (embryophores) passed out in dog faeces; hence the central role of the dog in the epidemiology of this disease. The dogs become infected through ingestion of the fertile cysts in the internal organs of sheep, camels and other animals.

Disease in Man and animals

Echinococcosis and hydatidosis are terms applied interchangeably to the infection of man with tapeworms of the genus *Enchinococcus*. Of the four recognized species of this genus, *E. granulosus* is widely distributed in the world and is the most important species from the public health point of view. Its hydatid is found in a variety of wild and domestic mammals of which sheep, camels, cattle and swine are important for continuation of the life cycle in dogs which are fed raw viscera of infected animals. Besides the dog, the adult tapeworm has been found in a number of canines (wolf, dingo, coyote, jackal, fox, racoon, dog, etc.) hyaenas, lions and leopards. Dogs are nevertheless the most important source of human infection. *E. multilocularis* with a fox-vole cycle in nature is locally distributed in temperate regions amd occasionally infects man. *E. vogeli* has been found to cause polycystic hydatidosis of the liver in man in Latin America but little is known of its prevalence. In nature, it uses the bush dog (*Speothos venaticus*) and the domestic dog as final hosts and the paca (*Cuniculus paca*) as an intermediate host. The fourth species, *E. oligarthus* is not known to infect man. The rest of this section, therefore, deals with the infection with *E. granulosus* only.

In man, liver and lungs are the more common sites of predilection of hydatids but in a small proportion of cases kidneys, heart, bone and the central nervous system may be involved. The cysts grow slowly and may not produce any observable symptoms for years or may degenerate and be detected only on radiographs or during surgery performed for other reasons. The cysts in the kidney, heart and brain may produce more serious symptoms than those in the liver and lungs. Rupture of the cyst can be dangerous and fatal because of the anaphylactic shock and pulmonary oedema caused by sudden reaction to the released antigens in the cyst fluid. If the patient recovers, the scolices in the fluid may grow into secondary cysts in the abdominal or the pleural cavity. Such growth can exert strong pressure on the viscera.

Among animals, the dog may suffer little inconvenience from the presence of *E. granulosus* in its intestine. Occasionally enteritis may occur if the infection is unusually heavy. In cattle, sheep, camels and pigs no definite signs and symptoms have been attributed to hydatids although general effects like loss of weight, debility and loss of wool has been ascribed to the infection. The most important economic loss in these animals results for the condemnation of infected livers and other viscera on meat inspection. Meat producing countries like Argentina, Chile and New Zealand lose millions of dollars worth of sheep livers every year.

Radiography is useful in the diagnosis of human hydatidosis but specific confirmation is obtained by immunological tests or by surgical removal and identification of the metacestode (cyst). Immunodiagnostic tests which have been widely used are latex agglutination, indirect haemagglutination, immunoelectrophoresis and enzyme-linked immunoabsorbant assay (ELISA). [For techniques see Eckert, Gemmel and Soulsby (1981)]. The intradermal (Casoni) test is less specific but is still used in many countries.

In dogs, the diagnosis is by examination of faeces for tapeworms or their eggs. The latter would be difficult to distinguish from those of other tapeworms of dogs. Usually, the faeces are collected after administration of arecoline hydrobromide and are examined for tapeworms. This procedure is however risky as a large mass of embryophores (eggs) of *Echinococcus* may be expelled. This procedure should therefore be carried out under professional supervision in a suitably isolated place. In domestic ruminants, the cysts can usually be detected in the slaughter house or on postmortem examination elsewhere.

Epidemiology

E. granulosus has a worldwide distribution but human infection takes place in certain endemic areas where exists a cycle involving dogs and domestic ruminants, particularly sheep and camels. Human infections are absent in areas of the dog-horse cycle and less frequent in some areas involving wild carnivores and herbivores. The infection is particularly important in the Mediterranean basin, in the Arctic and in parts of Australasia, although it has declined in the latter continent as a result of active control measures.

It is locally important also in parts of South America, Africa and Asia.

Sociocultural factors especially attitudes to dogs have an important influence on the risk of human infection. This is shown by the comparatively lower incidence of the disease among muslim populations in the eastern Meditterranean as compared to that in members of other faiths in the same area; the former consider the dog as an unclean animal and avoid handling it. Relatively high incidence of the infection among Eskimos, Basques and Amerindians in the USA, Turkana tribes in Kenya and Maoris in New Zealand has been attributed to socio-cultural factors (WHO Expert Committee on Parasitic Zoonoses, 1979).

Hydatidosis is an occupational disease among shepherds, camelmen and other pastoralists, whose families also run a higher risk than the rest of the population.

Surveillance

Surveillance of the infection is essential for establishing its importance in comparison with other diseases, for understanding the local process of transmission and for obtaining base-line data for control programmes. Prevalence of the infection in man is generally reported on the basis of hospital cases which is a relatively small part of the total prevalence in most countries. Autopsies provide additional information but special surveys have been carried out using miniature radiography and immunodiagnostic methods. A combination of some or all of these methods would be indicated in endemic areas.

In sheep, camels, cattle and pigs the prevalence can be measured by examination of livers and lungs during meat inspection or in other establishments where dead animals are available. Surveys of the prevalence of the adult tapeworm in dogs are of fundamental importance and are best carried out on autopsy but more commonly by examination of the stool (purge) after administration of arecoline hydrobromide.

Control

Theoretically, the control of this disease can be achieved by avoiding the feeding of viscera with cysts to dogs, a measure which presupposes proper meat inspection. In practice, however, there have been difficulties in the application of this simple measure in many areas. Furthermore, programmes based on the long-accepted treatment of dogs with arecoline hydrobromide have failed to achieve elimination of the infection.

A careful comparison was made of the successful control programmes carried out in some countries and the unsuccessful ones in others. The following factors conducive to success were identified:

(a) Intensive health education of the public, particularly of animal breeders, shepherds, butchers and other dog owners.

(b) Surveillance of dogs based on periodic examination of stool after administration of a taenifuge, such as arecoline hydrobromide, followed by isolation of infected animals and treatment with a taenicide (e.g. Praziquantel).

(c) Control of slaughter and proper meat inspection with destruction or sterilization of infected viscera as far as possible.

(d) Encouragement of cultural traits which lead to avoidance of contact with dogs in endemic areas.

Field control programmes conducted on the foregoing lines have been successful not only in temperate regions (New Zealand, Australia and Argentina) but also in Cyprus. For a full discussion of control measures see Eckert, Gemmel and Soulsby (1981).

The only successful treatment of hydatidosis in man is the surgical removal of cysts. Benzimidazole derivatives have been observed to cause damage or destruction of the cyst in sheep but in man the results have been variable so far (Schanz, van den Bossche and Eckert, 1982).

Toxocariasis (Syn. visceral larva migrans)

This disease is caused by the persistence and migration in the human body of the larvae of *Toxocara canis* of dogs and other related species notably *T. cati* of cats. Infection results from ingestion of eggs containing the infective second stage larvae which only rarely grow and develop in man but may migrate to various organs including the brain and the eye. The adult parasite is widely prevalent in dogs (and cats) throughout the world and there are indications that the human infection is a growing health problem which is particularly important in warm climates. Its importance and magnitude is not fully realized because of the difficulty of diagnosis.

Clinical manifestations depend on the number and location of the larvae, but they occur primarily in children in the age range 18 to 36 months. Mild infections may be inapparent but a blood count may show persistent eosinophilia. Continued reinfections result in formation of focal or generalized eosinophilic granulomas. There is marked debility associated with liver and lung disorders including coughing and asthma. More serious manifestations result from invasion of the brain (epileptic symptoms, paralysis) and the eye (chorioretinitis, occasionally blindness). The eye lesion may be mistaken for cancer and the eyeball removed by surgery.

Although clinical methods and biopsy of liver and lung tissue may help in the diagnosis, immunodiagnostic methods are of special value because of their sensitivity and specificity. These consist of indirect immunofluorescence, ELISA test and precipitation test using living larvae. A skin test has also been used and is valuable in surveys.

Epidemiology

Toxocara canis occurs throughout the world and in warm climates over 90 per cent of puppies below six months of age have been found infected. They can be infected *in utero*. The egg content of faeces of these animals can be as high as 10 000 to 15 000 per gram. The environment of infected animals therefore gets heavily contaminated and acts as a reservoir for human infection. Children play on infected ground or may handle dogs that carry infective eggs on their hair coat. Also the soil in public parks and streets where dogs deposit their faeces, has been found to contain eggs. Therefore, people who do not have dogs or cats in their homes are also exposed to the infection.

Prevention and control

Because of the high prevalence of infection in dogs, it is difficult to eliminate the risk entirely. Stray and pariah dogs should be eliminated. House dogs should be tested and given anthelmintic treatment at intervals. Because of the frequency of pre-natal infection, puppies should be treated two weeks after birth with piperazine adipate or other anthelmintic. Children and other dog owners should be made aware of the risk of infection and taught to observe rules of personal hygiene. Dogs should not be allowed into public parks and childrens' play grounds.

Chemotherapy of the disease in man is still unsatisfactory.

Linguatulosis

Linguatula serrata, a pentastomid, is parasitic in the nasal cavity of dogs, jackals, foxes and wolves, and is widely prevalent in the warm climates. The immature forms (nymphs) of the parasite are found in the lymph nodes, livers and other viscera of domestic and wild herbivores and occasionally man. The manifestations of this type of larval infection in man are not known.

In some Eastern Mediterranean and African countries infected livers and lungs of sheep and other herbivores are consumed raw on certain occasions, when the immature parasites contained in them lodge in the naso-pharynx causing a serious inflammatory (possibly allergic) reaction. It is called *halzoun* and may cause suffocation.

Prevention depends on avoidance of uncooked viscera.

Ectoparasites

A number of ectoparasites of dogs, cats and other companion (pet) animals attack man but are not considered as zoonoses by some epidemiologists. (See Macdonald Chapter 39).

Some of these, for example the dog tick (*Rhipicephalus sanguineus*), transmit an important rickettsial disease (boutonneuse fever) to man. The bites of this and other ticks may also cause tick paralysis. *Sarcoptes* of dogs and *Notoedres cati* may cause scabies-like disease in man. Fleas of dogs and cats (*Ctenocephalides canis* and *C. felis*) frequently attack man and are known to have replaced the human flea (*Pulex irritans*) in some areas. The chigoe or jigger flea (*Tunga penetrans*) attacks man and several species of animals in Africa and South America.

The control of the foregoing parasites has to be carried out in animals and their environments.

Toxoplasmosis

Human infection with the coccidian parasite *Toxoplasma gondii* may be congenital or acquired. Congenital infection occurs when the mother acquires a symptomatic or subclinical primary infection in the first or second trimester of pregnancy; in the third trimester the infection is generally inapparent. Congenital infection may cause death of the foetus or of the newborn or hydrocephalus, and other changes in the central nervous system as well as ocular disorders. Acquired infection is generally symptomless or mild causing general malaise, lymphadenopathy or chorioretinitis. The disease may flare up in acute and fatal form in patients receiving immunosuppressive therapy.*

The disease in animals is in general similar to that in man. It is usually asymptomatic but in sheep it may cause placentitis, abortions, encephalitis and eye lesions. In some sheep raising countries, toxoplasmosis causes serious economic losses.

Diagnosis:

In some cases of acute infection the diagnosis may be confirmed by isolating the parasite by intraperitoneal inoculation of blood or tissue fluids in mice. Some less sensitive alternatives to mice are the chick embryos or cell cultures (HeLa cells). Among serological tests, indirect immunofluorescence, indirect haemagglutination and Sabin-Feldman dye test are used. IgM antibodies detected in the newborn infant (by immunofluorescence test) are generally accepted as indicative of foetal infection since this type of immune globulin does not pass through the intact placenta.

The agent:

T. gondii is a coccidian sporozoan parasite of which the definitive forms occur only in the cat family and lynx (carnivore genera *Felis* and *Lynx*). The oocysts are produced by sexual multiplication in the alimentary tract of these animals only. The intermediate stages (tachyzoites and cystozoites) are found in a variety of mammals including man and in birds. Asexual multi-

---

* It has become particularly important as an opportunistic invader in the Aquired Immune Defficiency Syndrome (AIDS). D. Robinson.

plication takes place in the tissues of these intermediate hosts. Cats harbour intermediate forms in addition to the definitive stages of the parasite.

Epidemiology

Toxoplasmosis has a worldwide distribution and is one of the commonest of zoonoses. Cysts in the muscles, brains and internal organs of several species of animals are the source of infection in man and carnivorous animals which consume raw or undercooked meat. This is considered to be the commonest mode of infection in man. As stated above, transplacental infection of the foetus also occurs. The role of the oocyst passed out in cat faeces in causing human infection needs further assessment. However, sporulated oocysts in the soil are considered to be the source of infection of vegetarians and inhabitants of neotropical rain forests in Brazil. Furthermore, people living in homes with cats show a significantly higher seropositivity than those who are not in frequent contact with these animals.

Control

As the bulk of infection in man takes place through ingestion of raw or undercooked meat (mainly pork or mutton), it is obvious that uninfected (seronegative) individuals, especially pregnant women, should avoid eating insufficiently cooked meat. The cysts in meat can also be destroyed by keeping it frozen at $-15°C$ for longer than three days or by heating meat in all parts to $65°C$ for four to five minutes.

Contact with cat faeces and with sand or soil in which these animals have defecated should be avoided. The litter of house cats should be disposed of properly and preferably daily before oocysts have had time to sporulate. Polluted vessels and premises should be treated with boiling water.

REFERENCES

Eckert J Gemmel M A Soulsby EJL 1981 Guidelines for surveillance, prevention and control of echinococcosis/hydatidosis VPH/81.28 World Health Organization, Geneva
Kaplan M M Koprowski H (eds) 1973 Laboratory techniques in rabies, 3rd edn. WHO Monograph Series No. 23 World Health Organization, Geneva
Schanz P M van den Bossche H Eckert J 1982 Chemotherapy for larval echinococcosis in animals and humans: report of a workshop. Zeitschrift für Parasitenkunde 67: 5–26
WHO Expert Committee with the participation of FAO 1979 Parasitic zoonoses Technical Report Series No. 673 World Health Organization, Geneva
WHO Expert Committee on Rabies 1973 Sixth Report Technical Report Series No. 523 World Health Organization, Geneva

Infections from agriculture

INTRODUCTION

This group of infections constitute a special risk not only for those who come into direct contact with animals but also for those who handle animal products (meat, hides, wool et cetera). As an extremely important source of foodborne diseases they also constitute a hazard for a very large number of people. beyond those who are occupationally exposed. Included in this group are some of the most economically ravaging diseases such as brucellosis and salmonellosis. Their control and elimination from foodstuffs is one of the most important of the joint tasks of the public health and veterinary services.

Brucellosis (Malta Fever, undulant fever)

Brucellosis is a very costly zoonosis with highly variable clinical features. In most human cases the disease manifests itself by continued, intermittent or irregular fever, general weakness and a feeling of tiredness. There may also be sweating, chills and pains in joints and other parts of the body. The disease is markedly incapacitating and interferes seriously with the working capability and with the quality of life of the patient.

In animals it causes, among other manifestations, abortion and sterility. The organism is excreted in the genital discharges and milk thus exposing animal attendants and consumers of raw milk to serious risk of infection.

Control of brucellosis depends on its elimination from animals. Test and slaughter methods have been applied successfully in developed countries but their cost for the developing countries is prohibitive. In these areas the infection should be reduced by human or animal vaccination as a first step and, when the level of animal disease has been brought down, radical methods can be applied to eliminate the sources of infection.

Disease. in Man and animals

Brucellosis presents in Man as a diverse spectrum of disease varying from sub-clinical serological conversion to severe life threatening sickness. The clinical form usually starts as continued, intermittent or irregular fever, headache, general weakness or feeling of tiredness, profuse sweating, chills and joint and other pains. It may last for several days, many months and even for years and may have locomotor and nervous complications. It is one of the most incapacitating of diseases.

In animals the infection tends to become localized in the genital organs and in the mammary glands. Abortion is one of the common and important manifestations. At this time the placenta and genital discharges are heavily loaded with *Brucella* which also continue to be excreted for variable periods in the milk. Some animals become sterile and males may develop orchitis.

The agent

Of the six recognised species of *Brucella*, four are known to infect Man. These are *B. melitensis, B. abortus, B. suis* and *B. canis*. Of these *B. melitensis* and *B. suis* are, for Man, the more virulent species. For descriptions and classification of *Brucella* see Corbel and Brinley-Morgan (1981).

Epidemiology

As mentioned above the placenta, genital discharges and milk of infected animals are the main sources of human infections. Persons who handle or look after these animals or their newborn (including stillborn or aborted) are likely to be infected. Infectious materials and discharges dry on the ground and infectious dust may be inhaled. Drinking of raw unpasteurized milk or of products made from it are other important ways in which humans may be infected far from the animal source. *B. canis* infections have occured in laboratory workers and in persons directly in contact with infected dogs. Transmission through insects and other arthropods, as also transmission between human beings, does not ordinarily occur.

Among the animal reservoirs of brucellosis sheep and goats carry the more virulent species *B. melitensis*. It is widely prevalent but important foci have been identified in the Mediterranean basin, Central Asia and Latin America. Bovine infection caused by *B. abortus* is widespread throughout the world but has been reduced to a very low level in Europe and North America. In warm climate countries, important foci have developed in town dairies and cattle sheds around large towns. Swine infection caused by *B. suis* is important mainly in some parts of the New World. Elsewhere, there are local foci of infection. Certain biotypes of this species are the cause of reindeer brucellosis in the Far-North and others infect hares in nature. *B. canis* is known largely from North America but foci have recently been found in Europe and in other parts of the world.

The diagnosis of brucellosis in man and animals cannot be made from its vague and variable clinical picture alone. Cultivation of *Brucella* and serological tests (agglutination, complement fixation and Coombs tests) are employed. In animals, certain simplifications of the agglutination test (Rose-Bengal and milk-ring tests) as well as allergic tests are used for surveys and screening. For a description of these tests see Alton, Jones and Pietz (1975). Interpretation of the tests in man is discussed by Elberg (1981), who also deals with other aspects of human brucellosis.

Surveillance

This is mainly carried out in animals on a herd basis by using the screening tests mentioned above. Surveys in man using allergenic tests have not been very useful. However, cases of obscure fever should be tested for brucellosis especially if there is a history of contact with possibly infected animals or animal products.

Control

Radical control and prevention of brucellosis in man depends on its elimination from the reservoirs. In cattle, elimination of herds which contain reactors to the sero-agglutination test has proved effective in reducing the infection to an extremely low level in the industrially developed countries. In developing countries, economic factors make it difficult to apply this method, especially for the more virulent *B. melitensis* infection in sheep and goats which are generally owned by the poorer section of the population. In such cases, and especially if the rate of infection is high, vaccination of exposed persons and of animals should be considered. In the U.S.S.R. and China live vaccine has been used for several years to protect occupationally exposed individuals, with marked reduction in the number of cases. Animal vaccines, both live and inactivated, have been used for vaccinating female animals at a young age. Vaccination of older animals makes them react positively to diagnostic tests thus making it difficult to distinguish them from naturally infected animals. Recently, vaccines free from this handicap (i.e. non-agglutinogenic vaccines) have been prepared. One such vaccine prepared from Strain 45/20 is officially accepted for use in unvaccinated cattle in the face of an outbreak.

Control measures have to be applied on a planned basis so as to achieve the objective without undue interference with animal husbandry and at a cost which the community can afford. If the measures include elimination of infected animals a source of replacement should be assured beforehand.

Heat treatment of milk, including pasteurization, is vital for the prevention of milk-borne brucellosis.

Treatment

Spontaneous recovery of infected humans is not infrequent. However, antibiotic therapy, notably with tetracyclines, is used with or without supporting therapy with corticosteroids. For details see Elberg (1981).

Anthrax (Malignant pustule, Wool sorters' disease)

Each year between 20 000 and 100 000 persons are reported to suffer from anthrax. Most cases occur in rural populations but industrial areas are not exempt. The infection occurs throughout the world but it is most prevalent in warm, humid climates where control measures have not been undertaken.

Disease in Man and animals

The skin form is the most common. It begins as a local infection with *Bacillus anthracis* with an initial papule or vesicle which develops into a depressed black eschar with hard oedematous swelling of surrounding tissues. Untreated infection may become generalized resulting in septicaemia and death in from five to 20 per cent of patients. The inhalation and gastrointestinal forms resulting from primary infection of these systems are relatively rare but, the former is more frequently fatal.

Anthrax is primarily a disease of herbivorous animals both domestic (goats, sheep and cattle) and wild (hippopotamus, elephants and other game). Although it is endemic in most parts of the world the prevalence and consequent losses among livestock are highest where the animal industry and veterinary services are not well organized. In such areas diagnostic facilities are lacking. The epizootic may not be recognized in its early stages when the atypical, hyperacute or 'apoplectic' form is frequent especially in sheep and goats. Animals sick of anthrax are often left to die in the fields and this perpetuates and spreads the infective agent as the anthrax spores remain viable in the soil for many years. Furthermore, there is a tendency to salvage the hides, hair, wool and bones of dead animals which are handled by unsuspecting persons and may reach the world market. Not infrequently a sick animal is butchered and the meat used as food. Consequently persons in an endemic area are at hazard from infection from all the products mentioned while trading in skins, hair, wool and bone meal carries the infection to distant parts of the same or other countries. Human infection with anthrax is, therefore, frequently linked with economic activities. In Africa several outbreaks in Man have been traced to wild animals used for food.

Diagnosis

This depends upon demonstration of anthrax bacilli in smears from the skin lesions and from blood (of animals) soon after death. Serological methods for detecting the infection in hides are also available. Recently a fluorescent antibody test has been developed. Animal inoculation is used to detect infection in hair and wool.

Control

In endemic areas control of anthrax depends upon the provision of adequate local facilities for diagnosis and for proper disposal (incineration or burial of carcases at least two metres deep, covered with quick lime) and for free or low cost vaccination of livestock at regular intervals. Experience has shown that annual vaccination is necessary, but in badly affected areas this may have to be performed twice each year. Compulsory disinfection of animal products potentially contaminated with anthrax has been advocated but, unfortunately, there is no known satisfactory, inexpensive method of disinfecting hides and skins or of treating effluents from factories. Hair and wool can be disinfected but here again the process is not cheap. Irradiation of bales and other new processes may provide a solution to this problem.

Promising results have been obtained in protection by vaccination of individuals who handle potentially contaminated material. Ampicillin, tetracycline and other broad spectrum antibiotics are used in the treatment of human anthrax.

Salmonellosis

Zoonotic salmonellosis (which excludes typhoid and paratyphoid fevers of man and infections limited to animals) is a widespread infection. Its incidence in warm climate countries is, however, difficult to assess because of the absence of epidemiological surveillance and inadequate use of laboratory services. In the developed countries salmonellosis is at the top of the list of foodborne infections and its incidence is increasing. There are reasons to believe that in rapidly developing countries, for example some Gulf states, zoonotic salmonellosis increases as the incidence of typhoid fever declines.

Disease in Man and animals.

In man the symptoms usually appear suddenly from eight to 48 hours after ingestion of the infected food. They consist of gastroenteritis, fever, abdominal pain, diarrhoea and vomiting. Dehydration is pronounced especially in infants. In some cases the infection may develop into enteric fever and rarely abscesses or inflammation occur in different parts of the body. Death is rare, except in infants, in the elderly and in debilitated individuals.

In animals the infection may be asymptomatic with the organism localized in the lymph nodes and viscera. This is the usual form in dogs and in many wild animals and birds. In other cases there is fever and gastroenteritis. Pregnant animals may abort. In young animals and birds there may be high mortality and serious losses. On recovery some animals become carriers and excrete *Salmonella* in the faeces.

The clinical diagnosis in Man is confirmed by isolation of *Salmonella* from the faeces and blood during the acute stages, and by serological and, if necessary, phage typing.

The agent, *Salmonella enteritidis* has some 2000 serovars, some with different host specificities, the commonest being *typhimurium* which is sometimes classed as a separate species. Many of the 300 serovars of *S. arizona* (*Arizona hinshawii*) are also able to infect Man.

Epidemiology

In warm climates sporadic cases and familial outbreaks occur. Sometimes also large outbreaks are observed in homes for children, hospitals, restaurants and camps of pilgrims or among visitors to shrines. Food, especially that of animal origin, is the usual vehicle. It may be contaminated at its source or during handling or processing. Certain types of food stored at ambient temperatures may act as culture media for the growth of a few *Salmonella* which may be present, to dangerously high numbers.

Wild animals and birds may maintain the infection in the environment but in warm countries, where human and animal excreta and other wastes are left untreated or are used as field manure, the environmental contamination is heavy. Surface and coastal waters are also usually contaminated so that fish and shellfish caught there may act as a vehicle of transmission. Insanitary abattoirs and poultry slaughter houses are important sources of infection. The water used for the cooling of poultry carcases is often contaminated.

Pet animals, such as dogs, cats, rodents, tortoises and snakes have been reported as sources of infection in the home, especially among children. Occasionally large outbreaks have been traced to contamination of the water supply of the community. The danger of such contamination is increased during heavy rains, floods and other natural disasters.

Among animals the infection may spread from carriers to others but the most important sources are contaminated food and water. Animals grazing on polluted pastures and those receiving contaminated feed supplements, such as fish meal, suffer a high rate of infection. Chickens foraging on village manure heaps are similarly frequently infected.

Of the large numbers of serovars of *Salmonella* only a few are prevalent at a given time in a particular area. New serovars which appear in animals turn up in Man also eventually, and vice versa.

Occasionally outbreaks of human salmonellosis have been traced to unusual sources. These have included chocolates and weight reducing (thyroid) tablets.

Surveillance*

Epidemiological and bacteriological investigation of cases of food poisoning will indicate the common sources of infection. The typing of strains from various sources helps in this work. Foodstuffs should be monitored at a suitable critical point in the chain of production, processing and distribution.

Investigation of animals may be done also for veterinary purposes. Certain environments, such as food processing establishments, slaughter houses, common kitchens and restaurants may be investigated. Many *Salmonella* strains are showing resistance to antibiotics. This aspect should be considered in the surveillance program.

Control

Because of the multitude of sources, in domesticated as well as in wild animals and in the environment, it is not practicable to eliminate the infection. Although methods of breeding *Salmonella* free animals have been developed, they are so expensive that even the rich, industrialized countries cannot afford them. In the circumstances, the emphasis should be on food hygiene, particularly on through cooking of food, especially that of of animal origin. Food handlers and housewives should be reminded of the necessity of washing hands before and after food preparation, of maintaining a clean kitchen and of protecting prepared food from contamination with dirt or through flies and rodents. Where refrigeration is available it should be used in storing food.

Public health measures include adequate supervision of abattoirs, various food establishments and food markets. The veterinary services should supervise animal production establishments and those dealing with animal feeds. Rodent and insect control measures should be undertaken.

Pets liable to transmit the infection should be supervised where possible and children should be taught to wash their hands after handling them.

Treatment of clinically ill persons need not be more than rehydration where necessary. In case of prolonged fever and septicaemia, antibiotics (ampicillin, chloramphenicol, et cetera) should be given if the strain concerned is not resistant to them.

Animal tuberculosis

Human tuberculosis of animal origin is generally caused by the bovine tubercle bacillus (*Mycobacterium bovis*) and rarely by the avian type (*M. avium*). Infections with the so-called Battey bacillus (*M. intracellulare*) observed in both man and animals are apparently of environmental origin and are not interchangeable among them as a zoonosis.

---

* See: WHO guidelines for organization and management of surveillance of foodbourne diseases. VPH/82.39, World Health Organization, Geneva.

The disease in man and animals

The clinical and pathological manifestations of M. *bovis* infection in man do not differ essentially from those caused by the human type (M. *tuberculosis*). In areas where consumption of raw milk or milk products is the mode of transmission, a large proportion of cases develop extra-pulmonary lesions such as cervical adenitis, bone and joint lesions and meningitis. Pulmonary airborne infection with the bovine bacillus occurs principally in areas where people share dwellings with infected cattle (e.g. in parts of Africa) or among attendants in cow sheds. The avian type (*M. avium*) causes adenitis and only rarely pulmonary lesions in man.

In cattle the majority of cases show lesions in the chest cavity (lungs, pleura, lymph nodes) but many other organs including the uterus and the udder may be affected. Tubercle bacilli may be excreted in milk with or without visible udder lesions. A generalized (miliary) infection has also been observed. In poultry, the lesions are geneally found in the intestine, liver, spleen and bone marrow.

The diagnosis of the disease in man by the usual methods has to be supplemented with the isolation and typing of the tubercle bacillus, to determine if it is of one of the animal types. In cattle, the diagnosis is largely made by tuberculin test using a purified-protein derivative (PPD) tuberculin. In many cases, smears of mucus collected from the larynx can be used for microscopic diagnosis.

Epidemiology

Bovine tuberculosis has low prevalence in warm climates but foci of high prevalence may be found in places where cattle are housed or closely herded together. Human infection with (M. bovis) is also rare in warm climates but locally high prevalence has been found in parts of Africa. The mode of infection in man is by inhalation where people work or sleep in quarters shared with infected cattle. Infection through the digestive tract may take place where raw milk is consumed, especially by children.

Control

The principal method of control is the elimination of the infection in cattle. The most successful method has been the identification of infected animals by tuberculin testing and their elimination by slaughter. Repeated tuberculin tests in an area are essential for elimination of the disease. Chemotherapy of bovine infection is not recommended as a method of control.

Heat treatment (including pasteurization) of milk and BCG vaccination of children should be used as preventive measures.

Taeniasis and cysticercosis beef and pork tapeworm infections)

The beef and pork tapeworms (*Taenia saginata* and *T. solium*) are widely distributed in meat eating populations of the world. The beef tapeworm is more widely prevalent with areas of high endemicity in Africa, the eastern Mediterranean and in parts of the USSR. Elsewhere the prevalence is moderate but foci of heavy infection exist here and there. The pork tapeworm is prevalent in central and southern Africa, in Mexico, in central and South America and in southern Asia. The two species co-exist in many areas.

Disease in Man and animals

The adult tapeworms in man usually cause no clinical manifestations but some infected persons may suffer nervousness, insomnia, loss of appetite and weight and sometimes abdominal pain and digestive disturbances.

The larval stage of the pork tapeworm may invade human tissues and cause serious disease if localized in the heart, eye or central nervous system. Epileptiform seizures are indicative of involvement of the brain and this form usually ends fatally. Cysticerci located in the peritoneal cavity and in the subcutaneous tissues usually cause no clinical symptoms except palpable nodules under the skin.

In cattle and pigs, the larvae (cysticerci) occur in the muscles and do not usually cause any manifest disease.

Diagnosis

Infections with the adult tapeworms are diagnosed by examination of the proglottids in the faeces and by microscopic examination for eggs. In case of *T. saginata* a rectal swab or anal impression smears on adhesive tape are preferable to examination of faeces. Parasitological examination of the gravid proglottids helps in specific identification of the tapeworm.

Human cysticercosis can be diagnosed by radiography or by serological methods such as indirect immunofluorescence, passive haemagglutination and precipitation tests. In animals, medium to heavy infections with cysticerci can be detected on meat inspection and by serological tests but light infections may escape detection.

Epidemiology

Man becomes infected by ingesting raw or insufficiently cooked beef or pork containing viable cysticerci. When the worms mature, gravid proglottids containing embryophores (eggs) are passed out with the stool. When they disintegrate, the eggs spread on the pasture or on the ground and cattle and pigs ingest the eggs with grass or soil which eventually develop into cysticerci in the muscles. Unlike other zoonoses, man is an essential link in the life cycle of these parasites.

Inadequate processing of sewage or the use of raw sewage and human manure in cultivation or their discharge into streams increases the chances of infection in animals and many highly endemic areas indeed show this practice. Travellers and campers have been known to infect pastures, and birds which pick up tapeworm segments (e.g. sea gulls) also spread the eggs onto the grazing grounds.

Human infection results from ingestion of the eggs of *T. solium* in conditions of poor personal and environmental hygiene, *T. solium* cysticerci may also develop in dogs but this is of little importance except in areas where undercooked dog meat is consumed.

Surveillance

Infection rates in representative samples of the population may be determined by visual and microscopic examination of stool or anal impression smears. More commonly, the infection of cattle and pigs detected on meat examination is taken as an index of prevalance of this zoonosis. This is also one of the important aspects of control measures.

Control

The most important methods of control are the detection and exclusion or destruction of cysticerci on meat inspection. Unfortunately, present methods of inspection are unable to detect light infection. Another important approach is to induce people to cook meat thoroughly. This requires well conducted health education.

Detection and mass treatment of infected persons has been tried with varying degrees of success but at present this method is beyond the resources of many developing countries.

Adequate sewage disposal and sanitization of the environment is also expensive but proper housing of pigs has a marked effect on the incidence of *T. solium*.

Recently, anthelmintics have been found to be remarkably effective in the treatment of cysticerci in cattle. A single oral administration of 50–100 mg per kg bodyweight of Praziquantel has been found to be sufficient to kill mature cysticerci. This method is still not practicable in the field because of the high cost of the drug. It does nevertheless raise hopes of control by chemotherapy as cheaper drugs are developed. The effect of these drugs on human cysticercosis is not known. In most cases surgical excision is the only available treatment but the cysts in the brain and the eye are extremely difficult to remove.

For treatment of adult *T. saginata* infections, niclosamide (Yomesan) is widely used. For *T. solium*, quincarine hydrochloride (atabrine) is preferred.

MEAT INSPECTION

Official meat inspection is now compulsory in many countries although the coverage and efficacy of inspection is very variable. The two principal aims of meat inspection are to assure a safe and wholesome supply of meat to the community and to supply data on diseases encountered in slaughter animals to the animal disease control services. Thus, meat inspection plays an important role in the control of zoonoses of slaughter animals and interrupting in their transmission through meat.

Proper inspection starts at the farm of origin and reliable information on diseases and chemical residues gathered there can help to modify and often simplify subsequent inspection; this is the case particularly with intensively produced poultry and pigs.

Antemortem clinical examination of the animal is carried out shortly before slaughter and is aimed at detecting diseases and harmful residues transmitted through meat and those which reduce meat quality, for example debility, fever, skin disease.

Postmortem examination of the skeletal muscles and viscera is carried out to detect a variety of communicable and other diseases either by organoleptic inspection or by supplementary (laboratory) examinations. On the basis of the results of the foregoing examinations a judgement is reached as to the fitness (or otherwise) of meat for human consumption.

Meat inspection is generally carried out by an official veterinarian or by meat inspectors under his supervision. FAO and WHO have jointly published international codes of hygienic practice in this field and for judgement of slaughter animals and meat (CAC/RCO 11/13–1976 and CX/NH 82/3, August 1981).

PASTEURIZATION AND STERILIZATION OF MILK

Raw milk usually contains a variety of microorganisms derived from the milch animal, the milk handler or from the environment including containers. Some of these may be pathogenic to man and others may cause spoilage which occurs quickly in warm climates if milk is not refrigerated. In many communities it is customary to boil fresh milk and to keep it at a relatively high temperature (simmering) until consumed. This, however, imparts a 'cooked' flavour to milk and often a brownish tinge resulting from burning of milk sugar. In countries with warm climates, many groups have developed a taste for well boiled milk and they reject raw (and even pasteurized) milk. This habit should not be changed unless alternative methods of rendering milk safe become available and are applied properly.

Pasteurization

Methods have been developed for destruction by heat of the bulk of microorganisms in milk without reaching the boiling point and without changing the nutritional value as well as palatability of milk. Theoretically, this can be achieved by the application a large number of time-temperature combinations varying from about an hour at 56°C to a fraction of a second at 78°C. In practice, some half a dozen methods have been developed of which a few use a temperature of 60–65°C for holding milk for 30 minutes and then cooling it to 10°C or less. A variation of the 'holding' methods is 'in-bottle' pasteurization in which milk heated to 60–65°C is filled in bottles which are sealed hermetically and maintained at the holder temperature for 30 minutes before cooling. The foregoing methods are being abandoned as they are relatively expensive and slow although some dairies still use them.

The commonest method currently used in both industrialized and developing countries is the high-temperature short-time (HTST) process in which milk is rapidly brought to a temperature of 71–72°C at which it is held for at least 15 seconds (often 45 seconds) and then cooled rapidly to 10°C or below. The process is legally prescribed, giving the time-temperature combinations, in many countries and has to be carried out in officially approved dairy plants. A variation of the above process is the so-called 'flash' method in which milk is heated rapidly to 75–80°C and then cooled as soon as possible. This variant is much less commonly used than the HTST method.

Pasteurized milk should be stored and transported at temperatures lower than 10°C, preferably below 5°C.

Control

The milk received for pasteurization is examined for quality (composition) and its bacteriological content. After pasteurization, the milk is examined by the phosphatase test for efficiency of pasteurization, the methylene blue or similar test for keeping quality and the coliform test for re-contamination after pasteurization*. The sanitation of the plant, quality of water, washing of utensils and other hygienic aspects are controlled by inspection and appropriate laboratory methods.

Sterilization

Milk sterilized at high temperatures (up to 150°C) under pressure, is being used more and more in various countries because of its long storage life at room temperature. It is particularly suitable for warm climates and in the absence of cool storage facilities.

The ultra-high temperature process (UHT) consists of heating the milk in two stages (the second being under pressure) to temperatures ranging

---

* For these and other methods used in milk hygiene see: American Public Health Association — *Standard Methods for the Examination of Dairy Products*. New York, APHA.

between 135°C and 150°C for a few seconds and then cooling rapidly or bottling it hot (75°–80°C) before cooling. It is now customary to homogenize sterilized milk before cooling. In this process fat globules are split and any protein clusters which may have formed at high temperatures are broken up.

Sterilized milk can be stored at room temperature for two to three months, or even longer if the incoming milk was of high quality and the room temperature is moderate.

REFERENCE

Alton G G, Jones L M, Piez D E 1975 Laboratory techniques in brucellosis, 2nd edition. WHO Monograph Series No. 55. World Health Organization. Geneva
Corbel M J, Brinley Morgan W J 1981 Classification of the genus Brucella: the current position. WHO Momeographed Document WHO/Bruc/81.370: 1–8
Elberg S S (ed) 1981 A guide to the diagnosis, treatment and prevention of human brucellosis. VPH/81.31 World Health Organization, Geneva

See also list of references at the end of chapters 37 and 38.

Arbovirus

Transmission of true arthropod-borne disease is biological, for an essential part of the life cycle of the parasite takes place within the body of the vector, during which cyclical change, or multiplication, or both may occur. The host in which sexually mature forms are found is known as the definitive host and that in which only immature forms are found as the intermediate host. This differentiation cannot, of course, be made in some cases, such as, for example, viruses, where sexually mature forms are not known. The period of time occupied by the developmental cycle in the vector is known as the extrinsic incubation period and is important epidemiologically, for only after its completion is the infection transmissible. The transference of the parasite to the new host may result either from inoculation by the vector, from contamination of the skin or mucous membrane by infective faeces excreted by the vector, or by its infective body fluids when crushed.

Biological transmission of a particular infection is normally specific and confined to one vector genus, sometimes to a single species. In the case of ticks and mites which do not undergo a complete metamorphosis during development the infecting parasite may be transmitted hereditarily (transovarially) from one generation to another.

Transmission of a disease may take place purely mechanically without the vector acting as a host to the parasite. Mechanical transmission can occur as a result of contamination of the legs, body, or mouth-parts of any insect with the infecting organism, which may thus be carried to the person or food of another host. Mechanical transmission as opposed to biological transmission can be effected by widely separated genera.

Man plays an insignificant part in the life cycle of the arthropod-borne viruses (arboviruses) since in most of the diseases man is an incidental rather than a maintenance host.

The majority of arboviruses are zoonoses. Because infection usually produces prolonged immunity increased attack rates in all age groups indicate the introduction of a new arbovirus; while an increase in disease confined to children implies reintroduction of a virus or overflow from a continuous animal cycle to susceptible humans. A computer-simulated model has been designed to express in quantitative terms the factors which play a role in the transmission cycle of an arbovirus.

The medically most important arbovirus infections of warm climate countries are classified in Table 40.1.

I. ALPHAVIRUSES

a) Venezuelan equine encephalitis (VEE)

This is a disease of horses and mules which may affect humans of all ages. The incubation period is two to five days. The disease is marked by fever, headache, myalgia and mild central nervous system involvement — diplopia, tremors. The mortality is low. Most patients recover without sequelae. For endemic VEE a rodent-mosquito-rodent cycle is important and while horses play an important role in the transmission of epidemic VEE.

For high risk laboratory personnel an attenuated virus vaccine is available. Epidemics can be controlled by — a) large scale immunisation of horses, (b) vector control, and c) horse movement control.

In Central and South America VEE is called 'peste loca'.

b) Chikungunya

This has an acute onset with fever which may be diphasic; joint pains of excruciating severity which can immobilize some patients; an irritating maculopapular rash; bradycardia and leucopenia. Some patients develop enlarged and tender inguinal nodes as well as red swollen ears. In a small number of patients haemorrhagic phenomena occur. The disease derives its name from the Swahili word meaning 'that which bends up'.

Although a vaccine is available for human use, the low mortality of chikungunya has militated against its commercial production. Prevention essentially consists in avoiding exposure to mosquito bites, in areas where A. aegypti is the predominant vector, control measures are the same as for dengue.

c) O'nyong nyong
This is a mild disease, sudden in onset with fever, headache, rash, arthralgia and generalised lymphadenitis, most prominent in the posterior cervical region.

d) Ross River
(Epidemic Polyarthritis). This is a non-fatal disease with an incubation period of 10 days; fever is not a prominent feature. Lymphadenitis; a maculopapular or vesicular rash and arthralgia affecting the small joints occur.

Table 40.1 Medically Important Arbovirus (togavirus) infections of warm climate countries

Arbovirus Group	Disease	Reservoir	Vector	Geographical Area
I. Alphaviruses	a) Venezuelan equine encephalitis	Horses, rodents and other animals	Various types of mosquitoes	South and Central America
	b) Western equine encephalitis	Horses	Culex spp.	USA, Canada, Central and South America
	c) Eastern equine encephalitis (EEE)*		Aedes spp.	USA, Caribbean, Central and South America
	d) Chikungunya	Wild animals	Aedes and Culex spp.	Tropical Africa, India, South East Asia
	e) O'nyong nyong	Not known	Anopheles spp.	Central and East Africa
	f) Ross River	Wild and domestic animals	Aedes and Culex spp.	Australia, Western Pacific Islands, New Guinea.
II. Flaviviruses	a) Yellow fever	Monkeys	Aedes spp.	Tropical Africa, Central and South America.
	(b) Dengue	Monkeys/Man	Aedes spp.	Worldwide. Latitude 30°N to 40°S
	c) Japanese B encephalitis	Birds. Wild and domestic animals	Culex spp.	Far East, South East Asia, India.
	d) Murray Valley encephalitis	Birds/mammals	Culex spp.	Australia, New Guinea
	e) West Nile fever	Birds/poultry	Culex spp.	Africa, Asia
	f) Kyasanur Forest disease	Forest animals	Haemophysalis spp.	India
	g) St Louis encephalitis (SLE)*	Birds	Culex spp.	N and S. America, Caribbean
III. Nairoviruses	a) Sandfly fever	None	Phlebotomus sp.	Mediterranean, East Africa, Asia, South America
	b) Crimean haemorrhagic-Congo-fever	Horses, birds, cattle, sheep, hares, hedgehogs	Hyalomma spp.	Crimea, Africa, Asia
	c) Rift Valley fever	Domestic animals especially sheep	Aedes and Culex spp.	Kenya, Sudan, Egypt. South Africa

* The clinical features of WEE, EEE and SLE are very similar to those described for VEE

II. FLAVIVIRUSES

a. **Yellow fever** Yellow fever is a disease which is enzootic in certain species of forest monkeys in parts of both Africa and South America. The vectors are *Haemogogus* spp. and *Aedes leucocelanus* in South America and *A. africanus* and *A. simpsoni* in Africa, which can convey the infection to man. The disease usually appears sporadically in man in rural areas, but can assume severe epidemic form in urban areas, where it is spread by *A. aegypti*. *A. africanus* has also been observed to bite at ground level by day, and *A. simpsoni* is sometimes present at canopy level by night. These reversals of behaviour by the two mosquitoes offer further opportunities for the transmission of infection from monkey to man.

The endemic zone in Africa approximately covers that part of the continent which lies between 15°N and 10°S latitude. In South America the endemic zone stretches from south of Honduras to the southern border of Bolivia and includes the western two-thirds of Brazil, Venezuela, Colombia, and those parts of Peru and Ecuador which lie east of the Andes. Certain towns are considered as not forming part of these zones provided they maintain continuously an *Aedes* index not exceeding one per cent. This index represents the proportions of houses in a limited, well defined area in which breeding places of *A. aegypti* are found. Yellow fever does not occur in Asia or the Pacific region, though the urban vector is widespread.

Epidemic spread of the disease occurs only between 40°N. and 35°S. latitude, since a mean temperature of not less than 24°C is necessary for the developmental cycle in the vector. The extrinsic incubation period lasts from four to 12 days. The incubation period in man is three to six days.

There are two main epidemiological forms of yellow fever. In the *urban type*, the mosquito vector is *Aedes aegypti*, which is primarily a domestic mosquito which breeds in or near houses, with the female preferring to lay her eggs in water collecting artificial containers, such as old tins.

The virus cycle is man-mosquito-man; this method of spread requires large numbers of susceptible hosts and hence tends to occur in large towns. Villages, with frequent passage of people from one village to another, will also be suitable for this type of spread. Urban type yellow fever can be effectively controlled by anti-mosquito measures. *Jungle type* yellow fever may occur either in endemic or epizootic forms. In the endemic form, the disease, which is primarily one of monkeys, is almost constantly present, and sporadic cases of human infection occur from time to time. The primary spread of virus is from monkey to monkey, via *A. africanus* in Africa and *Haemogogus* sp. in South America; both these mosquitoes live in the tops of trees. *Haemagogus* sp. will occasionally bite man, for example when a tree is felled, and South American jungle yellow fever is thus maintained. In Africa, however, there is another way in which jungle yellow fever virus can be transmitted from monkey to man. Certain monkeys have the habit of raiding crops, particularly bananas; another mosquito, *A. simpsoni*, occurs on the edges of forests, and

AFRICAN YELLOW FEVER

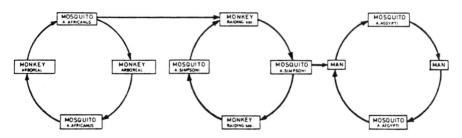

Fig. 40.1

becomes infected by biting infected raiding monkeys, and then later bites the farmer when he collects his crop. *A. simpsoni* thus acts as a so-called 'link-host' (Figs. 40.1, 40.2).

After an incubation period of three to six days the disease has an acute onset with fever and a rapid pulse at first. The pulse rate then drops dramatically while the fever remains high or rises (Faget's sign). Severe frontal headache, rigors, flushed face, congested conjunctivae, jaundice, oliguria and proteinuria develops. On the fifth day the patient's condition improves and in mild cases recovery follows. In severe cases the fever rises again; and terminal signs include severe prostration, anuria, uraemia, and widespread haemorrhages. Midzonal degeneration; Councilman bodies and Torres bodies are characteristic post mortem findings.

A life-long immunity follows recovery from the disease as well as from sub-clinical or unrecognised infections which comprise a large proportion of the total. There is evidence to suggest that the presence of extensive immunity to other group B viruses modifies the severity and spread of yellow fever. Clinical diagnosis should wherever possible be confirmed by laboratory tests.

SOUTH AMERICAN YELLOW FEVER

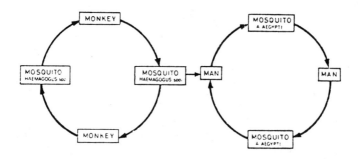

Fig. 40.2

The virus can be isolated from the blood during the first three days of the disease. After the third day the mouse protection test can be used. This test involves demonstrating whether or not mice are protected from a challenge dose of the virus by antibodies in the patient's serum. A second protection test should be made some five days later. A significant rise of titre in the second sample would confirm the diagnosis, while an unaltered titre would only indicate an immunity due to a past infection or vaccination. Neutralisation, complement fixation, or haemagglutination inhibition tests can also be employed, depending on the particular circumstances and the likelihood of previous exposure to other group B viruses. The interpretation of serological results is complicated by the cross-reactions that may occur with other members of group B. To confirm that the infection is due to yellow fever, the rise in HI, CF and N antibodies should be greater for yellow fever virus than for other group B arboviruses. In the event of death an autopsy should be performed and the liver examined for characteristic lesions. Where an autopsy is not possible a viscerotome may be used to obtain a piece of liver for examination.

Since the virus circulates in the blood during the first few days of the disease, a suspected case must be isolated for the first six days in a screened room or under a mosquito net. Steps should be taken at once to obtain laboratory confirmation of the diagnosis, but institution of control measures should not await results from the laboratory. Domestic contacts also should be isolated under screened conditions for six days, and the patient's house and all premises within a radius of 55 metres should be sprayed with a residual insecticide.

In densely populated areas elimination of vector breeding must be undertaken at once. A. aegypti is a peri-domestic mosquito and will breed in practically anything that will hold water. This includes water containers such as jars and cisterns, as well as innumerable objects which may hold rainwater: defective gutters, old tins, jars and coconut shells (often hidden in the grass), and the bottoms of small boats and canoes. These breeding foci should be reduced as far as possible by suitable measures — water containers covered or screened, tins and other rubbish buried, and so forth. This is unlikely to prevent all breeding, but it will simplify treatment of the remainder by regular oiling or by addition of insecticidal briquettes.

Residual spraying of the interiors of all houses and outbuildings or of all surfaces close to breeding places (peri-focal spraying) will reduce the Aedes population rapidly. Epidemic transmission will cease when the Aedes index is reduced to below five per cent.

Protection of scattered populations by vector control is, however impracticable, and recourse must be had to vaccination of the whole community. This will afford protection for at least ten years. Two vaccines are available: the 17D strain maintained by passage in chick embryo and the Dakar strain maintained in mouse brain. This latter is prepared in a form which permits administration by scarification and is very suitable for use in scattered populations in rural areas. *Infants under one year of age should preferably not be vaccinated*, since encephalitis follows vaccination in this age group more frequently than in adults. Some countries do not require vaccination certificates in the case of infants.

The spread of the disease is controlled by requiring all persons entering or leaving an endemic area to be in possession of a valid certificate of vaccination. Those not in possession of such a certificate may, on arrival in a non-endemic area, be subjected to quarantine for a period of six days from the date of last exposure to infection or until the certificate becomes valid. A vaccination certificate becomes valid ten days after vaccination and remains so for ten years. A certificate of re-vaccination done not more than ten years after a previous vaccination becomes valid on the day of vaccination.

To prevent introduction of an infected mosquito into countries where the disease is absent but conditions exist for transmission — receptive areas — aircraft coming from the endemic zone must be disinsecticized (by insecticidal aerosol) as specified by the World Health Organisation.

During epidemics mass vaccination must be initiated covering the majority of the population above six months of age, unless recent serological survey data are available to identify the portion of the population that has naturally acquired immunity.

b. Dengue

Dengue fever is widespread in urban areas in the tropics and sub-tropics and often appears in epidemic form. The virus, of which four main serotypes exist, circulates in the blood at the onset of symptoms and for a few days after. The incubation period is four to seven days, and transmission is through species of *Aedes*, usually *A. aegypti*, in which the extrinsic incubation period is eight to 14 days. Infection confers immunity to the homologous strain for about a year. Symptoms and signs include fever, severe frontal headache, retro-orbital pain, myalgia, arthralgia, infected conjunctivae, cervical lymphadenitis and a transient rash. After a remission the fever rises again giving the typical 'saddle back' pattern and signs recur followed by complete recovery after a prolonged convalescence often accompanied by depression.

In recent years epidemics of dengue with haemorrhagic manifestations have occurred in the Philippines, Thailand, Malaysia, Singapore, India, Burma, Indonesia, and the South Pacific Islands. During the past few years urbanization and rapid international travel are considered to have played a role in the re-introduction of dengue and its spread throughout South-East Asia and Western Pacific Regions. Dengue viruses have been isolated from *Aedes aegypti* during these epidemics. The outbreaks have an urban distribution with clinical cases clustered in the crowded poorer districts of cities. The disease is usually but not exclusively, seen in races of oriental origin, and the haemorrhagic fatal manifestations are usually confined to persons under 15 years of age, with a peak incidence in the three to six years group. The dengue shock syndrome (DSS) is the most severe manifestation of dengue haemorrhagic fever and it has been postulated that DSS occurs as a result of a second infection with a heterologous dengue virus and that an immunological mechanism is involved in the pathogenesis of the syndrome. Evidence is now available, however, that a *primary* dengue infection can also result in the dengue shock syndrome.

Aedes aegypti is a highly anthropophilic mosquito which breeds in artificial water containers in and around houses. The common practice of storing water in large jars provides abundant breeding sites.

The mortality from DHF is variable ranging from one per cent to 40 per cent; once shock has developed the prognosis is poor.

The only practical preventive measures are control of the vector by elimination of breeding places or insecticidal attack on the adults, or the prevention of mosquito bites by screening or repellents. Larvicides such as Abate have also been used in areas where water storage is mandatory as well as stressing the importance of tight fitting lids in such situations. Ultra-low volume (ULV) spraying of malathion or fenetrothion by truck or aircraft mounted sprayers rapidly destroys the adult *Aedes* population.

Health education aimed at alerting the population at risk on the breeding and biting habits of *Aedes* and motivating them to reduce breeding sources as well as legislation have met with success in Singapore. The advent of the Water/Sanitation Decade with the possible elimination of the need for water storage will hopefully have an added impact on the reduction of *Aedes* breeding sites.

c. Japanese B encephalitis

The majority of infections are inapparent or mild. The disease occurs in China, Taiwan, Korea, Japan, Malaysia, Singapore, India, and Sarawak. The most efficient vectors are *Culex tritaeniorrhynchus*, and *C. gelidus* and the preferred vertebrate hosts are birds and domestic animals, for example pigs: man being only an incidental host. The highest infection rates in man appear in populations which have close contact with both pigs and ricefields. The domestic pig is an amplifier host and is probably the main source of infection for man. The virus is spread from rural to urban areas by viraemic birds.

The peak incidence is in the summer in the Far East (Japan, Korea, Taiwan) while in South-East Asia (Sarawak, Thailand, Malaysia, India) transmission is endemically maintained throughout the year. Indigenous children are most susceptible as well as adult expatriates visiting endemic areas.

The disease develops after an incubation period of six to eight days with fever and headache soon to be followed by signs of meningeal irritation. Central nervous system symptoms and signs include mental confusion, difficulty in speaking, tremors, spasticity, exaggerated reflexes, delusions, drowsiness, convulsions and coma. There is a blood leucocytosis and the CSF contains protein and cells. Sequelae such as mental retardation are frequently seen and mortality can be high.

Control of the vector mosquitoes is not practicable on a large scale. Isolation of pigsties from human habitats reduces the mosquito/man contact. Vaccination of domestic pigs has been tried in Japan but the success of such a measure is highly debatable. Vaccination of children of target age groups (two to seven years) who received two doses of vaccine each year during April has resulted in a substantial incidence reduction in Taiwan. A large vaccine trial involving 40 000 school children (six to seven years) in Korea with a similar number of controls is being evaluated.

d. Murray Valley encephalitis

This acute and severe disease occurs in the Murray-Darling basin and in Northern Australia, as well as in New Guinea. It is a zoonotic infection involving birds and mammals and the virus is transmitted by *Culex*. The peak age specific prevalence is in children but occasionally a second peak in old age occurs.

Clinical disease manifests itself with all the symptoms and signs of an encephalitis — similar to Japanese B — case fatality rates have varied from 20 per cent to 60 per cent and serious neurological and psychiatric sequelae are common among survivors. Death or recovery usually occur within two weeks.

e. West Nile fever

West Nile virus has been reported from Africa (Uganda, Egypt, Central African Republic, South Africa, Zaire, Mozambique); Asia (India, Borneo) and Europe. The virus is maintained in birds and transmitted by *Culex* spp.

The incubation period is three to six days and the illness is characterized by fever, headache, sore throat, muscular pains, a rash, lymphadenopathy and occasionally meningoencephalitis. The severity of the disease is partially age-dependent being mild in the young and increasing in severity with age. Excephalitis is confined to the aged. Mortality is uncommon as are neurological sequelae.

f. Kyasanur Forest haemorrhagic fever occurs in the Kyasanur forest, Mysore State, India. The virus is maintained by ticks parasitic mainly on small and large mammals. The virus is maintained in mammals, monkeys acting as amplifiers and man becoming infected from the bites of infected ticks. The epidemic season of the disease coincides with the predominance

of nymphal forms of the ticks and with frequent occupational contact between man and forest.

The incubation period is three to seven days and clinical features include fever, frontal headache, severe myalgia, prostration, nausea, vomiting and confusion. The conjunctivae are infected, the palate covered with maculo-papular haemorrhagic spots. There may be a generalised lymphadenopathy, bleeding diathesis, bronchopneumonia and meningoencephalitis. Albuminuria, leucopenia and thrombocytopaenia are common laboratory findings.

A formalized tissue-culture vaccine can provide partial protection against KFD. Reduction of man/tick contact and tick control measures are other methods of combating the disease.

III. NAIROVIRUSES

a. Sandfly fever

This appears epidemically over much of the tropics and sub-tropics, where it is transmitted by *Phlebotomus papatasii*. Recovery from the disease is followed by a long-lasting immunity to the homologous strain of virus.

The disease has a short incubation period of three to seven days and an acute onset with fever, flushed face, severe frontal headache, infected conjunctivae, photophobia and aches and pains all over the body. It is a non-fatal disease but depression is common during convalescence.

Sandfly breeding can be controlled to some extent by clearing piles of rubbish and mending cracked and dilapidated walls. The insects are particularly susceptible to DDT, and have been drastically reduced in many places by residual house spraying employed for the control of mosquitoes.

b. Crimean haemorrhagic — Congo — fever

The disease occurs in the Crimea, East, West and Central Africa and in Asia (Pakistan, Iraq, United Arab Emirates) and is transmitted by ticks of the *Hyalomma* spp. Domestic animals probably act as amplifying hosts. The incubation period is seven to 12 days. The disease is characterised by fever, rigors, headache, flushed and puffy face and infected conjunctivae. There may be nausea, vomiting and diarrhoea. A generalised rash occurs and a haemorrhagic eruption in the oropharynx. A leucopenia and thrombo-cytopenia are found while haemorrhages which may occur from all orifices carry a bad prognosis. Mortality is variable.

Tick control and minimizing tick-man contact are basic measures for preventing CHC fever. A vaccine for high risk persons working in natural tick habitats, on farms, or in laboratories, is available.

c. Rift Valley fever This was first described in the Rift Valley in Kenya and human epidemics have also occurred in South Africa, the Sudan and

Egypt. It is primarily a disease of cattle and sheep and the infection is contracted either by handling infected animals or from the bite of an infected mosquito (*Culex* spp. or *Aedes* spp.).

The incubation period is three to 12 days and the disease is marked by fever, headache, rigors, arthralgia, myalgia, congested conjunctivae and haemorrhages. In the relatively recent Egyptian epidemic macular retinitis and encephalitis occurred.

Effective attenuated and inactivated vaccines have been developed in South Africa for veterinary use while an inactivated vaccine grown in monkey kidney cell cultures has shown promise for use in man.

DIAGNOSIS OF ARBOVIRUS INFECTION

Arbovirus infections are one of the commonest causes of 'short term fever' in the tropics and are often misdiagnosed as malaria, especially when clinical assessment is the only criterion used for such a diagnosis.

Good laboratory facilities are required for a definitive diagnosis of the arbovirus infections. Specimens of blood, throat washings, excretions, secretions, and body tissues for virus isolation and identification can be sent. The classical laboratory animal for isolation of arboviruses is the suckling mouse. Viruses can also be isolated from laboratory arthropods — Xeno-diagnosis while various tissue culture cell lines are also available.

Paired sera, that is serum taken as early as possible in the disease and a second specimen taken a week after, will show a diagnostic fourfold rise in titre in a variety of antibody tests — complement fixation, haemagglutin-ation inhibition, screen neutralizing and plaque reduction. Other useful tests in current use are fluorescent antibody, enzyme-linked immunosorbent assay, and radio-immunoassay.

PREVENTION AND CONTROL OF ARBOVIRUS INFECTIONS

Treatment of the arbovirus infections is essentially symptomatic and supportive, no specific chemotherapy is available.

Specific protective vaccines suitable for widespread public protection are available for yellow fever, chikungunya and Rift Valley fever.

General measures include a) personal protection against mosquito and tick bites, b) mosquito, tick and rodent control measures, c) control of the movement of infected domestic animals, and d) education of travellers, missionaries, teachers, forestry workers, survey engineers and others.

FURTHER READING

1. Handbook series in Zoonoses — James H Steele. Editor in Chief — Section B: Viral Zoonoses Volume I. George W Beran. Section Editor. CRC Press. Inc. Boca Raton, Florida. 1981.

Marburg and Ebola virus

INTRODUCTION

Marburg Virus Disease (MVD) was first described in Europe in 1967 when human infection occurred in laboratory workers exposed to infected Green Monkeys — *Cercopithecus aethiops*, imported from Uganda. Subsequent outbreaks occurred in South Africa (1975) and Kenya (1980). Ebola Virus Haemorrhagic Fever (EHF) was first recognised in 1976 following substantial outbreaks in the Southern Sudan and Zaire and subsequently in Southern Sudan in 1979. The viruses are morphologically identical, contain RNA and are filamentous and pleomorphic with frequent 'U' shaped and circular forms but are antigenically distinct.

CLINICAL FEATURES

The incubation period averages one week with a range of three to 16 days. The early clinical features are non-specific with fever, malaise and myalgia followed by diarrhoea, vomiting and pharyngitis. A transient maculopapular rash appears during the first week and subsequently desquamates. Haemorrhagic features, especially gastrointestinal and mucosal, occur in a high proportion a week after onset and are associated with progressive deterioration, shock and death. There is an early neutropenia and thrombocytopenia: liver cell enzymes are elevated although jaundice is unusual. Liver histology shows necrosis with inclusion bodies but no inflammatory response. Myocarditis, encephalitis and pancreatitis occur. The mortality in MVD has been 25 per cent. The higher mortality observed in EHF, from 50 to 90 per cent in rural outbreaks might be reduced with more sophisticated medical care including fluid replacement, blood transfusion and virus specific immune plasma. The differential diagnosis includes other causes of viral haemorrhagic fever (VHF) in Africa especially Yellow Fever, Lassa Fever (confined to West Africa) and Crimean Haemorrhagic Congo Hazara Fever (rarely recognised as a cause of VHF in Africa) as well as Falciparum malaria, Plague, Typhoid and Trypanosomiasis. The diagnosis is suggested when a cluster of febrile cases occur with haemorrhagic features in a high proportion and evidence of man to man transmission especially in a hospital situation.

Specific diagnosis requires the isolation of virus on Vero cells or guinea-pig inoculation of acute-phase blood or post-mortem liver tissue. Samples must be collected with full protection, packaged and transported to a laboratory with maximum security facilities.

A high convalescent titre or a rise in titre in paired sera with the virus-specific indirect fluorescent antibody test is of diagnostic value. Virus has also been isolated several months following clinical recovery from seminal fluid and from the anterior chamber of the eye.

EPIDEMIOLOGY

Marburg Virus Disease has originated from Uganda, Kenya and Zimbabwe. Ebola Haemorrhagic Fever has occurred in Southwestern Equatoria, Southern Sudan, and Equatoria Region, Zaire: more than 600 cases occurred in the first outbreaks. Man to man transmission requires close, intimate and usually prolonged contact with a case. Secondary attack rates are usually below 10 per cent except in those engaged in patient care either in hospital or at home. Whilst man to man transmission has been observed through only one generation in MVD, more than 12 generations have been observed in EHF. Explosive outbreaks of EHF have been augmented by syringe passage and one laboratory infection occurred in England following accidental needle puncture. In contrast to Lassa Fever, asymptomatic and mild cases do not appear common.

Both the origin and route of transmission to man in primary cases are unknown. Primates, incriminated in the original outbreak of MVD do not appear to be an important reservoir of infection.

CONTROL

In endemic areas of central and eastern Africa control is aimed at identifying cases and outbreaks. Routine surveillance should include the collection of acute-phase sera from suspects and post-mortem liver biopsy for virus isolation and electron microscopy. Laboratory investigation must be carried out only where bio-containment facilities are available, although treatable diseases especially Falciparum malaria should be excluded or treated expectantly. Fear may lead rural communities to suppress information and has caused both patients and staff to leave hospitals. Known cases and suspects should be nursed with full isolation. Personal protection of staff should include full face masks or Vickers positive pressure respirators. Careful handling and disposal of laboratory samples, excretions and fomites as well as cadavers is essential.

Primary contacts who have had close tissue contact should be placed in quarantine for 14 days or maintained under daily surveillance. Active surveillance and effective patient isolation have rapidly controlled extensive outbreaks of EHF.

While the risk of international spread of these virus infections as a consequence of air travel is perhaps less than the risk of transmitting Lassa Fever the management of suspects is the same. International reporting allows neighbouring countries and those in direct air communication to take appropriate surveillance action. The World Health Organisation is able to provide assistance with the control of outbreaks.

REFERENCES

Martini G A & Siegart R (eds) 1971 Marburg Virus Disease, Springler Verlag: Berlin
Pattyn, S R, (ed) 1978 Ebola Virus Haemorrhagic Fever, Elsevier: North Holland
Simpson D I H 1977 Marburg and Ebola Virus Infection. A guide to their diagnosis, management and control. WHO Offset Publ. No. 36. Geneva

Lassa fever

Lassa fever was first described in 1969 in the village of Lassa in north-east Nigeria. Although the virus is present in several West African countries, outbreaks have occurred only in Nigeria, Liberia and Sierra Leone.

THE AGENT

The virus — one of eleven members of the Arenavirus group — has the characteristic fine sand-like granules seen within by thin-section electron microscopy. Like all the other arenaviruses, it is a single-stranded RNA virus with a diameter of 60 to 350 nm.

Lassa fever virus seems to have a natural cycle of transmission in rodents and has been isolated from the multimammate rat — *Mastomys natalensis* — which acts both as a vector and reservoir. The rats are infected at birth, remain infective throughout their lifetime excreting the virus in urine and other body fluids.

EPIDEMIOLOGY

The early epidemiology of Lassa fever was predominantly based on the nosocomial infections that occurred in the mission hospitals at Jos (Nigeria) and Zorza (Liberia), and there is little doubt that close personal contact with infected secretions and excretions of patients is a source of human infection. The virus has been isolated from blood, pharyngeal and other secretions as well as from urine and tissues. It is equally probable that transmission to man occurs when he comes into close contact with rodents either by inhalation of dried infected urine or from the consumption of contaminated food or water. Accidental inoculation with needles or instruments have also been reported and occasional patients, for example, those with severe pulmonary involvement may be infective by the airborne route by droplets or droplet nuclei.

THE DISEASE

The clinical course is very variable ranging from asymptomatic infections to fatal disease. In children lassa fever seems to run a relatively mild course; there is nothing pathognomonic about the clinical presentation of Lassa fever but symptoms and signs that arouse a high index of suspicion are the following features:

After an incubation period of three to 17 days the patient presents with fever, lethargy, headache, puffy face and neck, conjunctivitis, lymphadenopathy, oropharyngeal papules and ulcers, nausea, vomiting and diarrhoea. The blood picture shows a leucopenia and thrombo-cytopenia with low prothrombin and raised serum enzyme levels. Proteinuria occurs.

Serious complications frequently leading to a fatal outcome include effusion in serous cavities; haemorrhagic diathesis, shock, cardiac and renal failure and encephalopathy.

Viraemia persists into the second week of illness and virus may be excreted in the patient's urine for many weeks.

The mortality in hospitalised patients is around 20 per cent except in pregnant women when it is significantly higher.

The diagnosis of lassa fever is carried out in maximum security laboratories by isolation of virus or a fourfold rise in antibody titre in paired sera. An initial IFAT titre of 1: 1024 is also generally accepted as diagnostic.

Treatment is supportive, if serum or plasma from convalescents or patients with asymptomatic infection and high antibody titres is available this should be administered as early as possible.

PREVENTION

The risk of community spread of Lassa fever has been exaggerated and it is the more real risk of hospital and laboratory spread that requires emphasis bearing in mind that in this context it is contact with infected material — blood, secretions, urine etcetera that is paramount.

Patients should be identified as minimal, moderate or high risk groups and managed accordingly ruling out common infections such as falciparum malaria.

Minimal risk patients or arrivals from major cities in West Africa, who have not worked in hospitals or laboratories should be cared for in isolation units and barrier nursed. Specimens can be sent to routine laboratories. No surveillance action is necessary.

Moderate risk patients, i.e. arrivals from rural areas or hospital and laboratory workers. These persons with a pysexia of unknown origin (within 3 weeks of arrival from an endemic area) should be seen by a specialist in infectious diseases before being considered a 'suspected case'. If confirmed as such, they should be admitted to a designated unit and surveillance of close contacts arranged. If pulmonary involvement has occurred more remote contacts should be traced. Laboratory examinations to exclude malaria and other diseases should be made in high security cabinets.

High risk patients, that is arrivals from places or hospitals where Lassa fever is known to be present at the time or persons who have had contact with known patients or have been handling specimens or materials likely to be contaminated. Arrangements should be made for admission to a designated unit, for virological examination of specimens in a high security laboratory and for surveillance of contacts as above.

Trexlor isolators are available in most designated units; failing this Vickers positive pressure respirators should be worn by all medical, nursing and laboratory staff. If neither of the above possibilities are available, strict barrier nursing in isolation units should be enforced with particular reference to avoiding direct contact with potentially infected material.

REFERENCES

Emond R T D, Smith H, Walsby P D 1978 Assessment of patients with suspected viral
    haemorrhagic fever: experience in a designated unit. Brit. med. J. I, 966
Galbraith N S, Berrie J R H, Forbes P 1972 Public Health Aspects of Viral Haemorrhagic
    fevers in Britain. Journal of Royal Society of Health, 98, 152

Spirochaetes and relapsing fever

Relapsing fever (Syns. Borreliosis, spirochaetal fever, etc.)

There are two forms of this spirochaetal disease which is characterized by fever in most cases lasting between four and seven days, ending with crisis and recurring after two to four days. The number of relapses varies between two and 12 depending on the variability of the organism and on the resistance of the patient. The first form, transmitted by human body and head lice (*Pediculus humanus*) is not a zoonosis but the second form transmitted by ticks of the genus *Ornithodoros* circulates in nature among small mammals and sometimes in domesticated animals, and ticks. Man becomes infected by entering the biotopes of the vector tick (caves, huts, animal dwellings, etcetera) and by being bitten by infected vectors. One species of the vector tick (*O. moubata*) in Africa has become adapted to human dwellings and may transmit the infection among humans without the intervention of other mammals.

The clinical manifestations of the two forms are similar although the louse-borne (epidemic) type tends to be somewhat severer with a higher mortality. The tick-borne form is characteristically endemic and is restricted to areas where the ticks are present.

The diagnosis is confirmed by microscopic demonstration of spirochaetes in the blood during the early febrile period, by dark-field or stained thick smear examination. The organism can be isolated by inoculation of the blood intraperitoneally into mice, rats or guinea-pigs.

The agent

Several strains of *Borrelia* have been given different names according to the transmitting arthropod especially ticks of which they are systemic parasites (The more frequent strains have been listed by Felsenfeld, 1979 and WHO, 1980).

The louse-borne *Borrelia* has been named *B. recurrentis* and some authors prefer to use this name provisionally also for the tick-borne strains until the status of the various 'species' has been clarified.

Epidemiology

Relapsing fever has been reported from all parts of the world except Australasia. Foci of the disease exist in Africa, Asia and Latin America. The tick-borne type is also distributed in these continents but not necessarily in the same foci. It extends into parts of Europe and North America.

Only about five to 10 per cent of lice feeding on an infected person are found to carry the *Borrelia* and they do not transmit it through their bites. Transmission occurs when a louse is crushed and its body fluid comes into contact with abraded (scratched) skin or a mucous membrane. The pubic louse (*Phthirius pubis*) does not transmit the disease. The tick-borne type is transmitted through bites during feeding. The tick acts also as a reservoir of infection as it may carry the agent for several years and pass it on trans-ovarially to the next generation.

It has been suggested that lice on persons having borrelaemia of tick-borne type may become infected and may transmit the disease further to healthy individuals.

Surveillance

In case of the tick-borne disease a search is made for the source of infection by looking for ticks in crevices in caves or walls of dwellings or in objects like wood or stones lying nearby. The spirochaete can be isolated from ticks by animal inoculation but tick control measures should start as soon as these arthropods are detected.

The search for lice is carried out in cooperation with the community and control measures are adopted.

In case of an outbreak, compulsory notification is enforced. In selected endemic areas also notification may be obligatory. The disease should be reported to WHO, under the International Health Regulations.

Control

This depends on appropriate louse or tick control. (See Macdonald chapter 36). Visits to or sleeping in premises infested with ticks should be avoided. Patients can be treated with antibiotics, particularly tetracyclines.

Leptospirosis

(Syns. Weil's disease, canicola fever, mud fever, swineherds' disease, etc.) This cosmopolitan zoonosis is particularly prevalent in warm climate countries with high rainfall and neutral or alkaline soil. For a long time, house and field rodents and dogs were considered to be the principal carriers but now all domesticated and a wide variety of wild animals are known to be possible sources of infection for man and other animals. Human infections are frequently traced to their origins in cattle, swine and other farm animals.

Disease in man and animals

The symptoms of the disease in man are variable and usually begin one to two weeks after exposure. There may be fever, headache, chills, malaise, vomiting, muscular pains, meningeal irritation and conjunctivitis. In severe cases, there may be jaundice, renal insufficiency, haemolytic anaemia and haemorrhages in the mucous membranes.

Most of the rodents and wild animals are well adapted to the infection and excrete leptospires in the urine without showing symptoms. A similar situation may be observed in farm animals but they are more likely to be mildly or severely sick. In cattle and sheep there may be fever, anorexia, drop in milk production and, in severe cases, abortion and haemoglobinaemia. In swine, the infection is generally sub-clinical, but occasionally fever, birth of weak piglets and even abortion may be observed. In dogs, the disease varies from sub-clinical to severe haemorrhagic form with myalgia in posterior limbs, haemorrhagic stomatitis, gastroenteritis and nephritis.

The diagnosis and surveillance of leptospirosis in man and animals requires the laboratory demonstration of the organism or of the serological reactivity induced by it. The methods used include direct examination of specimens by dark-field microscopy, direct culture from blood (acute phase) or from urine (convalescence). Guinea-pig or hamster inoculation and serum agglutination are also used.

The agent

The parasitic leptospires are grouped as a single species — *Leptospira interrogans* which has at least 180 serovars classified into 20 groups. The more important serovars are: *icterohaemorrhagiae, canicola, pomona, hardjo* and *grippotyphosa.*

Epidemiology

Infected animals often excrete large quantities of the organism in their urine which, when mixed with water or mud which is neutral or slightly alkaline, may remain infective for several weeks. Leptospires enter the body through cuts or abrasions in the skin or through the intact mucous membranes of the conjunctivae, nose or mouth. Rarely, the infection may be foodborne.

It has long been known that Weil's disease (*icterohaemorrhagiae* and *copenhageni* infections) may follow swimming or accidental immersion in contaminated water. In recent years, similar episodes involving other serotypes but having a common pattern have been reported from several countries. They occur in late summer or early autumn when ponds contaminated by infected animals are stagnant and streams slow-moving. Most such infections have been observed in children and young adults, with meningitis as a common manifestation.

Leptospirosis is also an important occupational hazard among animal attendants, for example veterinarians, slaughterhouse and packing-house workers, sewerage and canal workers, poultry and fish handlers, kennel men, swine-herds, plantation labourers and workers in rice fields and cane fields. Any occupation that involves contact with infected animal urine or contaminated mud or water is hazardous.

Prevention and control

For the prevention of leptospirosis, protective clothing such as boots and gloves worn by exposed persons is helpful but often impractical especially in warm climate countries. Contaminated water and bathing pools can be disinfected with chlorine, and pigsties, barns and other animal houses with cresol. Attempts at disinfection of rice fields and other tracts of land with copper sulphate or calcium cyanamide have been less successful.

Inactivated multivalent vaccines have proved useful in protecting exposed populations. Animal vaccination is liable to favour a sub-clinical infection with subsequent development of a shedder state; it could be justified only for preventing animal losses.

Antibiotic and serum therapy has been used in man and animals but the results are not very satisfactory. Moreover, antibiotics cannot be relied upon for eliminating the shedder state in animals.

REFERENCES

Felsenfeld O 1979 Borreliosis. In: Steele J H (ed) CRC Handbook Series in Zoonoses Vol I CRC Press Inc., Boca Raton, Florida
World Health Organization 1981 Approved names of biomedically important bacteria Terminology Circular TXB-1, TER/81.1

Malnutrition

INTRODUCTION

The background

Seventy years ago it was supposed that people would thrive on diets adequate in energy, protein and minerals. In 1912 Gowland Hopkins showed that some additional 'accessory food factors' were required 'in astonishingly small amount' and Casimir Funk introduced the concept of 'deficiency diseases' which 'break out in countries where a certain unvarying diet is partaken for long periods'. He attributed these diseases to deficiency of some essential substances in the food which he named 'vitamines'. The discovery of vitamins and their dramatic effect on deficiency diseases was a predominant influence on nutritional research and diet for many years. Nearly all malnutrition came to be considered in terms of some specific deficiency.

Twenty-five years later, Cicely Williams introduced the word kwashiorkor into the medical vacabulary. It is a word which a Ghanaian nurse told her was the word they used for a condition she had seen there, that followed a history of prolonged and eventually deficient breastfeeding, inadequately supplemented with watery gruels made from one staple root or grain.

Kwashiorkor was believed to be due to protein deficiency, and interest in this new concept of malnutrition was so great that nearly all malnutrition came to mean 'protein deficiency'. So the modern myth of the 'protein gap' became the target for international nutritional action until McLaren (1974) exploded the myth by calling it 'The great protein fiasco'. The problem of malnutrition is one of quantity rather than quality of food. The pathogenesis of kwashiorkor remains obscure. Sometimes it seems to be related to protein deficiency, at other times not.

There is a broad spectrum of malnutrition spreading from kwashiorkor to marasmus known as protein-energy malnutrition (PEM). PEM includes many intermediate forms of malnutrition as well as many undersized children without definite signs of disease, but who are presumed to show defects of growth (Waterlow and Payne, 1975). PEM is the most important health problem of communities in warm climates. By reducing growth and impairing the health of children, it has effects which extend throughout the population. It has to be given priority in any description of malnutrition in warm climates.

There is no one effective type of nutrient for the treatment of PEM. Skimmed milk or high protein foods cannot be used in its treatment with the precision and effectiveness of antibiotics in the treatment of infections. Nor can any special protective food act by itself to prevent PEM, in the way that a vaccine will prevent measles. A protective food of this kind is only useful as one factor in a general improvement in diet and social conditions. The organization of medical services to detect and treat PEM in its early stages, and of social services for the support and education of the family, are more important than the illusory pursuit of some new wonder-food to match the wonder-drugs.

EPIDEMIOLOGY OF FOOD

Man is omnivorous. This can be confusing for hundreds of different foods are used in different parts of the world, and any one person should eat several different foods. To simplify this confusion, foods are usually classified into a few groups, the foods within each group having similar nutritional properties. Food tables have been compiled which give details of the nutritional content of all commonly used foods, for example, the tables of representative values of foods commonly used in tropical countries, compiled by Platt (1962) give a list of some 350 foods classified into 16 groups. But for our purpose, to describe the broad principles underlying the dietary treatment of malnutrition nine food-groups shown in Table 1 will be sufficient.

Generally, the diet of a community is based on one or two staple foods which supply most of the energy. Other foods are contributory to the staple but they are equally important because they contain essential nutrients that the staple lacks, and may actually improve the nutritional value of the staple. In Table 1 cereals and starchy roots are shown as staples; other groups are contributory. The table is only intended as a general guide to show the necessity for supplementing the staples with food from other groups. More detailed information about particular foods is available in food-composition tables.

Historically, the geographical distribution of deficiency diseases has been related to the staple foods consumed by different populations. Pellagra was associated with maize, beri beri with rice. Mineral deficiencies such as iodine deficiency with endemic goitre may be associated with the geology of an inhabited area. The staple food-crops, themselves, depend on the geology and climate of the area in which they are consumed. With increasing knowledge of the causes and means of prevention, these geographical associations have become less obvious; but they still tend to appear in vulnerable groups within the historical geographical distributions.

Table 44.1 Food groups and their nutritional value.

Group	Energy	Protein[1]	Vitamins A[2]	Vitamins B[3]	Vitamins C[4]	Minerals Calcium[5]	Minerals Iron[6]
I Vegetable foods							
A Staples							
1 Cereal staples (wheat, rice, maize, millets, etc.)	++	++	-,	++,	-	++	++
2 Starchy staples roots, tubers and starchy fruits (yam, cassava, potato, plantain, etc.)	++	±	±,	-,	±	+	-
Contributory foods							
1 Legumes and pulses (peas, beans, groundnuts, soya, etc)	++	++	-,	++,	-	+	+
2 Green leafy vegetables (spinach, etc.)	+	+	+++,	-,	++	+	+
3 Fresh fruits	+	-	++,	-,	+++	+	-
II Animal foods							
1 Meat (including liver and offals)	++	+++	+++,	+++,	+	+	+++
2 Fish (fresh and canned)	++	+++	++,	++,	-	++	+
3 Milk, cheese	++	+++	++,	+++,	-	+++	-
III Special energy foods							
B Oils, fats, sugar and alcohol	+++	-	±,	-,	-	-	-

Values:
+++ means adequate for a growing child
++ means adequate for an adult
+ means inadequate for an adult
± means variable or doubtful
- means negligible

Notes:
[1] If two groups are combined in a diet the values given can be added up to a maximum of +++. A suitable mixture of cereals and legumes therefore gives a protein value similar to meat. This addition can only be made between staples and contributory foods in other groups.
[2] Carotene, the red-yellow pigment in coloured vegetable foods (e.g., carrots, and red palm oil), and in leaves, is the source of vitamin A in vegetables. The deeper the colour or the darker the leaf, the greater is the vitamin A value.
[3] The vitamin B group of vitamins can be removed by milling and may be lost in cooking.
[4] Vitamin C is destroyed by overcooking and exposure of prepared food to air.
[5] The absorption of calcium depends on vitamin D. This is dealt with in the text. It may not be well absorbed from vegetable foods.
[6] Iron is not well absorbed from vegetable foods.

Measurement of protein-energy values of food

Because protein is one of the energy-yielding constituents of food, the protein-value of a diet is inextricably mixed with energy-value and the full satisfaction of energy-needs. Protein-values of diets are best measured as the proportion of total energy in the diet contributed by protein. The available energy from dietary protein is measured by the 'Atwater factor' 17kJ/g (4 kcal/g). Protein-values of diets can be expressed as:

$$\frac{\text{Protein energy}}{\text{Total dietary energy}} \times 100$$

This is known as the P/E ratio per cent. As it is a ratio, the value is the same whatever units are used to measure energy; it has precisely the same value as the previously used P/Cal %.

For particular foodstuffs, a correction needs to be made for protein value; this can be expressed as the percentage-value the protein of the foodstuff has compared with milk protein, which has a value of 100. This is the protein score. Most human diets (with the exception of exclusively milk-fed infants) have a mixture of food proteins. The mixture enhances the protein score of the whole diet, even though the protein score of the staple may be very low.

Human milk from a well nourished mother is fully adequate for human growth. It has a P/E ratio of six per cent. Ordinary dietary protein in a good mixed diet has a protein score not less than 60 per cent. To ensure that a mixed diet has a protein value equivalent to milk the P/E must be raised to allow for the lower protein score:

$$6\% \times \frac{100}{60} = \text{P/E } 10\%$$

Most human diets, with the exception of some based on staples of starchy roots, tubers and fruits, have a P/E ratio of 10 per cent, or more.

Generally, if the total energy of the diet fully satisfies energy requirements, the protein value of the diet will be adequate. Insufficient dietary energy presents one kind of problem — growth faltering and marasmus. A low protein-value due to a low P/E ratio or protein score without so great a reduction in total dietary energy is less common, but may contribute to another kind of problem — kwashiorkor.

This is a simplified statement of the dietary background of PEM, but marasmus and kwashiorkor are diseases with profound metabolic disturbances which cannot be simply described in terms of dietary arithmetic. There are many other important contributory factors.

EPIDEMIOLOGY OF PROTEIN-ENERGY MALNUTRITION

In its severe forms PEM may affect up to five per cent of children before their fifth birthday in some countries, but moderate degrees of PEM may affect at least 40 per cent of children in many countries. De Maeyer (1976) gives incidences for the decade 1963–73 for children aged 0–5 years of three per cent severe and 29 per cent moderate, a total incidence of 32 per cent in Latin America, Africa and Asia. The Pan American Health Organization investigation of mortality (Puffer and Serrano, 1973) found that in Latin America and the Caribbean, PEM was directly (nine per cent) or indirectly (48.4 per cent) responsible for 57.4 per cent of total deaths of children in this age group.

These statistics of incidence can be misleading, for PEM is not a single clearly defined disease, like measles, malaria, or diabetes. Although it is the result of malnutrition, the causes of malnutrition are most complicated; they are a mixture of poverty, poor social conditions, a poor diet with many different deficiencies, bad hygiene and a high prevalence of infectious diseases. Malnutrition occurs in these conditions and as it occurs, reacts with them and aggravates them in a vicious circle. PEM is a general state of ill-health and failure to thrive, associated with many different diseases and deficiencies, causing a high mortality in young children before their fifth birthday and particularly before their second birthday. Scrimshaw, Taylor and Gordon (1968) have called this a synergism of malnutrition and infection. There is a combined contribution by each of these two promoters of disease to the final enhanced effect. There is, though, a contrary effect. Undernutrition of the host may restrict the metabolism of some parasites, particularly malaria. This was called antagonism by Scrimshaw, Taylor and Gordon. Mann (1980) suggested that competition for nutrients by host and parasite (and also the proliferating cells of malignant growths) might mean that anorexia and malnutrition could be part of a natural defence against invaders.

The weaning crisis

Weanling diarrhoea (Gordon, Chitkara and Wyon, 1963) is regularly associated with PEM, and is a principal cause of death. PEM and weanling diarrhoea occur particularly at this age because children, in common with all young mammals, face a weaning crisis when their mother's milk can no longer meet all their requirements. This normally occurs at four to six months of age and over the next 18 months there may be increasing undernutrition complicated by the greater exposure and susceptibility of children to infections. When breastfeeding stops prematurely and is replaced by inadequate and infective artificial feeds the crisis and its accompanying malnutrition occur earlier — often during the first six months of life.

Waterlow and Thomson (1979) have shown that the weaning crisis may occur earlier in breastfed children than was previously supposed. In the WHO Collaborative Breast-feeding study from 10 to 50 per cent of rural-breast-feeding mothers were giving supplementary food by two to three months; the commonest reason given for doing so was that mothers thought they had not enough milk. A study of faltering in infant growth in several tropical countries by Waterlow, Ashworth and Griffiths (1980) showed that the rate of growth falls off substantially between three and four months and in many cases earlier, and this was associated with increased mortality.

The inhibition of ovulation by prolactin in lactation is said to be a natural mechanism for birth control, in communities where breast-feeding of a child may extend over some two years. In conditions of rural poverty, women are engaged in the hard physical labour of cultivation and production of food. From puberty they go through a continuous cycle of pregnancy and lactation leading to premature aging and early death (Dobbing, 1982).

In Gambian mothers the lactational rise in serum prolactin is related as much to their undernutrition as to their lactation. A dietary supplement designed to match their energy intake with that of British mothers did not increase their low output of breast milk (Prentice et al., 1980) but shortened the duration of lactational infertility by at least six months (Lunn et al., 1981). There appears to be a risk that improving the diet of malnourished lactating mothers may cause a rise in birth rate. Dobbing comments that we should concentrate on feeding the mothers as well as the babies. We must find some less cruel method of contraception than maternal malnutrition.

The intense physical activity of pregnant Gambian women in the farming season, coupled with a general seasonal shortage of food with negative energy balance, is associated with striking falls in birthweight and a reduction in the quantity of breast milk during subsequent lactation (Paul, Muller and Whitehead, 1979; Roberts et al., 1982). Bleiberg et al. (1980, 1981) reported similar results in female farmers in Upper Volta. Both in The Gambia and Upper Volta the differences between energy expenditure and intake cannot be explained on the basis of present knowledge. There is some unexplained difference between women in communities where regularly occurring food shortage is normal and those whose food supplies are adequate. For these deprived women, FAO/WHO recommended energy intakes seem to be inappropriate.

Malnutrition in pregnancy is therefore a contributory factor to the weaning crisis in postnatal life. The foetus may thrive at the expense of the malnourished mother, but nutritional support for both mother and child should start in pregnancy. Supplementation of maternal diet from birth onwards through lactation is probably too late.

Mortality

Mortality statistics giving diseases of malnutrition as causes of death are very unreliable. The general death rates of children have been used as indicators of malnutrition, particularly the age-specific death rate of one to four years, between the first and fifth birthday and the one to two year death rate. High rates are due as much, or more, to uncontrolled diarrhoea and infectious disease, as to dietary malnutrition.

PRINCIPAL TYPES OF PEM

The two principal clinical types of severe PEM are kwashiorkor and marasmus. Many children have a mixture of the two types known as marasmic kwashiorkor.

Marasmus

Marasmus means wasting, and nutritional marasmus is starvation occurring in a child. It has usually been associated with failure in breast-feeding, or with the replacement of breast-feeding by bottle-feeding, or too early supplementation with additional feeds. With bottle-feeding, there is a greatly increased risk of infectious gastro-enteritis with diarrhoea; the feeds given are often dilute, being inadequate both in quantity and quality. In severe marasmus, the child may seem to be no more than skin and bones; the head and belly appear to be huge compared to the rest of the body.

In Gambia, supplementary feeds of bacteriologically contaminated watery gruel are given to infants at an early age (Rowland and McCollum, 1977; Rowland, Barrell and Whitehead, 1978). Because mothers' milk is lacking in quantity, marasmus with weaning diarrhoea occurs by about the age of three months. Marasmus and diarrhoea do therefore occur in breastfed children as well as in the artificially bottlefed.

Kwashiorkor

As in marasmus, there is a failure in growth, but the principal distinguishing feature is oedema. Other features of kwashiorkor vary greatly from place to place and do not occur universally. The cause of the oedema does not now appear to be dietary protein deficiency or hypoalbuminaemia as was supposed. Golden (1982) found that the rate of loss of oedema in Jamaican children treated for kwashiorkor was strongly related to dietary intake, not to protein intake. The oedema is indistinguishable from starvation oedema, but why some children suffering from PEM become oedematous and others do not, is still not explained.

Biochemical and metabolic changes

Serum albumin is reduced to between 20–30 g/litre in marasmus; there is a greater reduction in kwashiorkor to less than 20 g/1. Serum albumin returns to a normal value of 35 g/1 with successful treatment, and this is a good guide to the success of treatment. Changes in the amino acid content of plasma occur in kwashiorkor, but these are not consistent, and vary in different areas. Laboratory tests are of much less practical importance than the changes in bodyweight which may reflect changes in protein synthesis and rate of turnover. Anaemia, either iron deficiency type or dimorphic, is common.

Protein turnover

In life, there is a continual turnover of body proteins, from minute to minute. A simple model of protein turnover is:

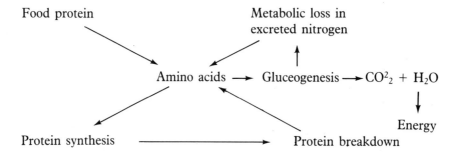

Protein in food replaces inevitable loss, and supplies the additional amino acids required for growth. Any amino acids which do not take part in protein synthesis may be used as sugar, to generate energy.

The chemical work of protein synthesis and turnover demands energy. The rates of turnover are variable and are closely related to metabolic rate. In malnutrition the metabolic rate and rate of whole-body protein turnover are reduced; they increase with catch-up growth during recovery from malnutrition or illness. The rate of whole-body protein turnover is the sum of rates in all tissues, the over-all rate may disguised changes occurring in the opposite directions in tissues such as liver and muscle (Waterlow and Jackson, 1981).

Generally speaking, reductions in rate of turnover mean reduction in protein synthesis below the rate of breakdown; conversely, increased turnover means increased synthesis in relation to breakdown. Different rates of turnover in different tissues govern the adaptation of the whole body to different levels of nutrition.

Marasmus

Gopalan (1968) considered that marasmus was an extreme example of adaptation to a deficiency of energy. The biochemical changes in marasmus, described by Coward and Lunn (1981) are mostly directed towards the maintenance of functions essential to life. There is a reduction in plasma insulin with a rise in plasma cortisol. Both these changes promote the availability of amino acids from muscles, for alternative protein synthesis and for energy needs. Other changes are directed towards the generation of energy from fatty tissue. These adaptive changes can be seen in children with faltering growth rates before they become clinically ill. In practice, any idea of adaptation breaks down when marasmus is associated with diarrhoea as, typically, it is. Diarrhoea causes dangerous deficiencies of water, base, sodium and potassium. The correction and control of these deficits is described later.

Kwashiorkor

If marasmus is an adaptation, kwashiorkor is a failure in adaptation. In India, Gopalan (1968) was not able to attribute the failure to a lack of dietary protein. Some additional stress of infection, hereditary disposition or psychological stress seemed to cause 'dysadaptation' of the biochemical mechanisms that maintain essential functions in marasmus.

The biochemical and hormonal changes which take place in kwashiorkor in two different African communities, in Uganda and Gambia, described by Lunn, Whitehead and Coward (1979) and Coward and Lunn (1981), show two contrasting types of the disease.

Ugandan kwashiorkor is believed to be of dietary origin; many children at risk received a low protein diet with a P/E ratio of only four to six per cent. In non-hospitalized children at risk, plasma insulin was high, but cortisol was not raised. These are precisely opposite to the changes in marasmus. A low protein diet prevents growth, this leads to a low expenditure of energy and a relative excess of energy with a distortion of normal protein synthesis leading to low serum albumin and oedema. There may be a genetic disposition to kwashiorkor in these circumstances. Coward and Lunn (1981) and also James and Trayhurn (1981) suggest a possible relationship to genetic disposition to obesity.

In Gambian kwashiorkor, the changes are quite different. As in marasmus, there is high cortisol with low insulin, but these marasmic changes are complicated by low serum albumin and oedema, typical of kwashiorkor. The oedema and low albumin appear suddenly and coincide with the occurrence of severe diarrhoea. This seems to be kwashiorkor, or marasmic kwashiorkor, caused by diarrhoeal infection. The upper small intestine is heavily colonized by the pathogens causing diarrhoea (Rowland and McCollum, 1977) and there is malabsorption. There appears to be a sudden loss of plasma protein through the intestinal wall into the gut.

Why some of Gopalan's Indian children 'adapted' with marasmus to malnutrition, while others showed the 'dysadaptation' of kwashiorkor has remained mysterious. Recently, Hendrickse et al. (1982) found that aflatoxins from contaminated groundnuts were associated with kwashiorkor in malnourished Sudanese children but not with marasmus. This may mean that greater exposure to aflatoxin was the precipitating stress causing the dysadaptation of kwashiorkor and that there was some fundamental difference in the metabolism of aflatoxins in the affected children. Whether the defect in metabolism is a cause or effect of kwashiorkor is an open question. Epidemiologically, a warm moist climate encouraging the growth of moulds in contaminated food, with the development of mycotoxins, is the kind of climate in which kwashiorkor occurs.

SURVEILLANCE

Targets for surveillance

Infants, children and adolescents

The growth rate is high at birth (actually highest before birth) and declines rapidly in the first year, slowly declining with a small rise at adolescence until it ceases in adult life. Nutritional requirements, generally speaking, follow the same course. Requirements are high in early childhood when there is high risk of malnutrition, a risk which is increased by susceptibility to infection. There is some increased risk of malnutrition at puberty.

Adults

In adult life, the highest risks are for women in pregnancy. Malnutrition or undernutrition in pregnancy is a threat to both mother and child. There are risks of vitamin deficiencies such as osteomalacia or xerophthalmia. Failure to achieve satisfactory gain of weight in pregnancy leads to a low postnatal maternal weight and a low birthweight. This and an inadequate diet lead to a poor milk yield, perhaps shortening the duration of lactaction. The resulting milk can be deficient in energy and, it is increasingly realized, in vitamins. The infant is already set on the road to PEM and possibly specific nutrient deficiencies.

People in care

Special risks are run by those who are not responsible for their own feeding and nutrition in boarding schools, and other residential institutions, or who are in disciplined organizations like the police or the army. Social change, even apparent advances in national economy, can cause malnutrition in these circumstances.

Accessibility

Some of the vulnerable groups receive attention because they are accessible. Schoolchildren, or attenders at Maternal and Child Health Centres, may be subjected to considerable, and often badly managed and ill-directed surveillance. Schools, if education is not universal and compulsory, may not include children most at risk. There is a serious gap between attendance at the post-natal and infants clinic and school age, but it is probable that in many places the greatest concentration should still be on the infant in the first year. There is no remedy for the schoolchild stunted from infancy — the child will never attain its full potential of growth. Surveillance must be aimed at the discovery of individuals at risk, particularly young children, before they become casualties of malnutrition. This means certainly before they are so ill that they need medical treatment.

Careful monitoring to detect in each social group of the community at what point in early childhood faltering in growth occurs, shown by a flattening of the growth curve for height or weight, is an important pointer to effective action. Equally important is monitoring of weight changes of pregnant women, to ensure that they store a sufficient reserve or energy to face the stress of lactation.

Anthropometry

Surveillance should start with the mother in pregnancy and the records of maternal weight change should be compared to birthweights. Birthweight is related to maternal height, which should be measured early in pregnancy; thereafter, ideally, the mother should be weighed at least monthly.

Longitudinal or serial measurements ideally taken from birth onwards in individual children are extremely useful if they are accurately made. A great deal of weighing and measuring is done in MCH centres, but it must be regularly and accurately done, at least three-monthly in the first year, to be useful.

Perhaps the crucial observation in planning measures for control is to identify the age at which growth faltering occurs. This must then be related to measurements or estimates of food intake, history of lactation and supplementary feeding. It is essential to determine whether the faltering is primarily nutritional or primarily due to infection, particularly to diarrhoea. The charting of serial measurements should be made on centile or standard deviation charts, as described below.

Cross sectional studies may be made from time to time, to establish a baseline for a programme or to monitor progress. Cross sectional studies may point to the crucial point of faltering. They are more likely to do so if the sample is stratified in social, environmental or economic classes.

Waterlow et al. (1977) made recommendations for the analysis and presentation of height and weight data in young children up to the age of 10 years, based on WHO recommendations. They advise the breakdown of data into much smaller age-groups than has been customary. Particular attention is needed in the first year. Start with birth weight, and thereafter 4×3-month groups should be used, but if numbers are less than 100 per group then 2×6-month groups are recommended. After the first birthday annual or 2-yearly groups should be used.

Under the age of one year weight for age is convenient and useful, for the length of babies is not such a simple measurement, though the length of babies should be measured in a stadiometer, if this can be arranged. After infancy both weight and height should be measured. Height for age is an indicator of past nutrition *stunting* and weight for height for present nutrition *wasting*. The recommended reference standards are data from the reference population of the U.S. National Center of Health Statistics (NCHS, 1976) which are very detailed (See Janes Chapter 54). Centile growth charts and tables of reference values, together with charts and tabulations of median values and standard deviations, are available from the Chief Medical Officer, Nutrition, World Health Organization.

Height and weight data of children from relatively well nourished groups are to be shown as centile distributions of height for age and weight for height. Relatively undernourished populations give values too extreme to be shown conveniently as centiles. Both stunting and wasting can be shown using a cross tabulation of standard deviation scores (Table 2). The standard deviation score replaces the percentage of reference weight formerly used. The score is the difference between the observed value and the median value in the reference population, divided by the standard deviation of the reference value. Since the centile and standard deviation for the reference population are all given the calculation is quite simple, and calls for no specialized statistical knowledge. If a computer is used appropriate programs are available, and WHO can advise about this.

Table 44.2 Example of cross tabulation in SD scores of weight for height and height for age, in a developing country, of children aged between 1 and 5 years (number in sample = 6482)

Grade	SD score of weight for height	SD score of height for age (percentage of population)				
		Grade 0 More than — 2.00	Grade 1 — 2.00 to — 2.99	Grade 2 — 3.00to — 3.99	Grade 3 — 4.00 or less	Total
0	More than — 2.00	24.3	24.8	21.3	15.1	85.5
1	— 2.00 to — 2.49	2.3	2.6	2.3	1.7	8.9
2	— 2.50 to — 2.99	0.8	1.2	1.1	0.7	3.7
3	— 3.00 or less	0.4	0.5	0.5	0.4	1.8
	Total	28.0	29.0	25.1	17.9	100.0

From Waterlow et al 1977 Bulletin of the World Health Organization 55: 496

Classification and assessment of PEM

The Wellcome classification (Table 3) has been used to distinguish kwashiorkor from marasmus for many years. It is based on a weight-for-age below 60 per cent of reference weight to designate marasmus. This is too severe for community studies, and the classification selects those who require hospital treatment.

Waterlow and Rutishauser (1974) proposed a graded classification for both stunting and wasting:

Table 44.3 Classification of PEM by bodyweight A using % standard weight B using SD score

A Percentage of standard weight*	Oedema Present	Absent	B SD score
60 — 80	Kwashiorkor	Undernourished	—2 to —3
under 60	Marasmic kwashiorkor	Marasmus	< — 3

* Standard = 50th percentile of Harvard weight for age

grade 0, normal; grade 1, mild; grade 2, moderate; and grade 3, severe. These grades can be used instead of SD scores and have been allotted to the appropriate categories in Table 2.

Where malnutrition is common, the precise age of children is generally not known. The difficulty is greatest in those classes of the community most at risk. It is less difficult to find the age in the first year of life than subsequently, and it is particularly important to know the age of infants at least within a month. Weight for age is then a satisfactory measure.

Dugdale (1971) produced an age-independent nutritional index for pre-school children after the first birthday. It is a valid measure of wasting, and correlates well with skinfold. For children in this age-group (first to fifth birthday) the ratio weight/height$^{1.6}$ is constant for the average (median) value of weight for age in the reference population at all ages. Measured in kilograms and centimetres

$$\frac{W}{H^{1.6}} = 100 \times 10^{-4}$$

This is multiplied by 10 000 to give the round figure of 100 as a reference value for a well-nourished child. A nutritional index of 87 corresponds approximately to the 5th percentile or -2 standard deviations in the NCHS reference population. Recently, Dugdale and Lovell (1981) have proposed another index for children aged 5 to 10 years.

Other anthropometrical measurements are detailed in Jelliffe (1966) and their use has been critically evaluated by Keller, Donoso and De Maeyer (1976). The reference standards for limb, head circumferences, skinfolds, etc., should be those given for the NCHS reference population.

The assessment of dietary intake and dietary surveys

Rutishauser (1973) has reviewed the practical applicability of different techniques of dietary assessment in Africa. There are four principal techniques:

1. Weighted food intake

Theoretically the most accurate. All items of food taken are weighed before consumption. This calls for reliable staff trained to work in people's own homes. It is a highly specialized undertaking.

2. Analysis of replicate diets

When a meal is served a precise replica is served for laboratory analysis, and the plate waste is analysed and subtracted.

3. Dietary recall

The mother of a child is asked to recall the amounts of food consumed in the last 24 hours. Rutishauser prepared a range of local foods used by Ugandan mothers and asked each mother at her clinic to say how much of each food had been given to her child. She achieved very satisfactory results.

4. Diary method

The mother, or other consumer, is asked to record the different dishes or types of food consumed over about a week. Again, Rutishauser made this method work with unsophisticated people by asking mothers to stick pins into squares for each day of the week placed under photographs of the groups of food that were in use. She obtained good records of the type of food consumed over a continuous period for some years.

Method 4 was a valuable qualitative check on the quantitative estimates of method 3.

Methods 3 and 4 are probably the most generally useful. They can be usefully supplemented, where accurate knowledge of some local food is needed by replicate analysis of method 2. The childlike simplicity of methods 3 and 4 is deceptive. The results obtained are of incalculable value and require a combination of knowledge, skill and friendly co-operation.

The energy content and nutrient content of foods are derived from the estimated weights with food tables. There are now many regional tables with reliable analytical values of local foods. There are always seasonal variations in intake, and four surveys each lasting a week in each quarter of the year are of more value than four weeks of survey in one month. Dietary measurements should be spread over the whole year.

Average nutritional values of the diet of a group presented without any measure of the range of values can be misleading. Whitehead et al. (1977) found that average protein: energy ratios in Ugandan and Gambian dietary surveys were about the same at P/E 8 to 8.5 per cent, but the 3rd centile of the Gambian diets was only reduced by 1 per cent to P/E 7 per cent whilst a much larger proportion of Ugandan diets below the 10th centile were below P/E 4 per cent — a value which put the children seriously at risk, many of them requiring hospital treatment.

NUTRITIONAL REQUIREMENTS AND RECOMMENDED INTAKES

Whether a diet is satisfactory or contains nutritional defects is determined by comparing the nutritional values obtained from a dietary survey with the *group requirement*. There is much confusion about such recommendations. 'Dietary requirements' 'recommended intakes', 'allowances' and 'safe level' for a nutrient have been used interchangeably, though 'requirements' and 'recommendations' are not the same.

There is a rising scale of standards, each of which has a useful purpose (Zollner, Wolfram and Kellner, 1977).

(i) The *average requirement* maintains nutrient balance in 50 per cent of a population and *no more*: it is a minimum figure.

(ii) The *group requirement* meets the physiological needs of nearly all people. It is the average requirement + 2 S.D. It is synonymous with *Safe Level*. This should be the intended meaning of such terms as 'physiological requirements' or 'needs', of a group for any nutrients.

(iii) *Recommended intakes* have a different, though related function. They are guides to dietitians, housewives and caterers to ensure that the diets they prepare are fully adequate. They usually exceed the physiological or *group requirement*, for a number of reasons. The recommendation may allow for extreme individuals, for common stresses of life, and often must be made realistic by matching the recommendations with the customary traditional dietary habits of a community, so far as this is compatible with (ii) *Group requirement*. They also allow for genuine differences of opinion concerning physiological requirements.

Recommended intakes, where they differ from *group requirements* ought not to be used as the criteria for judging whether or not a group is at risk of some nutritional deficiency; they are planning recommendations, not diagnostic parameters. The scale of measurement against which diets should be judged is the *group requirement*. Generally, the *group requirement* from which national *recommended intakes* are derived, is based on the reports of expert committees of WHO and FAO (WHO/FAO, 1967; 1973; WHO, 1974).

A PRACTICAL APPROACH TO SURVEILLANCE AND ASSESSMENT

Nutritional surveys and assessment extend from high grade expensive research to the District Medical Officer's need to assess the extent of malnutrition in his own area. For this purpose, the simplest observations are the best. Relatively simple anthropometry can yield information which should form the essential baseline of assessment. This can be made progressively more detailed if more complicated and sophisticated investigations are used for further investigations.

A quick cross-sectional survey is of very limited value as malnutrition is seasonal, but it may be useful if some assessment is needed when conditions are known to be bad. Repeated cross-sectional surveys over a year or more may give more information. These if well conducted become longitudinal surveys.

A good model is the survey conducted by Sommer et al. (1981) in six villages in West Java. All the families with pre-school age children were enrolled in the study after a preliminary census and for two years a trained clinical team visited homes every three months.

It is advisable to obtain statistical advice on sampling procedure, stratification of samples and sample size before undertaking any planned assessment.

Interpretation and screening

Birthweight

In all communities, both in developing and developed countries, there is an association between birthweight and maternal standard of living. Where malnutrition is common a large proportion of children have a birthweight less than 2.5 kg — the weight conventionally accepted as the low limit of normal. The proportion of birthweights below 2.5 kg might therefore be used as an index of malnutrition. Keller, Donoso and De Maeyer (1976) note this, but also draw attentiion to the many adverse factors, together with malnutrition, which affect birthweight. These include maternal stature, illness and toxic influences, including tobacco smoking in pregnancy. Paul, Muller and Whithead (1979) and Roberts et al. (1982) showed, however, that maternal energy-balance in pregnancy has a quantifiable effect on birthweight.

In some trials, small supplements to maternal diet in pregnancy (about 460 kJ or 100 kcal per 24 h) have increased birthweight. Average birthweight of a group — controlled for such variables as seasonal variation and maternal stature — could be used to measure the effectiveness of a planned intervention of a dietary supplement in pregnancy.

Wasting and stunting of children

A table of the type of Table 1 can be reduced to a fourfold table giving below –2 SD ($\equiv$ 5th centile or $p < 0.05$) as the limits for wasting and stunting. This serves as a plan for monitoring.

Wasted and stunted	Priority
Wasted but not stunted	Action
Not wasted but stunted	? Action
Not wasted not stunted	No action

Dugdale's index below 87 means wasting calling for action.

DEFICIENCY DISEASES

The classical deficiency diseases — xerophthalmia, beriberi, pellagra, scurvy and nutritional rickets are such clearly defined clinical syndromes that the vitamins were originally identified by the deficiency diseases caused by their absence and dramatically cured by their administration. They are the results of severe deficiency.

Three diagnostic methods are used to detect vitamin deficiency — therapeutic tests, biochemical and functional tests and dietary assessment. All three methods are used in group assessment.

Therapeutic tests are the oldest and still, perhaps, the most certain of all diagnostic measures. The instant restoration of physiological function when a deficient vitamin is administered leads to rapid recovery. This is diagnostic and may be lifesaving. In group assessment, controlled trials of vitamin supplementation may reveal protective effects of vitamins that were previously unsuspected.

Biochemical tests are often grouped into three categories: deficient, marginal or suspicious, and acceptable. A biochemical diagnosis must be based on experience — that findings at that level are associated with clinical signs, or some measurable loss of function. With greater knowledge of the function of particular nutrients it is now possible to detect large or small deviations from normality before the appearance of clinical disorder. A relatively low biochemical assessment of vitamin status may be associated with disease in ways that were not expected.

Dietary assessment is the least reliable method. The calculation of vitamin intake from food tables is subject to considerable error. Broad general descriptions of diet are useful as indicators of the possible cause of ill health. Deficiency diseases are often associated with a restricted variety of foods in a diet, with too much reliance on one staple that may be deficient.

Xerophthalmia — retinol (vitamin A) deficiency

Xeropthalmia is now the most serious vitamin deficiency in the world, causing blindness in thousands of young children every year. In West Java Sommer et al. (1981) estimated incidence at 2.7 per 1000 pre-school children per year. This means that in India, Bangladesh and the Philippines there are some 500 000 new cases with severe deficiency each year. Half of these become blind. It has its most serious effects in 'pre-school' children between the first and fifth birthdays. Retinol, a fat-soluble vitamin, the active form of vitamin A in animals, is only found in animal fats, particularly in liver and fish oils. All animal retinol is formed from carotene, the orange-yellow pigment found in coloured vegetable foods — carrot, red palm oil, or sweet potatoes — and green leaves. Vegetable carotene is the principal source of vitamin A in many warm climates. Vitamin A deficiency is called xerophthalmia, which means dryness of the eye — the chief symptom of the disease.

Xerophthalmia occurs in the same age group and is closely associated with PEM. Milder degrees of vitamin A deficiency together with PEM may account for much more childhood blindness (Dawson and Schwab, 1981).

It has long been known that vitamin A deficiency may cause epithelial degeneration or squamous metaplasia. It is now becoming clear that low serum retinol and low dietary carotenoids are linked with higher risks for epithelial cancers, particularly of the lung and gut.

Mild xerophthalmia — night blindness

The first sign to appear is inability to see in dim light. It is easily recognized in adolescents and adults but is difficult to discover in very young children. Examine children in a darkened room or hut; ask the mother to go away to a dark corner of the room to call her child. A normal child runs at once to mother. A child with night blindness cannot find her and is distressed. This condition is easily treated with prophylactic supplements.

Biochemical tests:

Blood levels below 20 μg/100 ml retinol and 80 μg/100 ml carotenoids suggest deficiency.

Plasma retinol will identify groups at risk of disease. Plasma carotenoids reflect the recent intake of vegetable carotenoids in food.

Beri beri. Thiamine deficiency

Without thiamine, sugars which supply the energy for cell-life and activity cannot be completely oxidised to yield their full potential energy, by conversion to carbon dioxide and water. The process stops half-way at the formation of pyruvic and lactic acids from glucose, and at a similar half-way stage in the breakdown of another important type of sugar — pentose. In thiamine deficiency, there is a high blood pyruvate and the degree of deficiency can be measured in well-equipped laboratories by the erythrocyte transketolase test.

Beri beri is liable to appear in times of crisis, particularly in rice-eating countries. It is often associated with bad catering in institutions such as schools, prisons or barracks. It most often appears in people doing hard physical work. In some rice-eating countries it is a disease of infants.

Mild malnutrition

Seasonal oedema of the legs occurring at the end of the dry season and before harvest is suspicious. Where infantile beri beri occurs, mothers should be given prophylactic supplements. Sporadic cases of unexplained heart failure with oedema are always suspicious.

Infantile beri beri

Infantile beri beri may occur in breast-fed children of mothers on a poor rice-diet at ages two to five months. The symptoms are similar to those of severe beri beri, passing into convulsions, coma and death. Laryngeal paralysis may cause a strange thin whining cry.

Biochemical tests

The most reliable test is the TPP (thiamine pyrophosphate) effect in the erythrocyte transketolase test. A TPP effect of 0 to 15 per cent is normal. 15 to 24 per cent shows mild deficiency. 25 per cent shows severe deficiency.

Pellagra. Niacin deficiency

Though pellagra is a vitamin deficiency its causes are complex; they are linked to protein deficiency. Niacin (syn. nicotinamide, nicotinic acid) can be made in the body from the essential amino-acid tryptophan. In a diet of high protein value there will be sufficient tryptophan to spare in the dietary protein for the synthesis of niacin, and pellagra will not occur. The amount of tryptophan in the dietary protein needs to be considerable for this to occur, as 80 mg of the amino acid are needed to produce 1 mg of niacin. Some food proteins, particularly the protein of maize, the staple cereal generally associated with pellagra, are deficient in tryptophan. Pellagra has tended to be endemic in areas where maize and sorghum are the staple cereals, but pellagra-like conditions may be seen anywhere in people taking an inadequate diet of low protein value. Some manifestation of pellagra is usually seen in severe undernutrition — in paupers, in protein-energy malnutrition in children, or during famines. It is not uncommon in residential institutions, particularly those for the mentally ill, in which catering is badly managed. The clinical condition of pellagra is due to a mixture of protein and vitamin deficiencies, niacin being the most important. It may occur in epidemic outbreaks in famine and disasters.

Mild malnutrition

The oro-genital syndrome is associated with multiple deficiencies of the vitamin B group described below. The most obvious sign is the condition of the skin which becomes red and inflamed where it is exposed to sunlight. The dermatitis stops where the skin is protected by clothing or shoes, and the ordinary clothing of the patient is clearly outlined, particularly at margins like the collars of shirts or singlets and the sleeves.

Patients admitted to mental hospitals, prisons or institutions for the aged or destitute should be regularly examined for pellagra; it may have been the cause for their admission or it may have occurred after admission with an inadequate diet. If it occurs in the institution it may be mistaken for a deterioration in the mental condition for which the patient was originally admitted. Even if the diet of the institution is satisfactory, mental illness may cause a patient to consume a deficient diet.

Biochemical tests

Excretion of a metabolite of niacin N-methylnicotinamide in urine is a possible group screening test. Urinary excretion below 2 mg per six hours or 0.5 mg per g creatinine indicates deficiency.

Riboflavine deficiencies and multiple deficiencies of vitamin B complex

Acute and chronic glossitis with conditions varying from fiery inflammation and soreness to chronic loss of epithelium of the tongue; cracked and peeling lips (cheilosis); inflamed sores with heaped up soggy epithelium at the corners of the mouth (angular stomatitis) and similar lesions at other mucocutaneous junctions at the nose, eyes and perineum: this collection of signs has been called the oro-genital syndrome. It is seen in pellagra with niacin deficiency, and also with deficiencies of other vitamins of the B group — riboflavine and pyridoxine. Treatment calls for prophylactic supplements and general improvement of diet.

Biochemical tests

The erythrocyte glutiathone reductase test can be used for measuring riboflavine status. In this test, activation co-efficients (or FAD effect) greater than 1.2 suggest mild deficiency; coefficients over 1.3 suggest severe deficiency. In Gambia, lactating women had a mean value of 1.8 with angular stomatitis and sore mouths. The riboflavine concentrations of their breast milk was only 0.22 μg/ml, about two-thirds that in U.K. mothers and well below the United States normal standard of 0.40 μg/ml. The babies were biochemically deficient by this test throughout lactation and weaning (Bates et al., 1982a). Whitehead (1980) considers that this mother-child deficiency is likely to occur elsewhere in communities that do not consume milk.

Scurvy: ascorbic acid (vitamin C) deficiency

Scurvy only occurs when there are no fresh fruits or fresh green leafy vegetables in the diet, or in infants who are artificially fed. It is likely to occur in infants who are bottle-fed on cow's milk, unless they receive prophylactic supplements. The clinical disease — scurvy — is not common in warm climates, but in Gambian villages Bates et al. (1982b) found that breast milk levels of ascorbic acid were reduced in the rainy season. This corresponds with low mean maternal plasma levels of 0.1–0.2 mg/dl in lactating mothers. They consider that the severely depleted plasma levels may have medical significance, as they occur in the rainy season, coinciding with the stresses of hard manual labour in food production on the farms in a hot humid climate with a high incidence of infections.

Ascorbic acid is concerned in the synthesis of collagen, and the integrity of connective tissue and basement membranes of blood vessels. This accounts for the haemorrhages of scurvy. Biochemical deficiency is associated with delayed healing of wounds and ulcers, while there is evidence that it may affect immunity to infections.

Biochemical tests

Ascorbic acid levels should exceed 0.4 mg/dl in plasma and 11 μg/10^8 white blood cells. Values less than 0.1 mg/dl or 2 μg/10^8 white blood cells indicate deficiency.

Rickets and osteomalacia: vitamin D deficiency

Vitamin D occurs naturally with the normal exposure of the skin to daylight. Most people in warm climates produce all they require in their skin apart from dietary sources.

Rickets in children and osteomalacia — the adult form of deficiency — do occur in slum conditions in warm climates, and with social habits which enforce the seclusion of women and children inside houses with inadequate exposure to sunlight.

Biochemical tests

Low serum calcium (< 10 mg/100 ml), low serum inorganic phosphorus (< 4 mg/100 ml) with raised serum alkaline phosphatase (> 25 King Armstrong units) are all suggestive of deficiency, but X-ray appearances of bones are the decisive sign to diagnosis. The competitive protein binding (CPB) assay for plasma vitamin D as 25-hydroxycholecalciferol (25-HCC) gives normal values for children of 15 to 37.5 μg/l and for adults, 18 to 80 μg/l. In rickets, plasma values are < 4 μg/l.

Nutritional anaemia

Anaemia is diagnosed by the measurement of haemoglobin and is said to exist if it falls below WHO (1972) standard:

	Hb concentration (Hb/100 ml blood)
Pregnant women and children aged 6 months to 6 years	11

Non-pregnant women and children   12
    aged 6–14 years
Men   13
There are two principal forms of nutritional anaemia:

Microcytic and hypochromic: is diagnosed by measuring packed cell volume
(PCV) with haematocrit and obtaining the mean corpuscular haemoglobin
concentration (MCHC). MCHC < 30 g/100 ml indicates hypochromic
anaemia. This diagnosis can be made in small peripheral centres if staff are
equipped and trained for it. The cause is lack of iron due to blood loss or
iron deficiency in the diet, or malabsorption of iron.

Megaloblastic anaemia: Accurate diagnosis requires the skill of a haematological laboratory, but a low Hb concentration with MCHC not less than
30 g/100 ml would suggest a megaloblastic anaemia. The cause is a
deficiency of folic acid or cobalamine (vitamin B_{12}). In malnutrition these two
hypochromic and megaloblastic anaemias are sometimes mixed due to
combined deficiency of iron and folic acid. The anaemia is then called
Dimorphic. Treatment of hypochromic anaemia with iron may then reveal
the megaloblastic anaemia of folate deficiency. Megaloblastic anaemias are
much less common than hypochromic anaemias.

Iron deficiency

Hypochromic anaemia due to iron deficiency accompanies most nutritional
deficiencies and is the commonest symptom of malnutrition. It is aggravated
by blood loss and malabsorption due to parasites. The measurement of
haemoglobin is therefore an essential procedure whenever malnutrition is
suspected.

Women of child-bearing age are particularly susceptible, as their intake
of dietary iron is smaller than that of men whilst their requirements are
higher because of menstrual loss. The children of anaemic women may have
small stores of iron at birth. A normal newborn child can flourish without
dietary iron for four to six months, and milk contains no iron. But after the
age of four months children must receive iron in the diet, preferably in
meat. Iron is poorly absorbed from vegetable foods and young children on
mainly vegetable diets run a serious risk of anaemia.

Folic acid deficiencies

In pregnancy

Folic acid deficiency commonly occurs in pregnancy and megaloblastic
anaemia is a serious complication. It should be prevented by giving supplements of folic acid and iron throughout pregnancy and the puerperium.

In children

Megaloblastic and dimorphic anaemia is a serious complication of PEM.

Cobalamine (vitamin B$_{12}$) deficiency

Pernicious anaemia is caused by an inability to absorb cobalamine and is rarely due to dietary deficiency. Strict vegetarians or vegans, who take no form of animal food whatsoever may develop megaloblastic anaemia, as cobalamines do not occur in plants. Nutritional neuropathies should always be treated with cobalamine and this is particularly important if any signs of neuropathy develop during treatment or prophylaxis with folic acid.

Trace elements

Including iron, 14 elements are required in quantities less than a few milligrams per day. Cobalt is considered under cobalamine (above). Iodine is well known as a component of thyroxine. Other trace elements, particularly zinc and possibly vanadium, play a part in PEM (Golden and Golden, 1981).

Nutritional neuropathies

A. Peripheral nervous lesions

Dry beri beri and other polyneuropathies. Chronic beri beri is associated with paralysis — wrist drop and ankle drop and other forms of motor nerve paralysis, with loss of tendon reflexes and disturbances of sensation. The principal deficiency is of thiamine but there are usually contributory deficiencies of the vitamins of the B group concerned with the metabolism of carbohydrates on which nerve cells are dependent.

Burning feet syndrome. It is not uncommon for patients on a poor diet to complain of severe burning pains in the feet — 'my feet are on fire'. The condition is extremely painful but is so odd that it may be disregarded as a neurosis. It has been attributed to deficiency of pantothenic acid, but is usually associated with multiple deficiencies.

B. Central nervous system lesions

Wernicke's encephalopathy. Double vision, nystagmus, mental confusion and coma may occur in acute thiamine deficiencies, especially with alcoholism.

Nutritional amblyopia. Vision becomes misty and indistinct. Literate patients usually complain that they cannot see well enough to read. Other cranial nerves can be affected, particularly the acoustic (eighth) nerve, causing singing in the ears and deafness. The condition is particularly common in cassava-eating areas in West Africa. It may be associated with spinal ataxia. It has been attributed to cyanogens in vegetable foods, particularly in cassava, which liberate cyanide when consumed. Cobalamines present in animal foods combine with cyanide, detoxicating it to form cyanocobalamin. The condition has been associated with diets with high vegetable and low animal content, but a similar amblyopia occurring in people of West African descent in the Caribbean and London has a genetic basis. Perhaps a nutritional stimulus may affect susceptible people (British Medical Journal, 1981).

Spastic paraplegia. A stiff paralysis, chiefly of the legs, leading to awkward stiff walking with crossing of the legs — the 'scissors gait', progressing to paraplegia and paralysis in a squatting position. In India and Pakistan the disease is caused by lathyrism due to the consumption of the pulse *Lathyrus sativus* used as a food crop in famine. But the condition may occur with many poor vegetable diets.

CONTROL AND PREVENTION

Deficiency diseases or qualitative malnutrition

The prevention, and in some areas the abolition of specific deficiencies of vitamins and minerals, though they are among the greatest successes of medicine, have generally accompanied economic and social progress. Examples are the prevention of endemic goitre with iodized salt, and the reduction of scurvy, pellagra, beri beri and rickets from major to minor problems, in Europe, USA and Japan, by suitable programmes of supplementation. Xerophthalmia is one such deficiency that awaits its own success-story.

As deficiencies are so often associated with a deficient staple and a lack of those foods that are particularly good sources of the deficient nutrient, the most satisfactory immediate answer may be a programme for supplementing the diet with a suitable food or preparation. The supplement, to be successful, must be acceptable and accessible to those most in need. The practical difficulties and possibilities have been described by Whitehead (1980) based on his personal experiences in The Gambia.

Some of the food-groups outlined in Table 1 may be poorly represented in the diet of those at risk of deficiency, and it may be possible by education, food supplementation, or marketing to make them more available.

To prevent the occurrence of mineral and vitamin deficiencies, pharmaceutical preparations or supplements may be administered prophylactically to vulnerable groups. This is common practice in maternity and child-welfare clinics, where vitamins and minerals which are likely to be deficient in the diet of mother or child are given in routine dosage. The deficient nutrients that would be present in a normally adequate diet may be given as prophylactic supplements of the kind shown in Table 4.

The prophylactic supplements shown in Table 4 are generally crude in

Table 44.4 Prophylactic supplements.

Deficiency	Supplement	Notes	Suggested daily dosage
Retinol and Essential fatty acids	'Eye Medicine' Cod liver oil B.P.	See text. 200 µg retinol per g + vit. D	Dosage of all supplements should give the following retinol equivalents approximately: Children under 7 yrs.,
	Shark liver oil* (Indian Pharmacopaeia)	2,000 µg retinol per g negligible vit. D	200 µg
	Other fish oils		7–10 yrs., 400 µg
			10–15 yrs., 500 µg
	Red palm oil	No vitamin D	over 15 yrs, 750 µg

* shark liver oil is ten times stronger than cod liver oil

Deficiency	Supplement	Notes	Suggested daily dosage
Vitamin B	Vitamin B compound tablets B.P.C.	15 mg niacin 1 mg thiamin 1 mg riboflavin	1–2 tablets daily
	Dried yeast tablets B.P.C. 300 mg	0.3 mg niacin 0.1 mg thiamin 0.4 mg riboflavin	6–12 tablets daily
	Meat extracts Extracts of brewers' yeast		
Ascorbic acid (Vitamin C)	Rose fruit B.P.C.	Contains up to 1% ascorbic acid with vit. A and vit. B complex.	One teaspoonful
Vitamin D	Exposure to daylight	In warm climates, ordinary daylight, even in cloudy weather, is prophylactic.	

their composition with a mixture of nutrients. They are examples of the sort of supplements that can be used and several alternatives are suggested. Other alternatives may be available that would be more suitable in particular places than those mentioned in the Table. This is a legitimate area for ingenuity and originality.

Acute diarrhoea and electrolyte balance

The diarrhoeal diseases are dealt with by Rohde in Chapter 20 but acute diarrhoea has so close a relationship with malnutrition, particularly with marasmus, that its control is an important factor, sometimes the principal factor, in the control of malnutrition. Programmes for home-based oral rehydration therapy (ORT) have greatly reduced mortality. The WHO (1977) recommended formula for the oral rehydration solution (ORS) contains in mmol/1: Na^+90; K^+20; Cl^-80; HCO_3^-30; glucose 110. Appropriate quantities of salts and sugar can be put up in packets or sachets to make a litre of solution. Packets of this kind distributed through village-leaders have successfully reduced case-mortality. Packets and sachets are expensive, but spoons, pinches of salt and scoops of sugar have been used. According to The Lancet (1981) ORT is effective, inexpensive, easily used and involves the mother in the child's care, but the MRC nutrition group in the Gambia which evaluated an electrolyte mixture of this kind found that these first aid measures could not replace the need for effective public measures in water supply and sanitation.

PEM or quantitative malnutrition

Gopalan (1968) working in India, found that there was no difference in the quality of the diets of children who developed kwashiorkor or marasmus. In India and elsewhere, in Africa and Central America (Waterlow and Payne, 1975) the main limiting factor in recovery from malnutrition was dietary energy-intake. One main fault in the maize and starchy paps which Cicely Williams originally found to be associated with kwashiorkor was that their large bulk and high water content when cooked made it difficult for a child to eat enough to satisfy energy-needs. Main targets in control will be to ensure that supplementary feeds in weaning, and meals for growing children are adequate for energy requirements.

An approach to a local problem of malnutrition should be to identify with the greatest precision possible the group that is most likely to respond. A close investigation may reveal that this is not necessarily the whole of the one to five year age group. If weaning troubles start within the first six months, start then. Find out which group of mothers yields the lowest birthweights and start supplemention in pregnancy there and measure the result. Identify as far as possible the cause of growth faltering or of clinical disease and attack that. Do not go for inaccessible targets.

An example is the 'MRC Supplement' used in the Gambia, a dry mix of wheat, soya, skim milk, ground-nut oil and sugar, similar in nature to the local traditional gruel. Prepared with water as a porridge it has an energy value, as consumed, of 4 MJ/kg (100 kcal/100g) at a P/E ratio of 18 per cent, a much higher protein-energy value than the local gruel. It was fed twice daily at a village centre to all children aged from three months to one year, for growth faltering began in that community from the age of three months. The supplement aimed to meet the calculated mean energy deficit of 625 kJ/day (150 kcal/day) at three months, rising to 1.25 MJ/day (300 kcal/day) by the age of one year. In spite of this daily provision of free food, the results in improved weight gain were disappointing. The nutrition unit reported that mothers with onerous domestic and agricultural duties found it difficult to fit in twice daily visits to the centre. 'Inadequate dietary intake cannot be automatically equated to lack of available food . . . The standards of day-to-day child care also influence feeding and the constraints imposed on many third world mothers, particularly during labour-intensive farming seasons, may be quite incompatible with adequate child care.'

Since 1945 malnutrition has been the target for an immense amount of international aid, medical and scientific research and programmes of nutritional intervention. Where the problem has been acute, as in the relief of famine following natural disaster or war, the results have been at least satisfactory, at best very good.

Where the problem is a long lasting persistence of endemic malnutrition, it has to be said that most programmes for prevention of malnutrition and improvement of nutrition have been only partially successful. Where there has been general success with improved growth rates and reduced death rates in children, these have usually been the result of economic improvement. The cost of petroleum oil and the swings of economic depression and recovery have had more influence than any planned programme of nutrition intervention.

One reason for this is that the problem is vast, and resources have been spread over too wide an area. When programmes have been aimed at a particular target, the target has been too large — covering a whole population or wide age-groups, or has been the wrong target — like the 'protein gap'.

Another reason is that the trained physician knows from knowledge and experience that many diseases, including malnutrition, can be easily and successfully treated, and just as successfully prevented if medical advice is taken. To the trained professional the solution seems simple. Putting the solution into practice may be extraordinarily difficult. Food habits and traditional practices in feeding children cannot change quickly. This has been called the 'myth of simple prevention and easy treatment' by Roger England (1978).

Malnutrition has its worst effects on the children of the poorest people. Any special food or supplement which adds to the total cost of food in the family budget will be self-defeating. It may make matters worse if a relatively expensive supplementary food is promoted, as a measure to prevent malnutrition, and the higher cost leads to a reduction in total energy intake. There is no easy answer. The problem must be tackled the hard way — by education, child welfare, the promotion and maintenance of breast feeding, improvement of the environment, and production of sufficient food of all kinds for the population. Limited resources should be concentrated upon an accessible vulnerable target. Much may be left undone, but to attempt everything is to dissipate resources and accomplish nothing.

REFERENCES

Bates C J, Prentice A M, Paul A A, Prentice A, Sutcliffe B A, Whitehead R G 1982a Riboflavin status in infants born in rural Gambia and the effect of weaning food supplement. Transactions of the Royal Society of Tropical Medicine and Hygiene 76: 253–258

Bates C J, Prentice A M, Prentice A, Paul A A, Whitehead R G 1982b Seasonal variations in ascorbic acid status and breast milk ascorbic acid levels in Gambian women in relation to dietary intake. Transactions of the Royal Society of Tropical Medicine and Hygiene 76: 341–347

Bleiberg F M, Brun T A, Goihman S and Gouba S 1980 Duration of activities and energy expenditure of female farmers in dry and rainy seasons in Upper Volta. British Journal of Nutrition 43: 71–82

Bleiberg F M, Brun T A, Goihman S and Lippman D 1981 Energy expenditure of male farmers in dry and rainy seasons in Upper Volta. British Journal of Nutrition 45: 505–515

British Medical Journal 1981 Bilateral amblyopia and race. British Medical Journal 283: 88

Coward W A, Lunn P G 1981 Biochemistry and physiology of kwashiorkor and marasmus. British Medical Bulletin 17: 19–24

Dawson C R, Schwab I 1981 Malnutrition's role in blindness. Lancet ii: 813–814

De Maeyer E M 1976 Protein-energy malnutrition. In: Nutrition in preventive medicine. WHO Monograph Series No 62. World Health Organization, Geneva. Ch 2, 23–54

Dobbing J 1982 Maternal nutrition, breast feeding, and contraception. British Medical Journal 284: 1725–1726

Dugdale A E 1971 An age-independent anthropometry index of nutritional state. American Journal of Clinical Nutrition 24: 174–176

Dugdale A E, Lovell S 1981 Measuring childhood obesity. Lancet ii: 1224

England R 1978 More myths in international health planning. American Journal of Public Health 68: 153–159

Golden M H N 1982 Protein deficiency, energy dificiency and the oedema of malnutrition. Lancet i: 1261–1265

Golden M H N, Golden B E 1981 Trace elements. British Medical Bulletin 37: 31–36

Gopalan C 1968 In: Calorie deficiences and protein deficiencies. McCance and Widdowson eds; Churchill, London p 49

Gordon J E, Chitkara I E, Wyon J B 1963 Weaning diarrhoea. American Journal of Medical Science 245: 345–377

Hendrickse R G, et al 1982 Aflatoxins and kwashiorkor: a study of Sudanese children. British Medical Journal 285: 843–846

James W P T, Trayhurn P 1981 Thermogenesis and obesity. British Medical Bulletin 37: 43–48

Jelliffe D B 1966 The assessment of the nutritional status of the community. WHO Monograph Series No 53. World Health Organization, Geneva

Keller W, Donoso G, De Maeyer E M 1976 Anthropometry in nutritional surveillance: a review based on results of the WHO Collaborative Study on Nutritional Anthropometry. Nutrition Abstracts and Reviews 46: 591–609

Lancet 1981 Oral therapy for acute diarrhoea. Lancet ii: 615–617

Lunn P G, Watkinson M, Prentice A M, Morrell P, Austin S and Whitehead R G 1981 Maternal nutrition and lactational amenorrhoea. Lancet i: 1428–1429

Lunn P G, Whitehead R G, Coward W A 1979 Two pathways to kwashiorkor. Transactions of the Royal Society ot Tropical Medicine and Hygiene 73: 438–444

Mann G V 1980 Food intake and resistance to disease. Lancet i: 1238–1239

McLaren D S 1974 The great protein fiasco. Lancet ii: 93–96

National Center for Health Statistics 1976 Growth charts. (HRA 76—a1120 vol 25: 3) United States Department of Health, Education and Welfare, Public Health Service, Health Resources Administration, Rockville, MD

Paul A A, Muller E M, Whitehead R G 1979 The quantitative effects of maternal dietary energy intake on pregnancy and lactation in rural Gambian women. Transactions of the Royal Society of Tropical Medicine and Hygiene 73: 686–692

Platt B S 1962 Tables of representative values of foods commonly used in tropical countries. Medical Research Council Special Report Series No 302. Her Majesty' Stationery Office, London

Prentice A M, et al 1980 Dietary supplementation of Gambian nursing mothers and lactational performance. Lancet i: 886–888

Puffer R C, Serrano C V 1973 Patterns of mortality in childhood. PAHO Scientific Publiation No 262. Pan American Health Organization, Washington DC

Roberts S B, Paul A A, Cole T J, Whitehead R G 1982 Seasonal changes in activity, birth weight and lactation performane in rural Gambian women. Transactions of the Royal Society of Tropical Medicine and Hygiene 76: 668–678

Rowland M G M, McCollum J P K 1977 Malnutrition and gastroenteritis in The Gambia. Transactions of the Royal Society of Tropical Medicine and Hygiene 71: 199–203

Rowland M G M, Barrell R A E, Whitehead R G 1978 Bacterial contamination in traditional Gambian weaning foods. Lancet i: 136

Rutishauser I H E 1973 Food intake studies in pre-school children in developing countries: problems of measurement and evaluation. Nutrition London 27: 253–261

Scrimshaw N S, Taylor C E, Gordon J E 1968 Interactions of nutrition and infection. WHO Monograph 57. World Health Organization, Geneva

Sommer A, Hussaini G, Tarwotjo I, Susanto D, Soegharto T 1981 Incidence, prevalence and scale of blinding malnutrition. Lancet i: 1407–1408

Waterlow J C, Jackson A A 1981 Nutrition and protein turnover in man. British Medical Bulletin 17: 5–10

Waterlow J C, Payne P R 1975 The protein gap Nature. 258: 113–117

Waterlow J C, Rutishauser I H E 1974 Malnutrition in man. In: Early malnutrition and mental development. Symposia of the Swedish Nutrition Foundation XII. Almqvist and Wiksell, Uppsala pp 13–16

Waterlow J C, Thomson A M 1979 Observations on the adequacy of breast feeding. Lancet ii: 238–242

Waterlow J C, Ashworth A, Griffiths M 1980 Faltering in infant growth in less-developed countries. Lancet ii: 1176–1178

Waterlow J C, Buzina R, Keller W, Lane J M, Nichaman M Z, Tanner J M 1977 The presentation and use of height and weight data for comparing nutritional status of groups of children under the age of 10 years. Bulletin of the World Health Organization 55: 489–498

Whitehead R G 1980 Use of food resources for infants and mothers In: More technologies for rural health. Proceedings of the Royal Society of London 209: 59–69

Whitehead R G, Coward W A, Lunn P G, Rutishauser Ingrid 1977 Comparison of protein-energy malnutrition in Uganda and The Gambia. Transactions of the Royal Society of Tropical Medicine and Hygiene 71: 189–195

WHO 1972 Report of a WHO Group of experts on nutritional anaemias. WHO Technical Report Series No 503. World Health Organization, Geneva

WHO 1974 Handbook on human nutritional requirements. WHO Monograph Series No 61. World Health Organization, Geneva

WHO 1977 Treatment and prevention of dehydration in diarrheal diseases. Guide for primary health care personnel. Scientific Publication No 336. World Health Organization, Geneva

WHO/FAO 1967 Requirements of vitamin A, thiamine, riboflavine, and niacin. WHO Technical Report Series No 362. World Health Organization, Geneva

WHO/FAO 1970 Requirements of ascorbic acid, vitamin D, vitamin B$_{12}$, folate and iron. WHO Technical Report Series No 452. World Health Organization, Geneva

WHO/FAO 1973 Energy and protein requirements. WHO Technical Report Series No 522. World Health Organization, Geneva

Zollner, Wolfram, Kellner (ed) 1977 The Second European Nutrition Conference. Round table on comparison of dietary recommendations in different European countries. Nutrition and Metabolism 21 No 4

Developmental disabilities

INTRODUCTION

During the last decade there have been major changes in the disability field. These have included changes in terminology, attitudes and policy on rehabilitation strategies. The two former have come about largely as a result of increasing public awareness of the needs and rights of the disabled, largely engineered by the disabled themselves or their advocates.

In spite of affirmative action, negative attitudes still continue to be the greatest obstacle faced by the disabled in their struggle to achieve their rights to live a normal life in the community. These attitudes relate to at least three main misconceptions of disability:

1. Ignorance of causes and consequent fear, superstition and rejection.
2. Shame and guilt of the stigma of disability leading to the person being isolated.
3. Under-estimation of the potential of the disabled person, leading to pity, overprotection and denial of opportunities; all of which result in under-achievement and apathy of the individual — the self-fulfilling prophecy.

Although there are local and regional variations in attitudes and superstitions, it is likely that the above misconceptions are pervasive in all societies. Lack of appropriate information in developing countries leads to even greater difficulties in shaking these attitudes and the models of expensive centralised and specialised western rehabilitation have made such services a difficult venture for governments of developing countries.

Changes in rehabilitation policy and strategy are beginning to emerge because of the increasing cost of health care in general and specialised rehabilitation in particular. Several international meetings in the past five to seven years have indicated new and more appropriate approaches. These are particularly relevant to developing countries which generally have very minimal provisions for the disabled.

This chapter will take the stand that disability prevention and rehabilitation are part of a spectrum of need which also incorporates social action as advocated by Acton (1979).

DEFINITIONS AND TERMINOLOGY:

The terms 'disability', 'handicap' and 'impairment' have recently been redefined during the International Year of Disabled Persons. The following is an appreviated terminology suggested by Rehabilitation International (UN, 1980):

'Impairment' is a permanent or transitory psychological, physiological or anatomical loss or abnormality of structure or function. Thus an impairment may be a missing or defective body part, an amputated limb, paralysis after polio, restrictive pulmonary capacity, diabetes, etcetera. It may be permanent, temporary, reversible or progressive.

'Disability' is any restriction or prevention of performance of activity resulting from an impairment in the manner considered normal. Disabilities as a result of an impairment may involve difficulties in walking, seeing, speaking, hearing, reading, writing, counting, lifting or taking an interest or making contact with one's surroundings.

A 'handicap' is a disability that constitutes a disadvantage for a given individual in that it limits or prevents the fulfilment of a role normally expected for the age, social and cultural situation of that individual.

A disability becomes a handicap when it interferes with doing what is expected at a particular time of one's life, such as caring for oneself, engaging in social interraction, communicating needs, learning in and out of school and developing a capacity for economic activity.

The term 'developmental disability' is also used here referring to any disorders of psycho-motor development occurring during the developmental period (birth to 18 years) and includes mental retardation, cerebral palsy, epilepsy, autism and other central nervous system defects. The American Association on Mental Deficiency (1973) defines mental retardation as follows:

'Significantly sub-average general intellectual functioning, existing concurrently with deficits in adaptive behaviour and manifested during the developmental period'.

Rehabilitation is the total process of restoring the disabled person to leading a normal life in the community. Traditionally, rehabilitation has been divided into several professionalised compartments:

1. Medical — concerned with medical and surgical treatment, aids and appliances.

2. Social — concerned with the daily living needs of the individual.

3. Psychological — concerned with the emotional and affective component.

4. Educational — dealing with schooling and training.

5. Vocational — the preparation for work and placement in an appropriate setting.

Western centralised rehabilitation facilities have developed whole cadres of rehabilitation professionals increasing the cost of rehabilitation. It has also taken the disabled person out of his home, family and community, and placed him in an artificial environment which has made resettlement more difficult (Acton, 1979).

In fact there are more cost effective ways of assisting the disabled by training in the community. Many disabled persons do not need outside help, their families have already rehabilitated them. The approach advocated by WHO (1980) in the manual 'Training the Disabled in the Community' avoids professionalised compartments and has the majority of rehabilitation tasks conducted by the family under the guidance of a community worker with the backing of community facilities.

This approach would save some of the costs of expensive institutions and is in keeping with principles of normalisation and integration, currently being accepted throughout the world.

CAUSES OF DEVELOPMENTAL DISABILITIES

It is true to say that a multiplicity of factors, sometimes operating singly such as the rubella virus, or in concert as in cerebral palsy, cause developmental disabilities. It is equally true that the effect of such agents can be multiple in that they may cause mental retardation, autism, deafness, motor paralyses or epilepsy.

Classification of etiology can be attempted from a number of standpoints, but the most useful one seems to be a developmental one. From this, epidemiological studies reveal varying prevalences of the different factors in different parts of the world which in turn lead to different priorities for prevention strategies. The phrase 'prevention is better than cure' is probably more appropriate for disabilities than almost any other disease group and the developmental approach is very helpful for timing and targeting prevention strategies.

The main agents causing mental retardation and developmental disabilities include infective (viral, bacterial, protozoal), parasitic, nutritional, traumatic, anoxic/asphyxial, toxic, genetic and socio/behavioural factors. Table 1 shows a useful developmental classification.

Since many of the factors listed are discussed in more detail in other chapters, attention here will be given only to the area of unidentified etiology and aspects of epidemiology and prevention that are relevant to disability.

Cases of unidentified etiology

A significant proportion of developmental disabilities especially mental retardation are of unidentified etiology. There are two main groups:

The first and smaller group includes the severely retarded biological cases which are undiagnosed because of lack of diagnostic facilities. Some of the factors listed in Table 1 may be causes.

Table 45.1 Developmental Classification

Timing	Factor
Pre-conceptual and at Conception	Genetic — single or multifactorial genes
	— chromosomal defects
	Infective agents — viral
	bacterial
	protozoal
	Anoxia
	Nutritional
Prenatal	Maternal disease
	Drugs
	Chemicals
	Physical agents (X-rays, ultra sound)
	Anoxia
Intranatal	Birth Trauma
	Prematurity
Neonatal	Severe jaundice
	Hypoglycaemia
	Infections — meningitis, etc.
	Anoxia
	Infections — Complications of common diseases (gastro-enteritis, measles, pertussis, poliomyelitis, parasites)
	Anoxia — due to inhalation of foreign bodies.
	·Meningitis, encephalitis
Post-neonatal	Poisoning — lead and others
	Head injuries
	Idiopathic Epilepsy
	Malnutrition
	Cultural-familial retardation
Other, Unknown	

The second and larger group making up approximately 75 to 80 per cent of all cases of mental retardation, are those due to socio-cultural-behavioural factors which can also be termed cultural-familial retardation.

Much controversy centres on the etiology of this syndrome concerning the genetic versus the environmental theory of causation (nature versus nurture).

Insinuations of racial and ethnic inferiority emerge. For the purposes of this discussion two major closely related environmental factors are of concern in etiology:

1. Lack of stimulation in the macro — and particularly the micro — environment of the young child and

2. Malnutrition.

In developing countries where malnutrition plays a major role in mortality, it has now clearly emerged as a factor in impairment of mental development. Hoorweg and Stanfield (1972) and Birch and Richardson (1972) showed significant impairment of general intelligence, learning ability and behaviour in children in Uganda and in Jamaica respectively who had previously been malnourished. Environmental deprivation is also involved as evidenced by deficiences in the micro environment provided for the young child by his mother (Cravioto and Delicardie, 1972, and Richardson, 1972).

In the United States, Heber et al (1972) showed a relationship between mild mental retardation in the mother and its development in the child. This may well be preventable in the latter by massive intervention at an early age. Providing a powerful argument against the genetic theory of etiology, striking increases in measured levels of intelligence and particularly language ability were demonstrated in children at high risk for mild mental retardation who were exposed to an intensive early stimulation programme as compared with control children who received no intervention.

A close interrelationship between maternal deprivation and the development of malnutrition with resulting withdrawal and decreasing responsiveness in the young child probably plays an important role in the genesis of learning impairment and low motivation for education. Other factors may include illegitimacy, illiteracy, high levels of unemployment, short spacing between children, loose family structure, inappropriate educational systems, late school entry and use of non-standard dialects when teaching is conducted in a standard language. Only massive social change and public education accompanying intervention in the environment of the young child could correct these problems.

EPIDEMIOLOGY

The causes of morbidity from disease are essentially the same as those causing mortality. Thus as a country's health and socio-economic resources improve, so will morbidity and disability patterns change. In poor countries with high infant mortality rates, the main causes of disability relate to the most prevalent infectious diseases such as poliomyelitis and malnutrition. In the more highly developed countries, developmental disabilities from these causes have disappeared and are replaced by cerebral palsy due to iatrogenic conditions resulting from sophisticated intensive care, and accidents, genetic disorders and congenital defects of unknown etiology.

Intermediate between these two are countries such as those of the Commonwealth Caribbean and some Latin-American countries who have infant mortality rates between 20 and 60 per 1000 and where poliomyelitis has been largely eliminated. Cerebral palsy due to inadequate maternal and child health services and mild mental retardation and middle-ear disease associated with poor socio-economic environment still exist.

Disabilities resulting from motor vehicle accidents and violence also take an increasing toll. Genetic diseases such as Down's syndrome become of increasing importance as malnutrition declines and more children survive the early years of life.

Prevalence

Exact prevalence figures of the types and causes of disability in developing countries are not widely available, though many surveys have been completed in Western countries.

Surveys are expensive and require a high level of expertise. Efforts are now being made to reduce this expense and complexity and to improve standards and terminology. Distinction needs to be made between different types and different causes of disability. Surveys usually examine the former, as the purpose is to determine the need for rehabilitation. This was the case in a Jamaican survey conducted in 1979 (Robinson and Sherlock) which estimated, from data collected in eight communities, that 80 000 of the one million children in Jamaica under 16 years of age had disabilities of various types. Eight per cent were estimated to be severely disabled.

To speculate and generalise a little, it seems probable that in least developed countries with a high infant mortality rate the disabilities which predominate due to high infection prevalence are physical, motor and visual disturbances. In intermediate countries, mental retardation and deafness come to the fore. In more highly developed countries, severe and multiple handicaps due to cerebral palsy, genetic diseases and learning disabilities become the main focus of attention.

Clinical studies, that is analysis of causes of disability in children presenting at clinics, are the main source of information and data from some of these are shown in Table 2. These are of limited value because of their

Table 45.2 Etiological factors in clinical studies of mental retardation.

	Jamaica (1)	(2)	Pakistan [3]	Singapore [4]
	%	%	%	%
Unknown	30.1	22.5	21.7	43.4
Genetic:	25.0	20.0	21.0	18.6
Chromosomal	18.0	12.6	4.2	16.2
Other		7.6	16.8	
Perinatal factors	19.6	18.3	14.8	10.0
Prenatal infections	4.2	7.25	0.5	
Post-natal infections	6.4	6.0	16.4	8.3
Seizure disorders (unknown cause)	7.2	6.5	8.2	4.3
Cultural-familial retardation	4.4	13.0		
Head injuries	0.8	1.6		
Period of study	1970–72	1975–78	1964–9	1963–71
Number of cases	500	1043	1000	2783

1. Thorburn, 1973
2. Thorburn, 1979
3. Hasan, 1971
4. Paul, 1972

bias towards the severer levels of disability which are in fact less frequent than the milder types. In mental retardation, for example, only the moderate and severe degrees tend to present at clinics due to the problems that they impose on the family especially in middle childhood when behaviour management problems emerge. The milder forms are not obvious, either because education is not compulsory or because classes are large and testing procedures do not exist to identify them.

Clinical studies also have a bias owing to the professional interest of the investigators. Even the level of awareness of the community and the availability of services will affect the age of referral and thus the severity of disability. For example, in a Jamaican study of this type (Thorburn, 1973) only 16 per cent of 500 referrals were under the age of four years. Six years later, 35 per cent were under four years with a concommittent increase in multiple handicap, especially cerebral palsy. A 1981 analysis showed 22 per cent under age one year and 67 per cent under age four.

Nevertheless, clinical analyses can indicate the principal causes of severe disability. Intervention in those amenable to preventive action avoids the high cost of rearing severely disabled children resulting in high cost benefits. This has been demonstrated in the French perinatal programme where preliminary research identified the perinatal period as the main target area. Prevention targets were clearly identified, measures carefully costed and specific programmes implemented (Lancet, 1976).

Developing countries that have eliminated poliomyelitis next need to look at the factors relating to perinatal care. In Jamaica with an infant mortality rate of approximately 18 to 20 per 1000, a recent perinatal study in 22 hospitals with 37 000 births (Thorburn, 1981a) revealed a mean perinatal rate of approximately 30 per 1000. The neonatal death rate was approximately half this and more than half of the infant mortality rate. Similar figures though somewhat higher, are now being found in the Eastern Caribbean countries (Boersma, 1982). Recent analyses of causes of disability in Jamaica in pre-school children (Thorburn, 1981b) indicate that at least 40 per cent of young childhood disability is of perinatal origin.

Clustering

Massive disability problems exist in many parts of the developing world which are caused by locally prevalent diseases, such as onchocerciasis in parts of Africa and vitamin A deficiency in India. Poliomyelitis is still widely prevalent either in endemic or epidemic form (see Dömök Chapter 24) and is proving difficult to eradicate. Even in relatively well developed health systems, such as in Jamaica, poliomyelitis recurred in epidemic form after a gap of 18 years in 1982.

There are also communities where specific deficiencies in iodine and thyroid problems exist. Consanguinity may lead to a high incidence of otherwise rare genetic conditions such as Cayman Disease, or Pendred's syndrome. Similarly there are racial differences in certain genetic diseases. The haemoglobinopathies are common while certain inborn errors of metabolism are rare in black populations. The whole subject of epidemiology of congenital defects is also extensive. For example, there is considerable variation in prevalence of neural tube defects with low prevalence rates in black populations and high rates in specific areas of European countries (Stevenson, 1966). The prevalence of these defects also changes across the north-American continent with the highest rates on the western coast.

SURVEILLANCE

Surveillance is limited by expense and by lack of international standards. In recent years intelligence tests are being less accepted because of labelling and discrimination and medical classifications have value only in prevention. The requirements of the disabled in planning for intervention necessitate classifications based on problems and needs such as those suggested by WHO (1980).

A major contribution would be more uniform methods of describing types of disability with acceptable classifications of etiology. Analysis of clinical case loads could then lead to development of a centralised registry serving the functions of placement, coordination and planning of services as well as prevention.

PREVENTION

This can be described at three levels: primary, secondary and tertiary. At each level, general and specific measures can be taken.

Primary prevention is directed at the elimination of etiological factors causing damage to the brain or sensory organs. General preventive measures include general improvement in health care, reduction of malnutrition, provision of safe water supplies, proper disposal of waste and refuse, improvements in childbearing practices, encouragement and maintenance of breast feeding and balanced diets.

Specific preventive measures will depend on locally prevalent diseases. Clearly the elimination of poliomyelitis, diphtheria, pertussis and measles by immunisation would be of the highest priority. Rubella and mumps immunisation assume greater importance in countries where infant mortality rates have been reduced.

Genetic diseases

The commonest single identified genetic cause of mental retardation in almost any country is Down's syndrome. The general frequency is approximately one in 800 births. In developing countries the prevention of genetic diseases by counselling and prenatal diagnosis has to be considered in the context of social practices in family planning. Most tropical countries have high birth rates and motivation towards family planning is low. Genetic counselling techniques must therefore be modified in the light of cultural practices and beliefs. Experience of genetic counselling in Jamaica relating mainly to chromosomal abnormalities has indicated that the vast majority of patients who request genetic advice are either from middle-class families or are older women who already have a large family. These factors need to be considered when embarking on other types of preventive services — prenatal diagnosis and newborn screening. Both of these are expensive and cost benefits must be carefully considered. Newborn biochemical screening requires several prerequisites including:

1. A readily identifiable population.
2. A favourable cost benefit analysis for undertaking screening.
3. A reliable test which is cheap and easily carried out.
4. A capacity to change the management of the disease being identified.
5. An ability to handle problems that may arise.

Many developing countries do not have the infrastructure to carry out such a programme. A very general approach to the prevention of genetic disease could include encouraging childbearing only between the ages of 20 and 35 years and discouraging intermarriage.

Prenatal infections

The prominent prenatal infections are rubella and syphilis, both preventable. There have been at least three epidemics of rubella in Jamaica since 1965. Unfortunately, it cannot be treated as can syphilis and immunisation is therefore an important procedure. Though expensive it can be shown to be cheaper than providing special education for the children affected.

One unknown factor is cytomegalic inclusion disease (CMV). This condition may be a common infection in the Caribbean as in other parts of the world. However, there is great variability in the extent to which the foetus is affected where the mother is infected with CMV. Unfortunately, development of a CMV vaccine is only in the early stage.

Post-natal infections

These are tragic and avoidable causes of mental retardation and other developmental disabilities which are directly related to poor health care both preventive and curative. Inadequate diagnosis and treatment of meningitis, complications of whooping-cough, measles, diphtheria and prolonged dehydration from gastro-enteritis are all common associates of high infant mortality rates.

Handicap of perinatal origin

A multipronged prevention programme will be necessary to reduce handicap of perinatal origin. Reports of the French perinatal programmes (Wynn and

Wynn, 1976) and analysis of the Jamaican situation (Thorburn, 1981) led to the following ten objectives being identified for a Jamaican prevention programme:

1. To reduce the number of births in mothers under 20 and over 35.
2. To increase measles and rubella immunisation.
3. To increase the quality and extent of antenatal coverage from 16 weeks of pregnancy to delivery.
4. To decrease the incidence of smoking and the use of alcohol, cannabis and other drugs.
5. To decrease the number of small-for-dates and premature babies.
6. To ensure minimum standards for delivery and newborn care including:
    a) proper resuscitation equipment;
    b) the means of keeping a baby warm;
    c) bilirubinometers in maternity units;
    d) simple devices for treating neonatal jaundice (phototherapy units).
    e) training in minimum standards of intranatal and newborn care.
    f) development of a minimum standards protocol.
    g) training all appropriate staff from primary to tertiary care.
7. To increase the bonding of mothers and babies at birth.
8. To promote the early detection and treatment of jaundice in the newborn.
9. To improve the establishment and maintenance of breast feeding.
10. To improve services for early detection and early intervention by the training of community personnel.

Some of the above are primary and others are secondary preventive measures and most would require public education in addition to improved and extended health care.

Secondary prevention is effected when a disease episode has already occurred but early diagnosis and treatment prevent permanent damage. Examples include the metabolic screening of newborn babies for early identification of phenylketonuria and dietary treatment and the provision of intensive care for newborn babies at risk due to insults such as prematurity or jaundice in the neonatal period.

Tertiary prevention must be applied when damage to the central nervous system has already occurred but early identification and intervention can result in amelioration of the effects of the damage and prevent the impairment from becoming a disability or the disability from becoming a handicap. This is perhaps the most controversial area of disability prevention and where it merges with rehabilitation.

MANAGEMENT

The role of the health services in the management of persons with disabilities is clearly an important one but not always readily assumed in developing countries. In the Jamaican survey (Robinson and Sherlock, 1979), only 2.8 per cent of the estimated disabled children in Jamaica were receiving services. This situation is fairly typical of developing countries (WHO, 1980).

Approaching the needs of the individual at various times during his lifespan, medical care although the first service usually received is not necessarily the most important one as the intervention most required will usually be in the area of training. The most important health roles are early identification, diagnosis, counselling and the initiation of intervention measures. The aim should be to keep the child developing as normally as possible in the mainstream of his family. It is the delays in acquisition of developmental skills that cause the negative reactions on the part of families and rejection and isolation of the child in his or her community. Fostering positive attitudes is a crucial role of health workers. The manner in which information is conveyed to the family and the practical usefulness of this information will make all the difference to the future of the child.

Specific programmes

Diagnosis and Evaluation: Early diagnosis is an essential prerequisite for effective rehabilitation. In medically untreatable conditions, early diagnosis should lead immediately to early intervention, counselling and parent training. These can be incorporated into maternal and child health or primary health care services or any other infrastructure serving the family. Developmental screening can be included among the general tools of assessment of growth, nutrition and development taught to primary health care workers. It can also be included in day care centres and preschool programmes.

A modified 'Road to Health' or 'Child Health Passport' showing developmental milestones could also be used for screening children at high risk from handicaps. Referral of screening failures could be made to a small team including a doctor, social worker or public health nurse or perhaps a teacher. More specialised personnel such as those in psychology, speech, physiotherapy and occupational therapy might be available for consultation at a regional level. For the older child, the educational system should provide a guidance service for learning and behavioural problems.

The importance of involving the community in rehabilitation work, as in primary health care, cannot be overemphasised. All persons who have any involvement with the child need to be informed as to how they can help.

Special education

Because of the numbers of children needing special education, specific professional training will be required for staff involved in this field if formal education is to be extended to all disabled as well as to all normal children. In many countries, special education was the primary target for parent action because of the concern about the inability of regular programmes to accept or effectively teach such children. Because of the magnitude of this problem, this responsibility has to be undertaken by government. Special education is, however, expensive and particularly in developing countries where regular education is not compulsory or widespread. Although the ideal situation of mainstreaming — including children with disabilities in the regular classroom — has been widely advocated and practised in western countries, it is still controversial. It may not be appropriate in the near future in some developing countries where classes may have fifty or more children. Units for disabled children placed in regular school settings would seem to be at least one feasible and less restrictive option.

Vocational rehabilitation and training:

It should be possible to incorporate vocational rehabilitation for all disabled individuals into an overall scheme. While the general aim is for integration of the disabled person into open employment, it is also recognised that developing countries have severe unemployment problems as well as negative attitudes which militate against the disabled in competition for jobs. Vocational rehabilitation therefore will not only have to provide training for disabled adults but will also be obliged to create employment opportunities through cooperatives and groups of disabled persons.

Social services:

Social welfare aspects tend to be the last to become financed in developing countries because of the expense involved. Here again a beginning could be an emphasis on community care, involving as far as far as possible, generic agencies in the community who can assist families.

There would seem to be only three justifications for removing a child from his home and into residential care:
1) Because parental care is inadequate;
2) Because special educational facilities are inaccessible;
3) Because the handicap is too severe for a family with poor resources to bear.

In choosing alternative forms of care, the first substitute for home care should be foster care. Where residential facilities are built, they should be limited to small units with a family structure and home-like appearance and integrated as much as possible into the community. They should be independent of schools or training institutions.

Manpower training aspects

The additional skills required by generic human service workers to handle the services described above can with some exceptions be provided by adding material to the regular training curricula or by giving short in-service training courses and seminars. Consideration can be given to the development of an indigenous worker trained specifically for screening abnormal development and/or home training, child rearing and behaviour management as described by Frankenberg et al (1970) and Thorburn (1981b). This is also the basis of the community based rehabilitation approach developed by WHO (1980). A major problem faced by developing countries lies in the delivery of health and rehabilitation services in the diffusely populated rural areas with poor communications. Indigenous health workers can be considered an acceptable alternative to the more expensive ideal of multidisciplinary services which could perhaps be provided in more densely populated areas. Supervision for primary rehabilitation workers is, however, vital and this requires increasing depth of knowledge and skills on the part of supervisory staff, whether they be the medical officer of health, public health nurse, social worker or a rehabilitation therapist.

The need for coordination and information

A wide diversity of service and training requirements is necessary if the disabled are to be fully served. As it is advocated that these should be integrated as far as possible into the regular services, coordination is vital. In many countries the delivery of services for the disabled have been started and continued by voluntary agencies. These need to be incorporated into an overall national plan. Several countries have attempted to develop national schemes, by establishing a council which uses the resources of voluntary, private, university and governmental agencies to help develop a national plan and to coordinate activities. The mode of operation of these councils varies from one country to another but often seems to be fraught with difficulties. Long established voluntary agencies seem to be reluctant to allow government to take over their services because of the loss of status that would result. There is also inter-agency rivalry and competition for resources. A more successful model seems to be an institute which devotes its activities to providing information, training and research and is not competitive with existing organisations in the provision of services (Roeher, 1978).

Another serious deficiency in developing countries is in the lack of appropriate information for all levels of society, from planners to primary health care workers. (Rehabilitation International report to UNICEF, 1980). WHO (1980) has made a major step forward in attempting to provide a rehabilitation manual for all types of disability, comparable to 'Where there is no doctor' (Werner, 1975). It is still being field tested. It will require modification and elaboration but will surely provide a basis for community rehabilitation along the lines of primary health care. In order to establish such a system, a network of community based home visiting workers of whatever type needs to be in place. The task of supervising a family member to train a disabled person requires time as well as training. Such a system would probably work best in conjunction with more sophisticated rehabilitation services at the regional level to which can be referred more difficult or specialised cases.

Finally, the newest and perhaps the most powerful resource which must not be neglected is the disabled individual. In many countries, groups of disabled persons are beginning to work together and to speak for themselves. They are often critical of the charity which has been meted out to them by well meaning voluntary organisations who perhaps have never previously consulted them. Such new trends need to be encouraged as it appears that the most serious barriers to the disabled, the attitudes of the public, are most effectively eliminated by disabled persons themselves.

REFERENCES

Acton N 1979 Address to the Symposium 'Disability and the developing World'. Rehabilitation International, 434 Park Avenue South, New York, N.Y. 10016.

American Association on Mental Deficiency 1973 Manual on Terminology and Classification in Mental Retardation. AAMD, Washington, D.C., Page 11.

Birch H G, Richardson S A 1972 The functioning of Jamaican school children, severely malnourished during the first two years of life. PAHO Scientific Publication 251, page 64.

Boersma R 1982 Personal communication.

Cravioto J, Delicardie E 1972 Environmental correlates of severe clinical malnutrition and language development in survivors from kwashiorkor or marasmus. IBID.

Frankenberg W K, Goldstein A, Chabot A, Camp C W, Fitch 1970 Training the indigenous non-professional: the screening technician. J Pediat 77: 504.

Hasan K Z 1971 Paper presented at the International Research Seminar on Vocational Rehabilitation of the Mentally Retarded. Figures obtained from final report: SRS Project, Department of Health Education and Welfare, United States.

Heber R, Garber H, Harrington S, Hoffman C 1972 Rehabilitation of families at risk for mental retardation. Progress Report Grant 16-G-56811. SRS, Department of Health Education and Welfare, U.S.A.

Hoorweg J, Stanfield P 1972 The influence of malnutrition on psychological and neurological development. PAHO Scientific Publication 251 Page 55.

Lancet Editorial 1976 October 30, Page 941.

Paul F M 1972 A statistical and clinical survey of mental subnormality in Singapore children. Paper presented at the First Conference on Special Education and Mental Retardation, Singapore.

Richardson S A 1972 Ecology of malnutrition: non-nutritional factors influencing intellectual and behavioural development. PAHO Scientific Publication 251, Page 101.

Robinson J, Sherlock H 1980 'Children at Risk'. A study to determine the number and needs of handicapped children in Jamaica. Jamaica Association for the Deaf, 9 Marescaux Road, Kingston 5, page 28.

Roeher G A 1976 International models for research utilisation. Research to Practice in Mental Retardation. Proceedings of Fourth Congress of the International Association for the Scientific Study of Mental Deficiency, vol. 1.

Stevenson A C, Johnston H A, Stewart M I P, Golding D R 1966 Congenital malformations. Supplement to Bulletin of WHO, vol. 34.

Thorburn M J 1973 An Analysis of 500 cases of mental retardation. Paper presented at the 18th Scientific Meeting of the Caribbean Medical Research Committee, Georgetown, Guyana.

Thorburn M J 1979 Long term needs of developmentally disabled children in Jamaica. A paper presented at the 24th Scientific Meeting of the Caribbean Medical Research Committee, Belize.

Thorburn M J 1981a Perinatal mortality in Jamaican hospitals. A paper presented at the Third International Conference of the Paediatric Association of Jamaica, Kingston.

Thorburn M J 1981b In Jamaica, Community aides for Disabled Pre-School Children. Assignment Children, 53/54.

U N Economic and Social Council 1980 Childhood disability: its prevention and rehabilitation. Report of Rehabilitation International to the Executive Board of UNICEF. E/ICEF/L1410.

Ward N 1979 Polio immunisation and travel. British Medical Journal, 2: 1072.

Werner D 1977 'Where there is no Doctor'. Hesperian Foundation, Palo Alto, California 94320.

WHO 1980 'Training the Disabled in the Community' An experimental manual published by WHO, Geneva.

Wynn M and Wynn A 1976 Prevention of handicap of perinatal origin. Foundation for Education and Research in Childbearing, London.

Mental illness

INTRODUCTION

The tendency for psychiatric disorders to be excluded from otherwise comprehensive descriptions of tropical medicine is only partially explained by the previous scarcity of epidemiological data. Other factors to be considered include the belief that certain mental illnesses, such as depression, only occur in Europeans and that a physical illness always has a greater priority for treatment than a mental illness; some physicians may believe that a psychiatric disorder is, in any case, best treated by a traditional healer and not by a physician at all.

This chapter attempts to modify these attitudes and to provide the reader with an introduction to the epidemiology of psychiatric disorder in a warm-climate country, as well as describing in outline the management of the more common mental illnesses.

Psychiatry may be regarded as a specialty of general medicine primarily concerned with the diagnosis and treatment of disorders of behaviour, mood or intellect. Some psychiatric disorders, however, are caused by malaria or epilepsy and it is often important, therefore, to establish whether or not a physical illness causes the mental illness.

The psychiatric disorders most commonly found in medical practice are the neuroses (anxiety and depressive neuroses, hysteria, and, more rarely, the obsessive compulsive neuroses and phobias). Physicians may also be consulted by patients with other difficulties such as alcohol dependence, drug addiction or because of marital or other relationship problems. The psychoses, such as schizophrenia, manic-depressive and organic psychoses, though less common than the neuroses, often require urgent treatment.

EPIDEMIOLOGY

In the last two decades, considerable advances in research methods have been made and the development of standarised clinical interviews, self report scales, and agreed criteria for psychiatric morbidity, have enabled a closer understanding of the epidemiology of mental illness. In a useful book by Leff (1981), entitled Psychiatry Around the Globe, the results of many such studies in tropical countries have been summarised. The frequency of schizophrenia in India, Europe or Africa is shown to be surprisingly similar, with an average of 2.4 per 1000; whilst the manic depressive psychoses, on the other hand, were somewhat less common (1.2 per 1000) (Table 46.1).

Closer agreement on the characteristic symptoms of mental illness has resulted in the diagnostic criteria now included in the International Classification of Disease or in the Research Diagnostic Criteria developed by Spitzer et al. (1975).

These semi-structured and standardised clinical interviews that are used in such community surveys are not the impersonal tools, described by some critics that dehumanize a patient, but on the contrary depend for their success on an interviewer having sufficient flexibility of clinical style both to relate to a patient as well as to rate defined symptoms. The Present State Examination (PSE) of Wing et al. (1974) is the standarised interview most widely used for determining the prevalence of psychoses, as well as the neuroses. Another schedule, the Standardised Psychiatric Interview (SPI) of Goldberg et al. (1970) is more useful when studying the neuroses, since psychotic symptoms are not always enquired after.

Self report scales, such as the 60 item General Health Questionnaire (Goldberg et al., 1972) are most valuable as screening devices to detect those subjects who score above a certain 'cut-off' point and so require a more lengthy personal interview. Visual Analogue Scales measure changes in mood over time and are useful when studying the response to treatment with an anti-depressant or when recording daily mood changes in the puerperium. They are also readily completed by subjects.

These questionnaires have already been satisfactorily translated into different languages for use in various transcultural studies. The PSE, for example, was translated into Yoruba, as well as into Hindi, for the International Pilot Study of Schizophrenia (World Health Organisation, 1974). It was found that, as long as participating psychiatrists were carefully trained, it was possible to obtain satisfactory reliability in the rating of psychiatric symptoms by psychiatrists within a research centre and also between psychiatrists at different centres. Some unexpected difficulties in translation were, however, found; 'the heart is weak' was the nearest linguistic equivalent to depression in the Yoruba language. The SPI has also been translated by Orley into Luganda and used by the author in a prospective study of postnatal depression in rural Ugandan women (Cox, 1983). Less difficulty was found translating 'depression' into the Luganda language, although 'depersonalisation' could only be translated in a very approximate way. Despite these difficulties, the reliability of the Luganda SPI, and also the accuracy of the interpreter, could be established by joint interviews with a bi-lingual corater present and found to be satisfactory.

Nevertheless, the use of such questionnaires in a culture different from the one in which the instrument was developed is open to the criticism that

Table 46.1: Prevalence Rates per 1000 from population surveys (Leff, 1981)

Population surveyed	Schizophrenia	Manic-depressive	Neuroses	Study
Taiwan Chinese	2.1	0.7	1.2	Lin (1953)
corrected for age over 15	3.7	1.1	2.1	
Taiwan aborigines	0.9	0.9	0.8	Rin and Lin (1962)
Taiwan Chinese	1.4	—	7.8	Lin et al. (1969)
Japaness	2.3	0.2[a]	3.0	Kato (1969)
N. Indians — Lucknow	2.5	1.1	27.1	Sethi et al. (1974)
N. Indians — Agra	2.2	1.3	12.6	Dube (1970)
corrected for age over 15	3.8	2.2	22.2	
W. Bengal	4.3	—	1.5	Elnagar et al. (1971)
corrected for age over 15	8.0	—	2.7	
N. Indians — Lucknow	1.9	1.9	20.4	Thacore et al. (1975)
corrected for age over 16	3.3	3.3	36.5	
W. Bengal	2.8	—	67.0	Nandi et al. (1975)
W. Bengal	2.2	1.5	16.8	Nandi et al. (1980)
Sri Lanka	3.8	—	25.2(60.0)[b]	Wijesinghe et al. (1978)
corrected for age over 15	5.6	—	89.0+	
S. African Cape Colored	—	—	54.0	Gillis et al. (1968)
Ethiopian town	—	—	41.7	Giel and Van Luijk (1969a)
corrected for age over 15	—	—	63.5	
Ethiopian village	—	—	51.4	Giel and Van Luijk (1969b)
corrected for age over 15	—	—	93.1	
Buenos Aires women (15)[b]	—	—	287.0	Tarnopolsky et al. (1977)
Buenos Aires men (15)[b]	—	—	94.0	
Ugandan women (18–65)	—	—	269.0	Orley and Wing (1979)
Ugandan men (18–65)	—	—	174.0	
Camberwell women (18–65)	—	—	106.0	Wing et al. (1978)
Camberwell women (18–65)	—	—	135.0	Bebbington et al. (1980)
Camberwell men (18–65)	—	—	58.0	

[a] Rate for 6 months only.
[b] Corrected for cases not interviewed.

any similarity in the frequency of psychiatric disorders might be an artefact of the instrument itself. A further criticism is that some questionnaires are not sufficiently sensitive to local variation in the presentation of mental illness and could even be a covert form of research imperialism.

Because of these and other limitations, Kapur et al. (1974) developed a questionnaire specifically for use in an Indian setting. In this questionnaire appropriate emphasis was given to the somatic presentation of mental disorder, the frequency of sexual worries, as well as including an interview with a relative and a physical examination. This interview also carefully distinguished between a possession state, as might occur in a religious ritual, and a delusion of control more characteristic of schizophrenia.

These and other questionnaires depend for their success on the interviewer obtaining a detailed description of recent psychiatric symptoms, as well as making careful observations of the mental state. The interviewers need careful training to establish good rapport with a respondent, as well as practice in the use of probing questions sufficient to enable accurate ratings to be made.

It is readily apparent that most of these interview schedules are based on familiar clinical methods whereby a psychiatric diagnosis is made from an accurate history and from the psychiatrist making systematic observations of the patient's behaviour. Thus, psychiatrists are nowadays less preoccupied with the more lengthy clinical methods that are derived from psychoanalysis. The 'analyst's couch' image of the general psychiatrist is perhaps a rather false stereotype. Furthermore those clinical skills that are required to diagnose a mental illness need also to be gained by doctors other than psychiatrists as well as by nurses or other health workers.

Community surveys

One of the first community studies of mental illness to be carried out in an African country was that by Giel and Van Luijk (1969) in Ethiopia. They personally interviewed a sample of 384 villagers and found 33 (9%) to have 'conspicuous psychiatric morbidity' that included 16 with a neurosis, six enuretics and yet only one subject had schizophrenia. Even more striking was the finding that of the outpatients attending a medical clinic at a General Hospital in Addis Ababa, 18 per cent had a psychiatric disorder and only 9 per cent an infectious illness. Furthermore, at a nearby rural health centre, psychiatric illness was again found to be a more common reason for medical consultation than an infectious disease.

Even if such findings are disregarded as biased observations made by European psychiatrists on atypical patients, other studies from Africa have generally found a similar rate of psychiatric morbidity. Orley interviewed rural Ugandans using the PSE and found 20 per cent of the villagers to have a psychiatric disorder; the majority being depressed (Orley & Wing, 1979).

Postnatal depression in Africans was no less frequent than that found in a similar study of Scottish women; 10 per cent of mothers had this disabling disorder (Cox, 1983).

Such high rates of psychiatric disorder are not particularly surprising since, in Britain, no less than 14 per cent of general practice consultations are because of a psychiatric problem (Shepherd et al., 1966). Nevertheless, for a psychiatric disorder to be as common as an infectious illness in a tropical country is of particular importance when planning medical services and establishing appropriate psychiatric training for doctors and paramedical personnel.

Even students at African universities are not immune to mental illness, and German and Arya (1969) found 10 per cent to have psychiatric problems. Indeed university students may be particularly vulnerable to any social or political change in a country. During the repression by the military regime in Uganda, for example, we found that the number of referrals to the Mental Health Clinic at Makerere University more than doubled and unexpected suicides also occurred (Cox & Muhangi, 1975).

Multi centre studies

(a) Schizophrenia

The International Pilot Study of Schizophrenia, carried out in six different countries, showed clearly that schizophrenia is recognised in cities as distant as Washington and Moscow and countries as contrasting as Columbia and Nigeria. Furthermore, certain symptoms such as delusions of control (when the will is experienced as being taken over by an outside force), hearing several imaginary voices (usually derogatory) talking about the patient, thought disorder or catatonia were also widely recognised as characteristic of this disorder (WHO 1974). Because schizophrenia may become a chronic illness that requires regular medication, the needs of such schizophrenic patients may even determine the clinical priorities as well as allocation of resources for the psychiatric services. Thus one third of a consecutive series of male admissions to Butabika Mental Hospital in Uganda were found to have schizophrenia (Cox, 1978) and a similar proportion of schizophrenic patients were also admitted to Harare Hospital in Zimbabwe (Buchan et al., 1981). The acute organic psychoses, such as delirium tremens, were the next most frequent diagnosis but manic depressive psychoses were found to be rare in these hospital series.

When the schizophrenic patients in the WHO study were followed up after five years, it was found that the prognosis was better than might be expected in a developed country. The explanation for this interesting finding is not clear but may be because of varying attitudes towards unemployment, different family infrastructures as well as different cultural determinants of stigma.

(b) Alcoholism

Another multi-centre study using standardised case finding criteria was that undertaken by WHO into alcohol related problems in Zambia, Scotland and Mexico (Ritson, 1983). Although high levels of alcohol related problems were found in all these countries, there were also important national differences. Both the Zambians and Mexicans, though having lower levels of annual per capita consumption than the Scots, when they did drink were much more likely to drink to drunkenness. This 'all or none' style of drinking gave rise to high levels of physical and social problems which were as evident in the rural areas as in the newly expanding towns. By contrast with the Scots, the Mexican women were more abstemious and were also much more distressed by their husbands' drinking.

The Royal College of Psychiatrists (1979) in Britain was sufficiently confident of the findings of surveys on alcoholism to provide a guide to the upper limits of daily drinking; adverse consequences were likely if more than four pints of beer, four doubles of spirits or a standard size bottle of wine was consumed daily. Much lower levels were thought safe for women.

(c) Primary care

For the general physician, perhaps the most important of the multicentre studies is that reported by Harding et al. (1980) in a collaborative investigation of 1624 patients who attended primary health facilities in four different countries — Columbia, India, Sudan and the Philippines. Using stringent criteria 13.9 per cent were found to have psychiatric morbidity but only a third were correctly detected by the health workers and many such patients had undergone unnecessary and also expensive investigations.

CLASSIFICATION OF PSYCHIATRIC DISORDER

Mental illnesses are often traditionally classified according to local beliefs about their cause. Thus among the Ganda they are divided into those that came by themselves or were caused by witchcraft, the strong and weak illnesses and those regarded as Western or non-Western (Orley, 1970). 'Madness' and epilepsy are examples of non-Western strong illnesses caused by witchcraft, whilst polio is a Western illness not caused by witchcraft and usually treated by Western medicine.

For the psychiatrist the major psychoses are customarily classified into schizophrenia, manic-depressive and the organic psychoses. The affective disorders are also further divided into the unipolar disorders, characterised by recurrent episodes of depression, and bipolar illnesses, in which depression alternates with mania. The precise classification of other major illnesses, such as schizo-affective psychosis, puerperal psychoses or the brief reactive psychoses is still more controversial.

These nosological debates are perhaps less relevant for a harassed physician who is confronted by a psychotic patient requiring urgent treatment and this doctor may prefer the more pragmatic scheme devised by Swift (1977) that groups patients according to their main presentation. Three such categories are described:

1. Agitated, restless or aggressive;
2. Withdrawn, mute or just sits;
3. Bizarre or strange behaviour.

The psychiatric diagnoses to be considered for each of these presentations are described in Table II, which also outlines the psychiatric management. These diagnoses are made by first obtaining an accurate personal and family history and then by making careful assessments of the patient's behaviour and mental state. The physician must also determine whether conflicts in the family may have caused stress and a knowledge of the sociocultural background is also necessary before deciding whether or not the patient has a delusion.

It is clear, therefore, that familiarity with the presenting symptoms of the major illnesses, such as depression, is essential for any medical officer. The most common symptoms of depression include a diurnal variation of mood, early morning waking, psychomotor retardation, as well as self-blame and suicidal thoughts and usually, but not always, the patients describe a low mood.

Schizophrenia is usually diagnosed from the typical deterioration over several years, as well as by the patients having certain particularly characteristic symptoms, such as delusions of control, thought broadcasting or certain types of auditory hallucinations. Other hallucinations or delusions are not usually diagnostic of a schizophrenic illness. Disorientation and clouding of consciousness only rarely occur in schizophrenia and are more typical of an organic psychosis. These differential diagnoses are by no means easy, and often only a careful follow-up of a patient may clarify the diagnosis further.

To be confident of these psychiatric diagnoses some physicians may require a refresher course in psychiatry. The textbook by Anderson and Trethowan (1979), which includes a glossary of psychiatry terms may therefore be useful, and if a more detailed description of mental illness is required then the Companion to Psychiatric Studies edited by Kendell and Zealley (1983) is also a valuable resource.

Several categories of psychiatric disorder, not included in Table II, are now described.

Puerperal psychoses

The puerperal psychoses are defined as those mental illnesses that occur within six weeks, and usually within two weeks, of childbirth. The family is often distressed by this illness that comes at a time of expected happiness; more especially if the mother has had an uneventful pregnancy.

Table 46.2: Modes of Presentation of Major Mental Illness (from Swift, 1977)

Mode of presentation	Differential diagnosis	Special Characteristics	Management Outpatient	Management Inpatient	Treatment if referred
Withdrawn, mute (can't or won't talk); just sits.	Schizophrenia (catatonic)	Withdrawal may be extreme; appear indifferent or may smile inappropriately; previous history variable (often personality has been mildly withdrawn with few friends); onset sudden or slow; if first episode, patient usually young	Inpatient treatment usually necessary.	Ensure hydration and nutrition. Activating tranquillizer (trifluoperazine). Nurses should be sympathetic but stimulate and arouse patient.	As under inpatient. ECT may be required.
	Depression	Patient usually responds in some way; appears sad, has lost interest, expresses hopelessness. History of anorexia, insomnia, perhaps weight loss, constipation, impotence. Duration often weeks, possibly previous episodes. Usually over 25 years of age.	Evaluate suicidal potential; ensure that responsible relative can supervise, or arrange for inpatient care. Give amitryptiline (or other antidepressant) (*not* chlorpromazine).	Ensure hydration and nutrition. Precautions to prevent suicide; drugs as under outpatient. Refer if no response in 2 weeks or if suicide precautions are inadequate.	Adequate suicide precautions. Antidepressant drug therapy. ECT if depression severe or does not respond to drug therapy.
	Hysteria	Sudden and short duration often in response to an upsetting episode; personality is attention-getting, dramatic, changeable. Commonest in adolescent girls.	Supportive psychotherapy; mild sedation; relatives advised to ignore symptoms.	Not usually necessary (or just overnight).	Explore frightening experience or troubled relations in family. These patients often derive help from traditional healers.

| Mode of presentation | Differential diagnosis | Special characteristics | Management | | Treatment if referred |
			Outpatient	Inpatient	
	Acute confusional state	Confusion; diorientation; frequent hallucinations; history of fever, illness, or special stress.	Determine and treat cause; control symptoms with chlorpromazine. Hospitalize if severe.	Same as outpatient. Refer for specialist care if no improvement in 2 weeks.	Treat underlying condition; maintain fluids diminishing dose of chlorpromazine or diazepam.
	Delirium tremens	Onset at night; confusion; extreme fear; vivid hallucinations (especially visual and tactile); tremors; history of heavy drinking (often discontinued a few days earlier).	Should hospitalize.	Hydrate, large doses of vitamin B (injection), sedate with chlormethiazole. (Avoid chlorpromazine, barbiturates). Check physical status carefully.	Sedate with Heminevrin for several days to prevent withdrawal seizures. If motivated give support in an abstinence programme.
Agitated Restless Perhaps Aggressive	Hypomania	Overactive, overtalkative, flight of ideas, possibly grandiose ideas, euphoria; usually no confusion or hallucinations; history of previous episodes of hypomania or depression; previous personality sociable; usually over 25 years old.	Control with chlorpromazine; psychotherapy; advice to relatives. If not possible to control, refer for inpatient treatment.	Same as outpatient; if no improvement in 2 weeks, refer for specialist attention.	May need Haloperidol if excitement persists. Sedation for some weeks to avoid early relapse. Consider Lithium therapy.
	Schizophrenia (paranoid or excited catatonic)	Often paranoid delusions, affect flat or inappropriate, hallucinations (usually auditory), self-neglect; often has history of previous psychotic episodes; young adult.	Treat as outpatient if no threat to self or others; chlorpromazine or other major tranquillizer; supportive psychotherapy. Refer to hospital if no improvement.	Same as outpatient. Refer for specialist attention if no response in 2 weeks.	In addition to major tranquillizer and psychotherapy, patient can benefit from occupational therapy and group living. Consider maintenance phenothiazine e.g. fluphenazine

	Hysteria	Sudden and short duration often in response to an upsetting episode.; personality is attention-getting, dramatic, changeable. Commonest in adolescent girls.	Supportive psychotherapy; mild sedation; relatives advised to ignore symptoms.		
Bizarre (strange) behaviour	Schizophrenia	Withdrawal may be extreme; appears indifferent or may smile inappropriately; previous history variable (often personality has been mildly withdrawn with few friends); if first episode, patient usually young.	Inpatient treatment usually necessary.	Ensure hydration and nutrition. Activating tranquillizer (trifluoperazine). Nurses should be sympathetic but stimulate and arouse patient.	Intra-muscular slow-release injection of fluphenazine decanoate (Modecate) or fluphenazine ethanthate (Moditen,) valuable for outpatient medication — at three week intervals.
	Post-epileptic automatic behaviour	History of seizures, bite-marks on tongue or scars from having fallen; symptoms disappear after sedation and rest.	Anticonvulsive therapy (phenobarbitone) and management of patient with epilepsy.	Not usually necessary	Enlist help of relatives to ensure regular taking of anti convulsant.

A depressive illness is generally the most common puerperal psychosis but, in a tropical country especially, a physical illness such as pelvic sepsis or breast abscess causing an organic psychosis must be excluded. The management may include the admission of the mother, as well as her baby, to a psychiatric unit where any physical illness is also treated. Electroconvulsive therapy is particularly effective if a mother is suicidal and unable to care for her baby. Phenothiazines or antidepressants may also be indicated depending on the diagnosis made. Once the acute illness is treated the mother will benefit from being able to talk about her guilt and describe any negative feelings she may have towards her baby. Contraceptive advice is mandatory since the risk of a further puerperal psychosis may be as high as one in four.

It seems likely that some women with a puerperal psychosis will consult a traditional healer in the first instance. Among the Ganda, for example, the illness is likely to be regarded as the traditional mental illness 'amakiro' caused by promiscuity during pregnancy and characterised by the belief that a mother may wish to eat her baby (Cox, 1979).

The range of emotional disorders in the puerperium is shown in Table 43.3 which also indicates the professional who is most likely to make the diagnosis and to undertake treatment. The possible contribution of a traditional healer to the management of a puerperal mental illness has not been established.

Attempted suicide

A patient who attempts suicide by taking a drug overdose or by wrist-slashing may evoke a strong hostile reaction from a physician. However, although overdoses are less common in a tropical than in a European country, they are more likely to increase because of the widespread availability of psychotropic drugs. Many patients who take an overdose have marked social problems and some have a depressive illness that requires urgent treatment. It is necessary therefore to recognise and to treat such depressed patients and in others it may be appropriate to answer the 'cry for help'. The risk of a completed suicide in patients from Western countries is highest in elderly depressed widowers. Alcoholics are also a particularly vulnerable group.

Epilepsy

In warm climate countries the psychiatrist is often regarded as a specialist in epilepsy; although not all psychiatrists regard themsleves in this way. It is, however, necessary for the general physician also to have expertise in the management of epilepsy. The disturbance of behaviour in an epileptic

Table 46.3: Spectrum of mood disturbance in puerperium

	Postnatal blues	Puerperal Neuroses	Puerperal psychoses
Frequency	50–70%	15%(13% — depression)	0.2% Affective psychoses — common Schizophrenia — rare Organic psychoses
Peak Time of Onset	4–5 days after childbirth	2–3 weeks after childbirth	1–3 weeks after childbirth
Duration	Usually 2–3 days	4–6 weeks if treated Up to 1 year if untreated.	6–12 weeks
	Severe 'blues' may →	Postnatal Depression →	Affective Psychosis
Profession of First Contact	Midwife (Hospital) Obstetrician	Midwife (Community) Health Visitor Medical Officer	Midwife Health Visitor Medical Officer Psychiatrist (rare)
Psychiatric Referral	Virtually never	Unusual	Common — especially if marked behaviour disturbance.
Treatment	Nil; but observation if severe	Counselling Antidepressants	Admit to mother & baby unit Phenothiazines; Lithium; ECT Counselling and advice on further pregnancies.

patient may occur during the aura or may be a manifestation of the seizure itself. It may also occur in the post ictal confusional state.

Temporal lobe epilepsy is especially common in a tropical country and this diagnosis is often missed. A history of brief episodes of altered consciousness, with motor automatism or a grand mal fit should alert the physician to this diagnosis. Only occasionally can uncinate fits, Lilliputian hallucinations or feelings of unexpected familiarity (déjà vu) be described. The electroencephalogram may show spikes in the temporal lobe and sleep-recordings or sphenoidal leads may sometimes be useful if the diagnosis is still in doubt.

Hysterical fits are considered in the differential diagnosis but generally occur in public places, and are never associated with a loss of consciousness. The 'advantage' (secondary gain) to the patient is usually obvious. A too hasty decision that a seizure is hysterical is rarely wise.

Acute psychotic reactions

Psychiatrists who work in tropical countries often describe patients with a sudden onset of perplexity, anxiety, paranoid delusions and auditory hallucinations that are precipitated by severe social stress and occur in a patient who has a good pre-morbid personality. These 'brief reactive psychoses' are particularly common in Africa and the Caribbean. Their initial presentation may be similar to schizophrenia but the prognosis is usually more favourable. The diagnosis of schizophrenia in such patients, because of its social stigma, should usually be avoided.

Most respond rapidly to treatment with phenothiazines but it is also necessary to understand and to alleviate any causal psychological stress. This latter task is often particularly difficult if an expatriate physician is unfamiliar with the local culture. However, a relative and interpreter/nurse can help considerably and can also advise whether or not a traditional ceremony should be carried out.

Alcohol dependence syndrome and other drug abuse

Delirium tremens and its treatment has already been described in Table II. Other mental illnesses caused by alcohol excess include dementia, depression and Korsakov's psychosis and they also require urgent treatment. A diagnosis of alcohol dependence is made by a history of morning shakes, with relief drinking and frequent blackouts. The social problems, however, are often disabling and include child abuse, aggression to the spouse, as well as social deprivation and road traffic accidents. Treatment may include warnings about the social consequences of drinking as well as informing the patient that alcohol is a poison that can cause serious heart and liver disease. Treatment with Antabuse is sometimes worthwhile and in some countries Alcoholics Anonymous gives valuable support.

When the medical resources are scarce, however, the physician may only have time to treat the complications of alcohol abuse and not the underlying cause. Some patients when shown their abnormal liver function test results or confronted by the prospect of social decline or death may stop, or substantially reduce, their alcohol intake themselves. Programmes of education about the consequences of alcohol abuse, restrictions on advertising and on easy availability are also a valuable part of preventive psychiatry.

Heroin and barbiturate drugs can cause a physical dependence syndrome; barbiturate withdrawal can also cause delirium tremens. The treatment of heroin addiction is best carried out in hospital but before admitting such a patient the risks of serum hepatitis must be assessed by screening for the Hepatitis B surface antigen. Methadone may prevent heroin withdrawal symptoms but itself causes physical dependence and large doses of Diazepam are therefore more preferable to control the withdrawal symptoms. Although the symptoms of an amphetamine psychosis are similar to those found in schizophrenia, restlessness and dilated pupils are particularly characteristic of amphetamine psychosis. Amphetamine substances can usually be found in the urine.

Cannabis

Cannabis abuse is common in most countries and, whilst often causing a state of transitory euphoria, may also aggravate an existing mental illness such as schizophrenia, or may possibly itself induce a psychosis. Overall, its harmful effects are increased if more concentrated extracts ('hash-oil') are taken but, unlike alcohol, barbiturate or heroin addiction, physical withdrawal symptoms do not generally occur.

Mental handicap

In all societies a proportion of the population have such limited intelligence that they cannot care for themselves. A small number of such individuals will also have epilepsy or other evidence of birth injury whilst a few will have a hereditary disorder such as phenylketonuria or a chromosome abnormality such as Down's syndrome. Some mentally handicapped individuals also have a co-existing mental illness.

In countries with limited medical resources it is difficult to determine whether special services for the mentally handicapped should be provided and there is a danger of raising an expectation of care that cannot be fulfilled. The causes of mental handicap are discussed by Thorburn in Chapter 45. The psychiatrist is involved when a mental illness develops or possibly if the family needs counselling. However nurses, clinical psychologists and social workers can also advise on the provision of services for the handicapped. Usually patients with mild handicap are best supported within their own families, and mental hospitais are not usually an optimum environment for long term care.

Psychogeriatrics

No account has so far been included in this chapter of dementia, which is one of the most pressing clinical problems in European countries at the present time. The problems to the provision of health services in Britain as a result of the increase in the proportion of the population over 65 years are considerable but are perhaps less pressing in many tropical countries. It is also not certain at the present time how these societies will meet the needs of their mentally ill elderly, as longevity increases.

GENERAL PRINCIPLES OF PSYCHIATRIC TREATMENT

Familiarity with the use of supportive psychotherapy is essential for the treatment of most mental illnesses and psychotherapy as a blend of art and technique is an important skill to acquire. Thus the docotor and nurse who are empathic and can give time without becoming over-involved will relieve much distress and also improve compliance with drugs (see Bloch,1979). For the expatriate physician such psychotherapy is particularly difficult because of language problems, racial discrimination or being unfamiliar with the local culture. Such difficulties need not necessarily be insurmountable and the author, for example, found that good rapport with a patient can be obtained even when an interpreter is present in an interview.

Before any psychiatric treatment is given however a provisional diagnosis must be made. A patient was once observed tied to his bed in the middle of the hospital compound and only approached by a nurse at meal times; no diagnosis of this patient's paranoid psychosis had been made and so treatment with phenothiazines that would have prevented this inhumane management had not been given.

Drugs

The drugs that are commonly used in psychiatry are few. All doctors therefore should be familiar with the indications, dosage and side effects of chlorpromazine or trifluoperazine, a long-acting intramuscular phenothiazine such as fluphenazine, flupenthixol and an antidepressant drug such as amitriptyline or imipramine. These antidepressants must be prescribed for at least three weeks at maximal dosage (usually 50 mg three times a day) before any improvement is to be expected and if the patient is warned of the likely side effects such as dry mouth or blurred vision their compliance will improve. The more recent tetracyclic antidepressants such as Mianserin are expensive but have fewer side effects and are possibly more safe if an overdose is taken.

The optimum storage of psychotropic drugs and their method of transport to up-country clinics need also to be carefully considered by pharmacists. Fluphenazine, Chlorpromazine, Stelazine and antidepressants must be constantly available at remote health centres to avoid relapse in some patients. Diazepam is only rarely indicated in the treatment of a neurosis and its use as a placebo is strongly to be discouraged.

The drugs most commonly used in Botswana at a time when the only psychiatrist was developing a community-based service are shown in Table IV. The medical personnel authorised to administer such drugs and the point in health care delivery where they are available is also indicated. A psychiatric nurse can usually prescribe psychotropic drugs but whether the village health worker can use chlorpromazine or phenobarbitone even in an emergency is more controversial.

Table 46.4 Suggested drugs and their possible use by health personnel

Health post
FAMILY WELFARE EDUCATOR OR ENROLLED NURSE
   possibly Chlorpromazine (oral)
         Phenobarbitone   *for emergency use only*
         Benzhexol

Health clinic
REGISTERED AND STATE ENROLLED NURSE
   Chlorpromazine (oral and IM)
   Phenobarbitone
   Phenytoin
   Benzhexol
   Vitamin C (Placebo)
   Flupenthixol Decanoate

District general hospital
PSYCHIATRIC NURSE
   Above drugs and
   Amitriptyline
   Imipramine
   Diazepam
   Haloperidol (oral, IM, drops)
   Perphenazine (oral, IM)
   Benztropine mesylate (IM and IV)
   Chlormethiazole
MEDICAL OFFICER
   Above drugs and
   lithium carbonate
   primidone
   clonazepam

SPECIALIST PSYCHIATRIST
   Above drugs and
   Thioridazine
   Dexamphetamine
   Carbamazepine
   Ethosuximide

The excited patient

In the management of an excited patient firm but not excessive restraint is important and a patient never needs to be tied down, handcuffed or treated like a criminal since he is not to blame for the illness and medical treatment is the priority.

It is unwise to argue with any delusionary beliefs a patient may have but to remain calm and ensure that adequate staff are available to give reassurance if the patient becomes excited or violent. The patient should be told that he is unwell and needs treatment in hospital. An explanation should also be given to the family about the nature of the mental illness and its likely response to treatment.

Electroconvulsive therapy

ECT is not commonly used in some tropical countries perhaps because patients with a serious depressive illness may only rarely attend for treatment. However, ECT is particularly effective in the treatment of severe endogenous depression especially when there is a high risk of suicide or if the patient has lapsed into stupor. Only rarely is ECT the treatment of choice for schizophrenia, unless a coexisting depressive illness is present or if the patient is catatonic.

Familiarity with the indications for ECT is essential and the psychiatrist or psychiatric nurse may need assistance from a general physician with its administration. A physical examination prior to ECT is mandatory to exclude recent cardiac disease or a severe infection, atropine pre-medication reduces the likelihood of cardiac arrhythmias, and oxygen is given prior to administering the anaesthetic and short-acting muscle relaxant. A mouth gag prevents damage to the teeth. ECT should usually be given unilaterally to the non dominant hemisphere to reduce the likelihood of any recent memory impairment. A modified grand mal fit must be induced for ECT to be effective but may only be apparent by observing small movements of the toes. Several ECT treatments are usually given before any improvement is noticed but only rarely are more than eight treatments necessary. ECT is given twice or three times a week but the patient's mental state must be carefully assessed between treatments. Permanent memory loss or brain damage does not occur when ECT is administered correctly but transient memory impairment and headache are common.

Although a psychiatric nurse should have had sufficient experience of the indications for ECT and its administration the co-operation of the medical officer is also helpful. If no anaesthetist is available, the physician may need to give the anaesthetic and only under exceptional circumstances should ECT be given without an anaesthetic or muscle relaxant.

Psychoanalysis

Intensive 'uncovering' psychotherapies such as psychoanalysis are rarely available in tropical countries and are also time-consuming and generally require highly trained therapists. Nevertheless psychoanalytic theory contributes substantially to the understanding of a mental illness and also provides an intellectual stimulus to any physician wishing to understand a patient's psychopathology in more detail. Unconscious defence mechanisms, such as projection, sublimation or denial, are valuable clinical concepts and will increase the physician's understanding of the patient, as well as enabling greater tolerance of the patient's anger. Psychoanalytic concepts may also enable some physicians to gain limited insight into the way they customarily react to their own patients and to their colleagues.

Behaviour therapy

Behaviour therapy based on learning theory is a less time-consuming treatment than other psychotherapies and is therefore often useful in the treatment of the anxiety neuroses, phobias or the more rare obsessive-compulsive neuroses (Wilkinson & Latif, 1974). Most physicians should understand the principles of relaxation therapy in the treatment of anxiety states and also be familiar with desensitisation in the treatment of agoraphobia. The more complex behaviour therapies such as 'flooding' when a patient has prolonged exposure to the phobic object or 'modelling' when the therapist handles the feared object require collaboration with an interested medical colleague or with a clinical psychologist.

Community services

Many neurotic patients seek help from traditional healers and the physician's tasks with such patients is also to prevent unnecessary or even dangerous medical investigations being carried out. Familiarity with the way neurotic patients present is often useful. In Botswana such patients are referred to as the 'palpitations people', whilst in Uganda they commonly complained of headache.

The physician needs to know where he fits in to the process of referral within the provision of a mental-health service. A psychiatrist may be available to advise a medical officer, but is more likely to be treating those patients who do not respond to therapy or who have developed a chronic illness. Some patients with acute mental illnesses may nevertheless be referred to the mental hospital even if it is very far distant and many such mental hospitals are overcrowded and understaffed. Furthermore these patients may be treated by doctors who cannot understand the patients' language and who may also be a long way from their relatives. It is therefore usually preferable for patients to be treated within their own community and then to educate other health professionals and the family in the management of the mental illness.

If a patient is referred to the mental hospital then detailed written information including the current medication should accompany the patient; a brief note 'this patient is confused; please see', or 'this patient is disturbed' is unhelpful and perjorative labels such as 'mad' or 'crazy' that belittle a patient's suffering and perpetuate stigma should also be avoided.

District hospitals

Many governments have a policy to build small psychiatric units in district general hospitals that are staffed by psychiatric nurses. These have been successfully developed, in Lesotho for example, but only flourish if the nurse is fully supported by the local general hospital administration as well as by the physicians and surgeons. A regular visit by a psychiatrist is therefore particularly important to discuss any difficult patients and also to authenticate the nurse's own professional skills.

The decentralisation of psychiatric services and their development at district and village level goes some way towards the provision of psychiatric treatment for patients who otherwise receive no treatment at all. In this way overcrowding of mental hospitals is also reduced and patients are treated closer to their own home communities. The development of half-way homes, hostels and rehabilitation villages for those with chronic mental illnesses such as schizophrenia or with mental handicap is often worthwhile. For this policy to succeed the integration of mental health care into primary care is essential so that all medical personnel are able to diagnose and treat the psychoses and to recognise the more common neuroses.

The physicians have a major influence on the development of mental health services by the encouragement they give to colleagues who treat the mentally ill as well as by their involvement in decision-making about the allocation of funds. A further task that involves the physician is to ensure that a country' mental health legislation enables humane psychiatric care. In a survey of such legislation, Harding and Curran (1978) showed how Senegal had promoted the community approach to mental health care by its legislation, whilst in other countries a voluntary admission to mental hospital would only be possible if the legislation were to be changed. Compulsory admission to a mental hospital may be an infringement of personal dignity and also perpetuates the stigma of mental illness.

The task of the psychiatrist

A psychiatrist's task in a developing country may be somewhat different from that elsewhere since the psychiatrist is more likely to work alone and to be overburdened by unlimited clinical work as well as by teaching demands. It is therefore necessary that these few psychiatrists develop their own professional interests and improve their skills as teachers. Whilst professional training should equip the psychiatrist for many such tasks, for those trained in a Western country some additional experience on return to the home country is often necessary. The ability to collaborate with others in the teaching, clinical and research tasks is also crucial; meeting colleagues from different countries also stimulates such collaboration and can also relieve professional isolation.

The development of a university department of psychiatry that encourages research and maintains high standards of clinical care increases the likelihood that psychiatry trainees are recruited as future teachers. Furthermore the training of nurses and medical students will also improve and so assist in the task of bringing psychiatric treatments to patients suffering from mental illness who may otherwise receive no treatment at all.

REFERENCES

Anderson F W, Trethowan W H 1979 Psychiatry, 4th edition, Concise Medical Textbooks, London

Bloch S 1979 Supportive psychotherapy. In: An introduction to the Psychotherapies (Ed S. Bloch) Oxford University Press

Buchan T, Nyasayswa R L, Futter G E 1981 Community psychiatric services in Mashonaland, Zimbabwe. Central African Journal of Medicine, 27: No 6, 111–116

Cox J L 1978 Psychiatric diagnoses of 94 Ugandan male patients admitted to Butabika Hospital, Uganda. African Journal of Psychiatry 3, 4, 103–107

Cox J L 1979 Amakiro: A Ugandan puerperal psychosis? Social Psychiatry 14: 49–52

Cox J L 1983 Postnatal depression: a comparison of Scottish and African women. Social Psychiatry 18: No. 1, 25–28

Cox J L Muhangi J 1975 Problems of mental illness among Makerere University students, with special reference to the period 1970–1973 East African Medical Journal 52: 615–618

German G A, Arya O P 1969 Psychiatric morbidity amongst a Ugandan student population. British Journal of Psychiatry, 121: 461–479

Giel R, Van Luijk J N 1969 Psychiatric morbidity in a small Ethiopian town. British Journal of Psychiatry 115, 149–162

Goldberg D 1972 Detecting psychiatric illness by questionnaire. Maudsley Monograph 22, Oxford University Press, Oxford

Goldberg D, Cooper B, Eastwood M R, Kedward H B, Shepherd M 1970 A standardised psychiatric interview for use in community surveys. British Journal of Preventive and Social Medicine 24: 18–23

Harding T W, De Arango M V, Baltazar J et al. 1980 Mental disorders in primary health care: a study of their frequency and diagnosis in four developing countries. Psycholigical Medicine 10: 231–241

Harding T W, Curran W J 1978 Promoting mental health through the law. World Health Organisation Chronicle 32: 109–113

Kapur R L, Maevika Kapur, Carstairs G M 1974 Indian Psychiatric Interview Schedule (IPIS) Social Psychiatry 9: 61–69

Kendell R E, Zealley A (Eds) 1983 Companion to Psychiatric Studies. Churchill Livingstone

Leff J 1981 Psychiatry around the globe: a transcultural view. Dekker: New York

Orley J H 1970 Culture and mental illness. East African Publishing House, Nairobi

Orley J H, Wing J K 1979 Psychiatric disorders in two African villages. Archives of General Psychiatry 36: 513–520

Ritson, E B 1983 Community response to alcohol related problems Report on WHO project (in press)

Royal College of Psychiatrists 1979 Alcohol and alcoholism. Tavistock Publications

Shepherd M, Cooper B, Brown A C, Kalton G W 1966 Psychiatric illness in general practice. Oxford University Press, London

Spitzer R L, Endicott J, Robins E 1975 Research diagnostic criteria. Biometrics Research. New York State Department

Swift C R 1977 Mental health: a manual for medical assistants and other rural health workers. African Medical and Research Foundation, Nairobi

Wilkinson, J C N, Latif K 1974 Common neuroses in general practice John Wright and Sons

Wing J K, Cooper J F, Sartorius N 1974 Measurement and classification of psychitric symptoms, Cambridge University Press

World Health Organisation 1974 Report of the International Pilot Study of Schizophrenia, Vol 1: Geneva

I am most grateful to Professor T. Buchan, Department of Psychiatry, University of Zimbabwe, and Dr. E. B. Ritson, Royal Edinburgh Hospital for their helpful comments on this chapter.

Cardiovascular diseases

INTRODUCTION

In the last few decades there has been an increasing awareness of the importance of cardiovascular disorders in the tropical and developing countries. A fascinating and complex pattern of problems has been revealed, involving many conditions previously thought to be peculiar to the temperate and advanced countries, as well as a variety of unusual conditions possibly peculiar to the tropics. The geographic distribution and the differences in the natural history of many cardiovascular problems in the tropics afford an important opportunity for research into aetiology and pathogenesis, and the findings could be of value to preventive medicine internationally. In this chapter only a few of the major problems will be considered and references will be given to other conditions occurring in the tropics but not discussed in this chapter.

RHEUMATIC HEART DISEASE

Rheumatic fever and its streptococcal antecedents have been covered in the chapter on 'Streptococcal Infections and their Sequelae'. Some reference will, however, be made to rheumatic heart disease as it probably remains the most important single cardiac problem in the tropical and developing countries today and there are indications that the incidence has not diminished. A great deal is written about differences in the clinical presentation of rheumatic fever (RF) and rheumatic heart disease (RHD) in tropical situations. Suffice it to say that there is no single standard natural history of rheumatic fever; there are a number of natural histories possible. Once rheumatic fever has developed, the presence or absence of extracardiac manifestations is of little importance. What matters is whether or not carditis occurs, for in the absence of carditis, RHD seldom if ever develops in patients with only arthritis or chorea, even during recurrences of RF in such patients. There is some suggestion that mortality may be higher during the acute attack in some tropical areas, and in a Jamaican study, 11 per cent of children admitted with acute RF died within a few weeks of progressive pancarditis. A further 11 per cent were dead within one to three years, mainly from cardiac failure. In other situations, for example Kuwait, acute rheumatic fever in childhood appears to be a mild condition. Chronic valvular lesions are undoubtedly present at a much earlier age than seen in Europe or America and the term 'juvenile' mitral stenosis is widely used. Many children presenting with acute RF under the age of 10 years already have well-established chronic valvular lesions.

Rheumatic fever and RHD have long been known to be diseases of poor socio-economic conditions but there is no convincing evidence to indicate that nutritional status is a factor determining individual susceptibility or determining prognosis. On the other hand, it seems clear that the attack rate of RF is determined by several factors. Firstly, by the duration of throat carriage of group A streptococcus, and by the failure to eradicate strepto-cocci which results in a high attack rate. The importance of this variable to tropical situations is devastatingly apparent. Where diagnosis is delayed and uncertain and where treatment is inadequate or absent the attack rate must inevitably be high. Secondly, the attack rate is influenced by the degree of immune response to the antecedent streptococcal infection. In Uganda, antistreptolysin O titres have been estimated in young children from birth to six years. Some 40 per cent of individuals at all age groups had ASO titres above 200 units. Titres of over 600 units appeared in the first six months of life and were present in 18 per cent of children aged seven months to two years. A high frequency of raised ASO titres has also been reported from Sri Lanka, Sudan, Thailand, Pakistan, Nigeria and Yaounde (Cameroon). These findings are consistent with the early age at which rheumatic heart disease is seen in the tropical countries.

Prospects for prevention

There has been a recorded decline in the incidence of acute RF in the developed countries over the past 70 years. The decline has been progressive and began long before the advent of antibiotics. We are clearly observing a socio-economic phenomenon and not one produced by modern thera-peutics. Given the present social and economic situation of many tropical countries, we may anticipate an increase in RF and RHD as urbanization, school attendance and group organization increase. Only in those tropical countries which have considerably improved their economic status has the prevalence of RHD markedly declined, for example Japan, Israel, Singa-pore, Hong Kong. Primary prevention of rheumatic fever with early detec-tion and treatment of group A streptococcus infection is not feasible in most tropical countries. Secondary prevention is more practical and aims at long term prophylaxis in those who have had rheumatic fever. A WHO inter-national study revealed sustained follow-up in half of the patients and regular prophylaxis is only half of these. There is little room for complacency in the public health management of this condition which is likely to remain a major problem for a long time to come.

BLOOD PRESSURE AND HYPERTENSION

The literature on blood pressure and hypertension in the tropics has been considerable in the past decade. Hypertension is clearly a widespread and common phenomenon in almost every tropical/warm climate country. The underlying causes of this hypertension, whether in the tropics or elsewhere, remain an intriguing but unsolved problem and we are probably no nearer an answer than we were a decade ago. In most populations the mean blood pressure level in males and females rises progressively with increasing age. This gradual increase in blood pressure is not a benign process and there is an increasing morbidity and mortality as the pressure rises. This general statement holds true for most communities in the tropical and subtropical countries but within these areas, there are communities in which blood pressure does not rise with age and in which the problems of essential hypertension appear to be virtually non-existent. These exceptional minorities are of considerable interest, for they may provide us with the information needed to unravel the aetiology of essential hypertension, and to prevent the damage which high blood pressure produces in the cardiovascular, cerebrovascular and renal systems.

Low-pressure communities

These include many relatively small and isolated communities such as New Guinea highlanders, Kalahari bushmen, Pacific islanders, Australian aborigines and East African nomads. Studies in these groups strongly suggest that blood pressure need not necessarily rise with age and we are faced with the problem of deciding whether these groups are normal, or whether they merely reflect the presence of such factors as chronic infection, parasitism or malnutrition which somehow prevent the usual rise of blood pressure with age. Critical to this problem is the question of whether these isolated, often tropical, communities are capable of developing higher blood pressures under changed environmental circumstances. There is some historical suggestion from studies in East Africa carried out in the 1920s, the 1930s and in the 1960s that communities in which blood pressure·does not rise with age may after a long period of time manifest the usual rising blood pressure pattern with age seen in most advanced countries. From studies carried out on young nomadic warriors in Kenya entering the army, there is evidence that a changing environmental situation may produce significant elevations in systolic blood pressure over a period of only two years. In New Guinea, the rural highlanders have low levels of blood pressure which do not rise with age, while an urban wage-earning group in Port Moresby show much higher blood pressures in the older age-groups, particularly among older women. Similar differences have been described between urban and rural Zulu subjects in South Africa. The obvious questions which arise from all these observations concern those features which these low-pressure groups might have in common and those factors which might possibly be concerned in producing an increase in their blood pressure levels.

Obesity

An obvious physical feature of all these low-pressure groups is their lean body build and their virtual absence of obesity. In situations in which the blood pressures rise consequent to environmental change there is usually an increase in body fatness. We still do not know, however, whether the observed rise in blood pressure with increase in body bulk is directly due to the accumulation of adipose tissue. The evidence suggests that the relationship is neither direct nor simple.

Salt intake

There is considerable circumstantial evidence to suggest a positive correlation between the level of salt intake and the prevalence of hypertension in a community. In almost all the low-pressure groups salt intake is very low, and in those groups in whom a rise in blood pressure has been associated with social and environmental change the salt intake has almost always increased considerably. There is also evidence that genetic factors may play an important role in determining which individuals are sensitive to salt ingestion.

Socio-cultural factors

A striking feature of the low-pressure groups is their social structure and its perpetuation by virtue of cultural or geographic isolation. The possibility that higher blood pressures represent a failure of adaptation to a changing environmental situation is fascinating and in the studies on Zulu subjects, the investigators observed that the 'individuals most likely to be hypertensive were those who maintained traditional cultural practices and who were unable to adapt successfully to the demands of urban living'.

Conclusions

From these studies of isolated communities it appears that ageing itself need not cause blood pressure levels to rise. It has been suggested that some trigger mechanism causes blood pressure to rise to a critical level at which the subsequent rate of rise is determined by the blood pressure itself. Any cause of minor but sustained rise in blood pressure could act in this way.

Obesity is such a factor but the relationship of blood pressure to weight seems indirect. Within this complex relation between body fatness and blood pressure may, however, lie the key to the story of essential hypertension, and salt metabolism which could possibly provide the additional factor linking body weight to blood pressure changes.

Hypertension and renal disease

In most tropical countries the majority of subjects seen with raised blood pressures are classified as having essential hypertension, particularly those individuals over 40 years of age. Some cases are associated with underlying renal disease and it is this group which produces most of the severe hypertension problems admitted to hospital. Thus impressions gained from hospital admission studies tend to over-emphasize the contribution of renal disease to the community pattern of blood pressure. Studies in several tropical countries indicate that *glomerulonephritis* accounts for a large proportion of those individuals diagnosed at necropsy as having had hypertensive heart disease, particularly in those under 30 years of age. The importance of glomerulonephritis is further emphasized by clinical studies in women found to have severe hypertension in pregnancy; in the majority of these subjects renal biopsy has revealed proliferative glomerulonephritis. The cause of the glomerular lesions is unknown, and both the streptococcus and malaria are considered to play important aetiological roles. *Pyelonephritis* is also of importance, particularly in male subjects in whom urethral stricture of gonococcal aetiology may be the underlying cause.

CORONARY HEART DISEASE

In earlier publications it was not unreasonable to state that 'CHD is excessively uncommon in most tropical and subtropical countries, except amongst those small sections of the community which are affluent and which follow the way of life common to most temperate economically advanced countries'. The situation has changed considerably, probably over the past decade, and hospital admission rates for coronary heart disease (myocardial infarction; angina pectoris) are now no longer negligible in many tropical countries. Reports from India, Pakistan, Egypt, Ivory Coast, Nigeria and China all indicate that there is a small but substantial number of hospital admissions for CHD and indeed, coronary care units exist in many of these countries. It is extremely difficult to be sure of the true size of the CHD problem either on the hospital scene or in the community and it is even more difficult to know the rate at which it might be increasing. Most reports are hospital-based and lack sufficient detail to allow conclusions to be drawn and the community surveys available are often of a limited nature. All that can be claimed at present is that it is no longer uncommon and that it is probably increasing in frequency. In general it would probably be reasonable to state that racial or ethnic factors appear to be irrelevant to the incidence of CHD, except insofar as they condition or determine social class and economic status. Thus, in South Africa, the white population has a rate of CHD higher than that obtaining almost anywhere else in the world, while it is uncommon in black South Africans. Nevertheless, some things do change, even in South Africa, and an autopsy study on black patients dying of cardiovascular disease in Johannesburg showed that 12 per cent of all cardiac deaths in 1976 were due to myocardial infarction compared with 1 per cent in 1959/ 960.

Aetiology

Virtually all CHD occurs on the basis of moderate to severe atherosclerosis, although not every person with severe atherosclerosis necessarily suffers from CHD. Epidemiological studies have shown clearly that populations with a high incidence of CHD have more atherosclerosis and higher blood cholesterol levels than populations with a low incidence of CHD. High blood cholesterols, moderate to severe atherosclerosis and high rates of CHD occur only where the usual diet is high in total fat, saturated fat and cholesterol and the marked international differences in death rates from CHD have been positively correlated with differences in nutritional intakes of saturated fats and cholesterol. In addition to this basic dietary-induced hypercholesterolaemia, it is well established that where CHD is endemic, it occurs with increased frequency in association with certain characteristics present in the population or in its environment. These 'risk factors' include hypertension, cigarette smoking and diabetes mellitus as well as physical inactivity, obesity and soft drinking water.

The coronary arteries, aortas and cerebral vessels of tropical communities are certainly not inherently immune to atherosclerosis and cases of CHD have been reported from many tropical/developing countries. In Ibadan, Nigeria, ten cases of myocardial infarction were seen among 8000 necropsies over a 10-year period; four of these were due to coronary embolism from bacterial endocarditis or EMF. In Johannesburg, South Africa, an intensive search of clinical and pathologic records for a 10-year period, in a hospital serving a population of 600–700 000 Africans revealed 30 cases with proved myocardial infarction. The African (Johannesburg) subjects with myocardial infarction showed a marked male predominance, more hypertension, diabetes and obesity and a higher educational, occupational and economic status when contrasted with a control group. They were less physically active and were more often habituated to a diet relatively high in animal protein and fat. In the majority of cases the blood lipid levels were elevated. Studies in Pakistan indicate a high prevalence of atherosclerosis and of myocardial infarction in medico-legal autopsies.

Prevention of coronary heart disease

At the present time, CHD is the major cause of death in most affluent, economically advanced countries of the world, whether in the temperate regions or in warm climates such as Australia or South Africa (white). There is considerable evidence that the essential prerequisite for the effective presence of CHD in a community is a way of life which includes a high intake of saturated fat and cholesterol as part of a general high calorie intake. If this is true, and the support for this 'nutritional-metabolic' concept is very well based on pathologic, experimental and epidemiological findings, then the developing countries of the tropics and subtropical world may expect an increasing incidence of CHD with increasing affluence. The coronary-prone dietary background is one which we have all been taught to regard as highly desirable and any attempt to present its disadvantages might well be misunderstood. Public health authorities and those concerned with agriculture and food production might do well, however, to keep in mind the nature of the problem when discussions are held on the patterns of food production and manufacture and on healthy eating habits in children and adults.

CARDIOMYOPATHY AND IDIOPATHIC CARDIOMEGALY

Over the past few decades there have been many reports from tropical and temperate countries of obscure forms of heart disease, primarily affecting the heart muscle. These cases are characterized by cardiomegaly and congestive heart failure and at necropsy, there is ventricular dilatation and hypertrophy, without any obvious cause and with no specific pathological features. To the pathologist the problem is one of *idiopathic cardiomegaly*; to the clinician it usually presents as a problem of primary myocardial disease or *cardiomyopathy*. The clinical term 'congestive cardiomyopathy' is used to describe any cardiomyopathy patient who presents in persistent congestive heart failure with a large heart, gallop rhythm and often with evidence of valvular insufficiency. Most cases of idiopathic cardiomegaly will present in this way, but not all cases presenting as congestive cardiomyopathy will have idiopathic cardiomegaly.

The term idiopathic cardiomegaly should only be used by the pathologist when he has excluded severe hypertension, valvular disease, ischaemic heart disease, intra-/or extracardiac shunts, cor pulmonale and systemic diseases affecting the heart and producing a secondary myocardial disease, for example amyloidosis, haemachromatosis and myocarditis. Idiopathic cardiomegaly may nevertheless be associated with certain clinical or epidemiological features such as the postpartal state and alcoholism or it may follow certain forms of myocarditis. In many cases, no aetiological factors or associations are apparent and it seems likely that idiopathic cardiomegaly or cardiomyopathy represents the end-stage of myocardial damage produced by a variety of possible agents.

A recent WHO/ISFC report on the definition and classification of *cardiomyopathies* defines them as 'heart muscle diseases of unknown cause'. They are classified as *dilated, hypertrophic* or *restrictive*. Heart muscle disease of known cause or associated with disorders of other systems is called *specific* heart muscle disease. This excludes myocardial disorder due to coronary artery disease, congenital abnormalities, valvular heart disease or hypertension (systemic or pulmonary).

Epidemiology

The restrictive cardiomyopathy seen in tropical countries is usually endomyocardial fibrosis. Hypertrophic (obstructive) cardiomyopathy is rare but authenticated cases have been described, for example in black South Africans. Dilated (congestive) cardiomyopathy appears to be not uncommon in many tropical countries and this may be due to a genuine increase in prevalence or it may merely reflect the inadequacy of diagnostic facilities which would allow a more specific diagnosis. A series of cases was described in Africans in Johannesburg and referred to as 'nutritional heart disease'. Later there was evidence which suggested that these were not due to malnutrition but were probably associated with alcohol ingestion. Series of cases have also been described from Nigeria, Jamaica, South India, Colombia, Venezuela and Brazil and there are also several large series from temperate countries such as the United States and Japan. In many of the North American reports, alcohol appears to be an important aetiological factor. The role of viral and parasite infections with associated myocarditis is uncertain, but this may well be the most important background factor in the tropical cardiomyopathies.

Pathology of dilated cardiomyopathy

Dilatation and hypertrophy of the ventricles are the characteristic features. In most series the minimum heart weight is given as 350 g or over for women and 400 g or over for men, but the heart weight should be assessed in relation to bodyweight in the individual case. The trabeculae carnae are stretched and the myocardium at the left ventricular apex may be thinned. The mitral and tricuspid valve rings are dilated producing a functional incompetence. The atria are usually dilated and mural thrombi are frequently present in the atrial cavities and in the atrial appendages. The endocardial surface of the ventricles often shows small areas of opacity or even scattered areas of endocardial fibrosis. Ventricular thrombi are usually apical and their frequency varies from five to 20 per cent of cases in reported series. The coronary arteries are usually normal and even in countries where coronary artery disease is prevalent, it is often reported that the vessels in dilated cardiomyopathy are relatively free of atherosclerosis.

Clinical

The clinical features and natural history of dilated cardiomyopathy are well described in the articles by Oakley (1978), Ikeme et al (1975) and Evans (1979).

POSTPARTUM CARDIOMYOPATHY

There is a well recognized syndrome of cardiomegaly and heart failure of unknown cause developing in women in relation to pregnancy and the puerperium. The earliest observations were made on black women in the Southern States of the United States and since then there have been many series of cases reported from the warm climate countries of the world. The condition has been reported in African women in South Africa, in Jamaica, in the Middle East, Korea and China. Postpartal heart disease has been described both in southern and northern Nigeria. Among the Hausa women in northern Nigeria, the condition appears to have a very high frequency.

Aetiology

The condition is more frequent in poorer groups in a community and it has been suggested that tryptophan deficiency is a causal factor. It has also been suggested that postpartal heart disease could be due to acute hypertensive heart failure or that it might be an expression of a primary myocardial disorder. However, studies in Nigeria (Zaria) strongly suggest that there is no significant underlying heart muscle disorder and that the primary event is probably fluid retention induced by traditional postpartum practices — a high sodium intake and lying on a heated bed.

Features

Mean age and parity tend to be higher than in the general population although some groups report a high frequency in young primipara. Twin pregnancies also appear to be an associated factor in many cases. Symptoms usually begin after delivery, the majority occurring about two weeks postpartum; only a small proportion of patients fall ill before delivery. Oedema and breathlessness are the earliest and commonest symptoms and systemic emboli may be a presenting feature. The physical signs are those of cardiac failure and the blood pressure is often raised. Rhythm disorders are unusual but transient murmurs are frequent. The heart is always enlarged. The blood pressure falls to normal on treatment for heart failure and the murmurs also tend to disappear. The electrocardiogram is usually abnormal but not in any specific way.

Prognosis

Response to treatment with digoxin and diuretics is usually dramatic and the heart size may return to normal. Death in the acute illness occurs in up to 20 per cent of patients in most published series but in northern Nigeria, this has been seen in only four per cent of cases. Subsequent pregnancies may be complicated by a recurrence of the heart failure. In Jamaica, the long-term prognosis was regarded as very good in a small series followed for up to 13 years; this is in marked contrast to the reports from the United States.

ALCOHOL AND THE HEART

Although there has been evidence linking the intake of alcohol to heart disease for almost a century, there remains considerable argument concerning the manner in which alcohol affects the myocardium. The situation has been complicated by the fact that many heavy drinkers are also malnourished and thus chronic malnutrition has often been regarded as the major cause of heart disease in alcoholics. There now seems good evidence that the myocardial disease found in many alcoholics is not due to thiamin deficiency and that the relationship between alcohol and beri beri heart disease is indirect. Alcoholic cardiomyopathy is now considered to be due to direct injury of the myocardium by alcohol.

Clinical

The patient is usually a male with a history of at least a decade of drinking prior to the onset of symptoms. Palpitations are often the first symptom, followed by symptoms of cardiac failure including dyspnoea on exertion, fatigue and peripheral oedema. The physical findings are in no way specific but the presence of a normal sized heart on radiography should make one question the diagnosis. A wide variety of electrocardiographic changes have been described; none are specific.

Prognosis

Complete abstinence from alcohol may turn the tide of events, but if the situation is advanced, then even this will not prevent progressive deterioration. The usual medical regime with digitalis and diuretics often produces improvement but may completely fail to do so. Anti-coagulants are indicated once embolic phenomena have occurred.

ENDOMYOCARDIAL FIBROSIS

The tropical endemic form of endomyocardial fibrosis (EMF) is character-ized in the established condition by endomyocardial fibrosis in the ventri-cular cavities, affecting in particular the apex and subvalvular regions. In the endemic areas it is a disorder almost as common clinically and at necropsy as rheumatic heart disease; it is not a tropical rarity. It is sometimes progressive and possibly recurrent and it can be thought of in the same general pattern of natural history as RF and RHD. Like RHD, it predomi-nantly affects children and young adults.

Epidemiology

EMF was first described in West African troops serving in the Middle East and in indigenous African subjects in Uganda. The main areas of endemicity appear to be Uganda and Western Nigeria but the condition has been described from the Sudan, Zaire (Congo), Kenya, Tanzania, Sri Lanka, South India, Thailand, Malaya, Ghana, Brazil and Colombia. There are convincing reports of EMF occurring in Europeans who have lived for long periods in Nigeria, the Cameroons and Zaire (Congo)and sporadic reports of EMF in subjects who have never been in any tropical situation.

Aetiology

The cause of EMF has not been established. Although it is predominantly a disorder of the poorer socio-economic groups, there is no evidence to suggest that malnutrition is a primary factor. Some attention has been paid to the possibility of EMF being produced by the serotonin content of bananas (plantains) but there is no acceptable evidence to incriminate this as a causal agent. A viral aetiology has been postulated but no positive evidence has been produced. Filariasis has been considered in Nigerian studies and arising from these studies there is an hypothesis that an eosino-phil leucocytosis, in a susceptible person, may cause endomyocardial fibrosis. There is a further hypothesis which regards EMF as a disorder similar to RHD, representing another form of hypersensitivity response to infection with the streptococcus. The reason for an individual developing EMF rather than RHD is considered to be the presence of an immunological syndrome induced by malaria or other parasitic infestations.

Natural history

In Nigeria, an acute febrile episode has been described as the earliest stage of the disease and from clinico-pathological studies it is evident that EMF is a pancarditis. There are probably recurrent inflammatory episodes, each accompanied by myocarditis and fresh necrosis. In the Nigerian studies, the initial illness usually began in the rainy season and relapses also tended to occur then.

Pathology

The characteristic involvement in EMF is fibrosis in the inflow tract and at the apex of one or both ventricles. The lesion affects the endocardium and the inner-third of the myocardium. The fibrosis may be localized to the apex or may involve the papillary muscles and chordae tendinae leading to atrioventricular incompetence. Pericarditis occurs in perhaps two-thirds of cases but does not produce constrictive pericarditis. Antemortem thrombi are extremely common but embolic phenomena in the absence of bacterial endocarditis do not occur more frequently than in RHD, possibly due to greater adherence of the thrombus to the endocardial surface. Bacterial endocarditis is an infrequent complication, unless EMF and RHD are concurrently present. In necropsy studies in Uganda, macroscopic lesions of both EMF and RHD occurred in the same heart far more frequently than would be expected if the two disorders were not in some way associated.

There are no abnormalities in the coronary arteries and unlike RHD the valves in EMF contain no vessels and show no evidence of inflammation, that is, the valves are not primarily involved. Myocardial scars are found throughout the myocardium in all parts of the heart and the distribution resembles that seen in healed cases of myocarditis.

Immunological aspects and eosinophilia

Histological studies suggest that EMF is probably a disorder of cardiac connective tissue and that the possible mechanism is one of hypersensitivity. Studies in Uganda of immunological factors in the blood reveal that an unusual syndrome may be present with undue frequency in patients with EMF and in groups susceptible to EMF. This immunological syndrome includes high levels of immunoglobulin-M, malarial antibodies, heart antibodies, thyroid and gastric parietal-cell antibodies and rheumatoid factor. These tissue autoantibodies may play a critical role in the pathogenesis of EMF.

In Uganda, it has been observed that there is a conspicuous preponderance of EMF among subjects originating from neighbouring Rwanda and Burundi; the local people around Kampala show a lower frequency than expected. RHD behaves in the converse way, affecting the indigenous people more than expected and the immigrant groups less than expected. It has been suggested that the unusual susceptibility of the migrants is associated with their movements from an area of low malarial endemicity to a hyperendemic area, with the resultant development of the immunological syndrome described. In a study of the familial occurrence of EMF, all nine subjects were of migrant origin and five of them had the tropical splenomegaly syndrome, a condition known to be associated with high titres of malarial antibody and immunoglobulin-M. From a study of patients with 'eosinophilic leukaemia', Roberts (1969) suggested that EMF might be a late or inactive stage of either Löffler's endocarditis or 'eosinophilic leukaemia'. This possibility has been examined with considerable enthusiasm by other workers and remains an interesting but unestablished hypothesis. Workers from the Ugandan scene maintain that eosinophilia is not a feature of EMF, which they regard as an entity distinct from Löffler's endocarditis and from the cardiac lesions seen in eosinophilic leukaemia or reactive eosinophilia.

Clinical features

The clinical diagnosis of EMF has been fully reviewed. (See references.) Survival in subjects presenting with EMF ranges from a few weeks to 12 years but is usually about two years. The commonest mode of death is progressive myocardial failure, frequently associated with acute pulmonary events, viz pulmonary oedema, bronchopneumonia or pulmonary infarction.

Treatment

There is nothing that is specific in the management of heart failure in EMF and on the whole the results of treatment are disappointing. There are no preventive measures possible at present and it may well be that this unusual condition may decrease in frequency with changing socio-economic conditions and may even disappear before its aetiology has been determined.

REFERENCES

General

Shaper A G, Hutt M S R, Fejfar Z 1974 Cardiovascular Disease in the Tropics. British Medical Association, London
Vaughan J P 1978 A review of cardiovascular disease in developing countries. Annals of Tropical Medicine and Parasitology 72: 101–109

Rheumatic Heart Disease

Agarwal B L 1981 Rheumatic heart disease unabated in developing countries. Lancet ii: 910–911
Editorial 1982 Prevention of rheumatic heart disease. Lancet i: 143–4
McLaren M J, et al 1975 Epidemiology of rheumatic heart disease in black schoolchildren of Soweto, Johannesburg. British Medical Journal 3: 474–8
Majeed H A, Khan N, Dabbagh M, Najdi K, Khateeb N 1981 Acute rheumatic fever during childhood in Kuwait: the mild nature of the initial attack. Annals of Tropical Paediatrics 1: 13–20
Shaper A G 1972 Cardiovascular Disease in the Tropics-I. Rheumatic Heart. British Medical Journal 3: 683–686
Strasser T, et al, 1981 The community control of rheumatic fever and rheumatic heart disease. Report of a WHO international cooperative project. Bull, WHO 59: 285–294
WHO 1980 Community control of rheumatic heart disease — I. A major health problem and — II. Strategies for prevention and control. WHO Chronicle 34: 336–345 & 389–395

Blood Pressure and Hypertension

Akinkugbe O O 1972 High Blood Pressure in the African. Churchill Livingstone, London
Akinkugbe O O, Bertrand E (Eds) 1975 Hypertension in Africa. Literamed Press, Nigeria
Sever P S, Gordon D, Peart W S, Beighton P 1980 Blood pressure and its correlates in
    urban and tribal Africa. Lancet ii: 60–64
Shaper A G (Ed) 1969 Symposium on blood pressure and hypertension in Africa. East
    African Medical Journal 46: 220–363
Shaper A G 1972 Cardiovascular Disease in the Tropics —. Blood pressure and
    hypertension. British Medical Journal 3: 805–807

Coronary Heart Disease

Atherosclerosis in Africa 1971. African Journal of Medical Science 2: No 3
McGill H G 1968 The Geographic Pathology of Atherosclerosis, Laboratory Investigation
    18: 465–653
Pedoe H Tunstall 1979 Atheroma. Medicine, 3rd Series 21: 1071–1080
Shaper A G 1972 Cardiovascular Disease in the Tropics — IV. Coronary heart disease.
    British Medical Journal 4: 32–35
Shaper A G 1975 Epidemiology of atherosclerosis and coronary heart disease. Medicine, 2nd
    Series 26: 1326–1335

Cardiomyopathies

Davidson N McD, Parry E H O 1974 Peripartum cardiac failure. In: Shaper A G, Hutt
    M S R, Fejfar Z (eds) Cardiovascular disease in the Tropics, British Medical Association,
    London, P 199–208
Evans T 1979 Heart muscle disease. Medicine, 3rd Series 20: 1042–1047
Falase A O 1977 Cardiomegaly of unknown origin among Nigerian adults: role of
    hypertension in its aetiology. British Heart Journal 39: 671–679
Ikeme A C, D'Arbela P G, Somers K 1975 The clinical features of idiopathic cardiomegaly
    in the tropics. Tropical Cardiology 1: 101–107
Lewis B S, Armstrong T G, Metha A S 1973 Hypertrophic obstructive cardiomyopathy in
    the South African Bantu. South African Medical Journal 47: 599–604
Oakley C 1978 Diagnosis and natural history of congested (dilated) cardiomyopathies.
    Postgraduate Medical Journal 54: 440–7
Rees P H, Rees M C, Fulton F M, Gichinga H N 1974 Cardiomyopathy in Nairobi: a
    follow-up study. East African Medical Journal 51: 863–8
Sanderson J E, Adesanya C O, Anjorin F I, Parry E H O 1979 Postpartum cardiac failure
    — heart failure due to volume overload. American Heart Journal 97: 613–621
Seftel H C 1973 Cardiomyopathies in Johannesburg Bantu. South African Medical Journal
    47: 321–4
WHO/ISFC Task Force 1980 Report on the definition and classification of
    cardiomyopathies. British Heart Journal 44: 672–3

Endomyocardial fibrosis

Oakley C M, Olsen E G J 1977 Eosinophilia and heart disease. British Heart Journal
    39: 233–237
Roberts W C Liegler D G, Carbone P P 1969 Endomyocardial disease and eosinophilia. A
    clinical and pathological spectrum. American Journal of Medicine 46: 28–42
Shaper A G 1974 Endomyocardial fibrosis. In: Shaper A G, Hutt M S R, Fejfar Z (eds)
    Cardiovascular disease in the tropics. British Medical Association, London, p 22–41
Somers K, D'Arbela P G & Patel A K 1972 Endomyocardial fibrosis. In: Shaper A G,
    Kibukamusoke J W, Hutt M S R (eds) Medicine in a tropical environment. British
    Medical Association, London, p 348–363

Pulmonary Heart Disease

Cavalcanti I de L, Thompson G, de Souza N, Barbosa F S 1962 Pulmonary hypertension in schistosomiasis. British Heart Journal 24: 363–371

Miller G J, Beadnell H M S G, Ashcroft M T 1968 Diffuse pulmonary fibrosis and blackfat tobacco smoking in Guyana. Lancet 2: 259–260

Obeyesekere I, de Souza N 1970 Primary pulmonary hypertension, eosinophilia and filariasis in Ceylon. British Heart Journal 32: 524–536

Padmavati S 1970 Chronic cor pulmonale. Cardiovascular Clinics 2: 128–136

Woolcock A J, Blackburn C R B 1967 Chronic lung disease in Papua and New Guinea. Australian Annals of Medicine 16: 11–19

Chagas' Heart Disease

Amorim D S 1979 Chagas' disease. In: Yu P N, Goodwin J F (eds) Progress in Cardiology, Lea & Febiger, Philadelphia 8: p 235–79

D'Alessandro A, Sanchez G, Dugue E 1973 Trypanosoma cruzi and virological studies in idiopathic cardiomyopathy in Cali, Colombia. American Journal of Tropical Medicine & Hygiene 23: 856–861

Marsden P D 1971 South American Trypanosomiasis (Chagas' Disease). International Review of Tropical Medicine Vol 4: 97–121

Puigbo J J, Nava-Rhodo J R, Garcia-Barrios J, Suarez J A, Yepez C Gil 1966 Clinical and epidemiological study of Chagas' chronic heart involvement. Bulletin of the World Health Organization 34: 655

Miscellaneous

Blankson J M, Christian E C 1975 Congenital heart disease in Ghana. An analysis of 210 clinical and necropsy cases. Tropical Cardiology 1: 5–12

D'Arbela P G, Patel A K, Grigg L G, Somers K 1972 Pericarditis, with particular emphasis on pyogenic pericarditis. East African Medical Journal 49: 803–816

Falase A O, Jaiyesimi F, Atlah F B 1976 Infective endocarditis: experience in Nigeria. Tropical and Geographical Medicine 28: 9–15

Jaiyesimi F, Abioye A A, Antia A U 1979 Infective pericarditis in Nigerian Children. Archives of Diseases in Childhood 54: 389–390

McLaren M J, Lachman A S, Barlow J B 1979 Prevalence of congenital heart disease in black schoolchildren of Soweto, Johannesburg. British Heart Journal 41: 554–8

Somers K 1967 Pericarditis. British Medical Journal 2: 423–425

Somers K, Patel A K, Steiner I, D'Arbela P G, Hutt M S R 1972 Infective endocarditis. An African experience. British Heart Journal 34: 1107–1112

Woodruff J F 1980 Viral myocarditis: A Review. American Journal of Pathology 101: 425–484

The sickling haemoglobinopathies

INTRODUCTION

Haemoglobinopathies result from abnormalities in haemoglobin structure and reach a high incidence in the tropics. The carrier state for HbE occurs in up to half of the population in South East Asia (Flatz, Pik, and Sringam 1965) and that for HbS in 40 per cent in some areas of Equatorial Africa (Lehmann and Raper 1956). The diseases resulting from these abnormalities are not only common clinical problems in a tropical environment but also cause significant mortality.

Haemoglobin, a large globular protein with a molecular weight of 68 000, is composed of two pairs of polypetide chains. Normal adult haemoglobin (HbA), composed of two α chains and two β chains, is designated $\alpha_2\beta_2$. A minor component of adult blood (HbA$_2$) has the structure $\alpha_2\delta_2$ and the principal fetal haemoglobin (HbF) has the structure $\alpha_2\gamma_2$. In normal development α chain synthesis is established early in fetal life and is initially associated with γ chain synthesis producing HbF (Fig. 48.1). Synthesis of β chain starts about the third month of foetal life and rises to a maximum in the year following birth, during which period, there is a progressive change from $\alpha_2\beta_2$(HbF) to $\alpha_2\beta_2$(HbA). Synthesis of δ chain commences shortly before birth but HbA$_2$ remains a minor component rarely exceeding 3.5 per cent in normal populations. A normal adult there-fore possesses the following three haemoglobins, HbA 96–98 per cent, HbA$_2$ 1.5–3.5 per cent, HbF < 1 per cent.

The polypeptide chains of haemoglobin are long unbranched structures which are intricately folded to form a globular subunit. The α chain contains 141 amino acids and the β chain 146 amino acids. The sequence of these amino acids is determined by the nucleotide triplets (codons) of messenger RNA according to the genetic code. The basic abnormality in the haemo-globinopathies is one base change in a nucleotide triplet resulting in the substitution of the incorrect amino acid. Some substitutions are well toler-ated without any apparent effects but in others there is a change in the behaviour and function of the molecule. The amino acid at position six from the amino terminus of the β chain is normally glutamic acid specified by

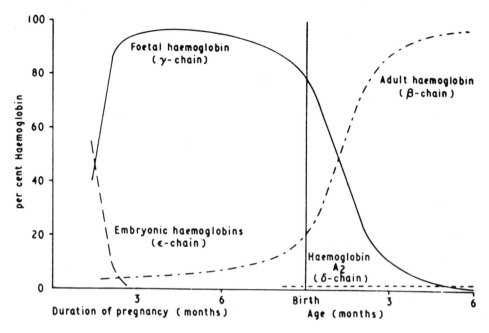

Fig 48.1 Pattern of polypeptide chain synthesis during foetal and early post natal life (Reproduced with the permission of Prof. Huehns and the Editor of the Journal of Medical Genetics).

the codon GAG which in sickle haemoglobin has been changed to GUG with the result that valine occupies this position. The introduction of a hydrophobic residue onto the surface of the molecule at this point is in some way related to the tendency to longitudinal polymerisation of deoxygenated molecules of HbS. The substitution of a neutral for a negatively charged amino acid results in the different electrophoretic mobility of HbS.

NOMENCLATURE

The term sickle cell disease covers a group of conditions in which significant pathology is attributed to the presence of HbS. Homozygous sickle cell (SS) disease is the commonest and most severe and results from the inheritance of the sickle cell gene from both parents. Sickle cell haemoglobin C (SC) disease which results from the inheritance of the sickle cell gene from one parent and that for HbC from the other, is the second commonest condition in populations of West African origin. The inheritance of the sickle cell gene along with that for β thalassaemia results in two forms of sickle cell-β thalassaemia. The β° thalassaemia gene which is associated with complete suppression of β chain synthesis results in sickle cell-β° thalassaemia, a relatively severe condition which resembles SS disease eletrophoretically, haematologically, and clinically. The β⁺ thalassaemia gene is associated with only a partial suppression of β chain synthesis and sickle cell-β^+ thalassaemia (in Black populations) with 20–25 per cent HbA is usually a mild condition similar to SC disease. Less commonly the sickle cell gene may be inherited along with that for another abnormal haemoglobin to produce a pathological condition as in SO Arab disease, SD Punjab disease, SE disease, and S/Lepore Boston.

The heterozygous state for HbS (the sickle cell trait) should not be classified as a form of sickle cell disease. Manifestations common to sickle cell disease may occur in the sickle cell trait, for example haematuria or splenic infarction under anoxic conditions, but these are uncommon under normal conditions. Inclusion of the essentially healthy sickle cell trait within the definition of sickle cell disease because of a few symptomatic cases would render the term almost meaningless. Inheritance of the gene for HbS along with other β chain structural variants may also result in totally benign syndromes even though normal haemoglobin is absent. These include the association of HbS with Hb Korle Bu, Osu Christiansborg, Ocho Rios, D Ibadan, D Iran, J Baltimore, and the gene for hereditary persistence of foetal haemoglobin.

Distribution of the sickle cell gene

There is a close geographical association between the distribution of the sickle cell trait and falciparum malaria in Equatorial Africa, the Mediterranean and parts of Asia. It is likely that this correlation has arisen because heterozygotes for the sickle cell gene have some protection against malaria and so are more likely to survive and pass on their genes. Foci of the gene with prevalences up to 30 per cent occur in Southern Italy and Sicily, parts of Greece and Turkey, the Eastern province of Saudi Arabia and in the Veddoid tribes of Southern India. However the greatest reservoir of the gene is in the Black population of Africa reaching the highest levels in Equatorial areas. The distribution of the gene in the Caribbean, and in the Americas follows population movements from West Africa during the slave trade in the seventeenth and eighteenth centuries and that in the United Kingdom and Europe from the recent pattern of immigration principally from the West Indies (Fig 48.2).

The wide distribution of the HbS gene contrasts with the distribution of HbC which is almost confined to areas of Northern Ghana and the Upper Volta where the prevalence may reach 20–25 per cent. The HbC gene has not been encountered in other areas of Africa except in cases of West African origin and its distribution throughout the Americas follows the same pattern as that for HbS.

It is important to realise that the sickle cell gene is not racially linked to Black populations but is found in a number of Caucasian groups where there is no reason to attribute its presence to Black genes. It seems likely that the sickle cell gene mutation has arisen independently in a number of areas, and

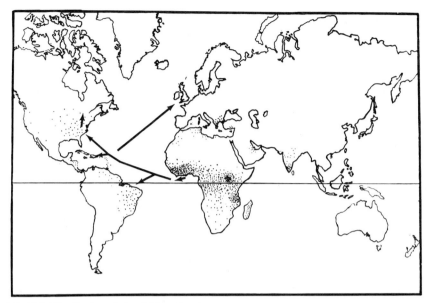

Fig 48.2 Distribution of the sickle cell trait.

been selected in those areas characterised by falciparum malaria. The most malarious area in the world is Equatorial Africa and hence there is a close relationship between the sickle cell gene and Black peoples.

Incidence of sickle cell disease

The incidence of the sickle cell syndromes at birth is determined by the prevalence of the different gene frequencies within a population. The gene frequencies observed during the screening of 100 000 consecutive deliveries in Jamaica are summarised in Table 48.1 and were used to calculate the

Table 48.1 Haemoglobin gene frequencies in 100 000 newborn infants in Jamaica

Gene	No. Observed	Relative Frequency
A	184904	0.924520
S	10941	0.054705
C	3918	0.019590
β thal	50*	0.000250
HPFH	8*	0.000040
Variants	179**	0.000895
	200000	1.000000

* The screening techniques employed do not allow detection of the β thalassaemia and hereditary persistence of foetal haemglobin (HPFH) traits and their incidence will certainly have been underestimated
** Gamma chain variants excluded

Table 48.2 Observed frequencies of some genotypes compared with values predicted from gene frequency

Genotype	Expected Relative Frequency	No. Predicted	No. Observed
AA	0.8547372	85473.72	85555
AS	0.1011516	10115.16	10941
AC	0.0362226	3622.26	3586
SS	0.0029926	299.26	319
SC	0.0021432	214.32	201
A/variant	0.0016548	165.48	167
S/variant	0.0000978	9.78	6
C/variant	0.0000350	3.50	6

expected genotype frequencies in Table 48.2. There is a close relationship between observed and predicted frequencies and the apparent excess of SS cases will be attributed in part to cases of Sβ° thalassaemia and S/HPFH not yet differentiated from SS disease.

The incidence of sickle cell disease in populations after birth will depend upon the relative mortalities in the different genotypes. Very little valid information is available on this since it requires long term follow up of a large representative sample of patients ascertained at birth. A cohort study of this type is under way in Jamaica but only eight years of follow up are currently available. Survival curve analysis of the first three years (Fig 48.3) indicates high mortality in SS disease in the second half of the first year of life with a substantial but decreasing mortality in the second and third years

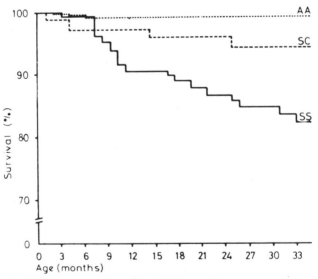

Fig 48.3 Survival in Jamaican children with AA, SC and SS genotypes diagnosed at birth.

(Rogers et al 1978). Overall mortality approaches 20 per cent by the age of five years even in a population diagnosed at birth which has received regular medical care, and therapeutic intervention where possible.

It is still clearly impossible to predict the length of survival but the high early mortality implies that expected survival must improve once the high risk period of early childhood is passed. Thus a five year old child would be expected to have a better average life expectancy than one at birth and it is probable in the Jamaican environment that once the age of 20 years has been reached, the chances of surviving to 40 years are good. However it will be many years before more reliable data are available.

Diagnosis of sickle cell disease

The differential diagnosis of the sickle cell syndromes is based on haemoglobin electrophoresis under alkaline and acid conditions. Conventional haemoglobin electrophoresis which is run at pH 8.4–8.6 using paper, starch gel or cellulose acetate as medium distinguishes haemoglobin bands according to their electric charge. Thus HbS which is positively charged relative to HbA, travels more slowly towards the positive pole, whereas HbC which is more positively charged than HbS travels even more slowly (Fig 48.4). Sickle cell-β° thalassaemia resembles SS disease and must be differentiated by family study, thalassaemic red cell indices (low MCV, MCH, MCHC) and the increase in proportional HbA_2. Sickle cell-β^{+} thalassaemia has the same major haemoglobin bands as the sickle cell trait (HbA and HbS) but whereas in the latter HbA always predominates, in Sβ^{+} thalassaemia, HbA never exceeds 30 per cent and HbS predominates. Agar gel electrophoresis conventionally conducted at pH 6.0–6.2 is a valuable

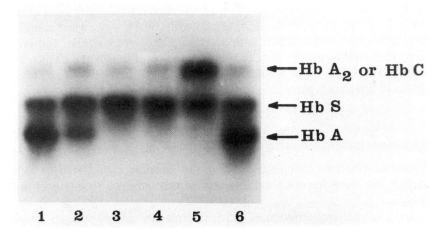

Fig. 48.4 Starch gel electrophoretic patterns in major genotypes of sickle cell disease: (1) AS control; (2) Sβ^{+} thalassaemia; (3) SS disease; (4) Sβ° thalassaemia; (5) SC disease; (6) AS control (photo courtesy of Dr. P. F. Milner)

confirmatory test since HbS and HbC have characteristic positions whereas most other abnormal haemoglobins travel in the position of HbA. Following the finding of a band in the position of HbS, the identity of HbS may be confirmed by either sickling or solubility tests.

Diagnosis at birth is complicated by the high levels of HbF normally present but techniques allowing the separation of HbA and HbS from HbF in cord blood samples are now well established. Large numbers of samples may be processed with relative ease using rapid methods with cellulose acetate and agar gel (Serjeant et al 1974). Cord blood screening has the advantages of accessibility of the population and is the optimum time if proper follow up and early intervention is to avoid the high risk period of the first year. Disadvantages of screening at this time are the difficulties of differentiating SS disease from $S\beta^{\circ}$ thalassaemia (which also needs specialised medical care) and from S/hereditary persistence of foetal haemoglobin (which does not).

During the past 10 years medical technology has advanced greatly allowing antenatal diagnosis at minimal risk to the pregnancy (Alter 1981). Fetal blood sampling at specialised centres carries a risk of less than five per cent and small samples of fetal blood may allow the diagnosis to be made. The recent discovery of a polymorphism of DNA linked to the sickle cell locus has allowed the diagnosis to be made from fetal DNA (Kan & Dozy 1978) in children where preliminary testing of both parents has confirmed this linkage (approximately 60 per cent of Black Americans). This has the great advantage that fetal DNA may be obtained by amniocentesis and does not require the technical expertise for direct puncture and sampling from fetal blood vessels.

Although feasible with sophisticated and elegant technology, the role of antenatal diagnosis remains controversial. It is most unlikely to be practicable, desirable or indeed indicated on a population scale but may be of great value in highly selected situations. Occasionally, in Jamaica, when couples have had one or two children with SS disease and severe clinical courses, there may be the desire for a further pregnancy in which the chance of another SS offspring can be excluded and antenatal diagnosis is a valuable option to offer such parents.

Early management following neonatal diagnosis

Several observations have emerged from the Jamaican cohort study which suggest that early diagnosis and intervention may improve prognosis of the disease.

Acute splenic sequestration in which the spleen suddenly enlarges, trapping the circulating red cell mass, and resulting in a rapidly falling haemoglobin level has emerged as the biggest single cause of mortality in early childhood (Topley et al 1981). The aetiology of such episodes is unknown but their clinical course may be precipitate sometimes taking only three hours for an apparently healthy child to become moribund. Making the mother or guardian aware of these episodes and teaching methods of detecting splenomegaly and pallor in the home has undoubtedly resulted in the earlier presentation of the complication giving time for successful intervention by blood transfusion. Attacks may be recurrent and mortality during repeat episodes may be prevented by splenectomy. Such postsplenectomy children clearly require special care to avoid infection but such care is probably needed by all children with SS disease because of their impaired splenic function.

It is well recognised that children with SS disease are prone to infections of which pneumococcal septicaemia is one of the most serious. The spleen loses its immunological competence early even though it may remain anatomically enlarged (Pearson et al 1969)and this functional asplenia may be temporally related to the onset of clinical splenomegaly. Data from the cohort study indicated that 12 out of 13 serious infections and 11 out of 12 pneumococcal isolations occurred in those children where clinical splenomegaly appeared in the first six months of life even though these children represented only one third of the total population (Rogers, Vaidya, and Serjeant, 1978). This observation means that early splenomegaly may be used to detect those children at highest risk from subsequent overwhelming septicaemia and prophylactic measures may be concentrated in this group.

The most appropriate methods of preventing infection in children with SS disease are still under investigation. Pneumococcal vaccine stimulates antibody formation to the serotypes within it but the antibody response is submaximal before the age of three. Yet it is at this time that there is the greatest risk of pneumococcal events. Pneumococcal infection with types represented in the vaccine (vaccine breakthrough) are not uncommon especially with types 6 and 23 which appear to be poorly antigenic and of course the vaccine is unlikely to be of value against pneumococcal subtypes not represented in it. Prophylactic penicillin appears to give more effective protection and no pneumococcal isolations have occurred in 162 children aged six months to three years receiving monthly injections of long acting penicillin (unpublished observations).

The aplastic crisis, in which transient bone marrow arrest is associated with a rapidly falling haemoglobin and very low or absent reticulocytes, may also be associated with mortality especially in young children. Such episodes have been suspected as having an infective aetiology because of the occurrence of epidemics and of clustering in families. Recent studies in a Jamaican epidemic of 38 cases in 1979–80 have indicated strong evidence for infection with a parvovirus-like agent in association with these attacks (Serjeant et al 1981a). Since recurrent attacks of aplastic crisis appear to be extremely rare or nonexistent it is possible that exposure to one attack confers immunity to subsequent attacks. This observation is compatible with parvoviruses being responsible for other epidemics of aplastic crises in

SS disease. If this hypothesis is confirmed by further studies, there may be the possibility of protecting children from this complication with vaccines.

Factors influencing the prognosis of sickle cell disease

Marked differences in the clinical course of sickle cell disease which occur between different geogrphical areas and between patients in the same areas must result from a variety of genetic and environmental factors.

1. Genetic factors

Persistence of γ chain synthesis with consequent high levels of HbF protects against sickling and results in a mild clinical course. The high levels normally present in the first six months of life render symptoms unusual during that period and examination of the clinical course in relation to the HbF level at one year has shown that children with low levels are more likely to suffer dactylitis, acute splenic sequestration, early splenomegaly, and death (Stevens et al, 1981). Increased levels of HbF persist in many adult patients and values above five per cent are usually associated with discernibly milder features. Factors determining the persistence of HbF are largely unknown although a genetic mechanism is implied in the observation that a mild elevation of HbF in one or both parents results in a marked elevation in an SS offspring (Mason et al 1982).

In the Caribbean, HbF levels above 10 per cent in adults with SS disease are unusual and levels above 20 per cent rare in contrast to observations in Saudi Arabia and Kuwait where levels of 10–40 per cent HbF are common and a very benign clinical course occurs (Ali 1970; Perrine et al 1978). The reason for the marked geographical variation is currently unknown.

The association of G6PD deficiency with SS disease has been suggested be beneficial (Lewis, Kay and Hathorn 1966; Piomelli et al 1972) but a recent study of patients in the steady state failed to show any haematological or clinical differences between SS patients with and without G6PD deficiency (Gibbs, Wardle and Serjeant 1980).

The association of α thalassaemia with SS disease has also been proposed as an ameliorating factor (Altay et al 1981; Embury et al 1982; Serjeant et al 1981b). The small cell size and lowered intra-cellular haemoglobin concentration induced by α thalassaemia might be expected to inhibit sickling and promote negotiation of the capillary bed by HbS containing cells. A study comparing the clinical and haematological features in age/sex matched groups of 44 SS patients homozygous for α thalassaemia 2 (α-/α-), 44 heterozygous for α thalassaemia 2 (α-/αα) and 88 with a normal α globin gene complement (αα/αα) has now confirmed these observations (Higgs et al 1982). Patients with homozygous α thalassaemia 2 had significantly higher total haemoglobin levels, red cell count, and proportional HbA$_2$ and a significantly lower mean cell volume, mean cell haemoglobin concentration, reticulocyte count, irreversible sickled cell count, bilirubin level, and HbF level (Table 48.3).

Clinically, patients homozygous for α thalassaemia 2 had a significantly lower incidence of leg ulceration and pneumonia and greater persistence of splenomegaly but no other clinical differences were apparent. These results are compatible with inhibition of in vivo sickling but the increase in haemoglobin may be disadvantageous because of its effect in increasing blood viscosity.

Despite DNA structural studies on nearly 300 patients with SS disease there was no evidence of an increasing association of homozygous α thalassaemia 2 and SS disease in older populations to support the hypothesis that homozygous α thalassaemia 2 had improved survival in the disease.

Heterozygous α thalassaemia 2 was observed in 35 per cent of the Jamaican SS population and homozygous α thalassaemia 2 in four per cent compatible with the Hardy-Weinberg hypothesis and also illustrating the high prevalence of these genotypes and the importance of their inter-action with SS disease in populations.

2. Climate

Cold or damp weather is a common precipitating factor in the painful crisis in sickle cell disease being well recognised in Ghana (Addae 1971), the United States (Diggs 1965; Amjad, Bannerman, and Judisch 1974) and in Jamaica (Redwood et al 1976). The pathology of the painful crisis is a bilateral and usually symmetrical limited form of bone marrow necrosis in the juxta-articular bones and the mechanisms of the relationship between skin temperature and bone marrow perfusion is entirely unknown. Recently dactylitis, which is the infants form of painful crisis, has also been shown to have a seasonal incidence (Stevens, Padwick and Serjeant 1981).

3. Diet

The increased haemolytic rate in SS disease is associated with increased folic acid requirements and a tendency to megaloblastic change especially in areas of limited dietary availability. Thus megaloblastic change is reported to be a frequent complication of young children with SS disease in West Africa whereas in Jamaica, megaloblastic change is uncommon in SS disease even at times of the additional demand associated with rapid growth in infants, adolescence, and during pregnancy.

4. Medical care

The availability of medical care influences the outcome of the disease through early detection of complications and the prompt and effective therapy of infections, thrombotic lesions, acute splenic sequestration, and

Table 48.3 Comparison of haematological features in the three subgroups of SS disease

Variable	αα/αα			α-/αα			α-/α-		
	n	mean	SD	n	mean	SD	n	mean	SD
HbA₂ (%)	88	2.78	0.36	44	3.11	0.34	44	3.87	0.38
¹HbF	88	1.84(5.3)	0.61	44	1.76(4.8)	0.51	44	1.58(3.8)	0.61
Hb (g/dl)	88	7.80	1.09	44	8.12	1.00	44	8.84	1.29
MCHC (g/dl)	88	34.8	1.7	44	34.3	1.6	44	32.8	1.3
RBC (×10¹²/l)	88	2.56	0.39	44	2.90	0.47	44	3.86	0.59
MCV (fl)	88	90.1	6.1	44	84.4	7.8	44	71.2	3.2
MCH (pg)	88	31.4	2.6	44	29.0	3.0	44	23.6	1.4
²Reticulocytes (%)	88	2.55 (11.9)	0.34	44	2.33(9.3)	0.27	44	2.00(6.4)	0.27
³ISC (%)	55	2.88 (7.7)	0.32	24	2.91(8.3)	0.28	29	2.60(3.5)	0.21
⁴Total bilirubin (mg/dl)	88	1.34 (2.8)	0.33	44	1.23(2.4)	0.36	44	0.93(1.5)	0.27

1–4 Means and SDs calculated after logarithmic transformations because of skewed distribution
$^1\log_{10}$ (HbF + 1), $^2\log_{10}$ (retics + 1), $^3\log_{10}$(ISC + 10), $^4\log_{10}$ (tot bil + 1)
Figures in parenthesis represent means re-expressed in original units.
All differences between α-/α- and αα/αα groups are highly significant (p < 0.01)

the aplastic crisis. Infections may not only be relevant in precipitating crises but may also result in death from overwhelming septicaemia especially with the pneumococcus. Gastro-enteritis and pneumonia are also likely to be common causes of death in early childhood, and other important infections include salmonellal osteomyelitis and tetanus secondary to leg ulceration in older patients. On a world scale, the most widespread and relevant infection is malaria. Although the heterozygote possesses some resistance to falciparum malaria, the combination of two severe haemolytic processes in the homozygote leads to a high mortality and the effectiveness of antimalarial therapy in improving prognosis has been well documented (Hendrickse, 1965). Regular vaccination and immunisation programmes should reduce the incidence of other infections and trials with pneumococcal vaccines are in progress. The role of prophylactic antibiotics is also being assessed.

5. Socio-economic factors

Improvement in the general standard of living, better medical care, better public health programmes, better nutrition, and a reduced exposure to infection all contribute to improving the prognosis of patients with sickle cell disease. These factors may largely account for the apparently milder course of the disease in the United States compared to Africa. In Jamaica this distinction is also apparent, middle class patients generally having more benign courses than their poorer counterparts despite a similar degree of haematological involvement. The influence of social class on the disease has also been recorded in Ghana (Konotey-Ahulu, 1971).

Control and treatment of the disease

Genetic counselling

The simple inheritance patterns of the sickle cell gene make it amenable to control by population screening and genetic counselling. If both parents are shown to have the sickle cell trait there is a one in four chance of as SS offspring for each pregnancy. Theoretically, creating an environment in which individuals with the sickle cell trait choose not marry or if married, decide not to have children would markedly reduce the prevalence of SS disease. Antenatal diagnosis in couples at risk with selective abortion of affected offspring would also reduce the prevalence in communities where such facilities were available.

The major problem with these approaches lies in the extreme clinical variability of SS disease. Homozygous β° thalassaemia as seen in Southern Italy results in a transfusion dependent individual with a more uniformly severe clinical course and in this situation, antenatal diagnosis may effectively prevent suffering in child and family. In SS disease in Jamaica, however, an affected person may run a complicated clinical course with death in early childhood or may be working full time and without clinical problems at the age of 60 years. A more logical requirement in the Jamaican situation might therefore be the ability to predict children destined to run a severe clinical course with selective prevention of such cases. Currently these prognostic factors are only beginning to be defined.

Haemoglobinopathy clinics

The management of sickle cell disease is best performed in haemoglobino-pathy clinics by physicians with specialised knowledge and experience of the disease. In the Jamaican clinic all patients are regularly reviewed at three to six monthly intervals in order to establish baselines for the steady state against which to judge acute and chronic complications. It may also be poss-ible to anticipate some clinical and haematological complications allowing earlier intervention.

The clinic is also a suitable environment for spreading information on the disease. In a suitably educated population, acute splenic sequestration will present earlier allowing effective therapy. Specialised vaccine programmes or antibiotic prophylaxis may prevent or reduce the prevalence of serious septicaemias. Chronic leg ulceration which is a major determinant of morbidity in the Jamaican setting compounds its effects by associated educational deprivation. At the onset of leg ulceration the child usually leaves school and there is a direct assocation between the age on onset of leg ulceration and educational attainment (Alleyne, Wint, and Serjeant 1977). Suitable information programmes should be able to ensure that the child continues to attend school despite ambulatory treatment for leg ulcers and so minimise this secondary effect. There are many similar ways in which simple procedures may have a marked impact on the life of affected patients.

Perhaps most important is the recognition that traditional concepts of the disease are based on grossly symptomatically selected population samples and do not truly reflect the pattern of disease in the community. It is increasingly recognised that SS disease may be compatible with mild clinical courses and the factors determining clinical variability are beginning to be understood. It is vital that research defining these factors continue since the influence of genetic and environmental effects profoundly determine the outcome of sickle cell disease.

REFERENCES

Addae S 1971 Mechanism for the high incidence of sickle cell crisis in the tropical cool season Lancet, 2: 1256
Ali A A 1970 Milder variant of sickle cell disease in Arabs in Kuwait associated with unusually high levels of foetal haemoglobin British Journal of Haematology, 19: 613–619
Alleyne S I, Wint E, Serjeant G R 1977 Social effects of leg ulceration in sickle cell anemia. Southern Medical Journal, 70: 213–214
Altay C, Gravely M E, Josephs B R, Williams D F 1981 Alpha thalassaemia 2 and variability of hematological values in children with sickle cell anemia. Pediatric Research, 15: 1093–1096

Alter B 1981 Prenatal diagnosis of haemoglobinopathies: a status report. Lancet, 2: 1152–1155

Amjad H, Bannerman R M, Judisch J M 1974 Sickling pain and season. British Medical Journal, 2: 54

Diggs L W 1965 Sickle cell crises. American Journal of Clinical Pathology, 44: 1–9

Embury S H, et al 1982 Concurrent sickle-cell anemia and α-thalassemia. New England Journal of Medicine, 306, 270–274

Flatz C, Pik C, Sringam S 1965 Haemoglobin E and thalassaemia: their distribution in Thailand. Annals of Human Genetics, 29, 151–170

Gibbs W N, Wardle J, Serjeant G R 1980 Glucose-6-phosphate dehydrogenase deficiency and homozygous sickle cell disease in Jamaica. British Journal of Haematology, 45, 73–80

Hendrickse R G 1965 The effect of malaria chemoprophylaxis on spleen size in sickle cell anaemia — in Abnormal Haemoglobins in Africa. Blackwell Scientific Publications, p. 445–449

Higgs D R, et al 1982 The interaction of alpha thalassemia and homozygous sickle cell disease. New England Journal of Medicine 306: 1441–1446

Kan Y W, Dozy A M 1978 Antenatal diagnosis of sickle cell anaemia by D N A analysia of amniotic fluid cells. Lancet, 2: 910–912

Konotey-Ahulu F I D 1971 M D Thesis, University of London

Lehmann H, Raper A B 1956 Maintenance of high sickling rate in an African community. British Medical Journal 2: 333–336

Lewis R A, Kay R W, Hathorn M 1966 Sickle cell disease and glucose-6-phosphate dehydrogenase. Acta Haematologica, 36: 399–411

Mason K P et al 1982 Post natal decline of fetal haemoglobin in homozygous sickle cell disease: relationship to parental HbF levels. British Journal of Haematology 52: 455–463

Pearson H A, Spencer R P, Cornelius E A 1969 Functional asplenia in sickle cell anemia. New England Journal of Medicine, 281, 923–926

Perrine R P, Pembrey M E, John P, Perrine S, Shoup F 1978 Natural history of sickle cell anemia in Saudi Arabs : a study of 270 subjects. Annals of Internal Medicine, 88, 1–6

Piomelli S, Reindorf C A, Arzanian M T, Corash L M 1972 Clinical and biochemical interactions of glucose-6-phosphate dehydrogenase deficiency and sickle cell anemia. New England Journal of Medicine, 287, 213–217.

Redwood A M, Williams E M, Desai P, Serjeant G R 1976 Climate and painful crisis of sickle cell disease in Jamaica. British Medical Journal, 1, 66–68

Rogers D W, Clarke J M, Cupidore L, Ramlal A M, Sparke B R, Serjeant G R 1978 Early deaths in Jamaican children with sickle cell disease. British Medical Journal, 1, 1515–1516

Rogers D W, Vaidya S, Serjeant G R 1978 Early splenomegaly in homozygous sickle cell disease : an indicator of susceptibility to infection. Lancet, 2: 963–965

Serjeant B E, Forbes M, Williams L L, Serjeant G R 1974 Screening cord bloods for detection of sickle cell disease in Jamaica. Clinical Chemistry, 20, 666–669

Serjeant G R, et al 1981a Outbreak of aplastic crisis in sickle cell anaemia associated with parvovirus like agent. Lancet 2: 595–597

Serjeant G R, Higgs D R, Aldridge B, Hayes R J, Weatherall D J 1981b Alpha thalassaemia and homozygous sickle cell disease. In : Brewer G J, ed the Red Cell: Fifth Ann Arbour Conference. New York: Alan R Liss, pp. 781–786

Stevens M C G, Hayes R J, Vaidya S, Serjeant G R 1981 Fetal hemoglobin and clinical severity of homozygous sickle cell disease in early childhood. Journal of Pediatrics, 98, 37–41

Stevens M C G, Padwick M, Serjeant G R 1981 Observations on the natural history of dactylitis in homozygous sickle cell disease. Clinical Pediatrics, 20, 311–317

Topley J M, Rogers D W, Stevens M C G, Serjeant G R 1981 Acute splenic sequestration and hypersplenism in the first five years in homozygous sickle cell disease. Archives of Diseases in Childhood, 56, 765–769

Malignant disease in warm climates

INTRODUCTION

Malignant disease is a major health problem in all countries of the world; once an individual has survived the first five years of childhood, cancer ranks as one of the three major causes of death in both developing and developed countries (WHO, 1980). Although there are certain features of malignant disease which are peculiar to warm climates, there are also enormous variations in the pattern of disease *within* the tropical zone. The size and nature of the health problem posed by cancer, and the control measures appropriate are therefore likely to vary widely from one area to another.

Statistics on cancer occurence are usually given as incidence (annual number of new cases of cancer) or mortality (annual deaths caused by cancer). When crude rates (new cases or deaths per 100,000 population of all ages) are studied, incidence and mortality appear to be much lower in developed than in developing countries. For example, the crude incidence rate of cancer in developing countries is approximately 50 to 150 cases per 100,000 population, compared to 250 to 350 in Europe and North America (Waterhouse et al, 1982); cancer deaths in the latter countries comprise about 20 per cent of all deaths, whereas in tropical Latin America and Asia cancer is usually responsible for 3 to 10 per cent of deaths (Segi, 1981). The major reason for this differing pattern is the relatively young age structure of the population in developing countries so that diseases which are common in young people, for example accidents and infections, are more prominent as causes of illness and death than cancer, which is largely a disease of the older age-groups.

Diseases are the result of the interplay of environmental factors and genetic susceptibility. It is of some importance to arrive at estimates of the relative contribution of each, since extrinsic environmental causes can presumably be modified and the occurrence of disease could be reduced. Several types of evidence from cancer epidemiology support the view that the great majority, perhaps up to 90 per cent, of cancers are due to potentially avoidable factors. This evidence comes from the study of cancer incidence rates in different communities throughout the world, the gradual divergence in cancer levels between migrants from a community and those who stay behind (rates in the migrants themselves tending to approximate to those of the host country (Kmet, 1970)), variations in time in the incidence of cancer in particular communities (Magnus, 1982), and the actual identification of many specific causes or risk factors. Two broad categories of malignancy might be defined (Higginson & Muir, 1979):

1. Cancers caused by well defined exogenous factors, usually personal habits such as smoking, sunbathing, betel quid chewing and excess alcohol consumption, but occasionally specific occupational or iatrogenic exposures. Such tumours generally occur in adults and for the most part are epithelial involving skin, respiratory organs and upper digestive tract (mouth and oesophagus).

2. Cancers, notably those of the gastrointestinal and reproductive systems, for which an environmental aetiology is suspected from the types of epidemiological evidence described earlier. The factors which have been found to relate to the occurrence of disease are, however, not the clearcut exposures referred to in (i), but involve elements of individual lifestyle, such as dietary and reproductive habits.

Figure 49.1 presents estimates of the relative contribution of exogenous factors in the causation of cancer in Bombay and Bulawayo based upon the relative frequency of different tumours in the population and current knowledge of causative factors. A comprehensive review of this kind has been also carried out to estimate the avoidable risks of cancer in the USA (Doll & Peto, 1981).

It is evident that malignant disease will pose an increasing health problem to developing countries in the coming decades. Table 49.1 shows some population projections for the year 2000, the population increase is most marked in developing regions, and it is the number of older persons, those most at risk of cancer, that shows the greatest rate of increase. Further, it is anticipated that the trend to urbanisation in developing countries will continue. Their urban populations are projected to increase 250 per cent between 1975 and 2000 compared with a 42 per cent increase in developed

Table 49.1 Projected world population growth, 1975–2000 (Source: UN, 1980)

	Population (millions)					
	Developed countries			Developing countries		
	1975	2000	(increase)	1975	2000	(increase)
Under 15	271	273	0.7%	1194	1694	42 %
15–64	706	831	18 %	1634	3005	84 %
65 +	116	168	45 %	112	227	103 %
All Ages	1093	1272	16 %	2940	4926	68 %

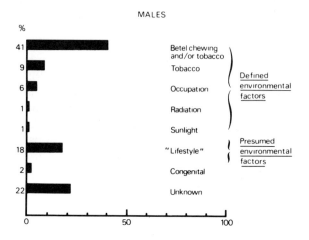

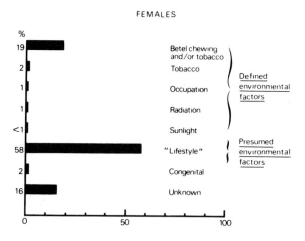

Fig. 49.1 Proportion of cancers attributed to causes listed (from Higginson and Muir, 1979)

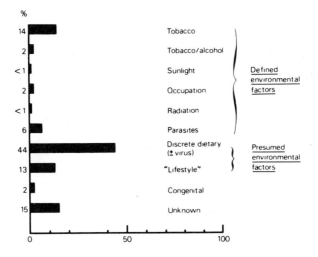

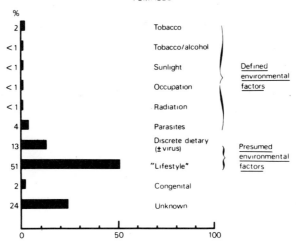

Fig. 49.1 Cont.

Table 49.2 World tobacco production and demand

	1962–64	ACTUAL 1972–74	1976	PROJECTED 1985	GROWTH RATES 1962–64 to 1972–74	1972–74 to 1985 (projected)
	average	average			% per annum	
PRODUCTION thousand metric tons (farm weight)						
World	4436.9	4948.6	5678.8	6308.9	1.1	2.0
Developing	2328.7	2864.6	3278.6	3973.3	2.1	2.8
Developed	2108.2	2084.0	2400.3	2335.6	-0.1	1.0
CONSUMPTION thousand metric tons (dry weight)						
World	3549.7	4458.0	4658.3	5544.3	2.3	1.8
Developing	1680.8	2137.7	2289.5	2978.3	2.4	2.8
Developed	1868.9	2320.3	2368.7	2565.9	2.2	0.8
CONSUMPTION PER CAPITA kg (dry weight)						
World	1.12	1.17	1.16	1.17	0.4	0.0
Developing	0.78	0.79	0.79	0.84	0.2	0.6
Developed	1.87	2.11	2.10	2.11	1.2	0.0

From: World Health
March/April 1980

countries. Wherever it has been possible to analyse cancer data by urban/rural residence, the evidence suggests that there are greater risks for the town dweller. The urban dweller is probably more exposed to cancer-causing agents, either at work or in his lifestyle. One potent carcinogen to which populations in developing countries are increasingly exposed is tobacco; Table 49.2 shows trends and projections in tobacco consumption.

Not only can an increased number of cancer cases be forecast, but the importance of cancer as a Public Health problem can be expected to grow. With increasing development the control of acute diseases such as infections is relatively easily achieved, so that the chronic conditions like cancer become more significant as causes of morbidity. This change can be quite abrupt. It has already occurred in China and Singapore in substantially less than one generation. Treatment (and frequently diagnosis) of cancer is expensive — it involves hospital care with surgery, radiotherapy or the use of costly drugs. Furthermore the enormous investment in expensive technology does not seem to have led to greatly improved survival from most common cancers (there are exceptions, however, such as some childhood leukaemia and choriocarcinoma).

Some of the geographical patterns of cancer are described below, together with brief statements about causative factors.

EPIDEMIOLOGY OF CANCER

Geographical distribution and causative factors

The brief descriptions below are confined to patterns observed in warm climate countries. A summary of the geographic occurrence of cancer is provided by Muir & Nectoux (1982) and a useful systematic presentation of cancer risk factors by Hirayama et al (1980). Incidence rates for the sites discussed below in five centres are shown in the Appendix.

1. Lip, oral cavity, and tongue

Cancer of the mouth is especially common where alcohol and tobacco consumption are high, or betel quid chewing or bidi smoking occur frequently. It is thus a common tumour in the Indian subcontinent, and where populations of Indian descent are found (Singapore, South Africa). Where emigrant Indian populations abandon the chewing habit, such as in Fiji, the risk decreases. Reverse smoking, with the lighted end of the cigarette or cigar inside the mouth, is practised in certain areas of India and Venezuela and is associated with cancer of the hard palate. The use of powdered tobacco, with or without lime, placed between lip and gingiva (khaini), also results in oral cancer.

2. Nasopharynx

This is a rare tumour except in southern China and persons originating from there, as in Singapore and Hawaii. The reasons for this striking racial occurrence are not clear. Raised frequencies have also been noted in the Maghreb, northern Sudan and parts of Kenya although the level is much lower than in southern China.

3. Oesophagus

Oesophageal cancer shows very striking geographical patterns with areas of high incidence around the Caspian Sea, in certain black populations of South Africa (Transkei), in several geographical locations in China and in the Asian Republics of the USSR. Adjacent areas within the same country may show markedly different rates. It is known that smoking and alcohol intake are risk factors in western countries. In such high-risk areas it is generally male rates that are elevated. There are exceptions as in Iran where, in high incidence areas, female rates are as high as those of males and neither alcohol nor tobacco can account for the geographical distribution. Dietary factors such as hot tea and deficiencies of trace elements or vitamins have been suspected but definitive proof is so far lacking.

4. Stomach

Stomach cancer is one of the major malignancies in many populations. In general the highest incidence rates are described in temperate climates, and there is an association with low social class or poverty. There may be underreporting of this internal, fatal disease in some tropical countries. High rates are found in Japan, China, and Korea. Latin America, as in Chile, Costa Rica, also contains areas of raised incidence and mortality. Various dietary factors have been suspected as causative, especially preserving practices, such as smoking, salting, pickling, and the use of nitrates. The almost universal decline of stomach cancer rates is ascribed to improved methods of food preservation and storage, including refrigeration, and in temperate zones it is also related to increased consumption of fresh fruit and vegetables.

5. Large bowel

Large bowel cancer is a disease of western society and is rare in tropical countries. Migrants to the USA and Europe acquire the high rates experienced by those born in such regions, which strongly suggests an environmental aetiology; lack of dietary fibre and high animal fat intake are suspected agents.

6. Liver

Primary cancer of the liver, which in terms of number of cases may be the commonest malignancy in the world today, shows enormous variation in geographical distribution. A high incidence is seen in sub-saharan Africa with very high rates in males in Mozambique and Zimbabwe. Areas of high incidence are also found in South East Asia, specifically Malaysia, Indonesia, the Philippines, Chinese in Singapore and coastal parts of China. This pattern coincides closely with the geographical distribution of serological evidence of infection with the Hepatitis B virus, particularly the HBsAg carrier state. Further study, both epidemiological and laboratory, has served to increase the suspicion that this virus is involved in the aetiology of liver cancer (Lancet, 1981). (See Zuckerman Chapter 26) Also suspected of playing a causative role is aflatoxin, which is known to be a powerful hepatatoxin and carcinogen for animals, and which is produced by moulds growing on grains and groundnuts where food storage and handling are not ideal. Aflatoxin levels in foodstuffs in East Africa (and Thailand) have been found to correlate closely with the incidence of liver cancer (Linsell, 1979). In developed countries, the occurrence of hepatic carcinoma is associated with alcohol intake, and the consequent alcoholic liver disease and cirrhosis.

7. Nasal cavity and sinuses

There is an excess incidence of these tumours in Japanese populations, and in some populations of African origin (Nigeria, Zimbabwe, South Africa, Kenya and Jamaica). Certain occupational exposures are known hazards such as those involving hard-wood dust, chromium and nickel.

8. Larynx/hypopharynx

Predominantly a disease of males, these cancers have been associated with the combination of alcohol intake and tobacco smoking. High frequency areas include Bombay, Assam, Burma and Chiang Mai (Thailand), where the increased risk is associated with combinations of betel quid chewing with smoking or with the use of various forms of local cigar. In such areas cancers are usually advanced when diagnosed and it is frequently not possible to assess the exact site of origin.

9. Bronchus and lung

Lung cancer is predominantly a disease of cigarette smokers. Males who are heavy smokers increase their rate of disease 10 to 20 fold, females somewhat less. It is particularly the squamous and oat cell varieties of the disease which are associated with the use of tobacco. To date, cigarette smoking has been more prevalent in western, developed nations, but the successful efforts of the tobacco companies to promote use of manufactured cigarettes (frequently of high tar and nicotine content) in developing nations has led to evidence of increasing rates of lung cancer. The role of air pollution has often been investigated though any effect is small compared to that of tobacco smoke but is greater in smokers. Certain occupational exposures are also dangerous including mining (uranium, haematite, fluorspar, asbestos), steel production, coal gas manufacture, nickel and chrome processing. Asbestos, in particular, interacts with cigarette smoking to produce very high risks, and exposure to this mineral, either during production or as an insulating material, is known to cause mesothelioma of the pleura and peritoneum.

10. Soft tissue tumours

Many relative frequency series from tropical countries contain a high proportion of such cancers. As they tend to occur at younger ages part of this apparent excess may be due to age distribution of the population in question. In East Africa soft tissue sarcoma is frequently reported, largely due to the high incidence there of Kaposi's sarcoma. Marked local variations occur. A viral aetiology has been suspected.

11. Melanoma

Malignant melanoma is a tumour which appears to be increasing in frequency in many parts of the world, especially where fair-skinned populations are exposed to strong sunlight as in Australia. Intermittent exposure, as in sunbathing, may be particularly hazardous. Lowest rates are seen in Asian populations. In Africans the disease is relatively common, especially on the sole of the foot, where it is claimed to arise from pre-existing pigmented spots.

12. Other skin tumours

Squamous and basal cell carcinoma of skin are amongst the least disabling or fatal of cancers, hence information on occurrence is hard to collect. Like melanoma they are particularly common in pale skins exposed to sunlight, and are rare in pigmented skin. In African and New Guinea populations squamous carcinoma arising in an ulcer, sinus or burn scar is not uncommon. Occupational exposure to sunlight, tar and arsenic may lead to skin cancer.

13. Breast

Cancer of the breast is predominantly a disease of European and North

American females. Although less frequent in developing countries, it is usually the second most common female cancer observed and it is the most common in certain countries of north Africa. Data from Latin America suggest a wide range of incidence or mortality between European and Asian experience. The incidence of this disease appears to be rising in many countries. Despite intensive study, the causes of breast cancer are still obscure. It appears to be associated with a late age at first pregnancy and nutritional features of the western lifestyle (? fat intake).

14. Uterus

In most warm climate countries carcinoma of the cervix uteri is the commonest form of cancer in females. Particularly high rates have been recorded in Latin America and the Caribbean, especially in groups of low socio-economic level. The observation of low levels of disease in Jewish and some Moslem populations led to the belief that circumcision of the male partner had an important protective effect. This is now largely discounted, for example Moslems in North Africa show high frequencies. Lack of penile hygiene may play a role in aetiology. Sexual factors shown to be of importance in the occurrence of cervix cancer are the age of first intercourse, and the number of sexual partners.

The geographical occurrence of tumours of the uterine corpus tends to be the reciprocal of that observed for the cervix. It is thus more frequent in western countries, where incidence is believed to be rising, and is common in the prosperous Parsi population of Bombay.

15. Chorionepithelioma

There are geographical areas of high risk in South East Asia (Taiwan, Singapore, Philippines), and particularly high rates have been reported for certain African populations (Nigeria, Zimbabwe). The tumour frequently follows molar pregnancy and incidence can be expected to decrease with better detection and management of this condition.

16. Prostate and testis

The highest rates for prostate cancer are recorded in Afro-Americans and a high incidence is seen also amongst black populations of the West Indies. African populations have lower rates equivalent to those in Europe, but since this is predominantly a disease of the old and is frequently only diagnosed on autopsy, there is considerable scope for under-detection in Africa. Low incidence rates are found in oriental populations. The causes of prostatic cancer are obscure.

Testicular cancer, by contrast, appears to be exceedingly rare in black populations of African origin.

17. Penis

Cancer of the penis is a rare disease in developed countries, but is not uncommon in several regions of Africa, Asia and South and Central America. There appears to be a relationship to circumcision, since it is a common cancer in Uganda where circumcision is not practised but rare in Kenya where it is; however this correlation is far from perfect. The incidence can be reduced by improvement in penile hygiene.

18. Bladder

This tumour is especially common in zones where Bilharziasis is frequent as in Egypt and Iraq, and in certain African populations such as Zimbabwe. The tumours here are predominantly of squamous cell type, unlike bladder cancers elsewhere which are usually transitional cell carcinomas. Expanded irrigation schemes in bilharzial countries are likely to result in increased numbers of cases. In East Africa there is an apparent association with post-gonococcal urethral stricture. Other causal factors include tobacco smoking, which increases risk two or three times and a variety of occupational exposures such as dye-stuffs, rubber industry, coal gas workers.

19. Malignant lymphomas

The most interesting entity in this group of tumours in warm climates is Burkitt's lymphoma. It occurs in children of both sexes and almost exclusively in tropical climatic conditions of high temperature, humidity, low altitude and in zones of malarial endemicity. It is found commonly in Nigeria, Uganda, South East Congo, West Malaysia and Papua-New Guinea, and may account for more than half of all childhood tumours in these endemic zones. An infectious aetiology is probable, the Epstein-Barr Virus is believed to play a role in combination with intense malarial infection.

Of the other lymphomatous tumours, Hodgkins disease shows interesting epidemiological features. In the western world this disease affects mainly young and middle aged adults, but in developing countries it is predominantly a disease of childhood, indeed it may be one of the commonest childhood cancers, affecting mainly males.

20. Leukaemia

There is relatively little international variation in the frequency of leukaemia. Chronic lymphatic leukaemia, a disease of the older age groups, appears to be very rare in such oriental countries as China and Japan.

Cancer surveillance: sources of data

The paragraphs above indicate the enormous diversity which might be found in tropical countries in the pattern of cancer. In order to plan services or to identify deficiencies in health care, it is essential to have an idea of the local relative importance of the different forms of cancer. The incidence of cancer is best measured by recording information on all new cases (registration). When this is done for all cancers in a defined area of which the population is known, incidence rates can be calculated. This is 'Population-based registration' and data from several such registries in developing countries are published regularly by IARC (Waterhouse et al, 1982). Collecting data on *all* cases is a difficult and time-consuming task, and cancer registration is frequently limited to patients attending a particular hospital, or data may be based solely on tissue specimens examined in a pathology laboratory. In these latter circumstances it is not possible to calculate rates of disease, cancer occurrence can only be tabulated as the 'Relative Frequency' of different tumours amongst the total. This may give an approximate idea of the local pattern of disease, although clearly patients attending hospital or receiving biopsies will not be truly representative of the burden of disease in the community. On occasion it may be possible to calculate a minimum incidence rate by relating, say, the histologically diagnosed cases to the population of a city or a country. Such rates by excluding clinical diagnoses underestimate incidence but the true rate can only be higher than that calculated — not lower.

When incidence data are not available, it may be possible to obtain statistics on cancer mortality. Mortality is related to the incidence of disease by the survival rate. Where the latter is known and relatively constant mortality is a useful proxy indicator of occurrence. Mortality data may be available from death registration, but this is likely to be incomplete or inaccurate to varying degrees for many developing countries. Statistics are published regularly by WHO and periodically consolidated by Segi (see Segi et al, 1981). A set of maps showing mortality rates or frequency ratios for common sites of cancer were prepared by Dunham & Bailar (1968). A unique example of the use of mortality statistics in the absence of a system for registration of deaths was recently observed in China, where information on almost two million deaths was collected by thousands of field workers, resulting in a detailed presentation of cancer mortality patterns for the whole country. The use of autopsy series as a guide to cancer occurrence requires great caution in interpretation.

CANCER CONTROL

The precise mixture of services which would make up an ideal programme for cancer control in a developing country is impossible to define, since our knowledge of the effectiveness of different preventive and treatment methods is quite imperfect. Furthermore, most health care developments are incremental in nature, adding or modifying the existing structure, rather than being tailor-made to meet a given set of health problems. Some of the interventions most likely to be effective in reducing the burden of cancer are discussed below.

Prevention strategies

The rapidly increasing cost and complexity of cancer therapy and, with minor exceptions, its limited success in providing cure have stimulated renewed interest in the possibilities of prevention. The term is used not only to describe measures to inhibit disease occurrence, that is primary prevention, but also embraces actions which lead to early diagnosis and treatment, that is secondary prevention.

The section on Epidemiology has outlined some of the agents suspected of increasing the risk of specific cancers. The potential for primary prevention of a given cancer will depend on the identification of such risk factors, and the ability to reduce exposure or susceptibility to them. There may also be factors which *reduce* susceptibility to cancer — vitamin A, for example, may protect against certain epithelial cancers. When the risk factors for a cancer are ill defined, as in breast cancer, or it is unlikely that Public Health measures would be able to effect a change in habits or lifestyle, as in cervix cancer, scope for primary prevention may be limited and early detection of disease may be a more suitable option.

Primary prevention

The most successful examples of Preventive medicine are provided by the control of infectious disease by immunisation. The potential for increasing host resistance to carcinogens is thus of great interest. A most promising future seems to lie with the use of Hepatitis B Vaccine in preventing infection with this agent and consequently in reducing incidence of hepatic cancer. The long latent period between infection and development of the hepatoma, and the relative rarity of this latter, will require comparative studies between large groups of vaccinated subjects and unvaccinated controls over a very long period before the benefit of vaccination to prevent hepatoma can be demonstrated. Such trials are currently only in the planning stage.

The other major preventive strategies involve alterations in exposure to potential carcinogens or risk factors. Some exposures primarily result from personal customs or habits, others from occupation, or from the wider geographical environment embracing air, water, etcetera. Cancer control methods can be hence grouped as those which involve personal action and initiative, and those which require community action to regulate the external environment, although in practice there is considerable overlap between them.

Dietary carcinogens

Although diet was mentioned in the Epidemiology section as a possible risk factor for several digestive and reproductive tract cancers, the potential problems identified relate mainly to 'western' diets high in animal fat and low in fibre. At present, no specific recommendations can be made for inhabitants of the developing world, although this situation may change as dietary habits alter.

The status of aflatoxin as a possible carcinogen for humans has already been mentioned. Peanut crops are especially liable to contamination, but other commodities are also susceptible (Table 3). The reaction of developed nations has been to set limits on the aflatoxin levels permissible in imports of groundnuts or other cereals (curiously, the prime concern seems to have been with animal rather than human foodstuffs). This has placed the producing warm climate countries in a difficult position, since a major source of export income is threatened, and one response has been to establish quality control so that exported crops are safeguarded. The result of this on the quality and contamination levels of crops remaining for local consumption must be guessed at. The prevention of contamination is a long term and difficult goal involving improvements in agricultural and storage techniques.

The role of other food contaminants or additives as possible carcinogens is much more uncertain. It is difficult to decide which, if any, should be subject to control regulations. For example nitrates and nitrites have been suggested as possible precursors of carcinogenic nitrosamines, but their value in food preservation, and in the prevention of botulism, militates against a bar on their use. Conversely, artificial sweeteners, such as cycla-

Table 49.3 World production and exports of selected agricultural commodities susceptible to mycotoxin contamination (1975)

Commodity	World production (million tons)	Value of world exports (million US $)
Groundnuts	19	622[a]
Copra	4	332[a]
Cottonseed	22	165[a]
Sesame seed	2	124
Tree nuts (pistachios, etc.)	2.4	—
Cocoa and products	1.6	2 350
Maize	322	6 998
Rice	344	3 318
Barley	155	1 777
Sorghum	54	1 000
Millet	47	10
Oats	49	141
Rye	24	70
Cassava	105	280

[a] Including the value of cake and meal exports

From Linsell (1979)

mate, or colourants serve a much less useful purpose, and low levels of suspicion may suffice to proscribe their use.

Tobacco smoking

Tobacco is, without doubt, the single most important avoidable cause of cancer in the world. Its relative importance may presently be greater in the developed nations, but the spread of the smoking epidemic to developing countries means that the rising trend of smoking related cancers, which is already observable, will continue.

There are several reasons for the increasing use of tobacco, especially in the form of cigarettes, in warm climate countries. Tobacco is a useful cash crop and production may form a valuable source of employment and export earnings for developing countries. Cigarette production may likewise be an important source of income or employment. The attitude of government is usually at best equivocal, since cigarette sales are often an important source of tax revenue. Finally, obvious in almost all countries, are the marketing efforts of the tobacco companies with a powerful mixture of promotional schemes, advertisements and sponsorships.

The measures required to control smoking and to prevent smoking-related disease are set out in a recent WHO publication 'Controlling the smoking epidemic' (WHO, 1979). At the level of the individual there is much that can be done by health education and persuasion such as providing information about the risks of smoking, attempting to prevent the young acquiring the habit, and assisting the established smoker to stop. *All this is made much easier, however, if there is a commitment to smoking prevention by the community and its representatives in government.* Health workers have a vital duty to press for the introduction of the necessary reforms; legislation and restrictive measures can be applied in:

1. Control of sales promotion
2. Health warnings on cigarette packets and advertisements
3. Product description showing yield of harmful substances
4. Imposition of upper limits for harmful substances in smoking materials
5. Ever increasing taxation
6. Sales restrictions
7. Restrictions on smoking in public places
8. Restrictions on smoking in places of work

The special problems of tobacco producing countries should be recognised; substitute crops should be sought and subsidies applied to encourage their planting.

Chewing

The chewing of tobacco, either alone or in association with betel nut or leaf, and other ingredients is associated with cancer of the mouth, oesophagus and pharynx. Research to identify the harmful components, and how they possibly react with saliva to produce carcinogens, is required with a view to producing a less harmful material for chewing. In the meantime broadly similar measures as have been applied to smoking prevention seem applicable, in order to reduce all tobacco use, since in areas where chewing is common so too are the use of clay pipes and cheap cigarettes or bidi. Public education in oral hygiene, for example cleaning the mouth after each chew, may be attempted in addition.

Parasitic diseases

Present evidence, based mainly on autopsy surveys, suggests a connection between cholangiocarcinoma (cancer of the intrahepatic bile ducts) and infestation with liver flukes (Clonorchiasis and Opisthorchiasis). The possible role of Schistosoma haematobium as a cause of bladder cancer has been discussed. Control measures for these parasites have been dealt with. (See Davis Chapter 29)

Solar radiation

The role of solar radiation in the induction of skin cancer, including malignant melanoma, in fair-skinned subjects has been discussed. Appropriate preventive measures include public education to reduce exposures of those most at risk (pale complexioned, with dysplastic moles) and the use of protective clothing and sunscreen lotions.

Sexual practices

The relationship of carcinoma of the cervix to intercourse has lead to the suspicion that a transmissible agent is involved. It seems highly unlikely that persuasive efforts by health workers could achieve any change in the sexual mores of a community. It has been shown, however, that the use of occlusive contraceptives (diaphragm, condom) provide protection against the disease where use of the pill or IUD do not. Improved hygiene may also be protective.

Occupational risks

A wide variety of agents used in industry, agriculture and medicine have been investigated for their carcinogenic potential. IARC periodically reviews the evidence available; Table 49.4 summarises the most recent results and conclusions (IARC 1982). Phoon in chapter 51 deals with specific occupational hazards and the regulatory mechanisms in their control. It is possible that in developing countries local manufacturing industries may carry risks — a problem little studied.

Secondary prevention

Secondary prevention includes the recognition of disease at an asymptomatic stage (screening) or very soon after the onset of symptoms (early diagnosis). The objective of secondary prevention is to attempt to start treatment for cancer at as early a stage as possible when chances of success are highest. Delay in seeking treatment means spread of disease, remote prospects for curative treatment, and often difficulties in providing palliative therapy. The seven warning signs for cancer, developed by the American Cancer Society,

Table 49.4 Chemical agents known to be carcinogenic

A INDUSTRIAL EXPOSURES

AGENT	PROCESSES	SITE OF TUMOUR
Aromatic Amines (4 aminodiphenyl, benzidine, 2-naphthylamine	Dye manufacture, rubber workers, coal gas manufacture	Bladder
Arsenic	Copper/Cobalt smelting; some pesticides	Skin, lung
Asbestos	Mining, insulation work, shipbuilding	Lung, pleura, peritoneum
Benzene	Working with glue, varnish	Marrow
Bis (Chloromethyl) ether	Making ion exchange resins	Lung
Cadmium (and certain compounds)	Cadmium workers	Prostate
Chromium (and certain compounds)	Chromate, pigment manufacturers	Lung
Isopropyl oil	Manufacture of isopropyl alcohol	Nasal sinus
Mustard gas	Poison gas manufacture	Larynx, lung
Nickel	Nickel refining	Nasal sinus, lung
Soot, tars, mineral oils	Coal gas manufacture, many occupations	Skin, scrotum, lung
Vinyl chloride	PVC manufacture	Liver

B MEDICAL EXPOSURES

AGENT		SITE OF TUMOUR
Alkylating agents:	Cyclophosphamide	Bladder
	Melphalan	Marrow
Busulphan		Marrow
Chlorambucil		Leukaemia
Chlornaphazine		Bladder
Diethylstilboestrol		Endometrium (vagina: if exposure transplacental)
Oxymethalone		Liver
Phenacetin		Kidney (Pelvis)

Seven Warning
Signals of Cancer

Change in bowel or bladder habits.

A sore that does not heal.

Unusual bleeding or discharge.

Thickening or lump in breast or elsewhere.

Indigestion or difficulty in swallowing.

Obvious change in wart or mole.

Nagging cough or hoarseness.

Fig. 49.2 The seven warning signs of cancer (American Cancer Society)

Figure 49.2 are a simple way of educating potential patients in the need to seek help at an early stage. These could easily be adapted to be more appropriate for local needs and cancers such as those of the nasopharynx and liver.

Screening

Screening is defined as 'the presumptive identification of unrecognised disease or defect by the application of tests, examinations, or other procedures which can be applied rapidly. Screening tests sort out apparently well persons who probably have disease from those who probably do not. A screening test is not intended to be diagnostic. Persons with positive or suspicious findings must be referred to their physicians for diagnosis and necessary treatment' (Wilson & Junger, 1968).

A variety of screening tests have been devised to detect early cancer, and many screening programmes have been introduced. The decision as to whether screening is worthwhile — producing improved results at reasonable cost — is far from easy in practice. The evidence for the effectiveness of the most widely used procedures has been recently summarised by the American Cancer Society (1980). Present consensus would seem to be that screening for cancers of the cervix and breast may be worthwhile, and for neither of these cancers are realistic primary prevention strategies currently available.

Cervix cancer screening is carried by cytological examination of smears obtained by spatula from the area of the cervical os. Women showing abnormal cellular patterns require further diagnostic procedures, usually some form of biopsy, and appropriate treatment for the lesions discovered. These may range from dysplastic epithelial change to invasive cancer. Before a screening programme can be contemplated, therefore, the adequacy of medical facilities for cytology, histology and necessary treatment must be ensured. Controversy rages over optimum ages and frequencies for screening: there is no single ideal policy. A law of diminishing returns applies, however, in that each additional test given to a woman costs about the same but the benefit resulting becomes smaller and smaller. A minimal programme might aim to examine women perhaps every five years between the ages of 35 and 60. A more ambitious one might envisage two tests at age 20 (or at onset of sexual activity) and one every three years thereafter.

Breast cancer screening by a combination of mammography and clinical examination at annual intervals has been shown to be effective in reducing mortality in women aged over 50. This is a costly programme and one that would be clearly beyond the reach of most developing countries. The potential benefit of breast self-examination, which does not involve expensive technology at the screening stage, is at present unknown. It seems plausible, however, that early diagnosis might be achieved in this fashion, and health education programmes demonstrating and assessing the technique of self-examination should be encouraged. Before doing so it is essential to ensure that medical personnel are available to examine and to evaluate any lumps that are found.

Other screening programmes have been introduced in areas with particularly high disease rates. In Japan there is extensive experience in searching for early gastric cancer by double contrast radiography or gastroscopy, in the Indian subcontinent schemes for detecting early oral cancer by regular examinations have been introduced, and in China there are programmes to search for early oesophageal cancer by cytological examination of specimens obtained by balloon cannulas. So far none of these procedures has been subjected to studies to evaluate the health benefit to the community in relation to the expenditures involved in mass screening.

Cancer therapy

Details of treatment methods for individual cancers are beyond the scope of this review. Some progress has been made in recent years with new chemotherapeutic agents in the treatment of certain cancers such as Hodgkins disease, childhood leukaemia and choriocarcinoma. An increasing range of drugs is used in conjunction with surgery and radiotherapy. Yet despite increasing cost and sophistication of chemotherapeutic and radiotherapy techniques, there has been little corresponding improvement in results. Furthermore, finance dictates that the latest drugs and equipment will be beyond the means of almost all hospitals in developing countries. An appropriate response is perhaps the establishment of a few specialized cancer institutes where a team approach by the disciplines of surgery, radiotherapy and oncology is possible. Such centres can act not only to provide treatment but also as foci of education for health workers in simple techniques of cancer management.

It is important that cancer treatment should be seen to comprise more than attempts at cure. For many cancers, much can be done to make life more comfortable for the patient by removal of tumour masses or by the relief of obstruction. An important component of any cancer programme is to ensure that health workers have a good knowledge of, and access to, methods for pain relief. This usually involves no more than a range of simple and inexpensive drugs. For the sufferer from incurable cancer a pain-free end to life with warm sympathetic human contact are perhaps the most important of all.

REFERENCES

American Cancer Society 1980 ACS Report on the Cancer — Related Health Checkup. CA — A cancer journal for clinicians, 30: 194–240
Doll R, Peto R 1981 The causes of cancer: Oxford, Oxford University Press
Dunham L J, Bailar J C 1968 World maps of cancer mortality rates and frequency ratios. Journal of the National Cancer Institute 41: 155–203
Higginson J, Muir C S 1979 Environmental Carcinogenesis: Misconceptions and limitations to Cancer Control. Journal of the National Cancer Institute 63: 1291–1298
Hirayama T, Waterhouse J A H, Fraumeni J F 1980 Cancer Risks by Site. UICC Technical Report Series Vol. 41, Geneva, UICC
Kmet J 1970 The role of migrant populations in studies of selected cancer sites. A review. Journal of Chronic Diseases 23: 305–324
Lancet 1981 Human virus, hepatic cancer. Lancet ii: 1394–1395
Linsell C A 1979 Decision on the control of a dietary carcinogen — Aflatoxin. In Davis W, Rosenfeld C (eds) Carcinogenic Risks: Strategies for Intervention. IARC Scientific Publications No 25. IARC Lyon
Magnus K (ed) 1982 Trends in Cancer Incidence; causes and practical implications. Washington, Hemisphere Publishing Corpn.
Muir C S, Nectoux J 1982 International Patterns of Cancer, In Schottenfeld D, Fraumeni J F (eds) Cancer Epidemiology & Prevention, Saunders, Philadelphia
Segi M, Aoki K, Kurihara M 1981 World Cancer Mortality. GANN Monograph on Cancer Research 26: 121–274
United Nations 1980 The World Population Situation in 1979. Population studies No 72. UN Publication No. ST/ESA/SER.A/72
Waterhouse J A H, Muir C S, Shanmugaratnam K, Powell J 1982 Cancer Incidence in Five Continents, Volume IV. IARC Scientific Publications No. 42, IARC Lyon
WHO 1979 Controlling the Smoking Epidemic. Technical Report Series No 636, Geneva, WHO
WHO 1980 Sixth report on the World Health Situation: I. Global Analysis, Geneva, WHO
Wilson J M G, Junger G 1968 Principles and practice of screening for disease. Public Health Papers No. 34, Geneva, WHO

Appendix overleaf.

APPENDIX

Incidence rates of solid tumours (around 1975)
Figures are age-adjusted incidence rates per 100,000 (World population standard)

SITE and ICD-8 NUMBER

		1 Mouth	2 Naso phar	3 Oes	4 Stom	5 Colon + Rect	6 Liver	7 Nose etc	8 Larynx	9 Lung	10 Soft tiss	11 Mela noma	12 Other skin	13 Breast	14 Cervix	15 Chorio	16 Prost	17 Penis	18 Bladder
		143/5	147	150	151	153/4	155	160	161	162	171	172	173	174	180	181	185	187	188
AFRICA																			
Senegal: Dakar (1969–74)	M	1.0	0.1	0.2	3.7	2.1	25.6	0.3	1.3	1.1	2.7	1.2	10.3	—	—	—	4.3	0.4	3.0
	F	1.3	0.0	0.2	2.0	1.7	9.0	0.3	0.1	0.1	1.5	1.3	7.9	11.8	17.2	0.9	—	—	1.7
CARIBBEAN/S. AMERICA																			
Jamaica: Kingston (1973–77)	M	2.8	1.7	7.1	17.7	12.4	6.1	1.3	4.6	19.8	2.4	0.7	10.1	—	—	—	28.6	5.7	8.5
	F	1.4	0.5	3.0	9.3	11.3	2.1	0.6	0.4	4.0	1.9	1.4	7.0	39.0	29.8	0.5	—	—	3.9
Brazil: Sao Paulo (1973)	M	6.8	0.7	14.1	45.7	19.3	1.2	2.2	15.8	31.1	2.7	2.1	53.6	—	—	—	22.2	2.1	15.4
	F	1.7	0.2	2.8	18.9	16.6	0.3	0.7	1.9	6.4	2.1	2.1	47.5	56.2	37.5	0.4	—	—	3.4
Colombia: Cali (1972–76)	M	2.1	0.3	3.1	46.3	7.9	1.9	1.7	6.5	19.5	2.6	2.6	47.5	—	—	—	22.3	2.0	9.8
	F	1.9	0.2	1.7	27.3	7.7	1.5	1.3	1.0	5.4	2.1	1.5	46.2	33.2	52.9	0.3	—	—	2.6
ASIA																			
Hong Kong: (1974–77)	M	2.8	32.9	18.6	22.5	26.6	34.4	3.2	11.2	55.5	1.8	1.1	5.8	—	—	—	5.1	1.5	17.1
	F	0.9	14.4	5.5	10.3	23.7	8.9	1.2	1.1	23.4	1.6	1.0	3.2	31.1	30.4	0.3	—	—	5.9
India: Bombay (1973–75)	M	5.8	0.7	15.7	9.7	8.0	2.7	1.3	12.9	14.2	1.2	0.2	2.8	—	—	—	6.8	2.0	3.5
	F	5.8	0.3	10.7	5.9	6.6	1.0	0.9	2.6	4.0	0.7	0.2	1.7	21.2	23.3	0.2	—	—	0.9
Israel: Jewish pop. (1972–76)	M	1.1	0.8	2.2	18.9	27.0	2.9	0.6	6.0	29.3	4.4	4.7	—	—	—	—	15.5	0.1	20.9
	F	0.6	0.5	1.5	11.4	25.8	1.3	0.4	0.6	9.0	2.8	6.1	—	59.9	4.9	0.4	—	—	4.5

Accidents and violence

INTRODUCTION

In much of the western world accidental injury has now replaced infectious disease as the major cause of death amongst persons in the first 40 years of life. Indeed accidents are now only exceeded by cancer and ischaemic heart disease in England and Wales as a cause of loss of years of working life. (Bull, 1979). This is, of course, not (yet) true for many of the developing countries, but the trend is already beginning towards a vastly increasing incidence of accidents and violence as causes of mortality and disability. Road accidents make up a very high proportion of the total, but domestic accidents contribute almost equally to the fatalities, and occupational accidents, while important, make only a small proportion (numerically) of the total.

The writer has worked as a general surgeon for five years in the university hospital in Uganda, and for six years in a consultant and reference hospital in Northern Tanzania. During this time he was much struck with the high proportion of accident cases among the surgical admissions. In the Kilimanjaro Christian Medical Centre, he found that sixty percent of the surgical beds were taken up with accident cases at any one time, and half the surgeon's time and energy was taken up in dealing with these as opposed to the non-accident cases. Tragically the same is true for children as for adults. Shija and Omar (1980) found that trauma accounted for nearly half of all admissions to the paediatric surgical ward in Dar-es-Salaam, Tanzania, and was the leading cause (45 to 55 percent) of death. Of the trauma cases in this paediatric series, fractures and dislocations accounted for 60 percent, and burns and scalds for 33 percent.

Archaeology bears mute witness to the fact that violence between humans has been present since our race began, and while Europe and North America have escaped the ravages of war for the last thirty five years, parts of the developing world have been less fortunate, and during wars and times of civil instability violence between humans dominates the traumatology scene. It compounds the damage by disrupting cemmunications and interfering with medical care.

ROAD TRAFFIC ACCIDENTS

Strictly comparable figures are not available from the different parts of the world, but such studies as have been made show an increase in the number of road accident fatalities per year as a proportion of the population in all countries. In the study made by Jacobs and Fouracre (1977), developing countries showed the greatest increases in this fatality rate, and among these, four (Kenya, Sabah, St. Lucia and Zambia), had a greater than 100 percent increase in the fatality rate over a ten year period.

It is probable that ten million people are injured in road traffic accidents each year, and about 250,000 die as a result of their injuries. Africa and Asia probably contribute between forty and fifty thousand of these deaths each year. The seriousness of these sombre figures is heightened by the fact that so many of those killed are drawn from the productive and educated sectors of society, and represent people who can ill be spared.

The importance of road accidents is such that transport and road research laboratories have been set up to study road accident statistics from many countries in the hope of learning where preventive action might halt or even reverse the steady increase in the toll on the roads of the world. An important paper by Smeed (1958) points out the value of such epidemiological research, and goes on to suggest the value of making 'Accident maps' whereby roads that had a very bad reputation for accidents could be distinguished from those that were relatively safe, and so allow preventive action to be focussed on the danger spots. Another important point made by Smeed is the multiplicity of factors that go toward the causation of any one accident — the mechanical condition of the vehicle(s) involved, the state of the road surface, negligence on the part of drivers, poor illumination of the roads and the presence or absence of adequate road signs. The implication was that improvement of any one of these factors might well have prevented that accident. The same writer (Smeed, 1968) in a study of accidents involving pedestrians revealed that certain types of vehicle were much more likely than others to injure pedestrians. In this respect, motor cycles were found to be the most dangerous, then public service vehicles, then the motor car, with the pedal cycle by far the least likely (per mile of road travelled) to cause such injury. He also confirmed that a pedestrian was three times more likely to become a casualty at night than by day, and much more likely to become a casualty at night if the roads were wet. In this important study evidence is quoted to show that the provision of illumination on roads at night reduces the number of pedestrian casualties by almost half.

For developing countries an important study is that of Jacobs and Sayer (1977) who showed that the accident rates in cities were considerably higher in developing countries than, for instance, in Britain for similar levels of vehicle flow. Thus rates in Nairobi and Surabaya were found to be respectively 35 percent and 140 percent greater than in Britain. Indeed at faster rates of vehicle flow these differences rose to 80 percent and 200 percent respectively. At a flow rate of 3000 vehicles per hour the risks to pedestrians were respectively 180 percent and 260 percent greater in Nairobi and Surabaya than in Great Britain. Why is there this difference? It is suggested that as vehicle ownership increases in a given community, so does the sophistication of the population and their awareness of the dangers that cars bring. With this awareness comes better discipline among road users together with road safety planning and legislation which introduce such devices as traffic lights, pedestrian crossings and segregated traffic schemes. With the increase in car ownership also comes a slowing up of traffic in major cities until, as in London at times, the vehicles travel at a crawl if at all and the danger to all concerned is proportionately reduced. Certainly the relationship between casualty rates and the numbers of vehicles on the roads is not a linear one, and Bull (1970) has pointed out that casualties are related not to the number of vehicles on the roads but to the cube root of that number.

Preventive measures

What can be done to bring the carnage on the roads under control? The first necessity is awareness on the part of those responsible for town planning, for legislation and for education, of the size of the problem. Here is the importance of proper epidemiological study. An analysis of the ten countermeasures that could theoretically be expected to reduce accidents and their results has been made by Haddon (1973) and this analysis repays careful study. Many of the countermeasures that his analysis suggests, for example multi-lane highways, crash helmets, speed limits, seat belts, and the setting up of accident centres, have already been tried and have been shown statistically to reduce mortality from road accidents. One of the most exciting developments in recent years has been the involvement of the road trauma committee of the Australasian College of Surgeons in active intervention to reduce fatality and injury on Australian roads (McDermott, 1978). This committee in 1970 began a nationwide campaign in support of legislation for the compulsory wearing of seatbelts in the front seats of cars. First public ignorance had to be countered by dissemination of adequate information based on firm statistical data, and parliamentary inertia had to be similarly overcome. Here were surgeons moving out of their conventional 'curative' role into a more unfamiliar 'preventive' role. (Should this not be so in many fields?) As a result very largely of the activities of this committee compulsory wearing of seatbelts was introduced, in Victoria at first and later in the whole of Australia. The result has been immediate, impressive and persistent reduction in the numbers of driver fatalities. Further activity is now being directed towards reducing injury to child occupants of cars and towards countering the very real menace of alcohol intake on the roads and the damage caused thereby. Although prosecution of drunken drivers has failed to bring the problem under control, a study using matched controls has shown a reduction (by 40 percent) of reconvictions for drunken driving when those convicted of drunken driving have been submitted to a re-education programme. As a result of their experience, the committee is suggesting a three-pronged attack on the drink-driving problem:— 1) Deterrence with increasingly vigorous law enforcement of deterrent breathalyser and random breath test legislation, 2) Improved education of drivers about the effect of alcohol on driving and 3) A national campaign directed at control of alcohol abuse, with (as part of the campaign) a total ban on all alcohol promotion and advertising.

Town planning plays a major part in preventing accidents. In Stevenage, a town in Britain, it was decided to segregate motorised traffic from the pedestrians and pedal cyclists, on the assumption that pedal cyclists were unlikely to inflict much harm on the pedestrians. The results (Hudson, 1978) have been impressive. Only nine accidents involving cyclists and pedestrians were recorded up to 1976, and no fatal accident has occurred on the pedestrian cycleway. Stevenage accident rates are only one third of the national average. As the rising costs of petrol drive greater numbers towards the bicycle as a means of transport, we would do well to heed the lesson of this important and imaginative piece of planning.

One countermeasure that has been found to reduce the number of accidents is the constant presence on the roads of police. These can not only detect and warn drivers of faulty driving habits, but also help in schools in the teaching of proper care on the roads. Smeed (1968) showed a significant improvement in the performance of drivers and pedestrians during and following a noticeable police presence.

BURNS

Of domestic accidents in warm climate countries burns must rate highly in consideration, not only because of the unduly high mortality, but also because of the severe disfigurement that so often follows the burn wound. Many victims are epileptic and it is tragic to note how few of them have had their seizures adequately kept under control and how few have even been warned of the dangers of sitting close to fires when on their own.

Fatal burn injuries may however also be sustained by those who are not epileptic, as when a voluminous dress, such as a sari, flares into conflagration as a result of an accident with an oil stove. Stringent regulations about the adequate safeguarding of electric, gas and other fires, are in force in countries such as Britain, largely because of the representations made by physicians who have studied and publicised the statistics of the results of burns (Colebrook et al 1956) (Bull et al 1964). It is now an offence to sell a portable heater that is not adequately safeguarded or to sell childrens nightdresses that are made of flammable material.

An epidemiological study of burns from Zambia (Sinha, 1978) shows that scalding was the cause of the injury in 73 out of 99 cases admitted to the wards of the teaching hospital. Tragically, 88 percent of the victims were under the age of 14 years, most of the children were, as would be expected, from the poorer sections of the population and most of the children had burns resulting directly or indirectly from an open fire. A lesson might be learned from the Ujamaa villages of Tanzania, where a preventive medical worker may go and visit a village at the request of the elders. He discusses their problems and answers their questions, but it is the villagers themselves who decide what action to take. It is their decision which is enforced. The penalty for non-compliance can be a fine of up to (the equivalent of) fifty dollars. Although medical professionals may have to be the initiators of the preventive process, decisions taken will have little effect unless it is the local community members who feel that they have made the decisions.

INDUSTRIAL ACCIDENTS

With the march towards industrialisation, the introduction of new, dangerous and often unfamiliar machinery often proceeds at a pace that outstrips the introduction of the necessary safety measures. The result is that lethal and crippling accidents occur at a quite unacceptable rate until the dangers become known and the necessary counter-measures are taken. The injuries of industrialised agriculture are perhaps the worst of all. (Robinson, 1978) In developing countries, the sophistication of the preventive measures often fails to match the sophistication of the industrial process, and disaster results. Even where factory safety practices are comprehensive and strict as many as 65 per cent of the accidents are due to infrigement, sometimes quite flagrant, of known regulations (Rea 1981). Britain is fortunate in having had several factories acts (Hunter, 1975) which require all accidents and mishaps in factories resulting in absence from work of more than three days to be reported to a factory inspector who visits the work and takes appropriate action. This action may involve fencing off heavy machines, providing guards to prevent hands getting inside power presses, providing padlocks on switchgear so that electrical machinery cannot be switched on while the equipment is being serviced, enforcing the wearing of toe caps in boots and the use of protective overalls and goggles where necessary. (Porter et al, 1981). Posters in factories should be specific in their warnings, as a warning 'danger within' may only introduce an atmosphere of nervousness. By contrast the words 'put out bare lights, extinguish cigarettes — explosives within' are more likely to result in appropriate action being taken. Medical staff, where they are aware of any factory or farm where accidents are taking a heavy toll, have the responsibility, not only of treating the patients, but also of advising the firm concerned, or the government's factories inspectorate, of measures that need to be taken. They may also advise on the contents of first aid boxes in such premises, and on the training of first aid workers within the workforce.

TREATMENT

One parameter that is measured in consideration of accident statistics is the 'severity index'. This is the proportion of casualties that are fatal. That for Singapore in 1968 was 3.26 (9576 casualties with 312 deaths) That for Pakistan in that year was 24.34 (Jacobs & Hutchinson, 1973). One of the many factors influencing this statistic is undoubtedly the availability, close to the scene of the accident, of adequate medical care and prompt attention. This does not necessarily mean that physicians are needed to give such early medical care. Paramedical workers, such as the Medical Assistants of East Africa, or the Assistant Medical Officers of Tanzania can be trained to give adequate care with simple yet reliable equipment provided that their training and the selection of equipment and methods is matched to the inevitable simplicity of their rural surroundings (Bewes, 1978). In many developing countries the selection and training of such cadres of personnel might well with advantage be given high priority. In far too many countries, those of the affluent West being no exception, the responsibility for the early care rests only too often upon the shoulders of junior and inexperienced staff, often working long hours quite unsupervised. Yet it is the early moments following injury that are often crucial in determining the outcome. It is not enough to provide physicians and surgeons in the urban centres only — accidents often occur out in the countryside far away from the sophisticated centres of modern medicine.

CONCLUSION

Epidemiology and appropriate action based upon the statistics studied are likely to play a crucial part in any attempts to halt the rising tide of accident fatalities and cripping injuries. Improvement in the present unacceptable situation is unlikely to be seen unless medical workers take the initiative in what is now proving one of the most challenging preventive opportunities facing medicine today.

REFERENCES

Bewes P C 1978 An appropriate technology for surgery in District Hospitals. Journal of Royal College of Surgeons of Edinburgh 23: 161–164
Bull J P 1970 Epidemiology of Road accidents. British Journal of Hospital Medicine, 437
Bull J P 1979 Accidents and their prevention. In: Hobson W (ed) Theory and Practice of Public Health, 5th edn. Oxford Medical Publications. ch 28, p 418
Bull J P, Jackson D M, Walton C 1964 Causes and Prevention of Domestic Burning Accidents. British Medical Journal 2: 1421–1427
Colebrook L, Colebrook V, Bull J P, Jackson D M 1956 prevention of burning accidents. British Medical Journal i, 1379
Haddon W 1973 Energy damage and the ten countermeasure strategies. Journal of Trauma 13: 321–331
Hudson M 1978 The Bicycle planning book. Friends of the Earth, London. ch. 6, pp 60–61
Hunter, D 1975 The diseases of Occupations. 5th edn. English Universities Press, London. ch. xv

Jacobs G D, Fouracre P R 1977 Further research on Road Accident rates in developing countries. Transport & Road Research Laboratory, supplementary report 270, Crowthorne, Berkshire

Jacobs G D, Hutchinson P 1973 A study of accident rates in developing countries. Transport & Road Research Laboratory report LR 546

Jacobs G D, Sayer I A 1977 A study of Road Accidents in selected urban areas in developing countries. Transport & Road Research Laboratory. Report 775

McDermott F 1978 Control of road trauma epidemic in Australia. Annals Royal College of Surgeons of England 60: 437–450

Porter R, Price J, Read R (eds) 1981 Trauma and after. Pitman Medical, London p 41–47

Rea E 1981 Mine accidents in Zambia. Proceedings of the Association of Surgeons of East Africa 4: 176–181

Robinson, D W 1978 Severe Farm injuries. Proceedings of Association of Surgeons of East Africa, 1: 78

Shija J K, Omar O S 1980 Trauma as a major paediatric surgical problem in Dar-es-Salaam. Proceedings of the Association of Surgeons of East Africa 3: 169–170

Sinha P 1978 Epidemiology of Burns. Proceedings of Association of Surgeons of East Africa. 1: 40–42

Smeed R J 1958 Road Accident Statistics in relation to Road Safety Activities. Reprinted from 'International Road Safety and Traffic Review' Vol VI, No. 4. World Touring and Automobile Association (O.T.A.) London

Smeed R J 1968 Aspects of Pedestrian Safety. Journal of Transport Economics and Policy, 2: No. 3

Smith R 1981 Preventing alcohol problems: a job for Canute? British Medical Journal 283: 972–975

Smith R 1982 Alcohol in the Third World — a chance to avoid a miserable trap. British Medical Journal 284: 183–185

Effects of industrialization

INTRODUCTION

Throughout warm climate countries, the process of industrialization is gaining momentum and is usually the cornerstone of national development. It has conferred great benefits upon the livelihood and prosperity of many people. Manual labour is often reduced. More jobs are created. With more money for the nation, more medical and social benefits are possible. With greater purchasing power for the individual worker, the nutrition, housing and health of his family and himself are often improved.

At the same time, new hazards to health could be introduced by industrialization or associated with it. The District Health Officer or community physician should have a good understanding of these possible hazards, so that the health of the community under his or her charge can be safeguarded.

COMMUNITY HEALTH PROBLEMS DUE TO INDUSTRIALIZATION

Lack of planning or zoning of industries

Sometimes there is insufficient co-ordination between the authorities responsible for approving and controlling industries and those responsible for health. Consequently, residential locations may be quite unnecessarily situated in the same immediate neighbourhood as industries which pose nuisance problems. In some warm climate countries, for example, modern and new housing estates have found themselves next to very dusty or noisy factories. Both the housing estates and factories were officially approved, but by different authorities acting in isolation from each other.

At other times, incompatible industries are placed side by side. For example, a soya-bean sauce factory was sited opposite one making mosquito coils. There was a danger of pyrethrum contaminating the sauce and hence food.

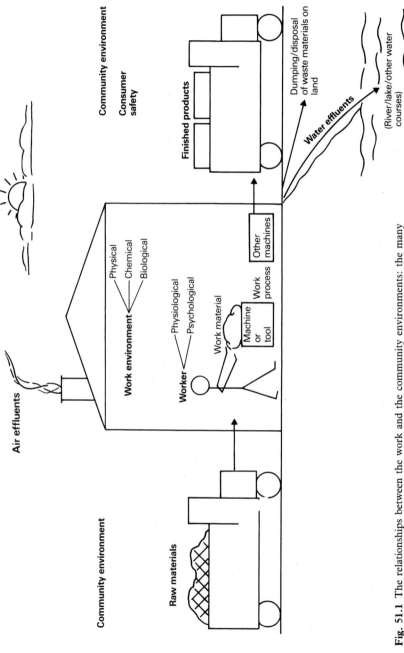

Fig. 51.1 The relationships between the work and the community environments: the many interfaces which could threaten health.

Pollution

The effluents from worksites could cause pollution of land, water and air. Notorious examples in developed countries have included 'Minamata disease', which was organic mercury poisoning owing to the discharge of untreated wastes from factories into Minamata Bay, Japan. Fish swallowed the mercury and humans became paralysed or blind as a result of eating contaminated fish. Smogs, a combination of fog and smoke, have arisen from air pollution due to industrial effluents, although in many cases the exhausts from automobiles and chimney flues have also been contributory factors. Warm climate countries usually have atmospheric conditions which do not favour the formation of severe smogs, but in many such countries there have been increasing levels of air pollution.

Ecological inbalances

In many tropical countries, insect-borne diseases, such as malaria and dengue haemorrhagic fever, are still prevalent. Large construction schemes are usual concomitants of industrialization. Sometimes, if sufficient care is not exercised, construction work may lead to disruption of normal drainage and may then create conditions favourable to the breeding of insect vectors. Epidemics of malaria have resulted from this cause. Epidemics of dengue haemorrhagic fever have occurred, following the proliferation of culicine mosquitoes in the puddles of water trapped in construction sites.

The control of community health and industrial health is often in the hands of different government ministries. As a result, the public health inspectors, responsible for community health, may not inspect the precincts of worksites. At the same time, the industrial health inspectors may be so engrossed with industrial health problems as to neglect the public health ones under their noses.

Rural-urban migration

Industrialization usually occurs in urban centres. Consequently, there is often a exodus from the villages and rural areas to the towns (Phoon 1975). The public health facilities are often subject to great strain as a result. Overcrowding of existing accommodation and the development of 'shanty towns' with their lack of sanitation, poverty and sometimes crime frequently follow. Many fail to realize their ambitions or to even find a job. They may drift into crime, alcoholism or drug-abuse.

OCCUPATIONAL HEALTH PROBLEMS

Often the terms 'occupational health' and 'industrial health' are used as synonyms. 'Occupational health' in recent years has gained more popularity, as many experts contend that the term 'industrial health' puts undue emphasis on industries. 'Occupational health' as usually understood, refers to the health of workers or the health problems arising from work. In occupational health we must always consider the following factors:—

(a) The worker
(b) The materials he uses
(c) The work process
(d) The work environment

The causes of occupational health problems can be grouped under the following headings:—

1. Accidents
2. Physical causes, such as light, heat, noise, changes in barometric pressure, electricity and dust hazards
3. Chemical causes, such as metals and hydrocarbons
4. Biological causes, such as anthrax and tetanus, which often occur in an occupational setting.
5. Mental causes, such as poor work morale or maladjustment to working conditions.

In a short chapter such as this, it is not possible to discuss in a comprehensive manner all these occupational health problems. We will confine our attention to those which are common to warm climate countries and of particular interest to a District Health Officer. Instead of giving lists of such problems, we shall deal with examples which illustrate important principles.

The introduction of new technology to traditional work situations

New chemicals

Probably one of the commonest examples is the increasing use of pesticides in agriculture. In many developing countries, poisoning from pesticides has become increasingly frequent (WHO 1979). Pesticide poisoning can be occupational or non-occupational. Pesticide sprayers and preparers could suffer from pesticide poisoning.

Accidental cases, especially among children, could occur from the careless disposal of half-empty containers. A minority of cases involves suicide. Obviously, the signs and symptoms vary according to the pesticide involved. Organophosphorus compounds are probably the commonest pesticides used. Their effects resemble those of exaggerated parasympathetic nervous activity.

Organochlorine derivatives, such as 'aldrin' and 'dieldrin' are also commonly used. Organochlorine compounds also tend to accumulate in the body, unlike organophosphorus ones, which do not. It is controversial whether they pose an imminent danger to human health. However, their use has been banned in several countries.

New equipment

In many developing countries, fishermen-divers abound. They are traditionally 'free divers', that is, they dive by holding their breath. In recent years, such workers have begun to use compressed air system with respirators. As a result, they can now dive to greater depths and for long periods of time. Their productivity is often enhanced. Now too they have begun to suffer from 'decompression illness', which is due basically to the formation of nitrogen bubbles in their tissues when they ascend too rapidly from the depths of the sea to the surface. These bubbles interfere with the blood supply to various organs. Along fascial planes and in the vicinity of joints, they may cause 'bends', manifested as pains in limbs. Similar phenomena in the coronary circulation may cause angina and in the brain 'staggers', which is in the form of ataxia. Hemiparesis, amblyopia, dyspnoea and syncope may also occur. A sequel to what is probably interference of the blood supply to bones causes 'osteonecrosis', a kind of aseptic necrosis affecting the long bones (Phoon et al 1976).

Another example is the introduction of electric drills and cutters into traditional trades such as stone masonry. In a village in a warm climate country, the carving of tombstones from granite blocks may have been a family occupation for generations. Previously, rather primitive tools such as hammer and chisel were used. During the last few years, electric-powered tools are used. The speed and finesse of work have improved. Unfortunately there is also now the production of more dust of fine particle size. The hazard to the workers' lungs of silicosis, due to the free silica in the granite, has multiplied many times.

It should be pointed out that environmental and health conditions are often worse in small than large worksites. In a study of 80 small factories, only nine were found to have satisfactory working conditions and work environment (Phoon and Tan 1975).

New processes

Many of the new processes introduced into traditional industries produce higher temperatures than the primitive processes they replaced. Sometimes the danger of heat stress, in the form of heat cramps, heat syncope or heat stroke, is thereby enhanced.

The introduction of new industries into the country or district

Importation of machines without guards

Many machines are imported without mechanical guards. In developed countries, and indeed in the laws of most developing countries, mechanical guards are required for all moving or cutting parts of machines within the usual reach of the operator. Hence many needless injuries have resulted, in the form of mangled or amputated limbs.

Importation of 'dangerous industries'

In developed countries, many hazards, especially chemical ones, are stringently controlled. For example, carbon disulphide was used extensively in the West in the vulcanization of rubber and later in the manufacture of viscose rayon. Partly because of stringent controls over this dangerous chemical and partly in order to avoid high wages, many such industries have shifted to developing countries, including those in the tropics. There is now a serious danger of carbon disulphide poisoning in those countries. Carbon disulphide can cause serious disturbances of the central nervous system, lungs and kidneys.

Another example is that of the industries concerned with asbestos. In developed countries more and more attention is now focussed on asbestos-related diseases, such as a higher risk of lung cancer, asbestosis (fibrosis of the lungs due to asbestos) and mesothelioma (cancer of the serous membranes of the pleura or peritoneum). Developing countries are now experiencing an increasing number of asbestos-related industries in their midst.

One of the newest chemical hazards imported into developing countries is vinyl chloride monomer. This chemical has been known for many decades to cause Raynaud's phenomenon, dermatitis and absorption of the bones of the fingers. It was also found to cause angiosarcoma of the liver in human beings only as recently as a decade ago. Many government in developed countries have imposed strict laws against this hazard. We now begin to see a few industries using this dangerous chemical in warm climate countries, often unaccompanied by adequate precautions.

Other common occupational hazards

In warm climate countries, there is a wide range of other occupational diseases. In mining countries, sillicosis is common. In all industrializing countries, noise-induced hearing loss, occupational dermatitis (also called occupational dermatosis) and metal poisoning occur frequently.

Noise-induced hearing loss is due to damage of the receptor cells for hearing in the cochlea from excessive levels of noise, usually above 85 or 90 decibels on the A scale. The process is insidious. At first the hearing loss is temporary and slight. Later on, usually after several years, permanent and severe hearing loss may ensue. Foundries, shipyards, bottling plants, boiler houses and construction sites are some locations where there is excessive noise.

Occupational dermatitis is often defined as inflammation of the skin of a non-infectious origin which arises from circumstances relating to work. It is a contact dermatitis which could be due to chemical or physical causes. Chemical causes predominate and the majority are 'primary irritants' (not causing allergy). Common causes of occupational dermatitis are acids, alkalis, mineral oils (such as kerosene and diesel oil), epoxy-resins, epichlorhydrin and fibre-glass. Other causes of occupational dermatitis include many kinds of wood-dust, cement dust, chromate compounds and nickel.

Metal poisoning is widespread in warm climate countries and is often undetected or misdiagnosed. Heavy metals, such as lead, mercury, arsenic and cadmium, are common causes. Different metals cause different signs and symptoms. Most of them cause disturbances of the nervous system as well as of other organs. The classical signs and symptoms of lead poisoning are anaemia, colic, fits and wrist drop. A well-known sign of lead absorption, with or without poisoning, is a bluish stippling of the gums. In many coloured races, patches of pigmentation in the gums and other parts of the mouth are common. They should not be mistaken for the 'lead line' suggestive of lead absorption. The latter is in the form of a fine interrupted line, in contrast to the usually large patches of natural pigmentation (Phoon 1977).

PSYCHOSOCIAL EFFECTS OF INDUSTRIALIZATION

This is a vast subject by itself. In this chapter, we shall be able to mention some of these main effects very briefly:—

Effects of urbanization

There are many positive effects of urbanization, such as a rise in the standard of living, improvements in health facilities and better amenities for education and welfare. Nevertheless, adverse effects can also occur from urbanization. They include an increase of traffic accidents (often due to greater congestion of vehicles and increased density of road users), intensification of noise levels in the community and overcrowding.

Mental stress

Mental stress can occur in any society. Industrialization additionally can lead to the erosion of traditional family ties, thereby depriving an individual of the moral support of the family, so vital especially in adversity. Moreover, individuals from rural areas migrating into a town may find themselves adrift in a very strange environment and a different life style. The regimentation of working hours and work organization, characteristic of modern industry, may also not be easily accepted by people more used to tribal or rural ways of life. The pace of modern life and the rapid transformation of society can pose additional threats to mental health.

In some warm climate countries, especially in the Southeast Asian region, numerous cases of 'mass hysteria' or epidemic hysteria' have occurred in recent years of (Phoon 1981). Most of the events occurred in young women working in electronic factories, where the work is usually light but boring and the pay is poor. Suddenly, a worker would fall into a trance-like state or become very violent. Often victims would claim that there was a 'bad smell' or that an apparition was haunting them. In a recent outbreak, several girls became hysterical, shouting and screaming, after one of their colleagues reported that she saw a woman with fangs licking the girl's used menstrual pad in the toilet.

INVESTIGATION AND CONTROL OF HEALTH EFFECTS OF INDUSTRIALIZATION

The investigation and control of the adverse effects on health caused by industrialization should follow epidemiological principles similar to those for communicable diseases.

'Agents'

Those which can cause ill effects should be prevented from entering the community whenever possible.

At the international level

We have already mentioned certain hazards which are being 'exported' from developed countries to warm climate countries. These hazards include carbon disulphide and vinyl chloride monomer. Through national governments and international agencies such as the World Health Organization, World Bank and International Labour Office, we could make sure that such hazards are not introduced into developing countries without stringent control and adequate safety measures.

At the national level

National authorities must make sure that health is not sacrificed for economic interests. All new enterprises should be properly screened for hazards before licensing and adequate safeguards should be insisted upon.

At the district level

The community medicine or public health professional staff must get to know all the worksites in their area and the processes and materials they used. Very often there would be no specialists in occupational health in the district. It would be the responsibility of the public health service to control both the occupational and public health hazards in such worksites.

The co-operation between the health and other authorities in charge of zoning, economic and industrial matters is vital to effective preventive action at the district, as well as at the national, level. It is necessary to hold regular consultations and to co-ordinate efforts between the various agencies responsible (Sofoluwe 1968).

Surveillance

Notification of cases

The notification of cases is an important aspect of disease control in the community (Colbourne 1978). Notification of both accidents and diseases arising from work (occupational accidents and occupational diseases) is often very incomplete, despite the fact that laws for such notification exist in most countries. In one warm climate country, researchers have found thousands of cases of pesticide poisoning among workers. Yet scarcely any of those cases had been notified to the government previously.

Registers of workers exposed to special risks

It is very useful to keep registers of workers subject to special risks, such as ionizing radiation, dangerous dusts, such as silica and asbestos, and high noise levels.

Regular examinations of workers exposed to special risks

Using the registers already mentioned, workers exposed to special risks can be traced and given clinical and laboratory examinations to detect early deviations of health or signs of absorption of noxious agents.

Monitoring of the work environment

Community health workers cannot expect to be able to do complicated tests to measure levels of physical or chemical agents in the work environment without further training in occupational health. Normally, such tests would be done either by an occupational hygienist or by an occupational health physician. The community health physician, however, could perform quite easily simple assessments of the work environment, such as measurement of noise levels with a sound-level meter, assessment of temperature and humidity with a hygrometer and testing for level of illumination with a photometer. With some extra training, the physician could also measure the approximate levels of toxic substances in the air with direct-reading indicator tubes. These tubes depend upon the principle of colour change. A measured volume of air containing the chemical in question is sucked into a tube containing reagents which react with that chemical.

Control

The scope of this chapter does not allow us to discuss specific control measures in detail.

Specific measures

For the individual worker, control measures could include use of protective equipment, such as respirators, aprons, boots, gloves, goggles, safety harnesses and helmets.

For the work environment, control measures could include exhaust ventilation and the enclosure of dangerous processes or machinery.

For the community environment, control measures, such as the installation of anti-pollution devices and the use of noise dampeners, could be implemented.

Non-specific measures

Individual workers should be educated regarding job hazards and how to control them. They should practise good personal hygiene, such as regular and thorough cleansing of their hands and bodies, to minimise absorption of noxious or irritating substances through the skin. They should be well-nourished, as ill-health or malnutrition predisposes to intoxication by chemicals in the work environment.

The community should ensure that its water drainage is not blocked by new construction and that its food and water supplies are not contaminated by industrial effluents. Proper heed should also be paid to mental health.

THE VALUE OF PRIMARY PREVENTION AND REHABILITATION

We have already referred to many undesirable consequence of industrialization. In some warm climate countries, where endemic tropical infections are rife, occupationally-related diseases have already overtaken such infections in prevalence. In an African country, cases of pesticide poisoning now outnumber those from schistosomiasis, which used to be the leading cause of severe morbidity in that country. The levels of air and water pollution, as well as of noise, are rapidly increasing in many developing countries. It usually costs far more to remedy established conditions than to prevent them, both in terms of economic and social costs. Moreover, there is no specific cure for many occupational diseases, most of which are preventable.

Rehabilitation of the victims of occupational accidents and diseases is essential for the well-being of the individuals, their families and the whole community. Industrial rehabilitation should be multi-disciplinary, planned according to the occupation, personality and socio-economic factors of the patient, and should be implemented as soon as possibe after the injury or disease. Neurosis or permanent physical disability may develop if rehabilitation is postponed for too long (Somerville 1981). The loss to the community could be severe, as often diseased or injured workers have been trained at considerable expense. Their inability to continue at work could affect severely the economic development of their community.

CONCLUSION

The health officer at the district or provincial level should be fully aware of the possible health consequences of industrialization. These include pollution, ecological inbalances, the strain on public health resources in the towns due to intense rural-urban migration and occupational health problems. Such occupational health problems may be physical, chemical, biological or psychosocial. These problems can be prevented or solved by applying epidemiological principles in the control of noxious agents, surveillance and the use of other specific and non-specific methods of disease control.

REFERENCES

Colbourne M J 1978 Interface between Public Health and Occupational Health and its implications. In 'Proceedings of the Regional Seminar on Occupational Health', Singapore, 3–5
Phoon W O 1975 The impact of industrial growth on health in South-East Asia. In 'Health and Industrial Growth', Ciba Foundation Symposium 32, ASP, Amsterdam, 107–126
Phoon W O, Tan S B 1975 Environmental and Health Conditions in Small Factories in Singapore. Singapore Medical Journal, 16, 3: 177–193
Phoon W O, Wan W P, Boey H K, Chao T C 1976 Health among Fishermen-Divers in Singapore. In 'Proceedings of 8th Asian Conference on Occupational Health', Tokyo, 263–267
Phoon W O 1977 Occupational Health in the Tropics. Journal of Occupational Medicine, USA, 19, 7: 458–463
Phoon W O 1981 Industrialization at a price. World Health, November: 26–29
Sofoluwe G O 1968 The Organization of Occupational Health Services — Nigerian Pattern. In 'Proceedings of the Lagos International Seminar on Occupational Health for Developing Countries', Lagos, 363–375
Somerville J G 1981 Employment of the severely disabled. In 'Recent Advances in Occupational Health I', (ed. J C McDonald), Churchill Livingstone, London, 239
WHO 1979 Safe use of pesticides, WHO Technical Report Series No. 634, 6–7

Disasters (Natural and man-made)

INTRODUCTION

Owing to the similarities in epidemiological approach and outcome of natural and man-made disasters, in this chapter the focus will be on natural disasters, but the same approach and general information are also applicable to man-made emergencies. It has to be stressed beforehand that the information and models given in this chapter cannot always be applicable to particular cases. Each disaster has to be considered in its own time and place. The approach and administrative models can, however, help in finding and planning the best way to manage any type of disaster.

DEFINITION

Several definitions of natural disaster have been made. One is: 'an ecological disruption exceeding the adjustment capacity of the affected community' (Lechat 1979). A more comprehensive definition is: 'An act of nature of such magnitude as to create a catastrophic situation in which the day-to-day pattern of life is suddenly disrupted and people are plunged into helplessness and suffering. As a result they need food, clothing, shelter, medical and nursing care and other necessities of life, and protection against unfavourable environmental factors and conditions'. (Assar 1971).

TYPES OF DISASTER

'It is possible to classify disasters according to their source:

1. Meteorological disasters: storms (hurricanes, tornadoes, cyclones, snowstorms), cold spells, heat waves, drought.

2. Topological disasters: floods, avalanches, landslides.

3. Telluric and tectonic disasters: earthquakes, volcanic eruptions.

4. Accidents: failure of structures (dams, tunnels, buildings, mines), explosions, fires, collisions, shipwrecks, train crashes, poison entering water supply systems. (Assar 1971).

These types of disaster are generally of sudden onset and imply unforeseen, serious and immediate threats to public health. Drought associated with famine, though it is predictable and develops slowly, may also be considered as a natural disaster since it creates similar problems requiring external assistance.

The magnitude and effect of a disaster can be found by evaluating some related results. These are:

a. loss of or damage to human and animal life
b. disruption of community services: electricity, gas, water supply, sewerage system, communications, food supply, public health et cetera.
c. spread of communicable diseases
d. disruption of normal activities
e. destruction of or damage to private and public property.

PRE-DISASTER ADMINISTRATION

The epidemiological evaluation of pre- and post-disaster periods is especially valuable for the administrators, enabling them to plan their activities to minimise the effects of future disasters. For example, knowing the age and sex distribution of those stricken may show the groups at risk that have to be given priority in taking preventive and administrative measures before, during and after a subsequent community emergency. These measures may include plans for first aid and emergency care services, training of medical and other manpower and use of resources. The indicators which suggest the severity of a disaster — the number of deaths in different types of construction in an earthquake, for example— may help the planners to decide on the best and most secure construction models.

Disasters can be managed by coordinated activities of different disciplines and sectors. The team operating in this field must include members from other related specialities as well as medical professionals. Coordination of activities in planning, organising and managing is essential. This would not be easy in many developing countries. In countries where job descriptions of different types of manpower and organisational planning are lacking, there will also be managerial confusion and chaos. To avoid disorganised activities the organisation and training of manpower beforehand are essential. The highest local authority must be responsible for directing and planning activities. Military resources must be taken into consideration and the army must be involved in planning to deal with civil emergencies. Predisaster planning activities can be considered under two headings: those concerning a) environment and b) people.

Activities concerning the environment are for sanitation and improvement of the physical and biological environment. Although these are not the duty of the health services in many countries, health units have responsibilities in assisting and supervising environmental sanitation activities. Further information on sanitation can be found in the relevant textbooks.

Activities to do with people include pre-disaster organisation, staffing, public education and personnel training and during a disaster activities such as medical treatment, patient referral and transportation of victims to places outside the disaster area. Pre-disaster activities can be expressed by the nomonic POSDCoRB which is made up of the initials of:

(P) Planning
(O) Organising
(S) Staffing
(D) Directing
(Co) Coordinating
(R) Reporting
(B) Budgeting

The items are not in order of importance so that the initials can form a pronounceable word. Each is explained below.

Planning

Planning is a vital part of pre-disaster activities. It has three steps:
1. Determining the available resources and the situation
2. Defining the objectives
3. Deciding the policy and action during a disaster

Determining the present situation and resources entails the evaluation of available manpower, materials, facilities and existing regulations. Certainly the experience of previous disasters can help the planners in this. The first step in planning has six major topics (Fig. 52.1). One is the determination of current regulations which will affect the action to be taken. The geographical location, transportation, communications and the characteristics of the population in a possible disaster area must be taken into consideration in planning. Two separate lists of materials should be made: materials already available and those which can be provided during a disaster. In many countries materials which can be commandeered and used by responsible bodies are defined by regulations. In some, the law permits the authorities even to commandeer privately-owned equipment. During this phase, the quality and quantity of available medical facilities and manpower and their possible extension should also be evaluated. Numerical analysis of past disasters is very valuable in estimating the type and magnitude of problems likely to be faced. Especially appropriate are the possible number of injured, the types of injury to be treated and the number of people to be transported to other places. These can be estimated roughly. Thus, the quality and quantity of required manpower and materials can be decided.

Information about previous disasters also helps to define the objectives of the work. It suggests ideas about the content of needed personnel and public education.

Every disaster threatens peoples' lives and affects their living conditions to some extent. Experience in the past shows that if pre-disaster planning

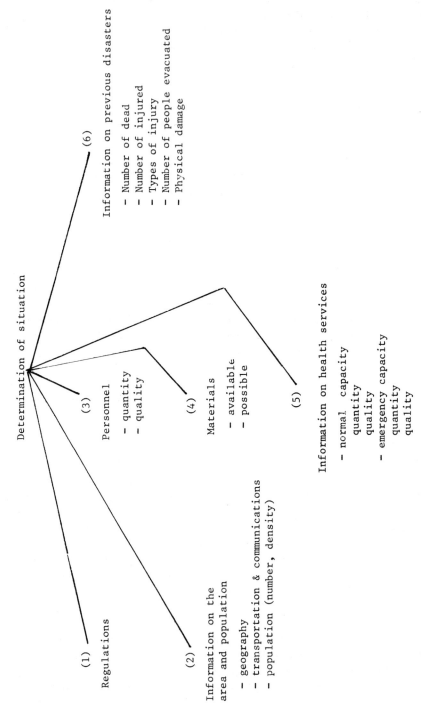

Fig. 52.1 Steps in disaster planning

is lacking or is not effectively undertaken, the damage caused is greater and more serious, and at the same time wastage of resources is maximised due to misuse of manpower and facilities. Effective planning will also facilitate management of the steps of pre-disaster activities, namely organisation, staffing, coordination and cooperation.

Organisation

In developing countries the lack of a body which is responsible for disaster activities, or for dealing with the damage caused by disasters is a fundamental problem. Its establishment under the direction of the highest local administrator should alleviate the difficulties. The head of the coordination body must be assisted by an administrator trained in disaster management and who is also the head of a civilian security organisation.

Figure 52.2 shows a modified organisation model for developing countries. As is seen, the coordinator has four assistants in four different service areas. It is important to delegate to each of the assistants one single task and to avoid giving them more than they can manage, unless there is an unexpected necessity. These four assistants must establish the units and train the personnel regarding their own tasks. The job descriptions of the staff must be clear. The four assistants must discuss each decision to be taken with the disaster coordinator. Another important point is to decide on the two way communication (warning, feed-back) between the highest and the lowest levels of the organisation. Other methods of communication in case of unexpected events, must also be considered. It should always be kept in mind during the planning phase that the most important factor for successful disaster management is communication.

Staffing

As a rule, the staff to be used must be selected from among people who perform similar work during their normal life. For example, the personnel responsible for warning the community may be selected from among newspaper correspondents or soldiers of the signals corps. Firemen may be authorised to carry out evacuation and rescue, health personnel may be selected for public health and sanitation work, disposal of the dead can be the responsibility of people working in cemeteries. The training of these staff must be continuous. The advance selection of personnel will improve their education and their work in general.

Since conditions in each country vary, it is difficult to define a standard model for staffing in terms of quantity and quality. Two points have, however, to be considered in deciding on the quantity: first that each task should be given to two persons, so that the work will continue if anything happens to one of them; second that the number of staff depends on the size of the area and the population. While deciding on the number of staff,

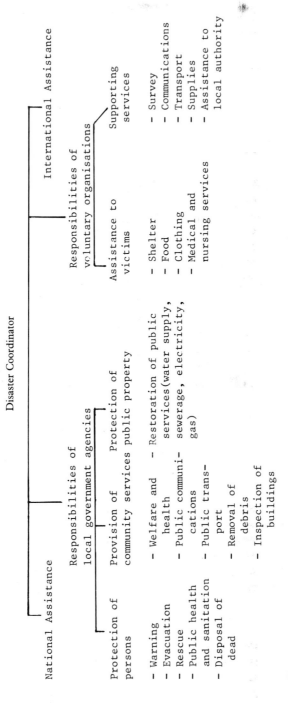

Fig. 52.2 Organization model for disasters.

Table 52.1 The number of environmental health personnel needed in an emergency.

Population affected	Number of personnel		
	Sanitary Engineers	Sanitarians	Auxiliaries
Less than 1000	–	2	2
1000–10 000	–	2	2–5
10 000–50 000	2	2	5–10
50 000–100 000	2	2–4	10–15
For every additional 100 000	2	2	10

it must be kept in mind that extending the service area of the team will probably create difficulties in management. On the other hand, the number of environmental health personnel needed in an emergency depends upon the nature of the community, the number of people affected, the extent of the area affected, the type of service required, the effectiveness of transport and communications, the training and efficiency of available personnel, et cetera. The figures presented in Table 52.1 are based on the experience of the author.

Direction

Each team member, including the chief who will be responsible for disaster control, has to be trained in leadership. The training must be practical and must be repeated frequently, (continuous training), and it must include subjects such as a) objectives, b) command and control structure, c) limits of authority and responsibility, d) duties and lines of communication, e) channels for requesting and supplying additional resources and f) operational details.

Coordination

Coordination in and between teams needs special attention. The staff may need some time to get to know each other and to adapt themselves to communication and coordination systems which may be new to them. They must be trained to work together. While doing this, it should never be forgotten that individuals may continue to believe that the system they know best is the most practical one for the new organisation they are working in.

Reporting

Both in natural and man-made disasters, correct information is needed in order to make mid-evaluation changes and to decide on future operations such as moving the teams from one place to another or devoting aid to different sections. Depending on the magnitude of the disaster and its severity, in some cases hourly reporting may be needed. It is advisable to standardise the reporting system beforehand. Information about previous disasters may be helpful in doing this.

Budgeting

Some of the main difficulties in obtaining or allocating funds in many developing countries are the bureaucratic procedures. In order to avoid such problems, and to save time when a disaster occurs, the necessary regulations have to be passed and funds and other supplies have to be ready beforehand. Taking into consideration the probable shortages in such countries, instead of setting aside funds and supplies possibly to remain idle for a long time, it would be wise to make regulations for mobilising them when they are needed.

SOCIAL REACTIONS FOLLOWING A DISASTER

Generally, the reaction of people affected by a disaster is one of panic with helplessness. Immediately after the first shock, unorganised, individual work begins and shortly after that people become organised to some extent. Although it may appear that this group work is to the benefit of the victims, further consideration suggests that this partly organised work in small groups and in particular areas may even lose time and waste resources. It is human nature for persons to delay effective help for others before being sure that their own families are safe. Rumours about the numbers of dead and injured and especially about diseases are common. These rumours can be eliminated by continuous announcements about the number of victims and by vaccination of the groups at risk against such infections as cholera or typhoid fever. Vaccinations, whatever their disease preventive value, have a beneficial psychological effect on the people and halt rumours. People do not always strictly follow the advice of the authorities. They may not want to leave their ruined houses after an earthquake or a flood. This attitude may be overcome by adequate pre-disaster education. Thus, they may be helpful in rescuing the injured and giving first aid. They can carry the injured to the medical centres and can build temporary shelters for the uninjured. If this is done, resources can be used in other areas where they are more needed. (Lechat 1976).

MAIN DUTIES OF A HEALTH TEAM

The main duties of a health team during a disaster are:
a) first aid
b) emergency care
c) ambulatory care
d) patient referral

These duties are similar to those of a primary health care organisation under normal conditions. After a disaster these responsibilities have to be supported by secondary and tertiary care units (hospitals).

The physicians who are or will be the chiefs of disaster health teams must train the other members of the team in first aid. This training must include at least the general principles of first aid. It must also include first aid in unconsciousness, shock, intoxication and in drowning. Training should also be provided for cardiovascular resuscitation and cardiac massage and in dealing with injuries and bleeding. Wound dressing and first aid in burns and in bone fractures must be included as well as training in the transportation of injured patients and in the appropriate referral techniques.

Past experience has shown that first aid is an important factor in reducing the number of deaths and disabilities. An adequate and effective first aid service will also help in better rehabilitation in the future.

Physicians are mainly responsible for emergency care and treatment. Nurses may also be used in emergency care services. Consequently emergency care must be a part of undergraduate training programs in both medical and nursing schools.

Health personnel must be careful about the recording of their services. Evaluation of these records and statistics will be used in future planning of manpower, training and other predisaster activities (Goyet et al 1976).

Vaccination is a routine service after many disasters. The preventive value of some vaccines, such as cholera and typhoid is, however, low. If the population is not immunised against diseases before the disaster, vaccination afterwards will not increase immunity in a short period of time. On the other hand, the most important preventive measure for potential waterborne and other communicable diseases is that of environmental sanitation. Any vaccination program must not preclude or delay necessary action for the environment, such as good sanitation, safe water, human and animal waste disposal and insect control. Healthy living conditions for the families must be assured. This includes housing, clothing and heating. Voluntary institutions and groups may be useful in assuring these conditions. It should always be kept in mind that there may be a heavy demand for such resources after a disaster. Means of locating these must be considered beforehand.

Once again the importance of public education has to be stressed. The people must at least know how and when to warn the authorities, how to do first aid and must have the necessary equipment ready for an emergency. This education can be carried out in collaboration with health and public (civil) security organizations. The education must be practical and continuous. Audio-visual aids can be used.

Burial of human and animal corpses and restoration of the physical environment must be done under the supervision of health personnel. Since these can be done later, there will be time to do them properly. All necessary measures must be taken to reduce the effect of disasters which may happen in the future. Since the sensitivity and motivation of both the people and the administrators are at the highest level immediately following a disaster such periods are the best time to make plans for future disaster control.

REFERENCES

Assar M 1971 Guide to Sanitation in Natural Disasters. World Health Organization, Geneva 1971
Goyet C V, Lechat M F 1976 Health Aspects in Natural Disasters. Tropical Doctor 6: 152–157
Goyet C V et al 1976 Earthquake in Guatemala: Epidemiologic Evaluation of the Relief Effort. Bulletin of the Pan American Health Organization 81: 199–215
Lechat M F 1976 The Epidemiology of Disasters. Proceedings of the Royal Society of Medicine 69 (6): 421–425
Lechat M F 1979 Disasters and Public Health. Bulletin of the World Health Organization 57 (1): 11–17

Population dynamics and family planning

INTRODUCTION

In recent years many textbooks have appeared on the subject of Population Dynamics, and the literature on Family Planning Programmes is vast. Summarising the relevant aspects of these subjects for a book such as this has inevitably resulted in considerable simplification of some very complex issues. The aim is, however, to provide physicians working in the Public/Community Health field with a basic understanding of population, and some practical information on the programmatic aspects of family planning. The subject matter should therefore be viewed in that context.

Ultimately, the process of family formation (and dissolution) is as unique for each person, as is the process of population change for each country. Yet, from the range of individual experience, and from the different socio-cultural, historical and economic conditions of each country, certain patterns can be observed. These patterns and the conclusions which can be drawn from them form the basis of this chapter.

POPULATION DYNAMICS

Population dynamics can be considered as the causes and consequences of population change. It is concerned with the size, composition and distribution of population, how changes in these come about and what effects such changes have. It comes under the broader heading of 'Demography'.

The historical growth of world population

It is convenient to begin a review of population dynamics by briefly examining a chronology of the world's population. This is shown in Figure 53.1, for the three century period beginning in 1700.

It took until about 1830 for the world's population to reach its first billion (one thousand million). Although the trend is shown as a smooth, gradual

* The views and opinions expressed in this chapter are those of the author and do not necessarily reflect those of the United Nations Fund for Population Activities.

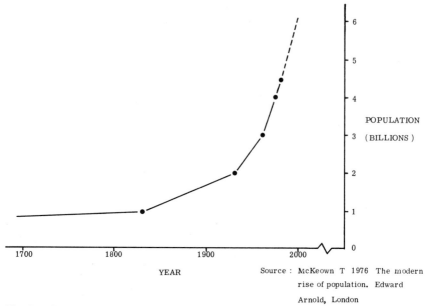

Fig. 53.1 World population 1700–2000 (. . . Projection)

Source : McKeown T 1976 The modern rise of population. Edward Arnold, London

increase, there was probably much fluctuation, particularly over short periods prior to the 19th Century, owing to such factors as epidemics and the availability of food. Also, it must be said that this figure of one billion is only an estimate, since, by 1830, only a handful of countries had taken a census. Even today, we do not have very accurate information for every country in the world, but we do have it for sufficient a number to make reasonable estimates.

Subsequently, an additional one billion people were added in the 100 years between 1830 and 1930, and a further billion accrued in the 30 years between 1930 and 1960. The addition of a fourth billion was completed a mere 15 years later, in 1975. In the remaining 20 years of this century, it is inevitable, major disasters aside, that two billion more people will be added to the world's population which will then reach six billion and still be growing.

This exponential growth of world population (known variously as the population explosion, population bomb, population problem, etcetera), especially its rapid rate of increase since 1900, has probably been the single major catalyst for the interest and concern generated in the subject of population in recent years.*

* Concern about population is not new. For example, Malthus (1798) voiced opinions about the imbalance between population growth and the growth of resources, particularly food. However, he did not foresee such things as the enormous increases in agricultural productivity that have taken place in the 19th and 20th centuries. (Today, we hope we are more aware of ameliorating factors that may emerge in the future.)

As might be expected, the historical pattern of population growth has varied greatly from country to country. For example, in England and Wales, population growth, which had been slow and erratic up until about 1750, suddenly began to increase very rapidly and continued to do so until about 1930. Since then, the population has continued to increase but at a slow rate, much as before 1750. On the other hand, Mauritius, a country for which quite good data is available, had a relatively stable population until as late as 1940. At that time, its population began a precipitous rise and by 1970, only 30 years later, it had doubled.

In general, most currently developed countries completed their phases of rapid population growth by the early part of this century, whereas, most developing countries are experiencing a period of rapid growth at the present time. Notable exceptions to this are: Japan, whose population growth rate was still high until the late 1940s; and China, whose birth rate has been substantially reduced in recent years, despite still being largely a rural, agrarian society.

The demographic transition

How have such changes in population size come about? A country's total population can only change through births, deaths or migration — the three major demographic processes. Migration is generally not a major factor in the historical process of population growth, though, on occasions, mass migrations have significantly affected the population size of of the countries concerned. The main determinants of population change are births and deaths, and population increase can come about either as a result of fewer deaths or more births, or a combination of both.

It appears that the phase of rapid population growth that most countries have experienced or are currently experiencing, is due to a fall in the death rate in the presence of a continuing high birth rate. This phase, which is part of what has come to be known as the demographic transition, is illustrated graphically in Figure 53.2.

Various writers have divided the demographic transition into a number of phases or stages; for simplicity, only three are described here. In the pre-transition phase, both birth and death rates are high. The death rate tends to fluctuate from year to year, but, on average, it is marginally exceeded by the birth rate. The result is slow population growth.

In the transition phase itself, the death rate falls to a much lower level, but the birth rate remains high. This large excess of births over deaths results in rapid population growth. In the later part of this phase, the birth rate declines, so that in the third, or post transition phase, the birth and death rates are once again roughly in equilibrium, but now at much reduced levels. Population growth once again is gradual, and short-term fluctuations occur more commonly now in the birth rate.

In summary, the demographic transition (the name given to the historical

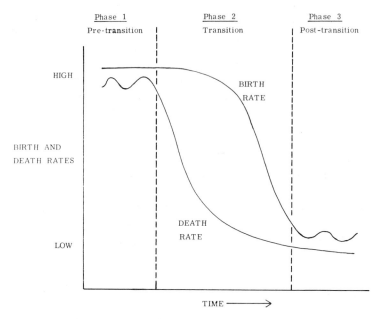

Fig. 53.2 Schematic representation of the demographic transition

process of population change that has been observed in many countries), is a transition from high birth and death rates to low birth and death rates encompassing a period of rapid population growth due to a large excess of births over deaths.

Current state of world population and future prospects

The recent, current and projected state of world population and its broad geographical distribution is given in Figure 53.3.

In 1950, developing countries made up about two thirds of the world's population, in 1980, about three quarters, and in the year 2010 are expected to make up more than four fifths. Thus the bulk of the world population is found in developing countries, and their proportion of the total world population is steadily increasing. Regionally, the bulk of population is to be found in Asia, which, in 1980 contained more than three quarters of all people in developing countries.

Finally, Table 53.1 summarises a number of differences between developed and developing countries in regard to the demographic transition and population size, distribution and growth.

Population structure and its consequences

The birth and death rates of a country determine not only its population

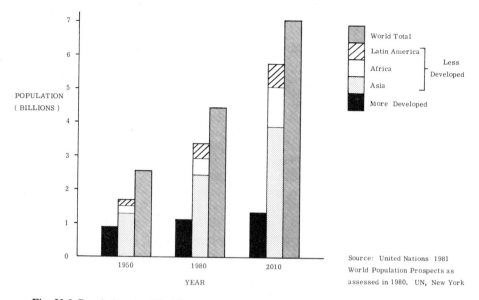

Source: United Nations 1981
World Population Prospects as
assessed in 1980. UN, New York

Fig. 53.3 Population size: World total, more developed regions, less developed regions, Africa, Asia and Latin America, 1950, 1980 and 2010, U.N. medium variant

Table 53.1 Population and the demographic transition — Some comparisons between developed and developing countries

	Developed	Developing
The demographic transition		
Began. . .	150–200 years ago	Within last 50 years
Current State. . .	Transition complete	Phase 2
Fall in death rate. . .	Took approximately 150 years	Similar falls in 30–40 years
Major causes of death, pretransition. . .	Communicable diseases	Communicable diseases
Causes of fall in death rate . . .	Improvements in nutrition, personal hygiene, public health, living conditions. Changes in biological factors in some diseases. Preventive and therapeutic medicine	The same as per developed plus mass disease control programmes
Knowledge of health and disease. . .	Acquired slowly during the transition	Available for instant application
Urbanization. . .	Gradual and largely complete	Rapid and continuing
Industrialization and economic growth	Going on at same time and rapid	Going on at same time but at a slower rate
Population		
Size in 1980 (billions)	1.13	3.30
Growth rate (crude birth rate minus crude death rate ÷ 10)	Less than 1%	Greater than 2%
Doubling time (70 years ÷ growth rate)	Greater than 70 years	About 35 years
Distribution	Mostly urban	Mostly rural

growth rate, but also its age structure. This structure can be demonstrated most simply by means of a population pyramid — a specially arranged double bar chart that displays the proportional distribution of total population by age and sex. The shape of any particular country's population pyramid results from the experience of that country with regard to births and deaths over many previous years. Mass migration, in or out of a country may also show up in the shape of the pyramid. Two such pyramids are illustrated in Figures 53.4 and 53.5.

Figure 53.4 is the population pyramid for Bangladesh in 1974 and is typical of the shape which developing countries generate.* The broad base reflects a long experience of high birth rates, and the sharply cut away sides signify a long experience of high death rates. The majority of individuals are found in the younger age groups — 63.2 per cent below the age of 25.

The population pyramid of Sweden in 1975 is shown in Figure 53.5, and, typical of most developed countries, looks more like a beehive than a true pyramid. The narrow base reflects a low birth rate and the roughly parallel

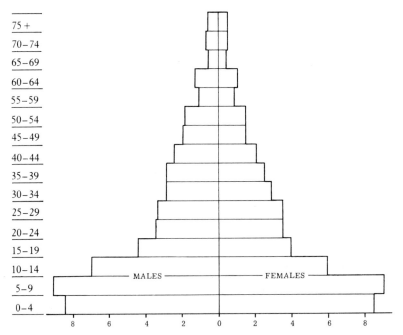

Age Group. PERCENTAGE OF TOTAL POPULATION IN EACH AGE/SEX GROUP

Source: UN Demographic
Yearbook 1979

Fig. 53.4 Population pyramid of Bangladesh, 1974

* It is also typical of the shape for a currently developed country back in the 19th century when it was experiencing, or had recently experienced high birth and death rates.

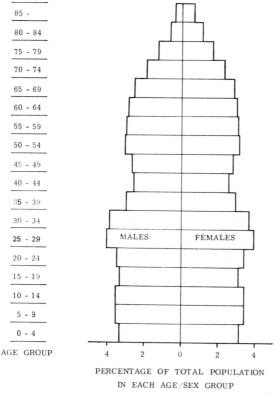

AGE GROUP

PERCENTAGE OF TOTAL POPULATION
IN EACH AGE/SEX GROUP

Source: UN Demographic
Yearbook 1979

Fig. 53.5 Population pyramid of Sweden, 1975

sides (until the older age groups) reflect the relatively low mortality. The age distribution is also quite different, with the majority of individuals, 66.2 per cent, now being aged 25 or over.

In order to look at age distribution more closely, Table 53.2 gives the percentage distribution of population in broad age groups for the sexes combined. There are two important points here.

First, the percentage of population aged under 15 is much higher for Bangladesh, 48.1 per cent, than it is for Sweden, 20.5 per cent. This situation is reversed in the age group 60+ with almost four times more in Sweden, 21.4 per cent, than in Bangladesh, 5.7 per cent. For such reasons, and in addition to the typically different patterns of disease found in developed and developing countries, it is vital that the health care planning process within a country should take account of the age distribution of the population it is serving. Developing countries tend to have 'young' populations and thus maternal and child health care (with a target population of maybe two thirds of the country total) is an obvious priority. Developed

Table 53.2 Age distribution of populations of Bangladesh 1974 and Sweden 1975, % (Both sexes combined), and dependency ratios

Age group	% in each age group	
	Bangladesh 1974	Sweden 1975
0–14	48.1	20.5
15–59	46.2	58.1
60+	5.7	21.4
All ages	100.0	100.0

Source: United Nations 1979 Demographic Yearbook, UN, New York

Dependency *Bangladesh 1974*   *Sweden 1975*
Ratios: $\dfrac{48.1 + 5.7}{46.2} \times 100 = 116.5$ $\dfrac{20.5 + 21.4}{58.1} \times 100 = 72.1$

countries, on the other hand, need to pay greater attention to their late middle and old age populations.

The second point is that from these figures we can calculate the dependency ratio. This is the ratio of those aged under 15 and 60 or over, to those aged 15–59. This ratio gives us a measure of the burden of dependence — the higher the ratio, the higher the social and economic costs which fall upon both those in the productive 15–59 age group and the state, in providing support for the dependent population.* The respective ratios for Bangladesh and Sweden are 116.5 and 72.1, indicating much greater dependency in Bangladesh, where for every 100 producers there are 116 dependents. Generally, dependency ratios are much higher in developing countries and they serve as further evidence of the adverse effects of currently high birth rates.

In summary, world population is rising very rapidly and this is largely due to high birth rates in developing countries. In addition, population has an in-built momentum, so that even if every couple were to have from this instant on only 2 children† (i.e. more or less replacing themselves), world population would still continue to grow for another 20 to 30 years because of the vast numbers of young people who have yet to enter the reproductive age group.

World population, of necessity, must stop growing at some stage in the future, the vital issue is whether or not this will be achieved in an agreeable and peaceful manner.

* Caution must be exercised in interpreting small differences in dependency ratios since some of those aged under 15 and over 60 may in fact be productive, whilst others in the 15–59 age group may be dependent. Also different age cut-off points are sometimes used.

† The difference between an average two and an average three child family may not seem very great, but its implications for the future are enormous. For example, in the U.S.A, an average two child family from now onwards would mean that the total U.S. population would stabilise at about 300 million in about 90 years time. If, however, the average was three children, the population would increase to 900 million in the same period (three times as high), and still be growing at a rapid pace.

The effects of rapid population growth

When we speak of rapid population growth in the world today, we are essentially talking about high birth rates, and thus large families in developing countries. What are the effects of a large family size?

These can be divided into effects on:
— The mother
— The family
— The community or country (some of which also act indirectly on the family)

The mother

Much evidence has accumulated in recent years on the effects of excessive childbearing on maternal mortality and morbidity.

Maternal mortality increases rapidly with birth order (Chen et al 1974, Tomkinson et al 1979), and may be as much as four times higher for fourth and higher order births as compared with first or second order births. The major causes of this mortality are haemorrhage, ante and post-partum, and toxaemia of pregnancy. Puerperal sepsis has also been found to be more common in older women (Nortman 1974).

Maternal morbidity also increases with birth order. The pattern of repeated pregnancies and short birth intervals exacerbates nutritional problems, anaemias, vitamin deficiencies and endemic diseases, and has come to be known as the maternal depletion syndrome. In addition, many pre-existing medical conditions such as hypertension, heart disease and renal problems are aggravated by pregnancy. Finally, in the absence of any alternative solutions, many women turn to illegal abortion which carries its own heavy toll of mortality and morbidity. Thus excessive childbearing undoubtedly affects the health and well-being of mothers, and close intervals between births, less than 24 months, only make their situation worse.

The family

Increasing birth order also affects foetal outcome. In addition to the primarily maternal conditions mentioned above, malpresentations, obstructed labour, prolapse of the cord and placental insufficiency are also associated with high birth order. Overall foetal mortality may be two to three times greater with fifth or higher order births as compared with first and second order births (Puffer and Serrano 1975). The difference in perinatal mortality, that is foetal deaths and deaths in the first week of life, may be even larger. A recent study in China (Lyle et al 1980) found a greater than fivefold difference in the perinatal mortality rate between first and second order births, and third and higher order births.

Birth weight, a very good indicator of infant survival is also associated with birth order. Beginning with the fourth birth, the proportion of low birth weight babies steadily increases.

Infant and child mortality are also found to be higher in large families and this may be attributed partly to such factors as overcrowding in the home, poorer nutrition and less supervision of children. Such differences exist irrespective of social class and have been clearly demonstrated with respect to deaths from infections (Adelstein et al 1980).

There seems little doubt, therefore, that excessive childbearing has adverse effects on the health of the family. Costs must, however, always be weighed against benefits. Those who desire large families must accept the higher risks to which they expose themselves. Ideally, such choices should be able to be made in a situation where couples are both fully informed and fully equipped to achieve their family size goals in the safest manner. Of paramount importance is the situation where undesired excess childbearing is taking place and women and their families are being subjected to risks, which are not of their own choosing, and are easily avoidable through the use of contraception.

The community or country

How does rapid population growth affect the community or country? There is a continuing debate on this subject particularly in regard to socio-economic development.

The traditional view is that rapid population growth interferes with socio-economic development by pre-empting a large proportion of national income for the non-productive, social service sector of the economy. Consequently, investment in productive industry is held back and rapid growth in gross national product (G.N.P.) is not possible. This is a very simplified account of the various forces at work, but it is nonetheless true that, other things being equal, slower population growth would result in higher annual increases in per capita G.N.P.

The practical effects of this relationship are that governments have to spend increasing amounts of national income in such areas as health, schooling, water and waste disposal services, housing, social welfare, transport services, urban renewal and food imports merely to maintain, let alone to improve, the conditions of life for their rapidly growing populations.

As a result there is constant economic pressure on governments to increase revenue (for example by taxation) or to decrease spending (for example by reducing services). The effects of these are felt sooner or later at the household level.

The alternative view of the relationship between population and socio-economic development is that family size decisions are fundamentally rational, particularly from an economic point of view, in any society. Family size is largely determined by the micro-social, cultural and economic environment in which people live. In many developing countries, according to this view, conditions are currently conducive to large family size because of the economic, social and political benefits which may accrue to large families. These conditions are ultimately determined by the international, political and economic order particularly the relationship between developed and developing countries. Not until this changes will the small family become a real desire for couples in the developing world.

Whatever the eventual outcome of this debate, and there are many other theories to be found in the middle ground between these two, the fact that it has occurred has had implications for family planning which will be dealt with in the next section.

Decline in birth rates in developed countries

Finally, it is useful to take note of Figure 53.6 which shows the fall in births (average family size) in a developed country, England and Wales, between 1865 and 1960.

Average family size fell in England and Wales from just over six to about two in the 60 years between 1870 and 1930. Since the 1930s it has remained relatively stable. What brought about this sudden decline? During this

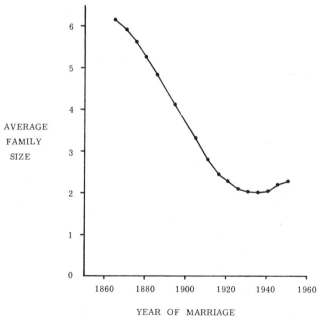

YEAR OF MARRIAGE

Source: Registrar General 1961, 1963 Statistical
Review of E. and W. HMSO London

Fig. 53.6 Average family size (number of liveborn children) for marriage cohorts 1865–1952, England and Wales

period, the status of women was relatively low (they were not fully enfranchised until 1928), there had been compulsory education for children since 1876, infant mortality was high (it was still over 100 per 1000 live births in 1900), industrial growth was progressing well and a decline in fatalism and an increase in secularism were also well underway (Banks 1981). All these factors may have contributed to the decline in family size, but, one thing that was not present during this period was modern methods of family planning. There were no steroids, no modern intra-uterine devices, no chemical spermicides, no widely available methods of sterilisation, and only a few primitive barrier methods. Presumably this large and rapid decline in family size was brought about by couples using traditional methods of family planning such as coitus interruptus, abstinence and abortion.

This is, therefore, an example of a population which managed to reduce its birth rate in the absence of modern contraception. Other examples also exist. The lesson is not that the provision of services and information on modern methods of family planning is unnecessary. Rather, that the provision of family planning methods may not of itself lead to smaller families unless the conditions of life are such that the desire for a small family arises. When these conditions are present, the availability of modern methods of family planning accelerate the spread of such a desire through a community and enable couples to reach their family size goals, whatever they may be, by more convenient and safer means than is possible without them.

FAMILY PLANNING PROGRAMMES

The international family planning movement

Up until the late 1940s family planning was largely left to individuals and national organisations. Since that time there has been a tremendous growth in international interest and concern with population and family planning (F.P.).

This movement was probably initiated in the United States through the Ford and Rockefeller Foundations and the Population Council (founded in 1952). The Population Council was largely responsible for carrying out the original knowledge, attitude and practice (K.A.P.) studies in regard to family planning. These demonstrated generally positive attitudes and moderate knowledge, but little practice of F.P., particularly in developing countries. They stimulated much interest and highlighted the need for much greater efforts in the F.P. field. The International Planned Parenthood Federation (IPPF) was also set up in 1952, and has continued to promote family planning through its national affiliates all over the world, stressing the importance of F.P. for human happiness, prosperity and peace.

In the years that followed, a number of countries began bilateral assistance in the Population and family planning field: Sweden in 1962, and the

U.S.A. in 1965. The latter quickly became the major provider of funding in the field, and remains so at the present time.

In the late 1960s, 30 world leaders signed a statement (United Nations 1968) recognising population and especially family planning as an important element in national planning.

In the early days, many family planning programmes were unipurpose and highly centralised, and their impact, particularly on birth rates was not in some cases, as great as had been expected. In response to this, programmes became less centralised, and more integrated, particularly, but not exclusively with health programmes. Greater attention was also paid to motivational aspects particularly information, education and communication programmes in support of F.P.

The United Nations Fund for Population Activities (UNFPA) which was set up as a trust fund in 1967 and became operational in 1969 has become the largest multilateral funding agency in the population field. Since 1969 it has provided more that $1 billion in population assistance to 147 countries and territories. Assigned the leading role in the United Nations system in promoting population programs by the United Nations Economic and Social Council (see UNFPA 1977), the UNFPA has been guided by three principles: 1. Neutrality: in not prescribing any particular approaches or solutions to population problems and providing assistance in those areas in which developing countries themselves attach importance. 2. Flexibility in the types of assistance provided, and 3. Innovation in its willingness to adopt new approaches whenever the need has arisen. The major part of UNFPA's budget has gone, and continues to go, in support of family planning programmes requested by governments for any or all of the following rationales: as a human right, for improvement in family health, for demographic change and as an adjunct to socio-economic development.

The 1970s also saw the World Population Conference, held in 1974 in Bucharest, which underlined the relationship between population and socio-economic development as being more complex than had been previously thought. This meeting also emphasized the relationship between resources, the environment and population; the status of women; and family health services.

In 1978, the Alma Ata conference confirmed Primary Health Care (PHC) as the main strategy for achieving 'Health for all by the year 2000'. Among the various components of PHC, 'maternal and child care, including family planning', was clearly identified as of great importance (see WHO/UNICEF 1978).

The World Fertility Survey (WFS), set up in 1972, continues its pioneering work in the field of demographic surveys in developing countries and over 40 have participated. Amongst its general findings are continuing gaps between the use of family planning methods and (a) those who know of a method, and (b) those who desire no further children (see Kendall 1979).

Findings such as these indicate the need for continued efforts in the family planning field, and the International Conference on F.P. in the 1980s, held in Jakarta in 1981 affirmed amongst other things that: 'Family planning is a basic human right. Governments should be encouraged to translate this right into realistic policies and programmes which meet the needs of their people.' (Population Council 1981).

The Context of Family Planning

Family Planning has been defined by the World Health Organisation in the following manner:

> 'Family planning refers to practices that help individuals or couples to attain certain objectives; to avoid unwanted births; to bring about wanted births; to regulate the intervals between pregnancies; to control the time at which births occur in relation to the ages of the parents; and to determine the number of children in the family. Services that make these practices possible include education and counselling on family planning; the provision of contraceptives; the management of infertility; education about sex and parenthood. . .' (WHO 1971)

Family planning can thus be used for both the spacing and limiting of births. Since most couples are initially interested in postponing a first birth or spacing subsequent births, this aspect is highly important in bringing about a general acceptance of F.P. methods and their use for limiting family size to that desired at a later stage.

Family planning should be an integral part of Maternal and Child Health (MCH) activities for the following reasons:

— The health benefits of F.P.
— The medical nature of many techniques.
— The general acceptability of F.P. within MCH care
— The preventive nature of F.P. (coinciding with the the preventive nature of much of MCH and PHC.)
— Accessibility through MCH care to the major target group for F.P.*

The health benefits of F.P. result from:

— The avoidance of unwanted pregnancies and the occurrence of wanted births that might otherwise not have taken place.
— A change in the total number of children born to a mother.
— The achievement of an optimum interval between pregnancies (at least two years).

---

* Adolescents, single and nulliparous women, and men may not receive adequate attention through conventional MCH services. These groups, which sometimes have special needs as regards both information and services, may thus have to be catered for outside regular channels.

— Changes in the time at which births occur, particularly the first and the last in relation to the age of the mother.

Although Health Services, particularly MCH care, are the main vehicle for family planning, there may be opportunities for integration with other programmes in certain countries. For example, F.P. may be delivered with agricultural extension programmes, nutrition promotion (including breast-feeding), community development, family life education, non-formal education and women's programmes. Finally, direct supply outlets in the private sector through social (subsidised) marketing schemes and community based delivery can also be very successful.

It is important to consider all possible means of delivery, whenever they are appropriate, in order to maximise both accessibility and acceptability — two crucial factors in the adoption of F.P. methods.

Factors influencing acceptance of the concept of family planning

Despite the great efforts to make family planning services and information widely available, there are a number of factors, acting often in combination, which may operate to deter use of F.P., as indicated earlier. These factors include:

Traditional	— Non-use may be a strong traditional norm.
	— Low status of women may work against acceptance.
Religious	— There may be a fatalistic attitude to family size — 'God decides'.
	— Some religions proscribe the use of most or all F.P. methods.
Political	Beliefs that . . .
	— An increase in numbers leads to an increase in political power and status at the level of the community (country) and family.
	— F.P. may be used with genocidal intentions.
Economic	— Children may contribute to family income from an early age in some societies and the belief that the chances of rearing one child who becomes a successful and important adult are maximised in a large family.
	— The belief that an expanding work force is needed to expand a country's economy.
	— Some research suggests that where socio-economic development is slow it is economically rational for couples to continue to have large families.
Educational	— Low educational status of parents, especially of the mother, is highly correlated with large family size.
Mortality	— The 'child survival hypothesis', which states that F.P. is unlikely to be used in situations where the probability of child survival is low, particularly where at

least one adult son may be required for parental security in old age

F.P. Methods — There may be particular problems with the use of
some methods of F.P. in certain societies.

Programmatic aspects of F.P., including choice of methods

Physicians, who are responsible for MCH/FP services, are unable to control
or take account of many of these factors. There are, nevertheless, ways in
which they can maximise the acceptance of family planning within a
community. This can be done through careful attention to the following
aspects:

Community participation and the user perspective

Since family planning is a sensitive issue, it is vital that the community be
involved in both the informational and service aspects of programmes. Only
in this way can needs be met appropriately and problems of acceptability
avoided as far as is possible.

Such involvement must take account of the way in which a community
is organised and might include initially discussions with the following:
village headmen, women's group leaders, community groups, religious
leaders, school teachers, local dignitaries, politicians and ordinary members
of the community.

Health personnel

It is important that all health personnel are involved in the family planning
programme at a level which is appropriate to their knowledge and skills.
This includes not only physicians, midwives and nurses, but also, for
example, auxiliary nurses and midwives, village health workers, and other
Primary Health Care workers, and traditional practitioners (e.g. Traditional
Birth Attendants) wherever appropriate.

In regard to this, the physician may find his or her main role to be that
of a trainer and supervisor of such personnel, delegating as much of the day-
to-day work to the various members of the health team, and dealing,
personally, only with such methods or problems which truly require his or
her technical expertise.

Community and clinic based delivery

In many situations, particularly rural areas in developing countries, it is not
sufficient to offer services only at clinics. The accessibility of these for the
vast majority of the population is often severely limited by distance, cost
and other factors. The solution lies in the use of Primary Health Care

workers (as mentioned above) who can give information and services vital to maximise community coverage.

Also, in this regard, F.P. information and services should not be restricted to particular times of day or days of the week. Because of the general infrequency of contacts between health personnel and clients all appropriate opportunities should be used to enquire about such a need. This is true integration of F.P. at the level of the family.

Appropriateness of information and methods

Western ideas continue to influence health service delivery in many developing countries. It is vital to avoid this pitfall particularly in the family planning area. What works, as regards both meaningful information and acceptable methods, in one place may not work in another. By involving the community (the user) it is possible to adapt information and to choose appropriate methods for each particular socio-cultural and economic setting.

The methods of F.P. to be offered depend upon a consideration of a number of factors amongsts which are:

Acceptability — Socio-cultural traditions and practices influence the broad choice of methods, but within this, individual preferences are important and must be met by a good variety of methods. In addition, minor side effects vary greatly from individual to individual. (For a comprehensive review of cultural acceptability see Polgar and Marshall 1976.)

Effectiveness — Including both method and user effectiveness.

Safety — General considerations and considerations of use in particular clients.

Cost — To both the government and the individual user.

Manpower — Personnel required for both initial prescription and follow-up visits.

Climate — Suitability of materials for storage in warehouses, clinics and the home.

Service setting — How this may affect the types of method which can be offered.

Purpose — A variety of methods for both spacing pregnancies and preventing any more when desired family size is reached.

Finally, the physician should be familiar with the various currently available methods of family planning, their relative advantages and disadvantages, their short and long term side effects and the guidelines for both prescription and follow-up of users. Physicians should also be available to give counselling and services (or at least referral) for subfertility, infertility, abortion and sterilisation where appropriate. It will also fall to them to collect some basic, useful data on family planning acceptors.

Table 53.3 Major methods of family planning and their characteristics

Methods	Theoretical[1] Effectiveness	Use[1] Effectiveness (Av.)	Cost per year[3] of protection US$	Main Medical Contraindications	Main Side Effects	Advantages/ Disadvantages
Steroidal contraceptives Oral pill	0.1	0.24	2.00	Breast cancer All genital cancers Liver disease History of cardiovascular disease Undiagnosed abnormal uterine bleeding Congenital hyperlipidaemia Aged over 40, or over 35 and heavy smoker Suspected pregnancy	Thrombo-embolism Hypertension Benign liver tumors Gall bladder disease	Highly effective Coitus unrelated Protects against certain diseases[4]
Injectable progestins	0.24	0.7	4.00	Breast cancer All genital cancers (except endometrial) Undiagnosed abnormal uterine bleeding Suspected pregnancy	Amenorrhoea Prolonged bleeding	Highly effective No oestrogen effects One injection gives 2–3 months protection
IUD Lippes loop Copper devices	1.9 —	2.7 2.2	0.04 0.40–1.20	Pelvic inflammatory disease Pregnancy Neoplasia of uterus or cervix	Pelvic inflammatory disease Perforation of uterus Menorrhagia/ Dysmennorrhoea Vaginal Discharge	Very effective Cheap Coitus unrelated One act to initiate High continuation

	Pregnancies per 100 woman years[1]		Cost (US$)[3]	Complications	Characteristics
Barrier methods					
Condom	3	12	5.00	—	Coitus related, Indpendent of health services, moderate effectiveness
Diaphragm and jelly	3	12	—	Prolapse, cystocoele	
Creams/jelly	4	20	6.00–10.00	—	
Aerosol foams	3	14	—	—	
Suppositories	14	22	—	—	
Periodic abstinence	2.5	20	0	—	Independent of health services, non-invasive, no continuing cost
Coitus Interruptus	8	18	0	—	
Lactation	—	6[2]	0	—	

[1] Pregnancies per 100 woman years. Source: Office of Technology Assessment 1982, World Population and Fertility Planning Technologies, U.S. Government, Printing Office, Washington.
[2] Mean percentage of women becoming pregnant before first post-partum menstruation, nine country study. Source: WHO 1981, Contemporary Patterns of Breast-feeding, WHO, Geneva.
[3] Approximate cost of consummable items-public sector bulk prices. (Office of Technology Assessment report cited above, estimates total cost per user per year to be US$15 on average in less developed countries, range US$6 to US$100.)
[4] Uterine and ovarian cancer, pelvic inflammatory disease, rheumatoid arthritis, various menstrual conditions, iron deficiency anaemia and benign breast disorders.

These subjects cannot be dealt with in the space of this short chapter, but the following references provide a selection of material on current methods and their programmatic aspects: Gray et al 1980, Hatcher et al 1980, Hawkins and Elder 1979, Kleinman 1980, Potts and Bhiwandiwala 1979, WHO 1976, WHO 1980, WHO 1982a and WHO 1982b.

Finally, Table 53.3 lists most of the currently used methods together with some of their more important characteristics. From Table 53.3 it can be concluded that those methods which are more effective (steroids and IUDs), also have more serious side effects. It is also important to weigh the risks against the benefits in any given situation. Where maternal morbidity and mortality are excessive, the benefits of non-pregnancy are bound to be greater than the risks associated with pregnancy. The importance of lactation, particularly in the spacing of births, has been underestimated in the past. Current research is revealing that this provides a high level of protection for women who are fully breast-feeding and are still amenorrhoeic in the post partum period. Finally, it should not be forgotten that abortion and menstrual regulation are used in many countries; and that many couples, who have attained their desired family size, opt for either male or female sterilisation as a permanent method.

SUMMARY

World population has been growing very rapidly in recent years. As a consequence of efforts in both the fields of family planning and development, this increase has decellerated somewhat in the last decade. In spite of this success, population growth rates in developing countries still generally remain in excess of two per cent — implying a doubling time of total population every 35 years. It is clear that there is no place for complacency. Greater efforts are needed to fund F.P. programmes, to develop new and modified contraceptives, and to improve accessibility and acceptability through greater attention to the socio-cultural and economic aspects of both F.P. methods and F.P. services.

It should, however, be recognised that these larger concerns will reap rewards only in that they support those dedicated individuals who are the direct providers of F.P. information, advice and services. The ultimate aim always remains to be to help couples to achieve their family size goals in the most reliable, convenient and safe manner.

REFERENCES

Adelstein A M, Davies I M M, Weatherall J 1980 Perinatal and infant mortality: Social and biological factors 1975–1977. Studies on Medical and Population subjects No. 41, H M S O, London
Banks J A 1981 Victorian values — secularism and the size of families
Chen L C, Gesche M C, Ahmed S, Chowdhury A I, Mosley W H 1974 Maternal mortality in rural Bangladesh. Studies in family planning 5: 11

Gray R H, Ramos R, Akin A 1980 Manual for the provision of intrauterine devices. WHO, Geneva

Hatcher R A, Stewart G K, Stewart F, Guest F, Schwartz D W, Jones S A 1980 Contraceptive Technology 1980–1981, 10th revised edn. Irvington Publishers Inc., New York

Hawkins D F, Elder M G 1979 Human Fertility Control. Butterworths, London

Kendall M 1979 The World Fertility Survey: current status and findings. Population Reports, Series M: No 3, Johns Hopkins University, Baltimore

Kleinman R L (ed) 1980 Family Planning Handbook for Doctors. IPPF Medical Publications, London

Lyle K C, Segal S J, Chang C, Ch'ien L 1980 Perinatal study in Tientsin 1978 International Journal of Gynaecology and Obstetrics 18(4)

Malthus T R 1798 An essay on the principle of population. Reprinted 1970, Penguin Books, Harmondsworth U.K

Nortman D 1974 Parental age as a factor in pregnancy outcome. Reports on population and family planning No. 16, Population Council, New York

Polgar S, Marshall J F 1976 The Search for Culturally Acceptable Fertility Regulating Methods. In Marshall J F, Polgar S (eds) Culture, Natality, and Family Planning, Monograph 21, Carolina Population Center, Chapel Hill

Population Council 1981 Family Planning in the 1980s — Recommendations of the International Conference on Family Planning in the 1980s, Jakarta, 1981. Population Council, New York

Potts M, Bhiwandiwala P (eds) 1979 Birth Control — an International Assessment. University Park Press, Baltimore

Puffer R R, Serrano C V 1975 Birth weight, maternal age and birth order: three important determinants in infant mortality. Scientific publication No. 294, Pan American Health Organisation, Washington D.C.

Tomkinson J, Turnbull A, Robson G, Cloake E, Adelstein A M, Weatherall J 1979 Report on confidential enquiries into maternal deaths in England and Wales 1973–1975. D H S S Reports on Health and Social subjects 14, H M S O, London

United Nations 1968. Department of Economic and Social Affairs, Newsletter No 1, UN, New York.

WHO 1971 Report of a WHO expert Committee on Family Planning and Health Services. Technical Report Series No. 476, WHO, Geneva

WHO 1976 New Trends and Approaches in the Delivery of Maternal and Child Care in Health Services. Technical Report Series No. 600, WHO, Geneva

WHO 1980 Female Sterilisation: Guidelines for the Development of Services, 2nd edn. Offset publication No. 26, WHO, Geneva

WHO 1982a Oral Contraceptives: Technical and Safety Aspects. Offset publication No. 64, WHO, Geneva

WHO 1982b Injectable Hormonal Contraceptives: Technical Safety Aspects. Offset publication No. 65, WHO, Geneva

WHO/UNICEF 1978. Primary Health Care, Alma Ata 1978. WHO, Geneva

World Leaders Declaration on Population presented at the United Nations on Human Rights Day December 1967. Population Council, New York

UNFPA 1977 Priorities in future allocations of UNFPA resources, UNFPA, New York

International comparisons in child growth and development

INTRODUCTION

Physical growth is becoming increasingly important universally to health personnel as an indicator of the well-being, health and nutritional status of both individuals and groups of people.

Growth is a product of the continuous and complex interaction of heredity and environment. The genotype determines the potential of an organism and the environment determines which or how much of those potentialities shall be realised during development. This interaction of heredity and environment causes differences among populations in body size and shape and tempo of growth in children. Knowledge of how they affect growth should be kept in mind when considering growth standards and interpreting results of growth studies.

GENETIC AND ENVIRONMENTAL INFLUENCES ON GROWTH AND DEVELOPMENT

Genes control both body size and shape independently and also the tempo of growth, or rate of development. Correlations between the size of parents and children are significant by 18 months of age in populations where the parents' size has not been affected by a poor environment. These correlations can be used to make standards for children's heights which allow for the height of the parents. The use of such standards increases the precision in diagnosing growth problems.

Genetic control in the tempo of growth is best seen in the inheritance of the age of menarche. Monozygotic twins reach menarche on average two months apart, dizygotic twelve months. Sister-sister and mother-daughter correlations are about 0.4. Similar correlations are seen in skeletal maturity and teeth eruption.

There are many general environmental factors affecting growth, probably acting through their influence on the more particular factors of nutrition and infection. These general factors include socio-economic status, numbers of children in the family, climate, urbanisation, level of hygiene, housing and cultural factors affecting child rearing practices.

In general, children from upper socio-economic levels and urban areas are larger and mature earlier than those from lower levels and rural areas.

The effects of malnutrition on growth depend on whether it is an acute episode or chronic state. Children can recover completely from an episode of acute starvation provided it is not too severe and does not go on for too long. Chronic malnutrition has a permanent effect on varying numbers of children in all populations.

Population studies in growth

Growth studies of many of the world's races have been carried out over the past few decades. There have been two recent publications which survey the more recent studies. One is entitled 'Worldwide Variation in Human Growth' by Eveleth and Tanner (1976). It reports on many growth studies and several parameters, comparing the results throughout the world. There are extensive appendices giving mean values for the growth parameters for all ages, for many populations. The second is a chapter by Eveleth on 'Population Differences in Growth: Environmental and Genetic Factors' in *Human Growth* (1979). The reader is referred to these publications for detailed reference, but a summary of the main findings is given below.

Summary of population differences in growth

Asiatics reach puberty earlier than Europeans on average, and pass through adolescence more rapidly. They are less tall at all ages than well-off Europeans and Africans. As adults they have shorter legs than Europeans.

Most Africans in Africa have their growth retarded by under-nutrition and infections, but well-off Africans grow very similarly to Europeans. Recent surveys in the USA have shown that Afro-Americans are taller and heavier at all ages than children of European descent, chiefly because from a young age they are maturing faster.

Africans have longer legs relative to length of trunk and narrow hips relative to width of shoulders. These differences are probably genetically influenced as they occur at all socio-economic levels.

Marked population differences are seen in both African and Asiatic groups. Australian Aborigines have extremely long legs from an early age, but only attain a small adult height.

GROWTH STUDY METHODS

A. Types of study

1. Cross-sectional study

Each child is measured once only. A large number of children is measured at each age and the means and variabilities are calculated. If the distribution about the mean is Gaussian, as is the case for height, the standard deviation is calculated and multiplied by the appropriate value to obtain centiles. When the distribution is skewed, as in the cases of weight and skinfold fat, the centiles are best estimated by direct counting. Such centiles can be used as standards (see Fig. 54.1). Ideally, about 1000 boys and 1000 girls are needed in each age group to obtain satisfactory standards, but about 500 for each sex produce acceptable standards.

2. Longitudinal study

Each child is measured at regular intervals from birth to maturity. This method of study is expensive and takes a very long time to complete. It is essential if rates of growth are required, although a modification (see 3 below) may produce satisfactory velocity charts.

3. Mixed longitudinal study

Velocity data may be obtained in this type of study, which involves sampling cohorts of children over the age range required and measuring them over a period of time. Another method is for children to enter and leave the study at different times. The means, standard deviations and centiles can be ascertained for the increments as for the cross-sectional data, size achieved. Growth rates in centimetres per year (velocity standards) can be obtained in a shorter time than by the standard longitudinal study.

To produce standards of height and weight, head circumference, etcetera, the cross-sectional method is satisfactory from birth to puberty. A longitudinal study for five years is needed to cover the adolescent period of the growth spurt, as well as measuring more children cross-sectionally at the same time, to increase the numbers.

B. Data analysis

It is best for the investigator, preferably with the help of a statistician, to decide how the data will be analysed before collection is begun. For mixed longitudinal data, methods are available which make the most of all the data collected (Tanner 1951). A computer programme LONGITS has been developed at the Institute of Child Health, London, for this purpose (Goldstein and Manning 1968). A full discussion on the 'Statistics of Growth Standards' by Healy is set out in *Human Growth* (1979). People wishing to construct national standards may also refer to the Cuban National Growth Survey, the methodology of which has been fully described (Jordan et al 1975).

C. Sampling

Advice is also needed on the precise method of sampling. Details are given in 'Sampling for Growth Studies' by Goldstein in *Human Growth* (1979).

D. Measuring techniques

These have all been standardised and a full description of the precise methods, together with recommended apparatus, is given by Cameron in *Human Growth* (1979). It is necessary for all personnel involved in measuring to have proper training before the study. Checks on measurements should be done throughout the study, to monitor inter- and intra-observer variation. It is hoped that prospective growth studies will all adopt the same techniques, to ensure international comparability.

CONSIDERATIONS IN THE CHOICE OF APPROPRIATE GROWTH STANDARDS

Choice of growth standards depends on the purpose for which they are needed and the particular population being studied.

Use of growth measurements

1. Growth data may be used as a screening device, to see whether a particular child is abnormal in relation to his peers, that is if his height measurement is below the 3rd centile for all children of his age. In this case, the centile standards to be used should be obtained by measuring representative samples of the total population to which the child belongs in a cross-sectional study. If it is found that there is a pathological cause for his small stature, appropriate treatment is given and serial measurements plotted on the same standards will monitor the outcome. Examples of this are hypothyroidism, growth hormone deficiency, and congenital adrenal hyperplasia. Examples of such standards are those of Tanner et al (1966).

2. Growth measurements may be collected and used as an index of the general health and nutrition of a population or sub-population. Representative samples from the population or group are measured and mean values of the population are compared with similar data from other countries. Comparison between them and similar data on the same population after some years or after some remedial action, either nutritional, social or medical, enables progress to be documented quantitatively.

Ideally, each population or sub-group needs its own particular ethnic standards using data from representative samples of the total population. In practice, there are still many countries without such a standard and there is some controversy about the best alternatives. The two main alternatives are the use of the measurements of the privileged or élite members of the population or the use of international reference standards. A full discussion is given by Goldstein and Tanner (1980).

Goldstein and Tanner point out that an élite group is living in a sophisticated environment, but not necessarily an optimal one.

> A better definition of optimal would be the level of nutrition and medical care which is associated with the greatest amount of health . . . since . . . there is not yet a satisfactory definition of positive health, we have to use a criterion based on lowest mortality and morbidity rates.

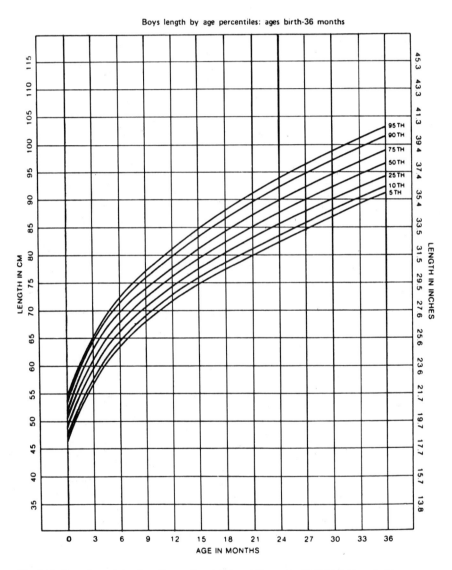

Fig. 54.1 Boys Length by Age Percentiles: Birth to 36 months N C H S Growth Charts 1976

Goldstein and Tanner think it only valid to use an élite group's measurements as standard if 'most healthy' can be substituted for 'most privileged'. It must be realised that . . .

> The minimum morbidity is not necessarily associated with the maximum growth rates, e.g. in a poor environment, a child who is small may have an advantage over faster-growing children in terms of morbidity and mortality. So he is performing as well as he can for his environment, but is still at a disadvantage because of the poverty of that environment, compared with the privileged children . . . . As the environment of the disadvantaged group is improved and morbidity and mortality rates approach those of the privileged group, so the definitions of optimal growth in the two groups will tend to coincide.

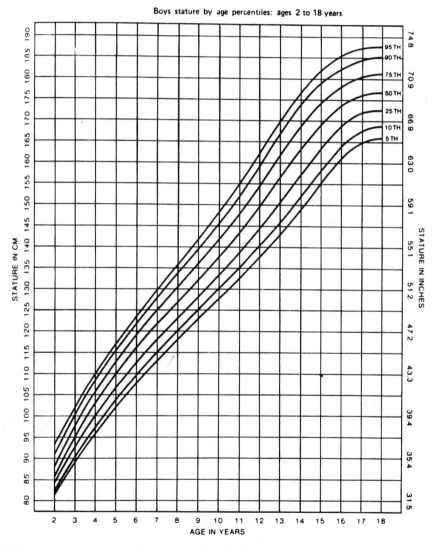

Fig. 54.2 Boys Stature by Age Percentiles: Ages 2 to 18 years N C H S Growth Charts 1976

They conclude:

> The percentile standards used should be those of the population of the environment which actually exists, rather than those of a privileged group, and should be updated as often as necessary.

Nevertheless, growth measurements of an élite group can give some idea of the 'ethnic' type of growth of a population (when environmental vicissitudes have not interfered significantly with the expression of the genetic potential). They also provide a 'target' towards which health personnel can

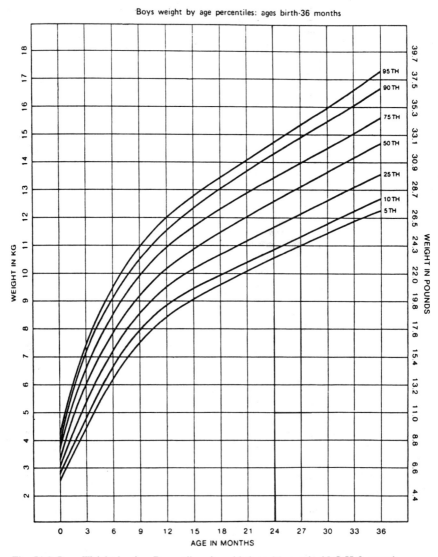

Fig. 54.3 Boys Weight by Age Percentiles: Ages birth to 36 months N C H S growth Charts 1976

work (Janes, Macfarlane and Moody 1981). It must be remembered that in countries undergoing rapid social and economic change, the élite group's measurements are also likely to change.

The other alternative to ethnic standards is the use of measurements of an international reference population. This allows data from different populations to be compared with each other or those from the same population at different times. For many years, the Harvard or Boston standards (Stuart and Stevenson 1960) have been used as a reference on an

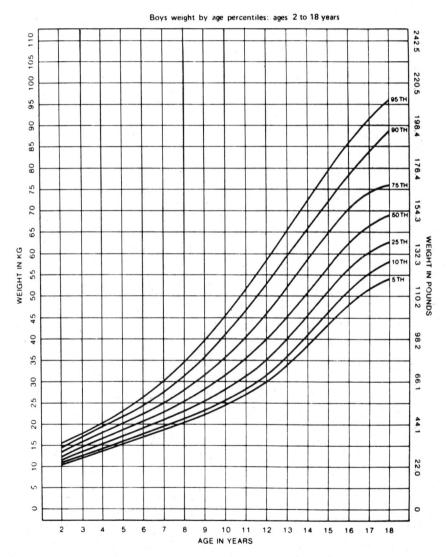

Fig. 54.4 Boys Weight by Age Percentiles: Ages 2 to 18 years N C H S Growth Charts 1976

international scale for the presentation of nutrition and other survey data and their use has enabled comparisons to be made between different countries. The data on which they are based were collected in the 1930s and were not representative of the general American population at the time. These Boston standards have now been superceded by more recent USA data (N.C.H.S. Growth Charts 1976) which have been recommended as a possible international reference population by an FAO/UNICEF/WHO Expert Committee on Nutritional Surveillance (Waterlow et al 1977). These authors

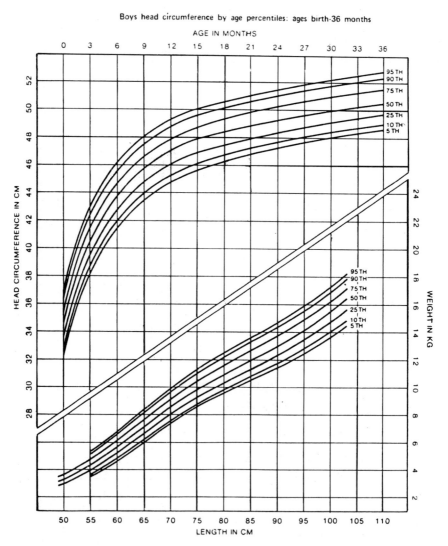

Fig. 54.5 Boys Head Circumference by Age Percentiles: Ages birth to 36 months Boys Weight by Length Percentiles: Ages birth to 36 months N C H S Growth Charts 1976

point out that a single international reference population is not suitable to be used as a target in all countries, as all ethnic groups do not have the same growth potential. It can be used for comparisons and until such time as there is a suitable local standard. The USA charts are shown in Figs. 54.1 to 54.6.

In the same paper they give details of the methodology involved in cross-sectional surveys made as part of nutritional monitoring or surveillance

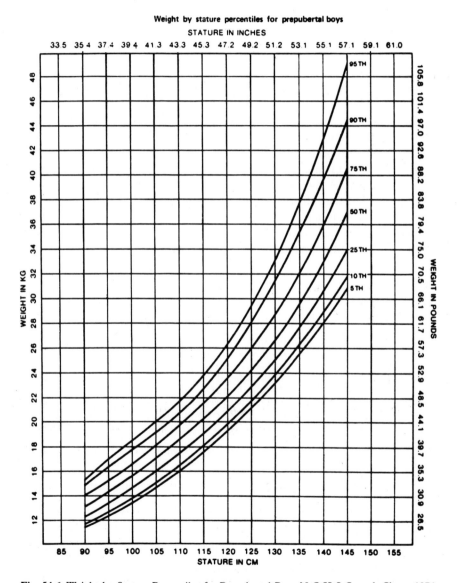

Fig. 54.6 Weight by Stature Percentiles for Prepubertal Boys N C H S Growth Charts 1976

programmes, using the American data as a reference. Indices to be studied are weight for height as an indicator of the present state of nutrition and height for age as an indicator of past nutrition. The results are expressed as centiles or in a cross-classification scheme using standard deviation scores. They conclude by expressing the hope that everyone working in the field will use such methods, to make international comparisons easier. In populations where the date of birth is not always known, an estimate of the nutritional status has to be made using the weight for height only. All countries should give priority to a policy of registration of births to overcome this problem.

CONCLUSIONS

Although it is true that children growing up in a satisfactory environment tend to grow in a similar way (Habicht et al 1974) there is now much evidence to show that there are differences in body size and shape between groups. It is no longer justified to continue to use growth standards which are based on European or American children for all populations.

Growth charts of suitable reference populations may be used for comparisons, and the USA data shown here (Figs. 54.1–54.6) are examples. For individual assessment the distance and velocity charts of Tanner et al (1966) are suitable. But the aim of health personnel concerned with growth monitoring should be to construct local standards obtained from a representative sample of the entire population, with regular updating.

REFERENCES:

Cameron N 1979 The methods of auxological anthropometry. In: Falkner F, Tanner J M (eds) Human Growth 2: Baillière Tindall, London, ch 3, p 35
Eveleth P B 1979 Population differences in growth: environmental and genetic factors. In: Falkner F, Tanner J M (eds) Human Growth 3: Baillière Tindall, London ch 12, p 373
Eveleth P B, Tanner J M (eds) 1976 Worldwide variation in human growth. Cambridge University press, Cambridge, London, New York, Melbourne
Goldstein H 1979 Sampling for growth studies. In: Falkner F, Tanner J M (eds) Human Growth 1: Baillière Tindall, London, ch 6, p 183
Goldstein H, Manning M 1968 Longitudinal survey program. Department of Growth and Development, Institute of Child Health, University of London
Goldstein H, Tanner J M 1980 Ecological considerations in the creation and the use of child growth standards. Lancet i: 582–585
Habicht J P, Martorell R, Yarbrough C, Malina R M, Klein R E 1974 Height and weight standards for pre-school children: are there really ethnic differences in growth potential? Lancet i: 611–615
Healy M J R 1979 Statistics of growth standards. In: Falkner F, Tanner J M (eds) Human Growth 1: Baillière Tindall, London, ch 5, p 169
Jordon J, Ruben M, Hernandez J, Bebelagua A, Tanner J M, Goldstein H 1975 The 1972 Cuban national child growth study as an example of population health monitoring, design and methods. Annals of Human Biology 2: 153–171
Janes M D, Macfarlane S B J, Moody J B 1981 Height and weight growth standards for Nigerian children. Annals of Tropical Paediatrics 1: 27–37
National Centre for Health Statistics 1976 Growth charts US department of health education and welfare, public health service, health resources administration, Rockville M D. HRA 76–1120: 25: 3

Stuart H C, Stevenson S S 1960 Harvard Standard. In: Nelson W W (ed) Textbook of
   Pediatrics, 7th edn. Saunders, Philadelphia
Tanner J M 1951 Some notes on the reporting of growth data. Human Biology 23: 93–159
Tanner J M, Whitehouse R H, Takaishi M 1966 Standards from birth to maturity for
   height, weight, height velocity and weight velocity; British children 1965. Archives of
   Disease in Childhood 41: 454–471, 613–635
Van Wieringen J C 1972 Secular changes of growth 1964–1966 height and weight surveys in
   the Netherlands. Leiden, Netherlands Institute for Preventive Medicine, TNO
Waterlow J C, Buzina R, Keller W, Lane J M, Nichaman M Z, Tanner J M 1977 The
   presentation and use of height and weight data for comparing the nutritional status of
   groups of children under the age of 10 years. Bulletin of the World Health Organization
   55: 489–498

Nomadic peoples, their health and health services

<hr>

NEGLECTED POPULATION GROUPS

'Health for All by the Year 2000' is the motto formulated by WHO. The main target for this drive, which aims at access for every individual to at least a village dispensary, will be the rural population in poor countries. Compared with urban populations, rural people are everywhere far underserved, especially in developing countries. In need of special consideration are the nomadic peoples of the world.

Characteristics of nomads include *scatteredness*, and *low average population density*. These two criteria, added to their *mobility*, create specific problems regarding health and social services, and education. Because of their migratory nature nomads constitute an extreme part of *adversely situated population groups* which also include refugees (about 16 million in 1984), Eskimos and other circumpolar peoples, countless families living their whole life on the coasts of the Far East, and inhabitants of Polynesian archipelagos. For all such groups difficulty of access requires specially designed health services.

Depending on *definition* there are between 50 and 100 million nomads in the world today. The vast majority are found in the 'nomad belt', from western Sahara through north Africa and the Middle East to central Asia, and ending in Outer Mongolia. Some regions in this belt have a total annual rainfall of less than 25 cm which means desert and empty areas. Around these barren lands there are marginal regions with a rainfall per year of 25 to 50 cm, which is enough for providing grazing to feed cattle and camels on the condition that the animals move seasonally from place to place for pasture and watering. This migration consequently forces the owners of the herds to a nomadic life. Pastoral nomadism is an ecological consequence in a traditional land, where a sedentary life and agriculture, without artificial irrigation, are out of the question.

Most nomads live in a hot and dry climate, scattered in small groups, and the average population density of their territories is usually below one per square kilometre. They have adapted their living to permanent migration, using mobile huts or tents, and carrying as few belongings as possible. A few nomadic tribes live in the Arctic, such as the 10 000 or so Mountain

Lapps of Scandinavia, with reindeer as their semi-domesticated animals. Their health service problems have been solved in an acceptable way. Other nomads include the small remaining groups of hunter-collectors living in the interior of Australia (Aborigines) and in the Kalahari desert (Bushmen).

HEALTH AND DISEASE AMONG NOMADS

When dealing with tribal people and especially with nomads, it is a matter of course to look at the *'total man in his total environment'*, and to consider all three components of the WHO definition of health: physical, mental and social wellbeing. Our knowledge of nomads' health is limited because few epidemiological studies have been carried out specifically on nomadic groups. A great number of observations and generalised statements of varying value have, however, been reported. In many countries popular opinion has it that nomads are malnourished and are heavily afflicted with diseases such as malaria, trachoma, syphilis and schistosomiasis. Yet no critical observations confirm this belief. They rather indicate to the contrary with better physical condition in nomads than in their sedentary neighbours. A wholesome diet with sufficient protein - meat, milk, blood all the year round combined with living outdoors result in physical strength and a certain resistance against diseases. In Kenya, the nomads suffer a milder form of trachoma than do the settled farmers who are poorly nourished during the dry seasons. Studies of Maasai men in East Africa have revealed unusually good physical condition as demonstrated in the maximal oxygen consumption per minute.

Accidents are frequent among people living in a harsh nature. Drowning is common among the Lapps. In the 1950s the author studied nomadic Lapps in northernmost Sweden, and found an average life expectancy for males of about 38 years, and for females of 44 years. Apart from accidents, high infant mortality figures explain these low figures. Eskimos in Alaska, Greenland and Canada present a similar pattern. In the past, and still in many poor countries, lack of access to health services contribute to the high mortality risk. Observations confirm, however, that on the whole (surviving) nomads are physically healthy and strong people. Not surprisingly nomads get their share of the endemic diseases prevalent in their provinces, such as trypanosomiasis, malaria and trachoma, but often their migratory routes avoid regions which are known for certain endemic diseases (Ghashghai in Iran). The perpetual movement of nomads eliminates much of the risk which might emanate from unsatisfying environmental sanitation, polluted water and food.

As could be expected, zoonotic diseases are relatively common among pastoral nomads. Hydatidosis (dogworm) has been common among reindeer herding Lapps, and the disease has today its highest known incidence in the enormous pastoral province and semi-desert Turkana in northwest Kenya. Brucellosis (undulant fever), causing abortions in cattle, has been responsible for great misery and economic loss in pastoral areas (Iran, Iraq), and WHO has run control programs in places such as Outer Mongolia. Brucellosis is spread to humans by raw meat and milk. Anthrax, especially important in Iran and the Sudan, also ravages pastoral regions as does viral foot-and-mouth disease.

A generation ago, tuberculosis was a devastating illness among Lapps and Eskimos, but is now almost eradicated. Unfortunately this disease is still uncontrolled in the tropics and among nomads (Tibetans).

There are no reports on nomads regarding psycho-social health. Psychiatry in such exotic conditions can only be studied as a science which mixes medicine and social anthropology, *transcultural psychiatry*, but this is still mainly an academic product. The author's impression from some 30 years periodically spent among nomads, is that the happiest and most harmonious people today are to be found among some nomadic peoples such as Lapps, Ghashghai and Ethiopian Shankella.

The most apparent mental disorder today seen in countries in transitional development is *acculturation* resulting from mixing of elements from native cultures and from western influences. This creates cultural gaps, 'lost generations' and split families, all characteristic of populations subject to a too rapid change. Nomads are traditionally conservative and resistant to ideas from outside, and acculturation phenomena do not hit them until they stop wandering and become settled.

HEALTH SERVICES FOR PASTORAL NOMADS

Health services in areas with low population density and scattered people, including mobile groups, are of interest to us in three ways:

1. They have the right to, and want primary health care services.

2. The extent to which a nation has developed its national health program can often be judged by the services offered to its adversely situated groups. The quality of front-line services can be used as *one* indicator of health development.

3. National public health programs against prevalent diseases may not reach people who are mobile. When a disease is thought to be under control unaccessible pockets of infection may remain among nomads. During their migrations they may carry the disease from province to province and from country to country. This has particularly seen the case with malaria and trypanosomiasis in some African countries.

Periodically during their wanderings nomads come closer to settlements provided with dispensaries. A complete chain of static front-line dispensaries or health stations is therefore the most important part of the services which they can use. In a few places trained nurse-aides (Sudan, Somalia) or midwives (Iran) follow the migration of their own tribes and are permanently available. They are provided with drug kits by the authorities. So far this system of care has not become widespread partly because of the high rate of illiteracy in the concerned groups. Most tribal people also have their own medicine-men and traditional healers practising native medicine. Native birth attendants are common and usually take care of the majority of rural deliveries (Jordan). In the absence of modern health services, these persons are of great value and have a high status within the group.

Dispensaries in the front-line chain of services should preferably be staffed with locally recruited personnel, who have graduated from primary school and have been trained as health auxiliaries. They must speak the local language and be accepted - and perhaps selected - by the people they are to serve. This system of 'bare-foot doctors' is practised with some variations in a great number of developing countries. Perhaps the most successful system is found in Alaska, where 205 Eskimo girls, selected by their own villagers, after 12 weeks of initial training as community nurse aides, return to their home area. They constitute a full coverage system and are frequently supervised and assisted by physicians and nurses. A well designed drug kit, an excellent manual and a foolproof radio-telephone make the equipment complete. At a fixed time daily the nurse aide *must* call her supervising nurse or physician for consultations. Transportation is mainly by air.

A basic problem for self-help systems in the poor world, the most tricky and expensive to solve, is transportation. Airplanes are hardly practicable under the usual circumstances but even with camel, mule and jeep as the only alternatives, the rest of the Alaskan system is worth copying. After that the great obstacle is illiteracy.

Any acceptable system for health services to scattered populations is bound to be expensive, because each day the number of patients is likely to be small. Consequently the per capita cost for services will be high. The national health budget of the poorest countries, where the nomads tend to be, such as Ethiopia, is about 2000 times lower (per capita) than in rich countries. Paradoxically the immunization of nomads (Mali) costs eleven times more than it would in the same number of sedentary, urbanised people. In poor countries, consequently, both nomads and distant rural groups are often neglected. It is simply not possible to provide cover with the available budget. In any case services would have to be specially designed for such regions including the training of health auxiliaries, the establishment of a reasonable transportation system and, hopefully, tele-communications. Occasional dramatic mobile units cannot replace small static, permanent health care units in areas with low population density and large distances.

EVALUATION/APPRAISAL OF PRIMARY HEALTH CARE

As reliable statistical information is seldom available in developing countries, and almost never from districts with scattered population, the evaluation of health programs is a delicate task and relies on estimations rather than actual measurements. First the District Health Officer will want to know the distribution of the population which it is aimed to serve. In Africa many rural settlements have no trafficable all-weather roads so that 15 kms walking distance has often been used as a criterion of *accessibility*. For nomadic people this term has almost no meaning.

Other information required concerns *acceptability* and *utilization rates*. Do people in the area like the services offered or do they prefer traditional healers. The mean number of visits per year per person is useful. From such information, the *effectiveness* of services, and also the *cost-efficiency*, can be calculated. In regions with low population density, with part of the population mobile, the daily number of patients may be as low as four or five, while in densely populated rural districts in Africa, a health unit can expect to provide up to 300 treatments per day. It is also important to get an idea of how services have influenced such indices as the birth rate, infant mortality, and life expectancy.

Obstacles to the development of services in distant rural areas include the ever present *shortage*, and *maldistribution* of medical and nursing personnel, favouring the capital and other urban areas. In Ethiopia, 95 per cent of all doctors are stationed in Addis Ababa, serving only five per cent of the population of the country.

For the development of rural primary health care cooperation with the local people is a fundamental necessity. It should be 'their' service.

An evaluation of the work of Alaskan Eskimo community nurse aides in 1980 discovered that they managed about 90 per cent of what a physician stationed in the same village could have done. The rather universal arctic figure for infant mortality of about 100 per thousand live-borne 25 years ago had dropped to below 20, near to the rest of the US. This in spite of being an extreme rural region with low population density and great scatteredness.

FUTURE OF NOMADISM

When dealing with development in foreign cultures, the observer often under-estimates the values of traditional life, rituals, religious beliefs, and native medicine. The first rule must be not to cause damage. It is important to 'hurry slowly' and to ask what are their priorities. Too rapid innovations from outside are likely to have harmful side-effects. In 'primitive' societies, acculturation is often an unexpected side-effect of well-intentioned international assistance. The eradication of tsetse flies in the Sahel region in Africa caused increased survival of humans and animals, and led successively to an ecological overpopulation and to the 'Sahel catastrophe'. A series of dry years played the role of trigger mechanism. Well-meaning medical measures likely to result in population increase, disturbance of the ecological balance and finally famine must not be introduced unless acceptance of birth control is guaranteed simultaneously. Marginal regions of the world, deserts and arctics, have resources which can bear only a finite number of inhabitants, human and animal. Surplus people seldom want to leave their native land and places for them to relocate to are increasingly difficult to find. There is also a risk of a 'brain drain', as the brightest youths are lost.

Like other peoples, nomads increase their population about two per cent annually, which means that some individuals have to leave. The alternative is overgrazing and ecological imbalance, with resulting desert. This has already occurred in several places (Sahel, Maasailand). Young people who leave the pastoral tribe must be ready to compete with other youngsters for jobs. For this reason primary school education is desired even by nomadic people. Because of the desire for education and access to primary health care services many bedouins (Jordan) become semi-nomadic. The whole family stays for part of the year in one place, or women and children stay all the year, often in their tent close to a village and near to a primary school and a rural dispensary. The herdsmen of the family continue to follow the herd and are nomadic most of the year.

The introduction of a monetary economy has occurred in many nomadic tribes. They sell cattle and meat and buy necessities and even food. This causes an increase of herds, overgrazing and a precarious ecological situation with irrevocable desertisation of large tracts of grazing land. In most of these regions one can confirm a gradual lowering of the subsoil water level.

Fortunately many nomadic tribes continue to live in ecological balance with nature, a traditional life with few elements introduced from outside and apparently happy, such as the Bushmen hunter-collectors of the Kalahari desert. It is important, like the case of the Botswana Bushmen, that they themselves choose if and when to settle down. In other places, nomads are encouraged or even forced, directly or indirectly, to become sedentary. In Arabic countries, where rich oil deposits have been discovered, under-developed countries suddenly become rich and try to hasten their development. Their policy often aims at getting nomads settled, as nomadism is apparently regarded as a sign of under-devlopment. On the contrary, pastoral nomadism should be seen as a source of national income from dry regions which cannot be utilised in any other way.

An American program, in which the author plays a part, deals with the 'least developed nations of the world' of which there are about 25. Each is characterised by three or four of the following: very limited natural resources, dry climate, land-locked situation (no access to the sea), natural catastrophes are relatively common (drought, earthquakes), and a rather high proportion of the population is nomadic. It goes without saying, that in these countries, such as Mauritania, Mali, Niger, Botswana and Somalia, it is important for the national economy to utlise even grazing as a modest source of income.

The total number of the world's 'full nomads' is steadily shrinking. Many are semi-nomadic, half way to a sedentary life. The demand for primary health care is a strong driving force in this event. It has to be realised that constantly accessible health services to people on the constant move are practically and economically unrealistic. Nomadic peoples have to compromise and rely on static health units on the outer border-line of the sedentary neighbouring population.

Most problems in the poor countries, including pastoral areas, are multifactorial by nature, and solutions, by necessity must be multidisciplinary. International sponsoring agencies and professionals must accept this, and medical professionals have increasingly to recognise *'non-medical solutions to medical problems'*, for example water supply. The high 'medical' priority in rural parts of developing countries is for primary education which then provides suitable young people for training as auxiliary health workers, and as links between professional health services and native people. This link is especially important when dealing with delicate commissions such as family planning and nutrition.

REFERENCES AND FURTHER READING

African Medical and Research Foundation (AMREF) 1978 and following. Annual reports Nairobi
Burkitt W R 1975 Jan Suggestions for the development of rural eye services in Africa, Tropical Doctor
Carriere E C de la 1979 The inadequate African road network. The Courier no 54
Dwyer J M 1973 Royal Flying Doctor Service of Australia. World Hospitals 9 (4)
Haraldson S R S 1962 Socio-medical conditions among the Lapps in northermost Sweden. Svenska Läkartidningan 59: 2829
Haraldson S R S 1972 Health problems of nomads. Working document for WHO, based on studies in the Sudan, Somalia, Iraq, Iran, Afghanistan
Haraldson S R S 1973 Health Problems of nomads. World Hospitals vol IX, edn no 4
Haraldson S R S 1976 Tribal people in transitional phase. The Ciba Foundation Symposium No 49, London
Haraldson S R S 1978 Planning of health services in sparesely populated areas (Eskimo regions in Alaska, Canada, Greenland). Oulu, Finland: Nordic Council for Arctic Medical Research
Haraldson S R S 1978 The approach to circumpolar health. WHO/EURO/N3/48/18
Haraldson S R S 1979 Socio-medical problems of nomad peoples. In: W Hobson (ed), Oxford, The theory and practice of public health. Oxford University Press
Haraldson S R S 1979 Alternative approaches to health services for the least developed countries. In: L Berry and R W Kates (eds) Making the most of the least: alternative development for poor nations. Holmes and Meier New York
Haraldson S R S 1981 Mobile health services. Program for International Development, Clark University, Worcester, Mass 01610
Imperato, Pascal J et al 1973 Mass campaigns and their comparative costs for nomadic and sedentary peoples in Mali. Tropical and Geographical Medicine 25: 416–422
Johnson Douglas L 1969 The nature of nomadism: a comparative study of pastoral migrations in southwestern Asia and northern Africa. The University of Chicago, Department of Geography, research paper no 118
Ormerod W E 1976 Drought in the Sahel: the credit side of development. Tropical Doctor, October 1976
Prothero R W 1965 Migrants and malaria, Longmans London
Prothero R W 1972 Problems of public health among pastoralists: A case study from Africa. In: McGlashan N E (ed) Medical Geography. Methuan London
Prothero R W 1977 Diseases and mobility: a neglected factor in epidemiology

Index